FUNDAMENTALS OF ATHLETIC TRAINING AND SPORTS MEDICINE

FIFTH EDITION

Lorin A. Cartwright, MS, ATC
Ann Arbor Pioneer High School

Kimberly S. Peer, EdD, AT, FNATA
Kent State University

HUMAN KINETICS

Library of Congress Cataloging-in-Publication Data

Names: Cartwright, Lorin, 1956- author. | Peer, Kimberly S., author.
Title: Fundamentals of athletic training and sports medicine / Lorin A. Cartwright, MS, ATC, Ann Arbor Pioneer High School, Kimberly S. Peer, EdD, AT, FNATA, Kent State University.
Description: Fifth edition. | Champaign, IL : Human Kinetics, [2025] | Includes bibliographical references and index.
Identifiers: LCCN 2024028300 (print) | LCCN 2024028301 (ebook) | ISBN 9781718215887 (hardback) | ISBN 9781718215894 (epub) | ISBN 9781718239272 (pdf)
Subjects: LCSH: Athletic trainers. | BISAC: MEDICAL / Sports Medicine | MEDICAL / Allied Health Services / Physical Therapy
Classification: LCC RC1210 .C365 2025 (print) | LCC RC1210 (ebook) | DDC 613.7/11--dc23/eng/20240627
LC record available at https://lccn.loc.gov/2024028300
LC ebook record available at https://lccn.loc.gov/2024028301

ISBN: 978-1-7182-1588-7 (print)

The web addresses cited in this text were current as of May 2024, unless otherwise noted.

Acquisitions Editor: Bethany J. Bentley
Managing Editor: Derek Campbell
Copyeditor: Michelle Horn
Proofreader: Leigh Keylock
Indexer: Beth Nauman-Montana
Permissions Manager: Laurel Mitchell
Graphic Designers: Joe Buck and Nancy Rasmus
Cover Designer: Keri Evans
Cover Design Specialist: Susan Rothermel Allen
Photographs (cover): © Human Kinetics (front cover; back cover, left and right); Clive Brunskill/Getty Images (back cover, middle)
Photographs (interior): © Human Kinetics, unless otherwise noted
Photo Asset Manager: Laura Fitch
Photo Production Manager: Jason Allen
Senior Art Manager: Kelly Hendren
Illustrations: © Human Kinetics, unless otherwise noted
Printer: Walsworth

Printed in the United States of America

2 3 4 5 6 7 8 9 10 WPC 29 28 27 26

The paper in this book was manufactured using responsible forestry methods.

Human Kinetics
1607 N. Market Street
Champaign, IL 61820
USA

United States and International
Website: **US.HumanKinetics.com**
Email: info@hkusa.com
Phone: 1-800-747-4457

Human Kinetics' authorized representative for product safety in the EU is Mare Nostrum Group B.V., Mauritskade 21D, 1091 GC Amsterdam, The Netherlands.
Email: gpsr@mare-nostrum.co.uk

E8799

To my parents, who were the best teachers and instilled the passion to reach for goals that may not seem obtainable. Your pride in me is a lasting gift I will always treasure. To Kim, for taking the challenge of writing. You are a guiding light during some of my toughest challenges. I cannot thank you enough for saying yes—and the impact we continue to make for years to come. Last but never least, Barb Hansen, for her smile, encouragement, and belief in me—my world changed for the better when we met.

Lorin A. Cartwright

If you love what you do, you will never work a day in your life. To my parents, who taught me from an early age that having a passion and pursuing it will provide rewards beyond measure. My journey has allowed me to travel with amazing colleagues who motivate, inspire, and challenge me to go further. Lorin, thank you for your lifelong leadership and commitment to advancing the profession and mentoring those around you. I'm a better professional and person for traveling this path with you. To Michelle, Braeden, and Connor, you complete me and are the best part of my world. Thanks for keeping me humble and providing me balance in my life!

Kimberly S. Peer

CONTENTS

UNIT II

Basics of Human Anatomy and Physiology 77

UNIT III

Athletic-Related Injuries to the Head, Spine, and Axial Region 107

UNIT VI

UNIT VII

LIST OF ANATOMICAL DRAWINGS

BASIC HUMAN ANATOMY

Bones

Muscles

AXIAL REGION

Head and Face

Throat and Thorax

Abdomen

UPPER EXTREMITY

Spine

Shoulder

Elbow

Wrist and Hand

LOWER EXTREMITY

Hip, Pelvis, and Thigh

Knee

Foot, Ankle, and Lower Leg

PREFACE

In 2020 it was found that more than 54 percent of youth had participated in sport in the previous year (Black, Terlizzi, and Vahratian 2022). More than 3 million children aged 14 and younger are injured annually in sporting or recreational activities (Stanford Medicine 2024). The impact of any injury long term is based on early intervention and great care. An athletic trainer can provide care before a person participates and in the early stages after an injury. This care can minimize effects of an injury and provide opportunities for continued participation in sport or recreation. In this textbook, the foundations of athletic training are laid out in an easy-to-follow sequence that supports the essential learning about the field of sports medicine.

The practice of athletic training changes daily. The members of the Athletic Training Strategic Alliance, specifically the Board of Certification, address new entry-level education for athletic trainers every five years. The fifth edition of *Fundamentals of Sports Medicine and Athletic Training* includes some recent changes and features that will enable the reader to develop a more comprehensive understanding of the field of sports medicine, specifically athletic training.

Five goals have been established for this edition:

- Provide updated information that is relevant for student aides.
- Expand content to include fundamental skills, medical conditions, and equipment.
- Feature activities that will support classroom instruction.
- Provide teachers with test questions, PowerPoint presentations, and end-of-chapter scenarios.
- Provide students with flash cards (located in the web resource), chapter reviews for determining level of understanding, and chapter treatment tips.

This book is specifically written for high school, community college, technical college, or first-year college students. It will help them become familiar with the practices of the athletic trainer and understand their role as student assistants.

Student assistants must understand the limits of their role and learn as much as possible to be at their very best. Certified athletic trainers must perform the tasks as designated by their certification, but students can gain invaluable experience observing and participating in daily routines and asking questions about things they are experiencing. We encourage students to be active participants in the learning process while abiding by the state law, which defines the skills you are able to perform.

We present key concepts about medical terminology, the interaction of medical professionals and interprofessional practice, anatomy and physiology, preexisting conditions, illnesses and injuries, medical emergencies, body types, nutrition, exercise, and working with people with disabilities and other special populations. Our final goal is to have students get the "bug" and decide that the medical field, especially athletic training, is a career worth pursuing.

HOW THIS BOOK IS ORGANIZED

The text is organized so that each unit can stand alone. We suggest, however, that units II through VI be covered in order so that students obtain a solid understanding of anatomy and physiology before reading about various injuries. Likewise, prior learning about bodily injuries and their associated anatomy is necessary for understanding rehabilitation and treatment strategies.

The book is divided into nine units:

- Unit I provides an overview of the athletic training profession, athletic training education, interaction between medical professionals, leadership, training room design, technology, insurance, and the administrative tasks important to being successful in the field.

- Unit II is a discussion of the body's anatomy and the physiology of injury and tissue healing.
- Units III, IV, and V explain the head-to-toe specific anatomy, injuries for each area of the body, medical conditions and illnesses, treatment, and referral for injured or ill athletes.
- Unit VI discusses the fundamentals of rehabilitation and returning an athlete to competition, including the psychological aspects of that return.
- Unit VII explains how to plan for and deal with emergency situations.
- Unit VIII explains preventing injury by taping and wrapping, the theory of protective padding, and protective equipment for an athlete. It also covers diagnostic testing and imaging techniques used in the evaluation and diagnosis of injured athletes.
- Unit IX covers various conditions, illnesses, disabilities, mental health issues, communicable diseases, common drugs, and nutritional aspects that affect athletes.

SPECIAL CHAPTER ELEMENTS

The textbook has several special features:

- A list of all anatomical drawings and their locations in the book is provided for quick reference.
- A list of objectives to be met by completing the chapter helps students focus their attention when reading the material.
- The Real World stories in the chapters share actual experiences of athletic trainers.
- What Would You Do If . . . segments act as discussion openers and allow student assistants to prioritize their thinking about situations.
- FYI (for your information) boxes give background about topics that may be particularly challenging.
- Understanding Diversity segments help students begin to think about issues of culture and race that they will encounter in the field.
- Red Flags indicate how to identify emergency situations that require immediate attention.
- At the end of each chapter is a wrap-up section, which includes a summary, key terms, and critical thinking scenario.

NEW TO THIS EDITION

In this edition we have added or expanded content on many topics, including the following:

- Nerves and ligaments
- Neurological conditions
- Genitourinary conditions
- Injuries of the thorax, head, and face
- Bandaging and casting
- Medical equipment and technology
- Diagnostic testing
- Crisis incident stress management
- Pandemic planning
- Drugs
- Popular diets

Many other topics have updated discussions as well. The websites and content related to current NATA position statements and other resources such as ATs Care are also fully updated.

TEACHER RESOURCES

The athletic training profession requires a foundation of knowledge and practical skill application. The book is intended to give the student the foundational knowledge required to attain the appropriate skill set. Each chapter builds on the previous one to help students feel confident using new skills. The practical skills are found in the ancillaries, and each chapter has a set. The ancillaries will ease day-to-day teaching and make the course interactive and dynamic.

The authors suggest that this textbook be used for a 15- to 18-week course in athletic training. The teacher can use the provided PowerPoint presentations, worksheets, and practice skills each week to maintain a diverse presentation format to keep excitement and interest high. Teachers have access to a full array of ancillary materials.

- ***Teacher guide.*** The teacher guide is organized into four sets of materials: introduction and supplements (including lesson plans, guidelines, index-card anatomy, sports medicine challenge questions, and various answer keys), activities for reinforcement or group work, a semester-long project, and guides for each chapter (including objectives and teaching outlines). We include materials for students to complete to ensure they are engaged and self-directed in their learning.
- ***Presentation package and image bank.*** To fine-tune teaching presentations, teachers also receive an image bank with the art and photos featured in the text. This will allow teachers to use graphics in PowerPoint presentations and help link information they wish to convey to the text the students have read. The presentation package includes more than 600 slides that provide detailed lecture notes. Teachers can modify these slides as needed to best fit their classes and lecture format. The image bank contains most of the art, photos, and tables from the text, which can be used to create custom presentations, student handouts, and other materials.
- ***Test package.*** Questions are organized according to chapter, with more than 600 questions available. Answers and immediate grading are provided.
- ***Chapter quizzes.*** These ready-made quizzes allow teachers to test students' understanding of the most important chapter concepts.

STUDENT RESOURCES

The web resource has exercises that will help students take their knowledge further.

- ***Vocabulary term review.*** Students will be able to study vocabulary flashcards and take vocabulary review quizzes to support their learning of the materials.
- ***Understanding Check worksheets.*** Each chapter has a printable worksheet containing matching, fill-in-the-blank, and short answer questions related to key chapter concepts. These worksheets work well as study guides, or teachers may use the worksheets as graded assignments. Answers for the worksheets are in the teacher guide.
- ***Extension activities.*** We challenge the student who wants to dig deeper to go above and beyond with suggested projects.
- ***Resources and forms.*** Printable materials, such as the assumption of risk form, athletic injury and accident reports, and concussion tools are provided. Several worksheets take students through a step-by-step process of how to perform a task (e.g., shoulder pad fitting).

Access the web resource: http://ancillaries.humankinetics.com/FundamentalsOfAthleticTrainingAndSportsMedicine5E

Unit I

Introduction to Sports Medicine and Athletic Training

chapter 1

Athletic Training as a Profession

Objectives

After completing this chapter, the student will be able to do the following:

- Define athletic training.
- Describe the roles of the certified athletic trainer.
- Understand and appreciate the domains in athletic training.
- Describe the roles of other health care providers and the sports medicine team.
- List the requirements for becoming a competent certified AT.
- Understand and apply the concept of medical ethics and how it relates to the certified AT.
- Describe the job opportunities and salary potential for certified ATs.
- Understand the role of the NATA position statements and critically appraised topics as guides for clinical practice.

Sports medicine is an expanding field that encompasses many different disciplines related to the care of athletes. Disciplines within the sports medicine field include, but are not limited to, nutritionists, physical therapists, physicians, strength and conditioning specialists, biomechanists, and athletic trainers. **Athletic training** is a profession dedicated to maintaining and improving the health and well-being of the physically active population and preventing athletic-related injuries and illnesses. Athletic trainers are defined as follows:

> *Athletic trainers (ATs) are highly qualified, multi-skilled health care professionals who render service or treatment, under the direction of or in collaboration with a physician, in accordance with their education and training and the states' statutes and regulations. As a part of the health care team, services provided by ATs include injury and illness prevention, wellness promotion and education, emergent care, examination and clinical diagnosis, therapeutic intervention, and rehabilitation of injuries and medical conditions. (National Athletic Trainers' Association n.d.)*

The NATA website provides a valuable resource to those interested in athletic training, and the link to the NATA website is provided in the online resources. This site has videos, infographics, and other information regarding athletic training.

The credential for a **certified athletic trainer (AT)** is the **ATC**. When *ATC* appears after one's name, it means that the person has the appropriate education and training to work as a certified AT. Although people have provided health care to injured athletes for centuries, it was not until 1991 that the American Medical Association formally recognized athletic training as an allied health care profession. **National Athletic Trainers' Association (NATA)**, which is the professional membership organization for ATs, was formed in 1950. The **Board of Certification** is responsible for conducting the national certification process.

ROLES OF THE ATHLETIC TRAINER

Domains in athletic training are critical because they provide the foundation for professional practice. Every five years, the BOC performs a practice analysis to review and update professional knowledge and skills to ensure the most relevant applications for the profession. In 2022, the BOC once again revised the various roles of the AT, which include the following practice domains (BOC 2022):

- ***Risk Reduction, Wellness and Health Literacy.*** Preventing athletic injuries and illness includes educating athletes and their families about the potential risks of athletic participation and how to reduce those risks. Managing risk includes preparticipation physical exams; proper strength and conditioning programs; proper equipment and equipment fitting; taping, bandaging, and bracing; and good nutrition.
- ***Assessment, Evaluation and Diagnosis.*** The AT must be able to recognize the type of injury and its severity so that they will know how to treat it or when to refer the athlete to a physician.
- ***Critical Incident Management.*** When an athlete is injured, the AT must be ready to respond with the standard of care appropriate for the emergency presented. The AT must be able to communicate with various providers and family under stressful conditions. They must maintain first aid and cardiopulmonary resuscitation (CPR) certification through such organizations as the **American Red Cross** and the **National Safety Council**.
- ***Therapeutic Intervention.*** After initial treatment, the AT directs the athlete through exercises and treatments to help them return to normal function. This is called **rehabilitation**. **Reconditioning** is getting the athlete back into physical shape for athletic participation.
- ***Health Care Administration and Professional Responsibility.*** ATs are often responsible for managing state-of-the-art facilities, so they must have the administrative skills necessary for preparing work orders and purchase orders and for scheduling staff. Additionally, injuries, treatments, and rehabilitation progress must be documented accurately.

Although somewhat different from the Practice Analysis 7 domains, the newest practice analysis document provides a more refined depiction of the roles and responsibilities of the AT (see table 1.1).

Table 1.1 Comparison of PA7 Domains and PA8 Domains

PA7 domain names	PA8 domain names
Domain 1: Injury and Illness Prevention and Wellness Promotion	Domain 1: Risk Reduction, Wellness and Health Literacy
Domain 2: Examination, Assessment, and Diagnosis	Domain 2: Assessment, Evaluation and Diagnosis
Domain 3: Immediate and Emergency Response	Domain 3: Critical Incident Management
Domain 4: Therapeutic Intervention	Domain 4: Therapeutic Intervention
Domain 5: Health Care Administration and Professional Responsibility	Domain 5: Health Care Administration and Professional Responsibility

Reprinted by permission from "BOC Practice Analysis, 8th Edition May Impact Your Education Program," Board of Certification, Inc., posted February 15, 2023. https://bocatc.org/newsroom/boc-practice-analysis-8th-edition-may-impact-your-education-program.

The Real World

We had a freshman football receiver who was unable to catch the ball. He was fast, but he dropped everything. The position coach recommended an eye exam and was sure that the results would be subpar and that we would recommend glasses or contacts to improve performance. The exam revealed the player's vision to be 20/10, which is much better than average. I recommended that the coach work with him on the skills necessary to perform well at the position. The player became one of the school's all-time statistical leaders and has had a long and successful career in the NFL as a receiver.

Paul W. Schmidt, MS, PT, ATC

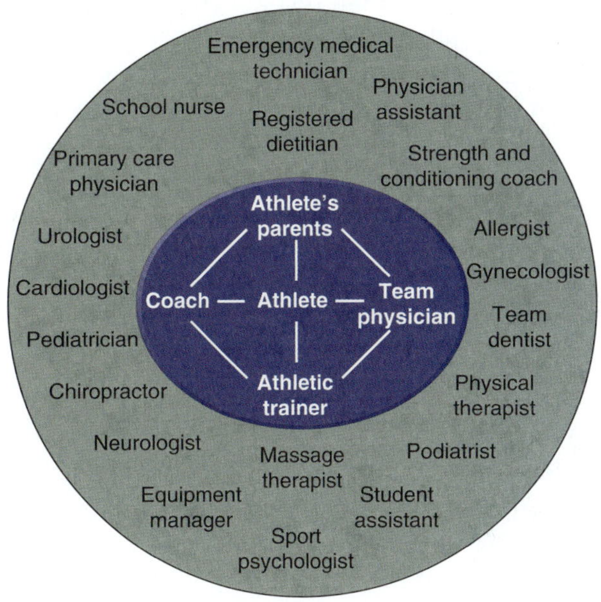

Figure 1.1 The sports medicine team has central and peripheral members, each with specific responsibilities and areas of expertise.

THE SPORTS MEDICINE TEAM

In this book, **sports medicine** refers to the care of physically active people who have suffered athletic-related injury or illness. The sports medicine profession includes ATs, medical doctors, physical therapists, dentists, chiropractors, coaches, sport psychologists, strength and conditioning specialists, school nurses, sport nutritionists, and student assistants (see figure 1.1). A sports medicine team may include any or all of these people.

As with any team, the sports medicine team must work cooperatively. If a football running back runs wherever they want with the ball regardless of where the blockers are, the team will never win. The team must coordinate its plays if it is ever to be successful. This is how an effective sports medicine team works.

Central Team

Ideally, the central team is composed of the injured athlete, the athlete's parents or guardians, the AT, the team physician, and the coach. The central team works together to make initial decisions about injuries, illness, and even sport performance.

- ***The athlete.*** The athlete is the center of the team. They provide other members with vital information about the injury and previous medical history.

- ***The athlete's parent or guardian.*** Because the sports medicine team is concerned about making decisions in the athlete's best interest, both

PRINCIPLES OF MEDICAL ETHICS

Physicians supervise and direct ATs and are critical sports medicine team members. A physician's care is guided by the principles of medical ethics. A direct link to these medical principles can be found at the AMA website found in the online resource (American Medical Association 2016).

1. A physician shall be dedicated to providing competent medical care, with compassion and respect for human dignity and rights.
2. A physician shall uphold the standards of professionalism, be honest in all professional interactions, and strive to report physicians deficient in character or competence, or engaging in fraud or deception, to appropriate entities.
3. A physician shall respect the law and recognize a responsibility to seek changes in those requirements that are contrary to the best interests of the patient.
4. A physician shall respect the rights of patients, colleagues, and other health professionals and shall safeguard patient confidences and privacy within the constraints of the law.
5. A physician shall continue to study, apply, and advance scientific knowledge; maintain a commitment to medical education; make relevant information available to patients, colleagues, and the public; obtain consultation; and use the talents of other health professionals when indicated.
6. A physician shall, in the provision of appropriate patient care, except in emergencies, be free to choose whom to serve, with whom to associate, and the environment in which to provide medical care.
7. A physician shall recognize a responsibility to participate in activities contributing to the improvement of the community and the betterment of public health.
8. A physician shall, while caring for a patient, regard responsibility to the patient as paramount.
9. A physician shall support access to medical care for all people.

Although physicians are bound by these principles, athletic trainers also have a code of ethics they must follow in providing care for their patients. You will notice the overlap between the National Athletic Trainers' Association's code of professional ethics and the American Medical Association's code. As a team, these members must uphold the highest standards. Athletic training most recently has established a set of shared professional values to help guide the behaviors of those within the profession. Shared professional values unite athletic trainers and support the tenets of the Code of Ethics. The NATA Professional Responsibility in AT (PRAT) committee carefully researched NATA members and came up with the following shared professional values (figure 1.2):

- ***Caring and Compassion:*** an intense concern and desire to help improve the welfare of another
- ***Integrity:*** a commitment that is internally motivated by an unyielding desire to do what is honest and right
- ***Respect:*** the act of imparting genuine and unconditional appreciation and value for all persons
- ***Competence:*** the ability to perform a task effectively with desirable outcomes
- ***Accountability:*** a willingness to be responsible for and answerable to one's own actions

C

Caring & Compassion is an intense concern and desire to help improve the welfare of another.

Sample behaviors include:
1) **Listening for understanding and a readiness to help.**
2) **Focusing on achieving the greatest well-being and the highest potential for others.**
3) **Spending the time needed to provide quality care.**

I

Integrity is a commitment that is internally motivated by an unyielding desire to do what is honest and right.

Sample behaviors include:
1) **Providing truthful, accurate and relevant information.**
2) **Abiding by the rules, regulations, laws and standards of the profession.**
3) **Using applicable professional standards and established policies and procedures when taking action or making decisions.**

R

Respect is the act of imparting genuine and unconditional appreciation and value for all persons.

Sample behaviors include:
1) **Engaging in active listening when communicating with others.**
2) **Acknowledging and expressing concern for others and their well-being.**
3) **Acting in light of the belief that the person has value.**

C

Competence is the ability to perform a task effectively with desirable outcomes.

Sample behaviors include:
1) **Thinking critically, demonstrating ethical sensitivity, committing to evidence-based practice, delivering quality skills and effective collaboration.**
2) **Making sound decisions while demonstrating integrity.**
3) **Ongoing continuous quality assessment and improvement.**

A

Accountability is a willingness to be responsible for and answerable to one's own actions.

Sample behaviors include:
1) **Acknowledging and accepting the consequences of one's own actions.**
2) **Adhering to laws, codes, practice acts and standards that govern professional practice.**
3) **Assuming responsibility for learning and change.**

Figure 1.2 Shared professional values.

Reprinted by permission from NATA, "Athletic Training's Shared Professional Values," National Athletic Trainers Association, accessed September 6, 2024, https://www.nata.org/sites/default/files/prat_5infographichandout-final.pdf.

the athlete and their parent or guardian must be involved in the central team.

- ***Team physician.*** The **team physician** is the medical authority who oversees the sports medicine team effort. To help determine the athlete's problem, the physician performs tests such as **X-rays** (electromagnetic waves used to make a picture of a body part); **magnetic resonance imaging (MRI)**, which uses radio waves and a magnetic field to make a picture of the body; or blood tests. The AT acts under the direction of the team physician, who is typically an orthopedic specialist. **Orthopedists** deal mostly with injuries to the musculoskeletal system.
- ***Certified AT.*** The AT communicates with the injured athlete, the athlete's parent or guardian, the team physician, and the coach. The AT is on-site at a game or practice and often makes the initial injury assessment and provides emergency care and follow-up treatment or referrals to other sports medicine team members as needed. Because of these multiple roles, the AT is a critical link in the chain of professionals on the sports medicine team.
- ***The coach.*** Daily contact with the athletes means the coach may know them better than the rest of the sports medicine team does. Because of their close contact with the parents or guardians of the athletes, the coach has a vital role in communicating with the injured athlete and their parents. When an athlete returns to competition following rehabilitation, the coach, in consultation with the AT, can modify the training, exercises, and drills the athlete performs so that they can safely progress to peak performance.

Peripheral Team

Although members of the central sports medicine team work together to manage an athletic injury, they often rely on peripheral team members to provide specialized care or assistance.

Many injured athletes have a **primary care physician**. Because this doctor has worked with the athlete before, the sports medicine team must include the primary care physician in their decisions. The primary care physician may refer the athlete to a specialist such as a podiatrist, allergist, urologist, gynecologist, cardiologist, neurologist, or pediatrician.

Understanding Diversity

Athletic Training as a Profession

Implicit bias is an internalized stereotype that can affect one's perception action or decision making and contributes to the unequal treatment of people based on certain characteristics. Those characteristics can be race, social economic status, marital status, age, religion, ethnicity, gender, sexual orientation, gender identity, disability, and educational status.

- A **podiatrist** examines and diagnoses problems below the knee and performs foot surgeries. They can prescribe corrective devices such as orthotics (shoe inserts).
- An **allergist** determines whether someone has an allergy and, if so, how to treat it. An **allergy** is an immune response such as red, swollen tissue or a runny nose to a substance that normally should be tolerated.
- A **urologist** treats problems of the urinary tract.
- A **gynecologist** diagnoses and treats the feminine reproductive system and provides sexual health services.
- A **cardiologist** treats heart disease and heart abnormalities.
- A **pediatrician** specializes in the medical treatment of children.
- A **dentist** may be involved if the athletic injury is to the facial area. The team dentist may also provide properly fitting mouth guards to prevent dental injuries.
- A **physical therapist** provides rehabilitation for bone and joint injuries, head injuries, and muscle injuries and imbalances so that patients may return to normal physical function and active daily living.
- A **physician assistant** works under the supervision of a physician and conducts examinations, orders diagnostic tests, writes prescriptions, and diagnoses and treats injuries and illnesses. Assistants typically specialize in a particular form of medicine. They free physicians to deal with more critical patients.

• A **neurologist** specializes in conditions of the nervous system and may examine an athlete who has suffered a head injury.

• A **student assistant** helps the AT with many daily tasks. For example, a student assistant may enter treatment data into a computer program, tape athletes before practices and games, stock medical cabinets and bags, organize the sidelines before games, hydrate the athletes during practices in hot weather, and prepare for rehabilitation procedures (e.g., organizing weights, whirlpools, and equipment). Also, because they are often the same age as the athletes, student assistants can identify with the athletes and may develop strong bonds with them. This can be especially helpful because the athletes often feel comfortable enough to ask questions and clarify information they have received. It is important to remember that *student assistants can function only under the direct supervision of an AT.* In some states, the student assistant is called an *athletic trainer aide.* Also, student assistants must not violate state practice acts or attempt to act in the capacity of an AT.

• A **chiropractor** is a health professional who takes a holistic approach to patient care by focusing on spinal misalignments. Although chiropractors are not physicians, they may treat musculoskeletal disorders and restore normal function by manipulating bones, specifically at the spinal column.

• The **school nurse** is a health care professional trained to identify and care for illnesses and disorders. The school nurse is a valuable educational resource for the AT and can help the athletic training team deliver safe, effective health care.

• A **dietitian (registered)** is a nutrition specialist who can help an athlete, and sometimes the entire athletic team, construct a proper diet based on activity level and dietary needs. They can also tailor meals for athletes who have specific conditions, such as diabetes.

• An **emergency medical technician (EMT)** is an emergency medical service (EMS) specialist who is certified to provide acute care for those who have a critical injury or illness. EMTs often also transport a victim to a nearby hospital. The National Registry for Emergency Medical Technicians (2023) recognizes varying levels of certification. These include EMT-Basic, EMT-Intermediate, and EMT-Paramedic (www.nremt.org/).

• A **massage therapist** is a health care professional who specializes in working with muscles and tendons. This role is important because tissue that is in spasm, needs to be warmed, or needs improved circulation can be aided by massage techniques.

• A **sport psychologist** works with athletes who may need help with goal setting, anxiety, frustration, self-esteem, family issues, and more. This work is essential to help athletes mentally prepare to participate at their best.

• A **strength and conditioning coach** works with athletes to ensure that each is in shape to meet the demands of athletic competition. Programs are designed to be sport-specific and to improve the athlete's areas of weakness.

• The **equipment manager** purchases and maintains appropriate protective and supportive athletic equipment. This is a significant role because many athletic injuries can be prevented with proper equipment. Equipment managers stay current on the latest and best types of padding, headgear, and clothing.

What Would You Do If . . .

An athlete was hit in the head during practice. The AT and the team physician evaluated the athlete and both wanted another opinion. The athlete complains to you, saying, "I don't understand why I have to see a neurologist. I've already been seen by our team physician."

BECOMING A CERTIFIED ATHLETIC TRAINER

Athletic training education has changed in recent years. To become an AT, you must now earn a master's degree from a college or university that has an athletic training program accredited by the **Commission on Accreditation of Athletic Training Education (CAATE)**. All athletic training programs will be entry-level master's degree programs (Commission on Accreditation of Athletic Training Education 2020). Bachelor degree programs have been phased out. Students enrolled in an entry-level athletic training program are expected to receive clinical experiences that provide supervised, hands-on experience, including a clinical immersion experience as well as specified courses related to athletic training. After graduation, a student must pass the BOC ATC exam and earn the ATC credential before practicing as a certified AT. Many states require state licensure in addition to national certification. Practicing without a license or certification could result in legal action, including arrest. The regulations for athletic training vary greatly from state to state. Three common forms of credentials are licensure, certification, and registration.

States that have **licensure** requirements generally specify who is allowed to practice athletic training and what duties they are allowed to perform. **Certification** ensures that an individual has achieved basic knowledge and skill to practice athletic training, and **registration** requires an individual to register with the state before practicing athletic training.

When a student enters an athletic training program, they must receive formal instruction in specific subject areas. The CAATE Standards for the Accreditation of Professional Programs in Athletic Training for 2020 define the required subjects. In addition to programmatic and administrative requirements, the core competencies and curricular content include the following:

1. Patient-centered care
2. Interprofessional practice and interprofessional education
3. Evidence-based practice
4. Quality improvement
5. Health care informatics
6. Professionalism
7. Patient or client care
8. Prevention, health promotion, and wellness
9. Health care administration

Each of these subjects is further clarified next by Institute of Medicine (2003).

- ***Patient-centered care.*** This means that an AT cares about patients' differences and needs, includes patients in the decision-making process, and educates them in wellness and disease prevention.
- ***Interprofessional practice and interprofessional education.*** This is the ability to work collaboratively with other health care providers. Providers can learn from one another in the best interest of the patient.
- ***Evidence-based practice.*** This means using clinical skills that have proven patient outcomes.
- ***Quality improvement.*** ATs need systems in place to improve their skill set and patient care.
- ***Health care informatics.*** This means that the educational program has the latest health care data. ATs must have access to the latest evidence-based information. It includes electronic documentation and data security of patient records.
- ***Professionalism.*** The AT agrees to behave in a way that is characteristic of others in the profession. The NATA Code of Ethics (2016b) defines the professional characteristics needed to be successful.
- ***Patient or client care.*** The AT will meet athlete needs, including being able to evaluate, properly examine, and diagnose all injuries and illnesses. The AT must be able to create a plan with the patient and educate them.
- ***Prevention, health, and wellness.*** The AT must prepare the athlete for lifelong health and wellness.
- ***Health care administration.*** This refers to the management aspects of athletic training. Many ATs develop policies and procedures for operating various facilities, financials, strategic planning, health insurance, and standards of practice that are supervised by the team physician.

Although these standards and competencies change regularly to ensure the most up-to-date content, they generally reflect emerging practices in the profession. Athletic training has created a strategic alliance of the key organizations involved in athletic training education and practice. NATA, BOC, CAATE, and NATA Research and Education Foundation (table 1.2) all collaborate to move the profession forward through advocacy and action (nata.org/about/strategic-alliance). Each member organization has its own role and works to advance athletic training.

An AT must recertify every two years by obtaining emergency cardiac care certification and participating in at least 50 hours of continuing education activity. Ten of the continuing education hours must come from evidence-based practices. Continuing education can take many forms, but the most common methods are workshops, online classes, and conferences that offer educational content. Both the BOC and state licensure agencies require continuing education independent of each other, so it is important to understand the role of each in maintaining your credentials.

The Real World

Although I originally went to college to become a physical educator, I have always been interested in health care. I selected athletic training as a health profession because it deals with sport and because it is one of the few health professions where you are trained to prevent injuries, give immediate care to an injury, and rehabilitate an injury. We have the privilege of working with people from the moment they are injured until the moment they return to their sport. This is a claim that few health professions can make.

Bill Pitney, EdD, ATC

ATHLETIC TRAINING CAREERS

ATs have a variety of opportunities for employment. The following describes various job settings, such as organized athletics and clinical and industrial venues. Information from NATA about average salaries from 2021 is also presented. The average 2021 salary across settings was $61,998, with ranges from $43,924 with one year of experience to $84,313 with 25 plus years of experience. Of course, academic degree completion influences average salaries as well, with those having a bachelor's degree earning on average $56,769, a master's degree $60,512, and doctoral degrees at $85,562 on average. As you can see, many variables contribute to the average salary and the good news is that salaries in athletic training continue to climb (NATA 2021).

Organized Athletics

Organized athletics are high schools, colleges or universities, professional or semiprofessional athletic teams, and youth sport leagues.

- ***High school environments.*** Considering that many high schools offer anywhere from 10 to 28 sports, these settings can be challenging. Some high schools have full-time ATs, but many high school ATs teach academic courses and receive a stipend for providing athletic training after school. Most high school ATs work 10 months of the year. Some ATs do similar work in middle school or junior high schools. In terms of salaries for this setting, the average range for ATs in high schools was $58,025 (NATA 2021).

Table 1.2 Athletic Training Strategic Alliance

Organization	Roles
Board of Certification for the Athletic Trainer (BOC)	Certification Consumer protection
Commission on Accreditation of Athletic Training Education (CAATE)	Accreditation Quality education
National Athletic Trainers' Association (NATA)	Advocacy Professional development
NATA Research and Education Foundation	Research Scholarship

- ***Universities and colleges.*** Nearly every college athletic program hires ATs to provide health care to its athletes. College athletic training contracts can be 9 to 12 months, and some college ATs also act as instructors for the athletic training education programs. Positions vary greatly in the college setting because programs come in many sizes, from large universities with many teams to small colleges with only a few athletic teams. The average salary for Division I college or university staff AT was $59,924, Division II was $52,289, and Division III was $52,290 (NATA 2021).

- ***Professional and semiprofessional teams.*** Although many students want to become an AT with a professional sport team, this goal is difficult to achieve. Compared with the number of positions in colleges, high schools, and clinical settings, there are few positions in the professional ranks. Also, ATs with professional teams often have a grueling travel schedule. The reward is the opportunity to work closely with elite athletes and coaches in an extremely competitive environment. The 2016 NATA salary survey is limited in the number of professional sports represented and the 2021 salary survey does not include this setting, but overall, the average salary range for this setting was $40,000 to $62,361. Professional football ATs averaged $137,993 annually (NATA 2021).

- ***Youth sport leagues.*** Some organized youth sport leagues have taken the initiative to hire full-time ATs to care for their athletes. The primary role of ATs in youth sport is the prevention and care of athletic injuries, and the reward is working with young athletes as they develop their athletic ability. Salaries for these positions are typically per diem or contracted as part-time event coverage. They are widely variable across the country.

Clinical and Hospital Settings

Clinical settings are sites such as outpatient rehabilitation or sports medicine centers. These positions are called clinical-outreach positions whereby an AT works in a sports medicine center part time and at a secondary school part time, or they can work full time in physician-owned clinics. Hospital settings involve ATs working in the emergency room, surgery, orthopedics, or even administration.

FYI

Medical Ethics and Legal Issues

The moral aspects of health care and legal statutes dictate what ATs are allowed to do as professionals.

Human Anatomy

This is how the body is organized; the study of bones, joints, muscles, and organs and their structure and location. The AT cannot recognize injuries unless they understand human anatomy.

Human Physiology

This covers human body functions. The treatments ATs render to athletes must be based on sound physiological principles. For example, after an athlete is injured, the tissue heals in several stages. The AT must understand what happens during each stage in order to prescribe exercises that will not reinjure the tissue.

Exercise Physiology

This refers to the processes that occur in the body during activity. When a person exercises, they place demands on the body and the body adapts to them. An exercising person's heart and breathing rates will be higher than when they are at rest. Understanding the changes that exercise causes in the body is essential for recognizing signs and symptoms of illness or injury.

First Aid and Emergency Care

This means systematically managing acute injury and illness in an emergency.

Strength Training and Reconditioning

This is preparing athletes for the demands of a sport or activity by helping them attain an appropriate level of strength, endurance, flexibility, and cardiorespiratory fitness. An AT must understand the principles and techniques of these programs.

Biomechanics

The science of movement mechanics, **biomechanics**, is also called **kinesiology**. ATs are responsible for teaching athletes how to properly perform exercises that will help them recover from injuries. In addition, ATs often apply tape and braces to prevent athletes from performing certain movements that might cause injury. These treatments cannot be effectively applied unless one first understands biomechanics.

Statistics and Research Design

This refers to how data are collected and analyzed. An AT must understand these fields to obtain accurate evidence related to injury treatment strategies, injury prevention programs, and so forth.

• ***Sports medicine centers.*** Although most ATs fill diverse roles ranging from emergency care to health care administration, the clinical AT tends to focus on rehabilitation. Many clinical ATs enjoy the one-on-one relationships they build with patients during their rehabilitation programs.

• ***Clinic outreach.*** Many programs have combined the traditional and clinical settings and created new positions and job opportunities for ATs. For example, it is not uncommon for a sports medicine center to have ATs who work part of a day (usually the morning) in a clinic and then go to a local high school in the afternoon to cover practices and events.

• ***Physician-owned clinics.*** Many physicians have found value in hiring an AT to examine patients, assist with medical procedures, and treat athletic injuries. Physicians hire ATs to provide durable goods care, meaning the AT fits patients with walking boots, splints, braces, and castings and performs other tasks. In 2021, average salary for ATs working in clinical and hospital settings was $59,919 (NATA 2021).

• Athletic trainers are also employed in the performing arts, military, occupational medicine, and other emerging settings.

Industrial and Occupational Settings

Industrial and occupational settings for ATs are health and fitness centers and industrial and manufacturing sites.

• ***Health and fitness centers.*** Many companies and health centers have come to realize that ATs are a business asset. Not everyone who enters a health center or corporate fitness program is completely healthy. Some may even be under a physician's care for a particular injury and may need an AT to get started on a safe fitness routine that will not aggravate the injury.

• ***Industrial, occupational, and manufacturing sites.*** Businesses spend billions of dollars annually for health care. To reduce health care costs, many companies see the advantages of having a full-time AT on staff to help prevent and treat worksite injuries. ATs can often treat these injuries at the workplace under the supervision of a physician, decreasing the amount of work time lost to the industrial athlete. This is a rapidly emerging area in the profession as companies see the value of an AT in an industrial role. Companies such as FedEx, Amazon, and others are opening internships and jobs for athletic trainers.

In the industrial setting, the supervisor replaces a coach and the employee replaces an athlete. The peripheral team may add an **ergonomics specialist** to the other allied medical professionals. An ergonomics specialist measures and adapts a work environment to prevent and treat musculoskeletal disorders. For example, rather than forcing workers to stand on a hard concrete floor and work at a bench that is so low they have to bend over for eight hours a day, executives may hire an ergonomics specialist to recommend changes in the physical environment that will reduce the wear and tear on workers' bodies. Such modifications may be as simple as providing higher workbenches, special chairs, and cushioned floor mats. The AT's job is to ensure that the employees work in ergonomically safe environments to prevent injury and save the company money.

Military, Public Health and Safety, and Law Enforcement Settings

An emerging practice setting for ATs is with the military and law enforcement. Administrators in

EMPLOYMENT SETTINGS

Many athletic trainers work outside the widely known settings. Some ATs have started their own businesses, such as owning physical fitness facilities, starting consulting firms, and creating and selling sports medicine or durable medical goods and equipment. ATs will continue to expand their roles and will have even greater opportunities as owners of health care facilities or businesses—the possibilities are endless.

these settings have recognized that many injuries suffered in combat are similar to what athletes suffer. Moreover, soldiers and law officers must make a quick recovery and return to their jobs in excellent physical condition; otherwise, their lives are at serious risk. Athletic trainers played an integral role in the COVID-19 pandemic as agents to support public health initiatives. This emerging setting has continued to develop as athletic trainers demonstrated their versatility and professionalism in a range of public health actions.

Job Outlook

Job Outlook 2020 documents show an expected 23% growth for athletic training jobs from 2020 to 2030. This job growth is much higher than average, with approximately 3,100 new jobs posted each year during this decade (Bureau of Labor Statistics n.d.). A direct link to the job outlook can be found in the online resources.

NATIONAL ATHLETIC TRAINERS' ASSOCIATION

The athletic training profession is directed by its professional association, NATA. This organization is composed of voluntary members, including ATs, athletic training students, and associate members. NATA guides the profession's advancement and sponsors the publishing of important information that affects how athletes are treated. Among these important publications are the *Journal of Athletic Training*, the *Athletic Training Education Journal*, and various professional statements that provide timely and important information related to injuries, illnesses, and diseases. NATA and the BOC also provide ethical guidelines that guide the practice of ATs. These are covered in chapter 2.

The NATA statements are important because they provide ATs with standards of care and guidelines for treating those in need. NATA position statements cover the following topics and continue to evolve annually:

- Management of acute skin trauma
- Preventing and managing sport-related dental and oral injuries
- Exertional heat illnesses
- Management of sport concussion
- Preparticipation physical examinations and disqualifying conditions
- Conservative management and prevention of ankle sprains in athletes
- Lightning safety for athletics and recreation
- Evaluation of dietary supplements for performance nutrition
- Anabolic-androgenic steroids
- Preventing sudden death in sports
- Heat illness treatment authorization form
- Consensus statements for heat illness guidelines
- Safe weight loss and maintenance practices in sport and exercise
- Prevention of pediatric overuse injuries
- Preventing, detecting, and managing disordered eating in athletes
- Management of athletes with type 1 diabetes
- Management of asthma in athletes
- Head-down contact and spearing in tackle football
- *Heads Up* video
- Fluid replacement for athletes
- Emergency planning in athletics
- Environmental cold injuries
- Acute management of the cervical spine-injured athlete
- Skin diseases

New position statements are written as health issues arise in the profession. Critically appraised topics (CATs), which are smaller evidence-based research projects based on a clinical question, support evidence-based practice. CATs are helpful in providing concise information on a range of clinical questions to gain insight about the clinical bottom line. For the full text of the position statements, visit the NATA website and search the web for critically appraised topics in the area of clinical interest.

Celebrating our profession is important. March is National Athletic Training Month. The purpose of this month is to make the public aware of the athletic training profession. NATA encourages all ATs to participate in the grassroots effort by sponsoring contests and doing presentations for parents, school boards, and legislative groups. Many students create signs and advertisements promoting the profession and others create websites to further describe what the profession is all about.

WORK–LIFE BALANCE

Athletic training is a wonderful profession. It requires a great amount of preparation clinically and academically to be successful in the broad range of settings. One area of recent development has been that of **work–life balance**. This line of research has encouraged athletic trainers to find a balance between the time-intensive nature of the work we do to make time for self-care. Burnout is a risk in any profession, and work–life balance helps athletic trainers have a long, successful, healthy career in the field.

Summary

The AT plays a vital role in providing health care to the physically active population. A successful AT recognizes that the best health care is given through a team approach that draws on the strengths of a variety of professionals. ATs provide health care in many places, such as high schools, colleges, professional sport teams, sports medicine clinics, and industrial settings. To become an AT, one must have a master's degree and study specific subjects, such as human anatomy and physiology, injury assessment, pharmacology, rehabilitation and reconditioning, and biomechanics. Programs are evolving to support and advocate for the athletic training profession.

Key Terms

Define the following terms found in this chapter:

- allergist
- allergy
- American Red Cross
- ATC
- athletic training
- biomechanics
- Board of Certification (BOC)
- cardiologist
- certification
- certified athletic trainer (AT)
- chiropractor
- Commission on the Accreditation of Athletic Training Education (CAATE)
- dentist
- dietitian (registered)
- emergency medical technician (EMT)
- equipment manager
- ergonomics specialist
- gynecologist
- kinesiology
- licensure
- massage therapist
- National Athletic Trainers' Association (NATA)
- National Safety Council
- neurologist
- orthopedist
- pediatrician
- physical therapist
- physician assistant
- podiatrist
- primary care physician
- reconditioning
- registration
- rehabilitation
- school nurse
- shared professional values
- sport psychologist
- sports medicine
- strength and conditioning coach
- student assistant
- team physician
- urologist
- work-life balance
- X-ray

As a student interested in athletic training, you are responsible for understanding the venues in which an AT can be employed. After you research the different employment settings, you attend a MSAT program and are now certified. What important steps will you need to take to ensure that you comply with ongoing credentialing standards as a certified athletic trainer?

To access supplementary material for this chapter, including the Understanding Check worksheet, vocabulary quizzes, extension activities, and chapter-specific resources and forms, visit the web resource: http://ancillaries.humankinetics.com/FundamentalsOfAthleticTrainingAndSportsMedicine5E

chapter 2

Administration and Professional Development

Objectives

After completing this chapter, the student will be able to do the following:

- Describe the concept of negligence and explain ways to prevent being negligent.
- Describe why insurance is necessary.
- Understand reimbursement for AT services.
- Understand the concept of professional practice in athletic training.
- Describe the standards of professional practice in athletic training and codes of ethics.
- Explain the importance of continuing education and the requirements.
- Explain the elements of leadership.
- Describe characteristics that are helpful to being a future professional.

In addition to caring for and preventing athletic injuries, ATs must perform a variety of administrative duties. Moreover, they must be aware of certain legal issues that will greatly affect how they choose to administrate their athletic training program.

LEGAL ISSUES

When athletes choose to participate in sport, they risk becoming injured or even permanently disabled. Because ATs may be legally liable because of athletes' injuries or illnesses, they must understand certain legal terminology and often carry their own personal liability insurance in addition to having liability coverage through their employer.

Duty of Care

Duty of care means that an AT has an official job responsibility to render treatment and follow procedures related to the health and well-being of an athlete. An AT's duty of care is often outlined in an official job description. If an AT has a duty of care but fails to perform that duty, negligence may be the result.

Negligence

Negligence is a legal wrong characterized by the failure to act as a reasonably prudent person would act in a similar situation. For example, if an AT provides care below the standard of the law, they may be found negligent in certain circumstances. Picture an AT who has noticed a large hole on the field a couple of hours before a field hockey game. A reasonably prudent person would think that this hole could cause an injury and would take reasonable action. For example, the AT could contact appropriate personnel, such as the grounds crew, athletic director, or maintenance department, to attempt to fill in the hole before game time, or they could place an orange cone in the hole to alert players of the danger.

Gross Negligence

Gross negligence has been described as a step beyond negligence; that is, an AT fails to provide even a slight amount of care when needed. To distinguish negligence from gross negligence, let's look at an example. In the case of basic first aid to care for a victim whose finger is bleeding severely, we would provide reasonable care for controlling bleeding by applying direct pressure, elevating the arm, using a pressure bandage if necessary, and applying pressure at a pressure point. If the AT only told the injured athlete to elevate the arm and eventually decided that perhaps a dressing should be put around the finger because it was still bleeding, the AT may be negligent. A grossly negligent AT, on the other hand, might fail to even provide instructions to the bleeding athlete. Although an AT may not want to come into contact with someone's blood for fear of disease transmission, they can at least give instructions so the athlete can start giving care to themselves, and the AT can also seek additional help.

Malpractice

Malpractice occurs when the AT causes an injury to the athlete by an act of omission or commission. An act of omission means that the AT failed to act prudently. An example of omission would be not doing CPR on a person who is not breathing and has no heartbeat. An act of commission would be to provide care outside the scope of practice or do something that should not be done. Making an incision into an athlete's trachea and inserting a tube is an act of commission because it is beyond the AT's scope of practice. In either instance, the athlete is injured; thus, there is legal malpractice.

Assumption of Risk

When an athlete participates in a sport, they have an **assumption of risk**. An athlete must fully understand that by participating in sport, they may be injured; that is, they assume the risk of being injured after being fully warned of the dangers. Thus, an organization such as a high school must warn athletes and parents of the dangers that are common in the sports that the athletes will play. To make sure that athletes and parents understand the dangers, many programs require athletes to read and sign an assumption-of-risk form. Many coaches and ATs go even further and have the teams watch movies that explain the rules of the game and potential consequences of playing, such as injury or death. In addition, they use well-organized practice plans that document the day, time, and names of athletes who were given specific instructions about rules and technique.

Go online to the Resources and Forms section in the web resource to find a printable assumption-of-risk form.

Informed Consent

Before an AT can perform any medical procedure, they must obtain the consent of the athlete (or parent or guardian if the athlete is a minor). Failure to do so may make the AT liable for negligence. Therefore, the athlete or parent or guardian must be given enough information to make an intelligent decision about granting permission for care. Many schools have rules addressing this particular issue and specific forms that must be signed before students can participate in a sport (i.e., **informed consent**). This example also includes a medical information card. Many ATs put the permission to treat and the medical information on opposite sides of an index card. If the information is organized in this manner, it is easy to transport in a file folder or medical bag. The hospital staff is often thankful to have this information as well.

Here are special circumstances that involve informed consent:

- It is presumed that an unconscious athlete gives permission to be treated, even if the athlete has not given consent before becoming unconscious.
- An athlete who is arrested and refuses treatment can still be treated under the law.
- An emancipated minor (underage but legally responsible for themselves) can make a legal decision for treatment without parental permission.

Go online to the Resources and Forms section in the web resource to find a printable permission-to-treat form.

What Would You Do If . . .

You are helping the team get ready for practice. You get to the football field and notice a large hole in the ground in the practice area.

Proximate Cause

Proximate cause is a close connection between the way an AT acted and the resulting injury to an athlete. Noticing that an action will lead to a certain result and potentially harm someone is a component of proximate cause. For example, suppose an AT evaluates an athlete's injured neck and determines that there is considerable weakness and a lack of movement when the athlete attempts to look up or down. Also, the athlete is in pain. If the AT allows the athlete to continue playing and this results in further injury and permanent neck damage, proximate cause could be shown. That is, the AT's action (letting the athlete continue playing) may be directly linked to the further injury (permanent neck damage).

Because ATs use many products to prevent and care for athletic injuries, they must be aware of the established guidelines for using them. For example, the sports medicine team should purchase only football helmets approved by the National Operating Committee on Standards for Athletic Equipment (NOCSAE). Failure to do so may lead to injury or even death. We recommend that an AT or an athletic program buy top-of-the-line products and research them to ensure that the products are high quality.

AVOIDING LEGAL PROBLEMS

Several authors in the literature on athletic training have offered suggestions for avoiding legal liability. These suggestions are summarized as follows:

- ***Have a written contract.*** ATs, coaches, and other pertinent personnel should have a detailed contract with their employer that includes a job description. Either in this contract or in a separate document, the relationship between the head AT and students or assistants should be explained. At the high school and college levels, student assistants are under the direct supervision of an AT, which means that anything a student does in the athletic training room should be monitored. Students are able to observe and learn, which is a valuable experience. They can also assist the AT with procedures if the AT deems it appropriate.

- ***Use equipment that meets established safety standards.*** Use equipment only for its intended purposes and be sure it is properly fitted. Equipment must be reconditioned and meet safety standards to be used. Certain equipment, like football helmets, must be destroyed after being used for a certain amount of time (e.g., 10 years). Equipment used in the athletic training room, such as whirlpools, compression units, and TENS units, needs to be checked to meet manufacturer standards to ensure it is safe.
- ***Identify risks and reduce them.*** The AT should monitor playing fields, both indoors and outdoors. They should report hazards and document problems. Things that can create injuries include falling goal cages, holes in fields, condensation on floors, and poor lighting. Having a checklist can be beneficial in staying on top of each area of participation.
- ***Require preparticipation physical examinations.*** Preparticipation exams help identify existing conditions that may lead to injuries. If these conditions can be identified, injuries can be prevented, which limits the chance of liability.
- ***Have all athletes and their parents or guardians sign an assumption-of-risk form.*** Participants must understand the risks involved with sport and know that the potential for injury or illness exists.
- ***Maintain CPR and first aid certifications.*** The AT should practice these skills regularly.
- ***Have a crisis plan.*** The AT must have an effective crisis plan in writing for all home and away contests. The crisis plan should explain the procedures to be carried out, and all who are involved should have a copy and know their roles.
- ***Control medications.*** The AT should have documentation for each athlete who uses prescription medication. Prescription medications are prohibited in most athletic training rooms according to state law. If they are permitted by state law to be in the athletic training facility, documentation with physician approval supports how the medication is to be used and stored. Over-the-counter medications need to be stored in a locked cabinet in individual packets if dispensed to athletes. The administration of over-the-counter medication must be documented, including type, dosage, date, time, and the person who administered it, and must comply with state regulations. Athletic trainers are prohibited from dispensing and administering prescription medication.
- ***Document all injuries and procedures.*** An AT should note in detail on the appropriate administrative forms not only all injuries that occur but also all rehabilitation procedures, treatments, and follow-up care.
- ***Maintain confidentiality.*** ATs are required by law to keep medical information confidential. The Health Insurance Portability and Accountability Act (HIPAA) of 1996 requires that personal health-related information be secured and kept private (see chapter 4).
- ***Build trust.*** An effective line of communication and good rapport within the athletic training team allows the AT to build trust and respect with everyone involved with an athletic injury.
- ***Stay educated.*** ATs have a responsibility to continue their education and stay current on the latest information in the allied medical field. An AT must also understand their qualifications and know their limitations. Moreover, because state laws differ, it is important for ATs to understand their state regulations.

Go online to the Resources and Forms section in the web resource to find a printable athletic injury and accident report.

INSURANCE

In most organizations, athletes are required to have medical insurance before participating in organized

> **RED FLAGS**
>
> When inspecting facilities before an athletics practice or game, report and document any of the following conditions:
>
> - Spills or dirty surfaces
> - Toxic smell or chemicals
> - Holes or divots in the surface
> - Equipment in ill repair
> - Heating or cooling system not functioning
> - Obstacles in or around the playing surface
> - Goal cages improperly secured to the ground
> - Bleachers improperly secured to the ground

sport. Many athletic programs require that insurance forms be kept with the informed consent (permission-to-treat) forms discussed earlier. Why is this necessary? Say that an athlete who is traveling with the team on the road gets injured. If their parents are not at the game, the injured athlete can still be treated at a local hospital because permission to treat has been granted and appropriate insurance information has been provided. Unfortunately, insurance coverage is becoming increasingly complicated—ask any AT about the paperwork involved with insurance and watch their reaction. However, insurance is necessary because medical costs can be substantial.

Athlete Medical Insurance

Medical insurance has been described as a written agreement between an insurance company and the person who buys it. This agreement clarifies the terms of reimbursement for medical costs after an athlete has been treated. Many athletic programs purchase supplemental insurance that covers the leftover costs not covered by the primary insurance. The insurance is usually for injuries that occur during athletic participation. Programs carry supplemental insurance so that an athlete's care is completely covered. Many athletic programs also carry a **catastrophic policy**, which is insurance for injuries that cause permanent disability, such as paralysis.

Several types of insurance exist. These include managed care plans, indemnity plans, and health savings accounts (Konin and Ray 2019).

Managed care plans include health maintenance organizations (HMOs) and preferred provider organizations (PPOs). Managed care plans have an agreement between the insurance company and a group or network of health care professionals. Essentially, restrictions are imposed on a patient, who must see a primary physician within the agreed-on network to receive health care. A copay is usually required at the time of service.

Indemnity plans are sometimes referred to as *reimbursement plans*. They are organized to have an insurance company fully or partially reimburse a patient for the cost of health care (Briscoe 2015).

A health savings account (HSA) is often created by having an employer or individual submit money to a fund used only for paying medical claims as they occur. Health care providers are often selected from a larger network. For that reason, HSAs are often similar to HMO or PPO plans.

Athletic Trainer Liability Insurance

Liability insurance helps protect the AT from personal financial loss in the event of a lawsuit. The insurance coverage should be for the types of services the AT provides; otherwise, the insurance will not protect the AT in the event of a lawsuit. If the AT is employed by a school or a private company, the employer will likely provide the liability insurance. If the AT is self-employed, they should purchase liability insurance.

Reimbursement for AT Services

An AT can get reimbursed for services provided to athletes if the educational institution, the state within which services are provided, and the insurance company agree to it. To get reimbursed, the AT must document their services and complete forms with coding so the insurance company understands the services. The insurance company will determine whether the service provided is covered.

When working with insurance companies, it is important to have a common way of talking about procedures that have been performed, which is called using *current procedural terminology codes*. Selecting the correct code has a direct effect on whether an insurance company will pay for a procedure.

Each insurance company has its own form that needs to be completed. An electronic version of insurance claim forms can be found online at the company website. When the AT is completing the form, the *Diagnostic Statistical Manual* can be useful in determining a code. Some online forms will generate codes that the AT can select.

There will be times when an athlete is injured and the AT needs to file forms to ensure coverage by an insurance company. The AT will work with the family of the student-athlete to obtain all the medical bills and proof of injury.

PROFESSIONAL DEVELOPMENT AND CONTINUING EDUCATION

Professional development is the ongoing responsibility of improving one's skills and knowledge to deliver appropriate health care to injured athletes. The successful AT will behave ethically, stay abreast of the latest medical issues and trends, display good communication skills, and be an effective leader.

The Real World

During an intercollegiate game, a goalie from a visiting soccer team received a blow to the head from a teammate while trying to scoop up a soccer ball. He was hit so hard that his skull was fractured. The host AT attended to the athlete and called for an ambulance immediately. The athlete's condition was worsening even as he was being taken to the emergency room, and a helicopter was called because the athlete needed to be transferred to a trauma center in another city. Unfortunately, the visiting team had no medical information about the athlete or any emergency contact information. Treatment was initiated because the athlete was unconscious; permission to treat was implied. Because the athlete had recently walked on to the team, even his full name was a mystery—thankfully, a rare occurrence. It took many phone calls to the school before the athlete's name was determined and then more detective work to figure out how to reach his parents. The moral of the story is to have appropriate medical information—complete with full name and emergency contact numbers—with the team at all times.

Phil Voorhis, MSEd, ATC

Standards and Codes for Professional Practice

Athletic trainers are governed by several organizations that have come together to create the Athletic Training Strategic Alliance. Each organization within the Strategic Alliance strives to move athletic training forward through individual areas of focus. As noted earlier, the Board of Certification (BOC) is the certifying or credentialing board responsible for protecting the public by ensuring athletic trainers are prepared to practice. They establish the domains for the profession of athletic training through the practice analysis document defining the knowledge and skills for athletic trainers. These are performed every five years and a comparison chart was provided for you in chapter 1. Information regarding the BOC Practice Analysis can be found at https://BOCATC.org.

The Commission on Accreditation of Athletic Training Education (CAATE) is responsible for ensuring that the educational programs prepare ATs to meet the expectations set forth by the profession and evaluated by the BOC entry-level certification examination. The National Athletic Trainers' Association (NATA) is the third pillar. It is the membership organization and provides member benefits and advocacy for the profession. The last pillar, Research and Education Foundation (REF), supports the advancement of the profession by supporting research and educational initiatives, including research grants and scholarships.

Through the collaboration of the Strategic Alliance members, athletic trainers are held to a high standard, and several key documents in the profession provide guidance. Athletic trainers are bound by state licensure or regulation and certification standards in most states. The state licensure acts vary from state to state but are the legal framework for professional practice in that particular state (BOC n.d.b). State regulatory information can be found at https://BOCATC.org. In addition to state regulation, ATs must comply with standards of professional practice the BOC set for the AT certifying agency. The BOC sets standards that each certificant is expected to follow as a matter of professional practice; these include professional standards and a code of professional responsibility.

BOC STANDARDS OF PROFESSIONAL PRACTICE

In addition to state laws, a certified AT must follow BOC standards of professional practice (Board of Certification 2022). The BOC has seven standards:

1. ***Direction.*** The AT renders service or treatment under the direction of or in collaboration with a physician, in accordance with their training and the state's statutes, rules, and regulations.
2. ***Prevention.*** The AT implements measures to prevent and mitigate injury, illness, and long-term disability.
3. ***Immediate care.*** The AT provides care in acute or emergency situations, independent of setting.
4. ***Examination, assessment, and diagnosis.*** The AT utilizes patient history and appropriate physical examination procedures to determine the patient's impairments, diagnosis, level of function, and disposition.
5. ***Therapeutic intervention.*** The AT determines appropriate treatment, rehabilitation, and reconditioning strategies. Intervention program objectives include long- and short-term goals and an appraisal of those that the patient can realistically be expected to achieve from the program. Appropriate patient-centered outcomes assessments are utilized to document the efficacy of interventions.
6. ***Program discontinuation.*** The AT may recommend discontinuation of the intervention program at such time the patient has received optimal benefit of the program. A final assessment of the patient's status is included in the discharge note.
7. ***Organization and administration.*** The AT documents all procedures and services in accordance with local, state, and federal laws, rules, and guidelines.

The BOC Code of Professional Responsibility includes patient care responsibilities, professional responsibility, research, social responsibility, and business practices. These areas define the expectations of ATs who practice in the profession.

Lastly, NATA, the national membership organization for athletic trainers, has a Code of Ethics for all members. The AT must treat people fairly to the best of their ability and do what is right. To help its members, NATA has updated its **code of ethics** (National Athletic Trainers' Association 2022).

The principles of this code are the following:

Principle 1: In the role of an athletic trainer, members shall practice with compassion, respecting the rights, well-being, and dignity of others.

Principle 2: Members shall comply with the laws and regulations governing the practice of athletic training, National Athletic Trainers' Association NATA membership standards, and the NATA Code of Ethics.

Principle 3: Members shall maintain and promote high standards in their provision of services.

Principle 4: Members shall not engage in conduct that could be construed as a conflict of interest, reflects negatively on the athletic training profession, or jeopardizes a patient's health and well-being.

The NATA Code of Ethics was recently changed to include the **Shared Professional Values (SPVs)** articulated by its members through the work of the Professional Responsibility in Athletic Training (PRAT) committee. These SPVs are known as CIRCA and represent NATA's five shared professional values of Caring and Compassion; Integrity, Respect, Competence; and Accountability, which were shared in chapter 1 as an infographic and are now part of the Code of Ethics. Each member of the organization is expected to adhere to these SPVs.

When an AT does not follow professional standards, the Code of Ethics, or state laws, there are checks and balances (see figure 2.1).

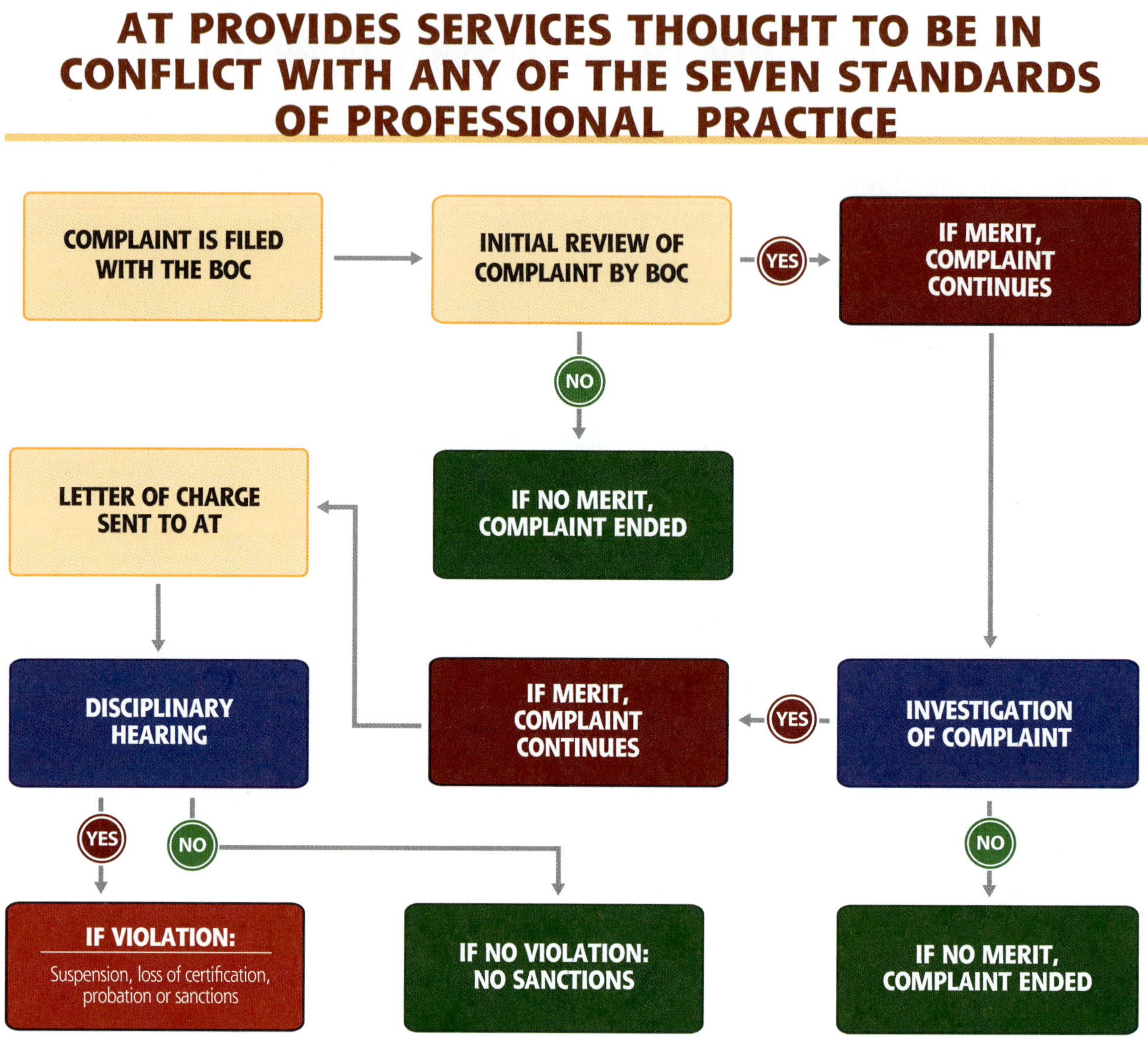

Figure 2.1 What happens if an AT provides services outside the BOC standards of professional practice?
Board of Certification 2022

NATA has created LERPS (laws, ethics, regulation, and professional standards) to help guide the AT in looking at all the different components that affect professional behavior. By understanding state laws, ethical standards, state regulation, and policies regarding professional practice, the AT can protect themselves and their patients by providing ethically sound care within their scope of practice.

Understanding Diversity

What Is Diversity, Equity, and Inclusion?

Diversity refers to a variety of people from different backgrounds. Equity is being impartial and providing everything anyone needs to make them equal. Inclusion is when those who are usually excluded have an equal opportunity to take part.

Staying Educated

If medical professionals do not learn to use anything new or fail to use the most up-to-date technology, an injured athlete will not get the best care. Therefore, once a person has earned the credential *ATC* after their name, they are required to continue their education. The BOC requires that an AT complete 50 continuing education hours, known as continuing education units (CEUs), every two years. In addition, states require continuing education to maintain licensure. You can use the CEUs from your state for the BOC and vice versa as long as they fall within the appropriate dates of the reporting period. These, however, are two different processes and require the AT to complete forms for both the state and the BOC.

CEUs are obtained in a variety of ways, such as by attending educational workshops, writing and publishing, taking college classes, and completing home study courses. In addition to these professional learning activities, an AT must maintain professional rescuer CPR certification (every two years, an AT must show proof of current CPR certification). Athletic trainers can be audited for CEUs and must be able to prove they have met requirements with documentation. Athletic trainers must retain their proof of CEUs for at least the next reporting period.

Communication

Whether an AT works at a high school, college, or sports medicine clinic, they must have good communication skills. ATs communicate daily with athletes, parents, physicians, coaches, and administrators at every level. Failure to send the right message can result in many anxious hours and negative consequences. In their book *Management Strategies in Athletic Training* (2019), Jeff Konin and Richard Ray offer many practical suggestions for ATs to enhance their communication skills. They suggest that when listening, you should devote your total effort and attention. To verify what the conversation has been, the active listener can repeat the conversation back. ATs must keep an open mind and refrain from passing judgment. Pay attention to your gestures; they send messages that can be interpreted in unintended ways. For example, if you cross your arms, someone may think you are impatient or angry.

Leadership

The athletic training profession has progressed and flourished, undoubtedly because of the leadership of its members. Several principles and qualities of leadership are important for ATs. Athletic training leaders come from all different backgrounds and practice settings. The professional organizations for the profession have many opportunities for athletic trainers to participate in initiatives and committees to advance the profession. Whether you are just getting started in the profession, mid-career, or late-career, there is a committee that would fit your needs. For example, NATA has committees ranging from the LGBTQ+ Advisory Committee to the Young Professionals Committee, with involvement opportunities to meet everyone's interests (NATA, n.d.). A full listing of NATA committees can be found at https://www.nata.org/membership/get-involved/volunteer-committees. Additionally, each state and district organization also has opportunities for involvement if you'd like to be involved at these levels of leadership. Leadership opportunities and involvement are very rewarding and help you advocate for the profession. Take the first steps to volunteer!

Athletic training is expanding relative to professional settings, interprofessional practice, and research and education. It is important to think about who you want to be as a professional in the field. Many models exist for leadership development, but the **PREMIER model** provides an easy way of thinking about being a future professional. This model is based on the authors' experience as professionals in athletic training. The acronym for this model can be found in figure 2.2.

- ***Promote a professional image.*** As a student assistant, you can project a professional image by the way you dress. An old saying states that you don't get a second chance at a first impression. Although wearing shorts, tennis shoes, and T-shirts may be fine during practice or game coverage for warm-weather activities, it is imperative that you be distinguishable and professional looking in case someone needs to find you for help.
- ***Remember your vision.*** You must have a good understanding of your career goals and objectives and what type of person you are striving

P	**Promote** a professional image
R	**Remember** your vision
E	**Engage** in learning
M	**Maximize** your strengths
I	**Innovate** and create
E	**Enlist** the help of others
R	**Reflect**

Figure 2.2 The PREMIER model gives helpful suggestions for developing yourself as a future professional.

to become. Some people write down their vision statement so they can continually be reminded of their purpose and set appropriate personal goals.

- ***Engage in learning.*** As a student and future professional, it is important to take initiative to learn new things daily.
- ***Maximize your strengths.*** We all have limitations. If you dwell too much on them, you may not learn and do the things that can make you successful. Cultivate your strengths and ask yourself how they can support your personal vision.
- ***Innovate and create.*** Over the past 10 to 20 years, technology has continually advanced. Today's problems cannot be solved with yesterday's solutions. As a future professional, it is important for you to develop new ideas. This will keep you excited about your work.
- ***Enlist the help of others.*** In the previous chapter, you learned about the role of the AT and the sports medicine team. The old saying that there is no *I* in *team* is absolutely accurate. Be a team player.
- ***Reflect.*** When you become a professional, it will be essential to think back on what you have done and consider the results, whether you are rehabilitating an athlete or taping an ankle. Get into the habit now of reflecting on your actions in the athletic training room to help you learn what you might do better in a similar situation in the future.

Tom Abdenour, ATC, states that you should *C* your way to success as a certified AT. The four Cs are conscientiousness, competency, courtesy, and courage. To be successful, be conscientious about the little things, such as following through with treatments, maintaining a clean and safe facility, and being available to the athletes. Being conscientious involves representing yourself, your organization, and your profession in a quality manner and being loyal to your staff and organization. Competency involves being good at what you do and continually learning to expand your horizons. Courtesy involves being a team player, interacting with everyone you work with in a positive manner, and treating people as you would want to be treated. Finally, to be successful, you must have the courage and fortitude to take on challenges.

REQUIREMENTS FOR CEUS (BASED ON THE REQUIRED 50 CEUS)

- Category A: (Level I): Attending workshops through a BOC-approved provider program: no maximum CEUs
- Category B: (Level II): Writing and publishing activities: maximum 33 CEUs
- Category C: (Level II): Post-certification college coursework: no more than 40 CEUs
- Category D: (Level II): Non-BOC-approved courses and workshops: no more than 28 CEUs

Board of Certification (n.d.a.)

Summary

ATs must follow the standards of professional practice that many professional agencies who work collaboratively to guide professional practice have set. These standards guide the AT in delivering professional health care. To maintain an acceptable level of knowledge, the AT is required to participate in 50 hours of continuing education every 2 years. ATs often find themselves in leadership roles and should conduct themselves with integrity, vision, inspiration, and competence. There are numerous administrative considerations for the AT, such as properly documenting injuries and treatments and considering the ethical expectations and legal liability inherent in the practice. Athletic trainers are held to a high standard because working with people is a serious responsibility. As a professional, it is your duty to know the laws, ethical standards, regulations, and policies that govern your practice.

Key Terms

Define the following terms found in this chapter:

- assumption of risk
- code of ethics
- duty of care
- gross negligence
- informed consent
- malpractice
- negligence
- PREMIER model
- proximate cause
- standards of professional practice

As an AT, you have been involved in a situation that ended in the catastrophic disablement of an athlete. Although you performed your duties as required by state law, a lawsuit is pending. What key elements do you need to consider as you defend yourself from this accusation?

To access supplementary material for this chapter, including the Understanding Check worksheet, vocabulary quizzes, extension activities, and chapter-specific resources and forms, visit the web resource: http://ancillaries.humankinetics.com/FundamentalsOfAthleticTrainingAndSportsMedicine5E

chapter 3

Design and Development of the Athletic Training Facility

Objectives

After completing this chapter, the student will be able to do the following:

- Understand the importance of careful planning in designing an athletic training facility.
- Communicate key elements for athletic training facilities with architects and administrators, including for gender-neutral facilities.
- Understand and evaluate an athletic training facility for key safety factors.
- Formulate and understand policies and rules that govern facility and modality maintenance to ensure proper, safe operations in the athletic training facility.
- Create technology and social media policies to ensure a professional and ethical athletic training facility culture.

An **athletic training facility** is a medical clinic required to meet specific health and safety standards to protect the patients. Formerly referred to as athletic training rooms, the contemporary terminology is *athletic training facility* to embrace the medical space in which athletic training services are provided, regardless of the setting. When it comes to evaluating athletes, conducting prevention procedures, treating injuries, and providing first aid, ATs fulfill their professional obligations in athletic training facilities that vary in size, design, and layout. As health care providers, ATs have an obligation to make sure the athletic training facility meets the patients' needs and allows for proper care. To ensure proper functioning and safety, athletic training facilities, regardless of their size and location, should comply with specific standards.

FACILITY DESIGN AND DEVELOPMENT

Athletic training facilities should be organized, clean, and well lit. Athletic training facilities should be at least 300 square feet (27.9 sq m), and college or university athletic training facilities should be at least 1,000 square feet (93 sq m). The BOC has created a document entitled *BOC Facility Principles* (BOC 2020) to guide the AT in understanding all aspects of the facility design and management.

The Real World

The new president at a Division I university made it a priority to upgrade the athletic training facilities. As the new space was being renovated, the head athletic trainer was asked about preferences for location, equipment, and accessibility features during construction. As the construction developed, adjustments needed to be made to ensure compliance with the safety and protection of the student-athletes who would use the facilities. Further, as new equipment was purchased and installed, new policies for the staff and student-athletes needed to be written to ensure proper safety and use. Although you may not expect it, you may be involved with major decisions regarding the design and development of an athletic training facility. Being informed is critical.

Kimberly S. Peer, EdD, AT, FNATA

The BOC provides information about accessibility; privacy and confidentiality; safety and infection control; display of licenses, certificates, and professional standards as well as information on regulations and Occupational Safety and Health Administration (OSHA n.d.). The full document can be found at www.BOCATC.org.

When designing a facility, each athletic training setting should consider the following essential areas:

- ***Private examination space.*** Team physicians will need a secure, quiet area to conduct examinations of athlete's injuries. If a private examination room does not exist, a section of a treatment area should be curtained off to ensure privacy.
- ***Treatment area.*** ATs will need plinths, or treatment tables, to treat athletes with ice or heat applications and other modalities.
- ***Game and practice preparation area.*** Game and practice preparation often involves taping and bracing limbs and applying protective padding. Because many athletes use this area alone (i.e., they do not receive other treatments), it should be located close to an entrance. This may not exist in industrial, medical office, and clinical settings.
- ***Wound care and first aid area.*** When athletes are wounded and need emergency care, they need an area with quick access to bandages, emergency equipment, and proper disposal containers for blood-stained items. Athletes should not have to walk through a treatment or taping area to access the wound care station. The wound care area should have a sink so ATs can wash their hands before and immediately after treatment as well as proper disposal containers (for biohazard waste) to ensure proper management of medical waste.
- ***Hydrotherapy area.*** Any whirlpools and ice machines should be sectioned off and located over an appropriate drainage area. This area should have a nonslip surface and be properly ventilated. A designated hydrotherapy area is necessary to prevent water from flowing into other regions of the room.
- ***Rehabilitation and reconditioning area.*** Athletes need a space to perform therapeutic exercises so they can regain strength, flexibility, balance, and range of motion. The rehabilitation space is often large because various types of equipment are needed to facilitate exercise.

- ***AT office or recordkeeping area.*** An AT must keep adequate injury reports and records of treatments. A quiet and secure location is necessary to complete the various forms and maintain the records in locked cabinets. If electronic records are used, proper security measures must be taken to ensure confidentiality and encryption, including for portable and cellular devices.
- ***AT storage area.*** Athletic training facilities require many supplies. These supplies are typically ordered in bulk to save money. A secure, dry, and easily accessible storage area protects the valuable supplies and helps control inventory throughout the year. Large equipment such as stretchers, splints, coolers, kits, and crutches can be stored here to keep the athletic training room free of clutter.

Not every facility has every area available for use, and adaptability will likely be necessary to adequately treat athletes and patients. The athletic training staff should supervise all athletic training facilities while it is open. Regardless of the size and quality of the facility, it should be kept organized and sanitized. Tables should be cleaned after an athlete or patient has been treated, and floors, whirlpools, and equipment must be disinfected daily with appropriate solutions. See figures 3.1 and 3.2 for sample floor plans for different sizes of training rooms.

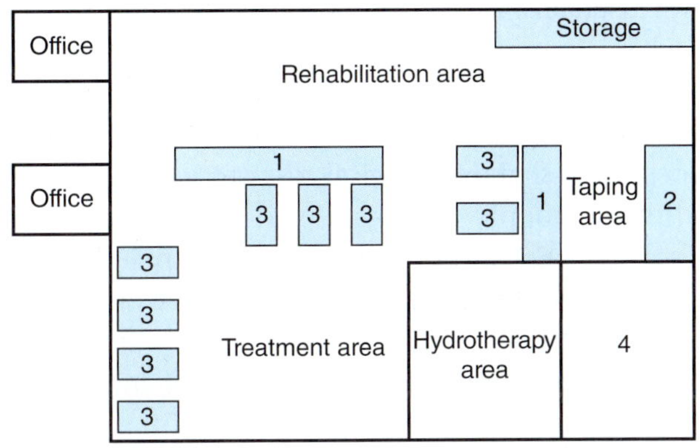

Key
1 Counter
2 Taping bench
3 Treatment tables
4 Therapy pool

Figure 3.1 Small athletic training facility.

Reprinted by permission from J.G. Konin and R.R. Ray, *Management Strategies in Athletic Training*, 5th ed. (Champaign, IL: Human Kinetics, 2018), 153.

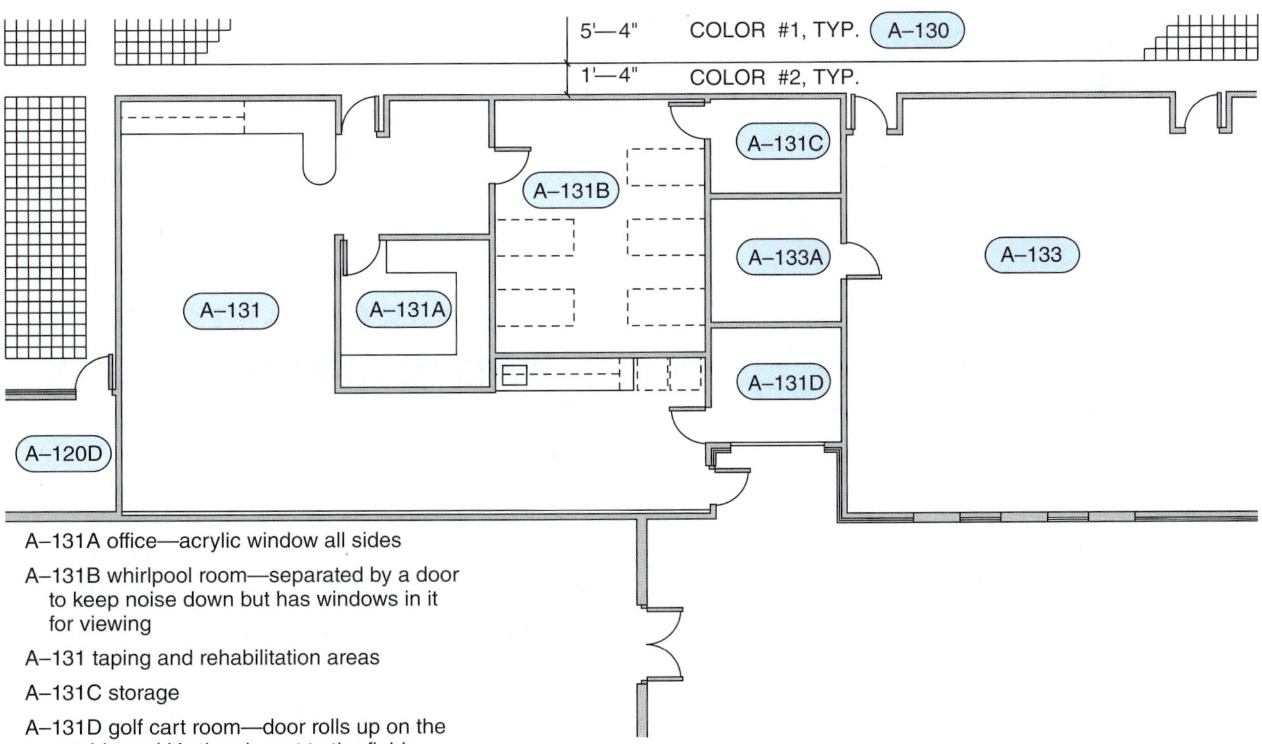

Figure 3.2 Large athletic training facility.

Sometimes, you will be required to set up a modified athletic training facility at a sideline or by using an outside tent. These are common at large events such as tournaments or even at cross country or golf events. Knowing what you need is essential because you will be away from your athletic training facility and will need to consider all the potential supplies and equipment you will need immediate access to. Although each event will vary slightly, a typical sideline tent will have first aid supplies, crutches and ambulatory aids, splints, AED and CPR equipment, a spine board, taping and wrapping supplies, a variety of braces, ice and heat modalities, coolers and water, cool water tanks and tubs (if appropriate), and communication devices.

An athletic training facility should be designed to create the best environment for serving the student or patient population. ATs often find themselves in a converted closet that was not made for the type of work they do. If you are able to design a new facility, research many articles, review *BOC Facility Principles*, speak with other athletic trainers, and look at other athletic training rooms to ensure you get what is necessary. If you must make do with what you have, add items as funding becomes available.

Facility Concept

Conceptualization is an important step in designing an athletic training facility. Regardless of the room size, proper planning will encourage optimal use of space and promote safe movement within the facility. A facility concept plan involves many different phases, including the actual design, architectural plans, environmental considerations, accessibility, and bidding. Consider all these elements in the conceptualization process. Although it can be tempting to go with the most extravagant plans, basic plans can be just as effective.

Planning Committee

The planning committee will vary depending on the setting. Most high schools have planning committees that include the athletic director, school board members, and the superintendent. Colleges and universities usually have university architects, athletic department leaders, and the athletic training staff involved in the planning. Hospital and clinic facilities include administrators and directors of AT services while occupational settings will include general managers and often occupational medicine physicians. Regardless of the setting, the AT should participate in the process and stay informed so that any recommendations are based on sound information, contemporary practice, and proper planning procedures. It is important to consider the LGBTQ+ community in designing facilities. NATA has created a resource to consider for athletic trainers in all settings; it is available at www.nata.org. You usually get only one chance to affect a facility design, so make sure you are prepared and clear when you communicate your needs.

Planning Process

The planning process can be long and tedious. It involves many different stages and often requires consultation with internal and external groups. If money is an issue, fund-raising may be necessary. This typically lengthens the planning process. Planning is a tedious but important process in facility design and management to ensure optimal outcomes. While planning, think short term and long term. You may be excited to get a new facility and think only about your current situation, but you should think five and ten years down the road as well to anticipate any changes. Documentation throughout the process will ensure consistent recollection of the discussions and decisions made along the way.

SAFETY FACTORS AND PLANNING ISSUES

Planning an athletic training facility allows for creativity; however, access and the safety and protection of the athletes are critical. Each athletic trainer should consider the following areas relative to safety and infection control: blood-borne pathogens, personal protective equipment, disposal of potentially hazardous or contaminated materials, hand hygiene, cleaning and disinfecting of surfaces and equipment, uniforms including closed-toe shoes, electrical safety, walking surfaces, patient supervision, reporting of adverse medical events, storage and handling of materials, emergency preparedness, and accessible entrance and exit routes into the facility. Being informed about these concerns allows the AT to work with the facilities design or management teams to ensure the optimal environment for all.

Location

The athletic training room should be centrally located near locker rooms and the gyms. With recent legislation regarding gender-neutral facilities in schools and medical facilities, your design considerations should integrate a gender-neutral restroom or locker room in the plan, with specific attention given to your state regulations. It is also best for the athletic training facility to have an exterior wall with an exit to the outdoors. If the athletic training facility has a golf cart, it should be located in a nearby storage room for easy access. Ideally, the athletic training facility should be on the first floor. If that is not possible, there must be an elevator to that floor where the room is located. All doors must be wide enough to allow EMS to bring in stretchers. The exterior door should allow EMS access and parking in proximity.

Electrical

The athletic training facility must have a **ground fault interrupter** for each outlet. This will prevent overload and electrocution. The outlets should not be lower than 3 feet (91 cm) from the floor (Konin and Ray 2019). Between each treatment table, there should be an electrical outlet for modalities. Outlets should be placed every 4 feet (123 cm) along the wall (Konin and Ray 2019).

Plumbing

Plumbing is essential in the whirlpool room. There should be a mixing valve (one that mixes the hot and cold water together to balance temperature) and a drain for each whirlpool. To ensure that whirlpools will work with the plumbing design, it's best to get the specifications for each whirlpool ahead of time. The ice machine requires only a water outlet and a drain. In some instances, the water will need to be filtered so the machine does not break. The hand-cleaning sink should have a sensor to start the water flow so that users do not have to touch the handles. Proper planning will promote safety for all.

Ventilation

A ventilation system must heat and cool effectively. The whirlpool area must have ventilation to reduce the **humidity** (moisture in the air) that may build up. Finally, the athletic training room must have its own thermostat to control the temperature and keep the room at approximately 40% to 50% humidity (Konin and Ray 2019).

Lighting

Konin and Ray (2019) suggest that 30 to 50 foot-candles (323-538 lux) are appropriate for the athletic training room. If natural lighting is available, the lighting should come from overhead. If natural light is available on the sides, appropriate window coverings should be installed to protect the patient and equipment. The lighting in the whirlpool room must be sealed to prevent humidity from entering the fixtures.

Acoustics

Because of the amount of traffic into and out of the athletic training facility and the equipment housed in the facility, it can quickly get very loud in an athletic training room. When designing the facility, ensure appropriate sound dissipation to control the volume in the room. The AT must be able to hear the patient and vice versa. Sound-reducing panels are often used to dissipate the noise and buffer the volume of the equipment.

Signage

Appropriate signage is important to guide athletes to the athletic training facility and through the facility to the proper areas once they arrive. Appropriate signage ensures optimal flow through the facility as it guides athletes to the appropriate areas. At least one sign is also needed on each level of the facility to guide athletes and patients to the athletic training facility itself. NATA has recommended using the term "athletic training facility" rather than "athletic training room" to accurately reflect the work ATs do. Signs outside each entrance door to the facility will provide clear access for all, especially during an emergency. In larger facilities, signs designating each specific area of the facility, including rehabilitation, storage, and hydrotherapy, are often used. Signs should also list the responsible personnel in the facility by name and title.

Office

The office should be big enough for all AT staff to have a desk space. It needs to be isolated so that ATs can take private calls without being overheard. Athletic files, records from physicals, and injury reports have to be stored in locked cabinets or saved on properly encrypted computers. Any windows should provide a view of the entire training room. Line of vision from the athletic training office to all other areas in the facility is critical. Reliable Internet and phone access should be available in the office.

Whirlpool Room or Hydrotherapy Room

The whirlpool room has to be large enough to allow space for all the whirlpools and the flow of traffic through the room. The room should be visible from as many areas of the athletic training facility as possible. In some cases, convex mirrors can be placed to reflect the whirlpool area to make it easier to see. The whirlpool room should be closed off from the rest of the athletic training facility to keep the noise level down and the water in the room. The floor must have an antislip surface and drains in the floor in the event of an overflow. The floor should have a small pitch so water flows toward the floor drain. Some athletic training facilities have in-ground hydrotherapy pools. The size of these pools means there are additional safety measures, such as specific supervision standards, the lifesaving qualifications of supervisors, security and access considerations, and maintenance and sanitation guidelines for a large pool area.

Rehabilitation

In a high school setting, there may not be enough space for a rehabilitation area in the athletic training facility. For some, the rehabilitation space may be the weight room. If the rehabilitation area is located in the athletic training facility, it's best to have either a rubberized or carpeted floor for safety and noise control. The area will have to be large enough to accommodate all machines, rehabilitation tables, mirrors, weights, and balls and provide open floor space for stretching and exercises.

Taping

The taping area is determined by the number of staff members who will be working and the number of students the AT will be dealing with at peak times. Because the taping area is the busiest, it should be located close to the door to provide quick entry and exit for athletes. Between each taping table or underneath each taping station, there should be storage for extra taping supplies.

Treatment

The treatment area is for athletes who require ice, heat, ultrasound, muscle stimulation, intermittent compression, or evaluation. Therapy equipment should be located on moveable carts between each treatment table. Some treatment tables are adjustable to ergonomically accommodate the AT's needs during treatment. If electrical modalities are used, safeguards must be in place to ensure that the athlete or patient cannot self-administer a treatment.

Storage

The storage room should be located close to the taping area. The size of the room will depend on whether supplies are ordered once a year (i.e., large amounts need to be stored) or delivered more than once a year. The availability of cabinets that can store supplies will also influence the size of the storage room. Tape should be stored in a cool, dry room. Expensive supplies should be held in a locked cabinet. If old injury files are to be kept in storage, they must be kept in locked file cabinets. If possible, the size of the storage room should be slightly larger than what was originally calculated.

RED FLAGS

Facilities with the following conditions should be considered unsafe:

- Electrical work is not complete.
- A whirlpool is not wired to a ground fault interrupter.
- An ultrasound therapy machine has not been calibrated in two years.
- An AT office does not provide direct line of vision to the athletic training room for supervision.

At the very least, 80 square feet of space is needed for storage.

Ergonomics

As an AT, you will be spending much time on your feet treating your athletes and patients. A facility that encourages proper **ergonomics** is essential. Consider the type of flooring you install so that it is easy to clean yet soft enough to tolerate hours of standing. Antifatigue mats may be used in areas where ATs stand for extended periods of time to reduce strain on the body. These mats absorb some of the strain from the hard surfaces. Many athletic training rooms have comfortable and slip-resistant mat floors. Consider the height of the taping tables you purchase. If you have to bend too far over or reach up high, your back will begin to hurt after long days. Treatment tables should have the capacity to move up and down (if possible) to allow for proper positioning of the AT during massage, manual therapy, and stretching. Alternatively, stools or bolsters can be used to raise or lower the AT or athlete. Additional ergonomic concerns involve variable seat heights through adjustable stools, appropriate computer stations, and properly designed storage space to avoid stooping and reaching.

MAINTENANCE OF FACILITY AND MODALITIES

Maintaining an athletic training facility is of the utmost importance. The athletic training staff can perform much of the work, but outside maintenance support may be needed. The athletic training room should be cleaned regularly. All used spaces should be disinfected after use, especially the whirlpools, tables, rehabilitation equipment, and modalities. Coolers and water bottles should be cleaned and stored upside down to prevent the accumulation of mold and bacteria. Trash bins should be emptied daily and biohazard waste disposed of on a regular basis as directed by the facility managers and the **Occupational Safety and Health Administration (OSHA)**. Floors should be vacuumed or swept or mopped daily to keep surfaces free from dirt and prevent accumulation of contaminants. After daily cleaning, athletic training room supplies should be restocked to ensure proper availability for the next day.

Modality maintenance is critical to prevent injury and ensure proper functioning. All therapeutic modalities, including whirlpools, electrical stimulation devices, ice machines, hydrocollator, and ultrasound machines should be inspected annually and calibrated by a licensed electrician. **Calibration** ensures safe and appropriate function of the modality. A sticker should be placed on the device to reflect annual review and proper functioning.

Clear and specific policy and procedures should be available regarding using any modality and all personnel operating the devices should be trained and licensed to do so. As an athletic training aide, you are not permitted by most state laws to administer therapeutic modalities to patients nor are athletes permitted to self-administer them. Be sure to understand your scope of practice and what you are permitted to perform as designated by your state law. Further, be sure to facilitate a safe environment by reporting any dangerous or inappropriate use of the modalities.

> **What Would You Do If . . .**
>
> Your budget has recently been cut. You had your modalities inspected last year, and all passed without any issues. The approximate cost of modality calibration for your school is about $1,500 annually. You are considering skipping the calibrations this year and getting back on schedule next year because you seldom use the electrical modalities, and they passed last year. Is this the right thing to do? Why or why not?

MATERIAL SAFETY DATA SHEETS

As part of the United States Department of Labor, OSHA has communication standards that discuss the safe treatment and disposal of potentially dangerous materials. In the athletic training room, blood-borne pathogens are a common occupational hazard since ATs deal with blood when caring for certain injuries. Guidelines must be shared with all workers who may be exposed to blood and are established by OSHA (2019). When managing material safety where potentially dangerous materials are possible, specialized training is often required. Material safety data sheets should be displayed in all athletic training facilities and reviewed regularly with all personnel. Personnel, volunteers, and students working in the facility should be fully trained and directed to the guidelines as soon as they begin work.

FACILITY RULES

Athletic training facilities should have rules posted and readily accessible. Rules and regulations help ensure the safety of all who use the facility and maintain order and cleanliness of the facility. Although athletic training room rules vary from facility to facility, the following are common rules.

- Athletes must sign in each time they enter the athletic training room.
- Shower before entering the athletic training room after practice or games.
- No food, drink, gum, or tobacco in the athletic training facility.
- No foul language or bullying in the athletic training room.
- Remove headphones or earbuds before entering the athletic training facility and turn off cellular devices.
- Leave equipment and gym bags outside the athletic training room.
- No cleats or spikes in the athletic training facility.
- Do not turn the whirlpools on or off without the supervision of the AT.
- Do not touch the therapeutic modalities.
- No horseplay.

Understanding Diversity

Creating a Culturally Competent Healthcare Facility

- Train in culturally competent healthcare annually.
- Post a nondiscrimination policy.
- Have culturally competent healthcare materials.
- Ensure cultural competency among professional referrals.
- Stop discriminatory language and jokes.
- Use preferred names and pronouns.
- Provide gender-neutral restrooms and changing rooms.
- Employ individuals from all races, age, and gender.
- Make sure electronic medical records are confidential.

Adapted from National Athletic Trainers' Association.

Although facilities may enforce many more rules, the premise is to have a safe, clean environment for athletic health care. Instituting these rules early and enforcing them will prevent problems down the road.

Technology is an emerging practice in all settings, so it is important to have specific policies regarding technology use and social media. It is prudent to limit technology use in the athletic training facility by athletes and patients. Further, athletic trainers and athletic training aides should use caution and good judgment when engaging on social media with those to whom they provide care. Social media has become a common source of ethical and legal violations for medical professionals, and it is best to err on the side of caution when establishing policy regarding its use. Remember, the safety of those you care for is the primary concern, and protecting yourself and others against ethical and legal issues is of the utmost priority. These rules help to provide a safe environment for all.

Summary

Athletic training facilities are health care facilities. They are governed and maintained by the highest standards to ensure the safety of the patients we serve. Design is a critical element in the proper functioning of the facility and can provide an optimal environment for providing the needed services. Many areas are preferred in an athletic training facility but are not essential if space is limited. However, ensuring adequate access and maintenance is nonnegotiable.

Key Terms

Define the following terms found in this chapter:

- athletic training facility
- calibration
- ergonomics
- ground fault interrupter
- humidity
- Occupational Safety and Health Administration (OSHA)

As an AT at a high school, you are responsible for creating a form that will highlight the proper management, containment, and reporting of any incident that involves blood or other potentially infectious materials. You access the OSHA webpage to discover the many criteria that are important for these situations. What are the key pieces of information that you need to post and enforce? What are the reporting mechanisms for an exposure? Lastly, how will you communicate this with your coaches, athletes, administrators, and staff?

To access supplementary material for this chapter, including the Understanding Check worksheet, vocabulary quizzes, extension activities, and chapter-specific resources and forms, visit the web resource: http://ancillaries.humankinetics.com/FundamentalsOfAthleticTrainingAndSportsMedicine5E

chapter 4

Documentation and Recordkeeping

Objectives

After completing this chapter, the student will be able to do the following:

- Identify key medical terms and use them appropriately in communication.
- Understand the important concepts of recordkeeping and note-taking and perform basic note-taking skills in an athletic training setting.
- Identify and understand the various records kept in an athletic training setting.
- Identify the key elements of the electronic medical record (EMR).
- Understand and practice good note-taking strategies to promote accuracy, brevity, and clarity in communication.
- Identify the concepts associated with medical coding and their role in athletic training.
- Use disablement models in athletic training in recordkeeping for athletic injuries.
- Understand and appreciate the important role documentation plays in athletic training.

The sports medicine team must document all the procedures they perform to prevent lawsuits and provide the best care possible. For example, ATs need to be able to compare current physical findings of an injured athlete with previous findings from a physical examination or injury report. Moreover, it may be essential to review past injury treatments to determine the best type of care for an athlete.

Understanding Diversity

Positives of Hiring Diverse Candidates

- Meets the needs of patients to see someone that looks like them.
- Diverse candidates have different ideas, knowledge, and ways to do things.
- Encourages greater appreciation of diverse skillsets.
- Leads to higher productivity.

Harvard (n.d.)

MEDICAL TERMINOLOGY BASICS

Medical terminology creates a common language for ATs to communicate with other health care providers. Understanding the fundamentals of medical terminology can help the AT communicate with precision and clarity and allow the AT to clearly demonstrate their knowledge of concepts related to athletic training to the larger medical community.

Medical terminology is divided into three parts: roots, prefixes, and suffixes. Root words are the foundational terms—they can stand alone and hold their own meaning (see table 4.1). Prefixes come before the root word and add additional meaning to the word. Often, prefixes are added to designate time, place, or number. Common prefixes are presented in table 4.2. Suffixes are located at the end of the word and can be combined with the root word or a prefix and a root word. Suffixes refer to conditions, procedures, surgeries, or techniques. Although there are many suffixes, commonly used ones are listed in table 4.3.

Table 4.1 Common Root Words

Root word	Meaning
cardio	heart
cephal/o	head
Chrom	color
enter/o	intestine
derm/o	skin
gastr/o	stomach
hem/o, hemat/o	blood
my/o	muscle
myel/o	spinal cord
onych/o	nail
oste/o	bone
Phag	eat or swallow
phleb/o	vein
pulm/o, pulmon/o	lungs
synov/i	synovial fluid, joint, or membrane
thromb/o	clot
vas/o	vessel or duct

Table 4.2 Common Prefixes

Prefix	Meaning
a-, an-	without, absence of
ab-	away from
ad-	toward, near
ante-	before
ec-, ect/o-	out, outside
end/o-	in, within
mon/o-	one
peri-	surrounding
poly-	many, much
post-	after, behind
trans-	across, through
supra-	above

Combining prefixes with root words often requires adding an "o" to the end of the prefix. *Ect-* and *-derm* would create the word "ectderm," which is not correct. Adding an "o" creates the correct word, which is "ectoderm."

Table 4.3 Common Suffixes

Suffix	Meaning
-algia	pain
-centesis	puncture, tap
-desis	binding, fusion
-ectomy	excision, removal (surgical)
-emia	having a substance in the blood, condition of the blood
-graphy	act of recording (i.e., data)
-pexy	fixation (as in surgery)
-plasty	surgical repair, reconstruction
-sclerosis	hardening
-tripsy	crushing
-uria	condition of urine, urination

Several examples combining root words, prefixes, and suffixes are as follows:

- arthralgia = painful joints
- transdermal = across the skin
- monochromatic = one color
- osteoplasty = reconstruction of the bone

Other important medical terms that are helpful to know are directional terms. Directional terms indicate where in the body we are referencing. They can demonstrate movement or simple location. Directional terms are typically referenced in respect to the midline of the body for a point of orientation. Commonly used directional and movement terms are presented in table 4.4 and further illustrated in chapter 7.

Table 4.4 Directional Terms

Term	Meaning
anterior	front of body
posterior	back of body
distal	away from the top of the body; farther away
proximal	toward the center of the body; nearer to
lateral	toward the outside
medial	toward the midline
cephalad	near the head
caudal	near the tail or bottom
abduction	movement away from the midline
adduction	movement toward the midline
flexion	bending or making the angle less
extension	straightening or making the angle larger
dorsiflexion	flexion of ankle to reduce angle
plantar flexion	flexion of ankle to increase angle
internal rotation	rotation toward the midline
external rotation	rotation away from the midline

Abbreviations are used in charts and among health care providers (see table 4.5). The common language is concise and mutually understood. Abbreviations also help to keep records consistent so that other health care providers can fully understand what was done to the patient. Finally, abbreviations help

Table 4.5 Common Abbreviations

Pt	Patient	PWB	partial weight bearing
ROM	range of motion	WWP	warm whirlpool
Ther ex	therapeutic exercise	CWP	cold whirlpool
US	ultrasound	FLEX	flexion
E-stim	electrical stimulation	EXT	extension
TKA	total knee arthroplasty	ABD	abduction
RC	rotator cuff	ADD	adduction
ACL	anterior cruciate ligament	PRO	pronation
PCL	posterior cruciate ligament	SUP	supination
MCL	medial collateral ligament	DF	dorsiflexion
LCL	lateral collateral ligament	PF	plantar flexion
WB	weight bearing	IR	internal rotation
NWB	non-weight bearing	ER	external rotation
FWB	full weight bearing	BID	twice daily

What Would You Do If . . .

You are an athletic trainer working in a clinical environment and receive the following note from a patient who recently saw the doctor and another physical therapist at the hospital postsurgery. Decipher the terminology and determine which area you are going to rehabilitate.

Pt reports 2 weeks post-op with L TKA. Pt is PWB, restricted FLEX/EXT, and distal to surgery. Treat with E-stim to decrease pain, progress to FWB as tolerated with gait training to support the functional movement. Treat patient BID as tolerated.

athletic trainers to keep their records brief. Recordkeeping is a critical aspect of athletic training, but it can be time consuming. Abbreviations help contribute to the ABCs of documentation: being **a**ccurate, **b**rief, and **c**lear.

Combining root words and directional terms will help the AT to be clear and concise in communication. For example, a patient with a medial meniscus who comes to the AT with a prescription for treatment after arthroscopy may need strengthening distal and proximal to the injury yet immediately need ROM performed at the knee.

MEDICAL DOCUMENTATION NOTES

Medical **documentation** is important because it is the permanent record of what happened. If an incident or injury is not documented, it technically did not happen. Many athletic training and medical facilities use the electronic medical record (EMR). Key information on an EMR is a problem list, procedures, diagnoses, medication list, allergies, demographics, diagnostic test results, radiology results, health maintenance information, advance directives, dispositions, and level of service. Whether electronic or on paper, these records are used to recall observations, inform others, teach students, and justify interventions. They must be legible. Think about some of the advantages of having electronic records as compared to handwritten or paper records.

In addition to having a formalized note-taking system, a standard format for notes helps health care providers communicate and understand information about the patient. It is important to document using the ABCs of documentation: **a**ccurate, **b**rief, and **c**lear. When documenting any event, keeping it short yet clear provides the optimal record. Too much information can cloud the details, so the AT should focus on the ABCs as they record the information. Two formats have been widely used in the medical fields: SOAP and HOPS.

SOAP is an acronym that stands for **subjective**, **objective**, **assessment**, and **plan**. The **SOAP note** was widely used in clinics for decades and is still the foundation of many electronic recordkeeping forms and programs. SOAP provides a short-term and long-term overview of the patient and can be used as an initial note or a follow-up note. Prompts from a SOAP note are shown in table 4.6.

Another helpful model that is commonly used in athletic training is the HOPS (or HIPS) method. Like the SOAP note, this acronym is widely recognized in the medical field. HOPS stands for **history**, **observation**, **palpation**, and **special tests**. (Some ATs replace "observation" with "inspection" for the acronym HIPS.) Prompts from a HOPS note are shown in table 4.7.

These two models of note-taking have similarities. Most health care programs will use a derivative of these templates. Many programs have moved online, with forms built into their database for ease of recording. As with all records, security is an issue and is of utmost importance. Many contemporary records also consider the elements of the International Classification of Functioning, Disability, and Health (ICF) **disablement model** in their templates. The model in figure 4.1 considers the unique needs of each patient and emphasizes an interprofessional approach to managing all injuries (NATA 2016).

Table 4.6 SOAP Notes

Element	Factors included
S = subjective	Anything the athlete tells the AT How do they feel? Where does it hurt? When did the injury happen? Where did it happen? Has it ever happened before? If so, when? Is there a time the pain is worse? Better? Does it radiate to another region? Does anything make it better?
O = objective	Anything the AT physically measures that generates a number or grade Rate the pain on a scale of 1 to 10. (Can be subjective, too.) Degree of laxity (grade 1, 2, 3) ROM (in degrees) Manual muscle testing (grade 1 to 5) Vital signs (BP, pulse, respirations, temperature) Height, weight Test results (X-ray, MRI, CT scan, blood work)
A = assessment	Diagnosis—what is it that is wrong with the patient? Prioritize the major issues Differential diagnosis if uncertain
P = plan	What the AT intends to do to the patient or for the patient Other tests that need to be ordered Treatments and rehabilitation Home instructions Referral to other doctors or services (such as meals, transportation) Medications

Table 4.7 HOPS/HIPS Notes

Element	Factors included
H = history	Anything the AT asks the patient All subjective information from the SOAP note would fall into this category
O/I = observation or inspection	Anything the AT sees Swelling Discoloration Bruising Skin changes Crutches Limited ROM Braces, casts, or bandages Infection signs Amputations
Palpation	Anything the AT can touch Skin temperature Crepitation (creaking in the bone) Bony landmarks Ligaments Muscles and other soft tissue Bursas
Special tests	Things the AT does to determine the degree of injury Range-of-motion testing Strength testing Gait analysis Stress tests for bones, ligaments, and others Functional capacity testing

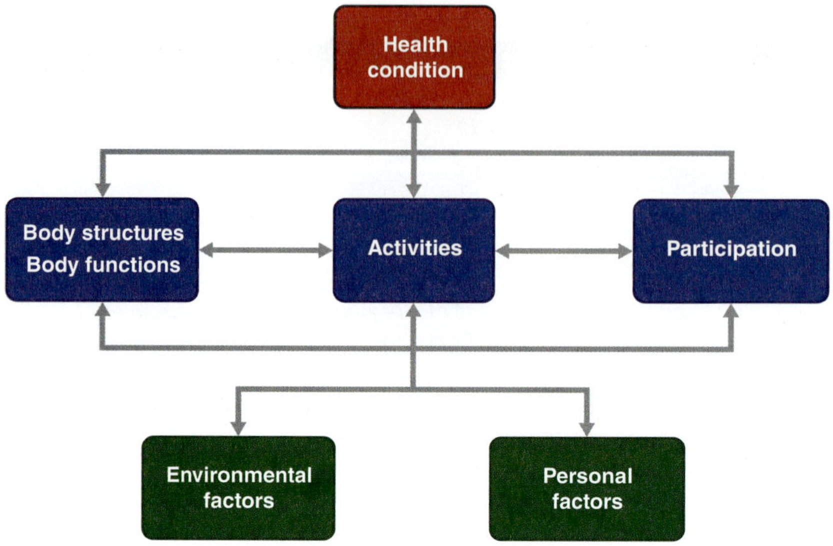

Figure 4.1 WHO International Classification of Functioning, Disability, and Health Disablement Model.

Reprinted by permission from National Athletic Trainers' Association.

DOCUMENTATION AND RECORDKEEPING

Data from injury reports should be recorded not only to reduce liability but also to track injury trends and help ATs make decisions about how best to treat these injuries. The benefit of electronic records is that they provide a database for future reference. These records can provide data regarding supply use, traffic flow in the athletic training room during peak times, specific injury patterns for each sport, rehabilitation equipment usage, and other valuable information that can be used to direct the functions in the athletic training room. In today's environment, numbers are powerful, and if the AT can prove that another staff member or a new piece of equipment is needed, the likelihood of acquiring support is stronger with numbers.

Records are also part of the legal system (see chapter 2). Documentation of everything that happens protects the AT throughout their career. That is why it is so important to have accurate, organized records that are prioritized and maintained regularly. Although one would hope to never need them in a legal case, records protect the AT and provide evidence of what was or was not done in a given situation.

Exactly which procedures must be documented is often debated. ATs should document any accident of which they are aware (even if it is not due to athletic participation), any treatment that an athlete receives, and the rehabilitation progress that an athlete makes. Many electronic documentation or recordkeeping systems are available to ATs. These systems make it easy to file injury reports, rehabilitation progress, and referral forms.

Records in paper form should be protected in locked file cabinets. Most systems require double locks, which means they are kept in a locked file cabinet behind a locked door. Electronic records should be secured through passwords, encryption, and other technical means. ATs should consult their technology experts to ensure appropriate security of all electronic records.

Accident and Injury Reports

Accident and injury reports contain vital information, including the athlete's name, the date of injury, the date of the report, the athlete's sport, the age of the athlete, and the body part that is injured. Additionally, the report must contain information about how the injury or accident occurred, whether it is a new or previous injury, and the AT's inspection and assessment information and signature. The report should also contain the AT's thoughts about the injury and record treatment such as ice application, splinting, or medical referral.

Go online to the Resources and Forms section in the web resource to find a printable injury report form.

Treatment Logs

Any treatment an athlete receives must be documented. Ice application, heat application, elastic wraps, stretching, strengthening, and so on must all be logged on a specific form. These forms also allow the AT to track how many treatments are being administered per day and helps to monitor compliance with prescribed treatment and rehabilitation programs.

Go online to the Resources and Forms section in the web resource to find a printable daily treatment log and treatment progress chart.

Rehabilitation Charts

Once an athlete has been injured, the injury assessed, and a proper rehabilitation program designed and implemented, the AT must document the athlete's progress. The AT must record the exact treatment the athlete receives, the date it was received, any problems or complaints, any changes in treatment, the athlete's response to treatment, and reevaluation data.

Injury-Tracking Systems

Injury-tracking systems have become popular in athletic training. As athletic trainers try to prove their worth by getting information from a national database, these records are compiled in computer programs. Whether they are used exclusively for the AT program or as part of a larger initiative, injury-tracking systems provide valuable information for the AT. Although new systems emerge regularly, several are quite popular in athletic training. Athletic Trainer System (ATS), SportsWareOnLine, Sports Injury Monitoring System (SIMS), SimTrack, NCAA Injury Surveillance Program, and Presagia Sports are the most prevalent software packages to date. When selecting a system, it is important to evaluate the following factors:

- Calendar
- Demographics
- Disablement models
- EMR
- Exercise flow sheet
- ICD codes
- Injury report
- Insurance information and claims
- Medication log
- Physician referral
- Price and annual fee
- Progress notes
- Report generation
- Treatment reports

Each system has specific strengths and weaknesses. If you want to learn more about injury-tracking programs, do an Internet search for "comparison of injury-tracking programs" and track the changes that have occurred over the years as technology has expanded. Selecting a program that is useful and appropriate for the AT's individual program is critical. Some systems are synchronized with insurance billing systems to expedite processing. International Classification of Disease (ICD) codes are universally used to provide diagnostic health information. Although commonly used in billing, you will want to familiarize yourself with the more common codes seen in your patient population. If you choose to become a medical biller as a career choice, these will be more important.

PATIENT CONFIDENTIALITY

Patient confidentiality is an important element in the medical field. Securing records is not only the AT's obligation as part of their role but also a legal responsibility. Two federal guidelines help us define our role in maintaining record security: HIPAA and FERPA.

The **Health Insurance Portability and Accountability Act (HIPAA)** defines what medical professionals, including athletic trainers, can share with others about a medical record of a patient they are treating. Among other controls, this act ensures that a patient has full access to their own medical record at any time. It is important to have policies that govern access and, in some cases, waivers that allow access by others. The patient (of legal age) or legal guardian (for minors) must formally agree to have medical records released to other health care providers or insurance companies. This allows the patient or their family to have control over the medical records. HIPAA release forms are common in medical practices, and you have likely seen one at your doctor's office. See figure 4.2 for a sample HIPAA release form.

Forms that are covered under HIPAA include physicals, rehabilitation plans, treatment logs, evaluations, treatment plans, and insurance information. So the information stays secure, all paperwork must be stored in a locked cabinet with controlled access. Electronic medical information must be encrypted and its access limited to only those who have permission. Even discussing an athlete's health with another AT who is not responsible for the care of that athlete can be a violation of HIPAA.

In other words, ATs can share information only if permission is granted. If an athlete is younger than 18, their parent or guardian must give permission to the AT to share information to necessary people such as coaches. The concept of confidentiality involves not only oral information but also written documents, such as injury reports and other forms used in the athletic training room. It is important not to divulge medical information to anyone who is

I, ______________________________ Date of Birth ____________

Authorize the release of my medical information including:

[ ] Diagnosis
[ ] Personal health information
[ ] Radiographs
[ ] Treatment and rehabilitation
[ ] Records

Information can be released to: (Print Name)

Relationship:

Do not disclose the following information:

[ ] Diagnosis
[ ] Social security
[ ] Radiographs
[ ] Address
[ ] Records
[ ] Payment information
[ ] Personal health information
[ ] Insurance
[ ] Treatment and rehabilitation

This authorization may be revoked with written notice. I understand I can refuse to sign and it will not affect my ability to receive services.

Printed Name: ______________________________

Signature: ______________________________

Date: ______________________________

Printed Name of Witness: ______________________________

Signature: ______________________________

Date: ______________________________

Figure 4.2 Sample HIPAA medical release form.

not authorized. For example, student assistants may be approached by a reporter looking for information about an injured athlete to print in a newspaper.

Another legislative measure to protect information about a person is the **Family Educational Rights and Privacy Act (FERPA)**. As the name reflects, this law deals with educational records rather than medical records. FERPA is similar to HIPAA in that an individual must release records for others to see if that is what they desire. Otherwise, school personnel, including ATs, do not have the right to view or release educational records without written consent from the student or guardian. See figure 4.3 for an example of a FERPA release form.

FERPA was put in place to ensure a family or student's right to privacy, especially as it pertains to educational information. Information that applies under FERPA includes health information, academic records, and behavioral records. The family or student who is of age has a right to review these documents and ask to have records amended if found to be incorrect. Student assistants may at times encounter private information, but they must respect the privacy of the family and student-athlete. Be sure to avoid disclosing any information regarding a student-athlete.

I, ______________________________ Date of Birth __________

Student Identification Number ______________________________

Authorize the release of my educational information including:

[ ] Transcripts [ ] Disciplinary records

[ ] National tests (ACT, SAT, etc.) [ ] Letters of reference

[ ] Other ______________________________

Information can be released to: ______________________________
(Print Name)

Relationship: ______________________________

Institution: ______________________________

Do not disclose the following information:

[ ] Transcripts [ ] Disciplinary records

[ ] National tests (ACT, SAT, etc.) [ ] Letters of reference

[ ] Other ______________________________

This authorization may be revoked with written notice. I understand I have the right to review my records at any time.

Printed Name: ______________________________

Signature: ______________________________

Date: ______________________________

Consent from parent or guardian needed for minors: ______________________________

Printed Name of Parent: ______________________________

Signature: ______________________________

Date: ______________________________

Figure 4.3 Sample FERPA release form.

RED FLAGS

- An athletic trainer leaves the record of a student-athlete lying on the treatment table in the athletic training room during treatment times.
- A college student requests that the AT speak with his mother regarding his medical condition without a written consent for the mother to view the record.
- A high school student posts pictures on social media of another student's injured ankle with a comment about the injury and the name of the student.
- A student aide reads though a student-athlete's file as part of the medical experience and tells a friend about a medication that the student is taking for depression.

What Would You Do If . . .

As an athletic trainer in a high school, you have centralized computers at the entry to your facility. One computer is locked and has security measures so that no one other than staff can sign into it, since it holds all medical records for each athlete. Although this system has been approved by legal counsel, an incoming freshman says that anyone can see his treatment protocol for the day and that the high school AT is violating HIPAA by allowing others to see his record when they pull up the team injury report for the day. How do you address this with the athlete? Do you need to change your protocol? Why or why not?

COMPUTER SECURITY

Many programs use computers, tablets, or other portable devices to grant mobile access to records. Once there is a decision to move to digital recordkeeping, the AT program must carefully determine how the computers will be used and how they will be accessed and supported. Backing up records regularly and designing a policy that governs the appropriate use of AT computers or portable devices is important on the front end of implementation.

The most common electronic records used in athletic training include injury reports, sign-in sheets, inventory forms (see figure 4.4), purchase orders (found in chapter 5), coaches' injury reports (see figure 4.5), preparticipation clearance forms, insurance forms, and doctor's notes. Although convenient, the level of protection of electronic medical records needs to be seriously evaluated to design a safe system. It is best to consult both the IT department as well as the legal department at your institution to ensure that record security is maintained. As discussed earlier, a breech in record security is not just inconvenient, it is illegal, since it violates HIPAA and FERPA.

Item no.	Description	Quantity	Location	Reorder at
44201	McDavid shin splint support	10	Main TR	4
48102	Medco high-intensity penlight pack	12	Main TR	4
46064M	Medique diotame tubes	2	Main TR	1
5551-18	Miltex utility scissors, 5-1/2″	3	Main TR	1
27680	Mission Pharmacal Super Cleaner	4	Main TR	1
99920	Mueller knee strap	10	Main TR	4
929436	QuikClot Nosebleed	2	Ice arena	1
69575	New-Skin liquid	3	Main TR	1
26002M	New-Skin liquid bandage spray	2	Main TR	1
261623	Omron automatic inflation blood pressure monitor	3	Main TR	2
5580136	Omron automatic inflation blood pressure monitor	3	Field house	2
39030M	Paper cups, 4 oz jazz 5,000/cs	5,000	Main TR	2,500
39032M	Plastic cups, 5 oz clear 2,500/cs	2,500	Field house	1,250
87700	Plastic goniometer, 12-1/2″ long	2	Main TR	1
37200	Powerflex 2″ 24/box	8	Main TR	96
37302	Powerflex 3″ 48/box	3	Main TR	72

Figure 4.4 Sample inventory form.

Coaches' Injury Report

Athlete	Sport	Body part	Progress	Status
Winifred Bailey	Basketball	Ankle	Scheduled for surgery	Out of season
Rahual Setty	Cricket	Shin	Icing daily	No lower-body workouts
Walsh Fredrickson	Ice hockey	Forearm	Sutures removed today	Full go

This report contains confidential information and is not to be shared. Any breach of this information is a violation of the Health Insurance Portability and Accountability Act.

Figure 4.5 Coaches' injury report.

Summary

Medical records are the foundation of providing medical care to any patient. Accurate, clear, and concise records help guide diagnoses, treatment, and rehabilitation. Electronic recordkeeping and medical records are efficient and can help provide valuable data to guide future needs and the growth of an athletic training program. It can also help the AT see trends in injury incidences programmatically or nationally, if participating in a national database. This will ultimately help the AT provide better preventive care for all. However, record confidentiality is critical for protecting the patient and the AT. Having good policies that govern medical records is essential for the AT. Legal considerations in recordkeeping cannot be underestimated, and appropriate measures should be taken to promptly and securely document all events that occur.

Key Terms

Define the following terms found in this chapter:

- assessment
- disablement model
- documentation
- electronic medical record (EMR)
- Family Educational Rights and Privacy Act (FERPA)
- Health Insurance Portability and Accountability Act (HIPAA)
- history
- objective
- observation
- palpation
- plan
- SOAP note
- special tests
- subjective

As an AT, you are designing a rehabilitation program for a factory worker who stands for 10 hours per day and has a family with small children at home where he is the primary caregiver. He has a low-back injury that requires an extensive stretching and strengthening regimen each day. The disablement models encourage the AT to infuse the life factors of each patient into their rehabilitation program. Based on this scenario, consider the limitations this patient might encounter with an extensive, time-intensive home rehabilitation program. How might you try to work with the patient to meet their needs at work and home while meeting the rehabilitation goals?

To access supplementary material for this chapter, including the Understanding Check worksheet, vocabulary quizzes, extension activities, and chapter-specific resources and forms, visit the web resource: http://ancillaries.humankinetics.com/FundamentalsOfAthleticTrainingAndSportsMedicine5E

chapter 5

Fiscal Management

Objectives

After completing this chapter, the student will be able to do the following:

- Understand basic concepts of budgeting for athletic training programs.
- Use the concepts to design a basic budget.
- Understand the importance of inventory management to the athletic training program.
- Evaluate purchasing models and determine the appropriate technique for various settings.
- Appreciate how fiscal management can promote fair, equitable, and reasonable use of resources.
- Understand the basic concepts of insurance billing in athletic training.
- Understand and appreciate the role of reimbursement for athletic training services.

What Would You Do If . . .

As an athletic trainer at a high school, you are charged with ordering supplies and equipment for the entire year. Since supplies are acquired at the beginning of the year, it is important to disperse the supplies and equipment so that sports at the end of the school year still have supplies for their teams. You are only halfway through the fall semester and have already exceeded your allocation for the football team due to a high number of unexpected injuries. What do you do?

A major problem facing today's athletic trainers is fiscal management. Athletic trainers are typically provided nominal budgets to provide services to all they treat. With often limited space and supplies, it is increasingly difficult to ensure appropriate care to athletes. The AT should be integrally involved in the fiscal management of the program because they know firsthand what the program needs to perform professionally and safely.

Fiscal management is a complex and challenging task for ATs, and it is but one of the daily tasks on their schedules. ATs must anticipate supplies and equipment needs throughout the year. When supplies are limited, they must make tough choices or find alternative ways of generating income to fund the supplies. Careful planning can prevent issues associated with limited supplies, but not all budgetary issues can be predicted. It is prudent for the AT to carefully evaluate and plan to ensure proper care and treatment. Sometimes, fund-raising initiatives support athletic training facility budgets, sometimes booster clubs or private hospitals or clinics donate supplies or equipment, and sometimes a private donor may contribute to the program. It is a huge responsibility to manage these resources and funds in a fiscally sound manner.

TYPES OF BUDGETS

Budgeting is an important role. Many programs do not have unlimited amounts of money, so budgeting takes on increased importance. Since most athletic training programs do not generate money, they are at the mercy of the administration to allocate specific amounts of money to purchase supplies, equipment, and other resources. The budget should closely reflect the mission of the program (Konin and Ray 2019; Harrelson, Gardner, and Winterstein 2016) and should be based on a **needs assessment** that defines the important elements of the program. Further, the budget must be evaluated regularly to determine if adjustments need to be made. Although it seems to be something that happens once a year, budgeting is a yearlong, ongoing process that is constantly being reevaluated and adjusted.

Several types of budgets are common in the athletic training profession. The type of budget a program uses depends on the circumstances of the program and often the overall budgeting process used by a larger entity such as a school system or athletic department. The common types are **zero-based**, **fixed**, **variable**, **lump-sum**, and **line-item budgets** (Konin and Ray 2019).

- ***Zero-based budgets.*** This budget process essentially starts at zero each year. There is no link to the previous year's budget. Each expenditure requires justification. In a zero-based system, priorities emerge as the rationale for need is expressed and when alternatives (or lack of alternatives) are presented for consideration. Zero-based budgeting is time intensive and requires attention to the fine details of each item requested.
- ***Fixed budgets.*** A fixed budget is an annual budget that is divided into months and summed together to reflect the annual expenditures and income (if any). This budget model works well when the athletic training program is financially stable and accommodates for variability in needs throughout the year (such as higher expenses during fall seasons). Although it is a good model, most programs do not use it because most athletic training departments do not generate revenue; therefore, the usefulness of this model is limited.
- ***Variable budgets.*** This model allows for adjustments based on the ebb and flow of the expenditures for the year. It allows the director to adjust the budget by evaluating revenues and modifying future expenses as needed. Since most programs do not generate revenue, this model, like the fixed budgeting model, is not used in many athletic training programs across the country.

- ***Lump-sum budgets.*** As its name implies, this model revolves around a lump sum that is spent at the discretion of the program director. This model has tremendous flexibility, but it requires careful attention to ensure fair distribution of resources throughout the year. Lump-sum budgeting has few restrictions or limitations, so it is a popular model. However, accountability is still important and necessary.
- ***Line-item budgets.*** This budget model divides expenditures into categories such as expendable supplies, equipment, insurance, and personnel resources. When the money is allocated to one line, it cannot be moved to another line (for example, money from supplies cannot be moved to buy a large piece of rehabilitation equipment). Although not as flexible as a lump-sum model, this model is specific and easy to understand (see table 5.1).

Although no model is perfect, most program teams will find a model that is comfortable to use, and they will become proficient at designing and managing the financial resources of the program. Often, that is decided in collaboration with the school board or district office or other administrator, depending on the organizational structure. The AT should be involved in the budgeting process whenever possible.

DESIGNING A BUDGET

Designing the budget is an important function and should be done with consultation from others in the organization whenever possible. Although the director or head AT may be ultimately responsible for creating the budget, input from everyone on the sports medicine team will provide a broader perspective to create a more useful, equitable representation of the program as a whole.

Creating a budget has several steps, but the first and most important is a needs assessment. A needs assessment identifies priorities systematically and helps direct the organization or program through the budgeting process. Konin and Ray (2019) identify three major steps in designing a budget:

1. ***Exploration.*** Identifying needs through various personnel and resources.
2. ***Information gathering.*** Collecting as much information as possible.
3. ***Decision making.*** Determining priorities and aligning them with the mission of the program.

Another common way to determine needs is through a **SWOT analysis**. SWOT is an acronym for **s**trengths, **w**eaknesses, **o**pportunities, and **t**hreats (see figure 5.1). A common protocol in the business sector, this strategy looks at both internal and external influences to help determine needs and assess strengths. Strengths and weaknesses are considered internal functions and are determined by evaluating the things the AT does well and the things they could improve. These are factors that the AT can control organizationally or programmatically. The external influences are the factors that challenge the AT, such as competition, workplace climate, and new collaborations. Opportunities are elements outside the organization proper that could help the organization in some way (such as collaborating with an area college to get part-time staff to help the head AT) or that threaten the program (such as a college program that sends students to help the AT as a clinical rotation where the program has lost its accreditation).

Table 5.1 Sample Line-Item Budget

Code	Description	2023-2024 budget	2024-2025 request	Difference
12333	Taping supplies	7,000.00	7,500.00	+500.00
12444	Therapeutic modalities	25,000.00	28,000.00	+3,000.00
12555	Travel	10,000.00	10,000.00	0.00
12666	Rehab equipment	4,500.00	4,000.00	−500.00
12777	Speaker fees	500.00	0.00	-500.00

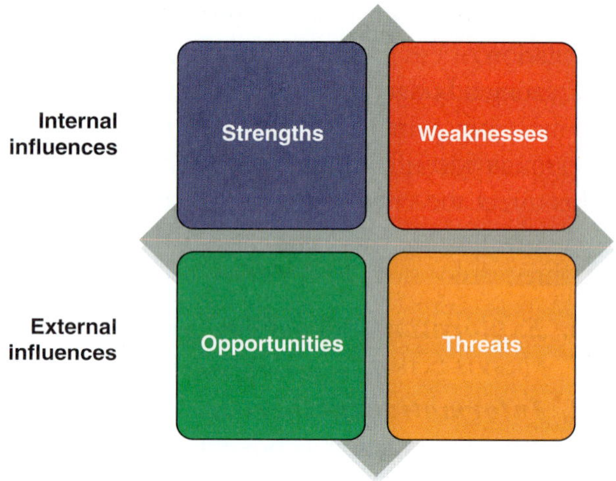

Figure 5.1 SWOT analysis.

Once the priorities are set, the program team needs to request what they need. Through the formal budgeting process, a budget model is selected, and the process begins. The first year of a budget is usually the most difficult because the athletic team is starting from scratch and often has little or no guidance. However, when the team knows its need, it should be clear what they should request. Sometimes, major equipment is needed on a one-time basis. These are called capital expenditures or improvements. Some capital equipment purchases can be spaced out over a 3- to 5-year span. However, others will be needed immediately, and it is the role of the AT to appropriately prioritize needs to serve the patient population. Therefore, the AT will likely not allocate funds for major rehabilitation equipment or modalities each year, like for first aid supplies or travel. In these cases, the AT will typically ask for a capital improvement, which often has a special process, or prioritize these purchases for a specific period in a carefully designed acquisition plan. Sometimes fund-raising is required to help support the major purchase; other times, funding is provided through specific groups such as boosters or parent groups. It is important to understand that these major purchases are necessary and must be planned for in advance. Starting the conversation early with the administration will help ease the process.

PURCHASING

After carefully assessing the needs for the program and designing a budget, the next step is purchasing. Purchasing involves the actual process of acquiring the supplies that the AT determined were needed in the planning phase. Purchasing is an important step in the fiscal management of a program and typically requires specific processes. The six basic steps to purchasing are as follows (Konin and Ray 2019):

1. ***Requesting a quotation.*** This is sometimes called the bidding process and requires certain vendors to set the price for each item needed so that the AT can evaluate who has the fairest price for each item. This is a good way to reduce costs because it encourages all vendors to offer their best price (see figure 5.2 for an example of a request for quotation form).

2. ***Negotiation.*** Negotiations help ATs secure capital equipment, insurance, and other fees such as ambulances and consumables. When negotiating, consider quality, price, supply, shipping, and other support such as warranty and service agreements. Remember, sometimes it is not best to go with the lowest price if the quality of product suffers. Do your homework—it is important to know what you are getting.

3. ***Requisition.*** After deciding what they want, the AT will need to complete a requisition to secure the supplies. This is a written internal request for permission to order the supplies through the vendor at a specific price (see figure 5.3 for a sample requisition form).

4. ***Purchase order.*** This is the actual order that is sent to the vendor that defines the terms and conditions of the purchase (see figure 5.4 for an example). Most **purchase orders** are now done electronically to expedite the process.

5. ***Receiving.*** Once the order is completed, it is shipped to the AT facility. It is important to list the full mailing addresses and identify where supplies are to be stored until the AT can access them in case they are not there at the time of delivery. ATs will need to verify receipt of the order and then complete the inventory as they unpack the supplies.

6. ***Accounts payable.*** Once the materials are received, the vendor will want to be paid. After ensuring all is in the prescribed order, accounts payable are notified to ensure proper payment of the bill. It is the AT's responsibility to ensure that the information is forwarded to accounts payable to facilitate efficient payment.

Understanding Diversity

Honorifics Are Important in Completing Requests and Payments

A title used that precedes a person's name conveys respect. Several commonly used honorifics are:

Title = Pronunciation

Mr. = Mister (used for men, married or unmarried)

Mrs. = Missus (used for a married woman)

Miss = Miss (used for unmarried woman)

Ms. = Miz (used for a woman but does not distinguish if they are married)

Mx. = Mix (gender-neutral title)

Sample Request for Quotation

All quotes are to be sent to:

Athletic Trainer
Laker High School
Laker Street
All City, All State
Contact the athletic trainer at 800-123-1234 with questions.

Date of issue: April 15, 2024

Quotes due on May 30, 2024, at 5:30 p.m. Late quotes will not be considered.

Bid opening on May 31, 2024, at 1 p.m.

Notifications:

1. Please quote itemized prices.
2. Please quote delivery dates.
3. Freight on board is for All City, All State.
4. Laker High School reserves the right to reject any quotations.
5. Only the Laker High School athletics director may assign the purchase order.
6. All quotes must be valid for 90 days from the due date.
7. Bidders may provide a substitute, with clarity as to the quality of that item.
8. *Taxes.* Laker High School is a federally constituted government body and is not subject to state or federal excise tax.
9. *Disclosure of conflicts of interest.* Bidder must disclose in writing whether, to its actual knowledge, any member of their organization is a Laker High School employee.
10. *Payment terms.* Payment shall be made by Laker High School within thirty (30) days of the last date of delivery.
11. *Warranty.* All equipment and supplies shall be warranted by the Bidder for a period of at least one (1) year against defects in design and workmanship.
12. *Default by Bidder.* If Bidder defaults by failing, at any time, to comply with these terms and conditions, Laker High School reserves the right to terminate any and all contracts with Bidder.

Figure 5.2 Request for quotation (RFQ) form.

Sample Requisition Form

Quantity	Item description	Cost	Total
4 dozen	Latex-free exam glove, large		
1,000 pieces	4″ × 4″ sterile gauze		
100 cases	2″ Zonas athletic tape		
24	Lace-up canvas ankle braces, medium		
200	Dip mouth guards, blue		
5	Hydrocollator cover 25″ × 18″		
1 dozen	6″ elastic wraps		
6 cans	Tuf-skin adherent, 4 oz		
6	Lister bandage scissors 5-1/2″		
1 dozen	Emergency penlights		
10 dozen	1″ × 3″ flexible adhesive strips		
1 dozen	.05 oz first aid cream		
6	16 oz hydrogen peroxide 3% solution		
1	AED with pads for adults and child		
1	AED cabinet with alarm to match AED		
1	Digital thermometer		
100	Digital thermometer covers		
2	Hollow-core contoured foam roller		
1	Shipping		
	Totals		

Quotations due by May 30, 2024, at 5:30 p.m.

All quotes are to be sent to:

Athletic Trainer
Laker High School
Laker Street
All City, All State

As the Bidder, I hereby certify that the bid amounts listed above are true and correct based on the specifications that are a part of the RFQ.

Company name: ____________________

Print name: ____________________

Signature: ____________________

Title: ____________________

Email: ____________________

Phone: ____________________

Fax: ____________________

Figure 5.3 Sample requisition form.

Sample Purchase Order

Laker Public Schools
To: Ninja Sports Medicine
Bill to: Laker High School, Finances
Laker Street
All City, All State

Purchase Order: 28368064

Deliver to: Laker High School
Laker Street
All City, All State

Account number: 147.510.1259.0775

Item #	Description	Quantity	Unit price	Total
28003M	3″ × 4-1/2 yd elastic bandages	48	$0.43	$20.64
82102	3M Scotchcast Soft Cast, 2″	2	$79.31	$158.62
36330	6″ × 10 yd elastic bandages	48	$2.35	$112.80
00301	Andover moleskin, 3″	2	$11.43	$22.86
68002	Bayer Multistix 10SG	1	$49.94	$49.94
47060	Guard for broken nose	2	$20.31	$40.62
69412	Cavicide 24 oz trigger spray	10	$6.18	$61.80
69410	Cavicide, gallon	2	$16.14	$32.28
45561	Cold therapy gel/brace	5	$12.50	$62.50
260772	Cooler, 10 gallon	4	$53.96	$215.84
20440B	Coverlet strips, 1″ × 3″	10	$2.75	$27.50
35140	Cover-Roll stretch adhesive, 2″ bandage	6	$7.03	$42.18
47295C	Cramer mouth guards, black (100/bag)	1	$22.50	$22.50
13534	Cramer OSI pads: shin	10	$9.56	$95.60
13545	Cramer OSI pads: square 5″ × 5″	10	$7.91	$79.10
47013M	Tooth-saver kit	2	$10.00	$20.00
46043M	ES Tylenol	3	$9.85	$29.55
17881	Exoclear	1	$27.10	$27.10
47053M	Flexi-Wrap	2	$30.28	$60.56
929432	Functional model of the knee joint	1	$218.50	$218.50
35008	Glutose 15	1	$10.24	$10.24
5569-76	Heavy elastic belts	1	$31.46	$31.46
28052M	Cramer heel and lace pads	1	$11.88	$11.88
65061	HydroChlor whirlpool antiseptic	6	$46.25	$277.50
			Total	**$1,731.57**

Approved by: ____________________ Date: __________

Figure 5.4 Sample purchase order.

Some programs will not have such an extensive process for acquiring supplies and equipment, but most will have a variation of these important steps. It is the AT's job to ensure proper ordering and payment for the supplies used. Be sure to understand the processes at your organization to follow the proper procedures.

INVENTORY MANAGEMENT

Once the AT has acquired all the equipment and supplies, they will then have to ensure that they are inventoried, stored, and managed properly. Each supply and piece of equipment should be logged and recorded to ensure proper inventory. Proper storage of supplies maintains the items and provides security so that they can be used as intended. Most programs will have a complete inventory process where supplies and equipment are counted every three to six months. This helps to monitor equipment use and supplies so the AT can plan for the next year's budget. If during the inventory the AT notices that supplies are low, they may also use this information to adjust current year supplies as needed. There are many ways to inventory equipment and supplies, both on paper and electronically, but the key is to do it regularly.

Storage of inventory is important to ensure control of the supplies and equipment. A clean, dry, and secure storage area is needed. To prevent misuse of supplies, only designated representatives of the athletic training staff should have access to this area. This is an important issue that will often create challenges, since coaches may want access to the supplies for times when the AT is not available. In those circumstances, it is advisable to provide a small kit supplied with basic first aid supplies rather than to give full access to all the supplies in the inventory (see figure 5.5).

? What Would You Do If . . .

Taping every athlete who requests to be taped for stability is a controversial topic. The literature reflects that bracing is equally as effective in preventing injury and protecting athletes from reinjury. Yet many athletic programs still have all athletes taped before games and practice. As an AT, a large portion of your budget is typically allocated to taping supplies. How do you educate the coaches and players about the true value of taping or the limitations of tape application so that you can use the limited resources you do have on equipment needed for all the athletes to use?

Item no.	Description	Quantity	Location	Reorder at
44201	McDavid shin splint support	10	Main TR	4
48102	Medco high-intensity penlight pack	12	Main TR	4
46064M	Medique Diotame tablets	2	Main TR	1
5551-18	Miltex utility scissors, 5-1/2″	3	Main TR	1
27680	Mission Pharacal super cleaner	4	Main TR	1
99920	Muellers knee strap	10	Main TR	4
929436	QuikClot bleeding control gauze for nose bleeds	2	Ice arena	1
69575	New-Skin liquid	3	Main TR	1
26002M	New-Skin liquid bandage spray	2	Main TR	1
261623	Omron automatic inflation blood pressure monitor	3	Main TR	2
5580136	Omron automatic inflation blood pressure monitor	3	Field house	2
39030M	Paper cups, 4 oz. jazz 5000/cs	5,000	Main TR	2,500
39032M	Plastic cups, 5 oz. clear 2500/cs	2,500	Field house	1,250
87700	Plastic goniometer 12 1/2″ long	2	Main TR	1
37200	Powerflex 2″, 24/box	8	Main TR	96
37302	Powerflex 3″, 48/box	3	Main TR	72

Figure 5.5 Inventory sheet.

What Would You Do If . . .

- You have to decide to buy either more tape of poorer quality or less tape of greater quality due to changes in athlete numbers for your program. What are the issues with compromising quality for quantity?
- You have a friend who is the owner of a medical supply company, and he wants to be considered in the bidding process for the supplies at your school. What could happen in this situation?
- A major sponsor of the athletic booster organization at your school will maintain their level of sponsorship (which is significant) only if you agree to post signs for their medical bracing company in the stadium. Is this a problem?

INSURANCE AND REIMBURSEMENT

Athletic trainers are often responsible for insurance billing and are eligible for reimbursement for their services in some states. Both insurance and **reimbursement** can be considered fiscal management components since they deal with the financial functions of the organization. Insurance is a complicated system, but these basics will help you to understand how it works overall. Most athletes will have private or public insurance as a medical coverage. These insurance policies will be coordinated by the parents, guardians, or the athlete themselves if they are old enough to have their own insurance coverage. Insurance will typically pay for medical services, prescriptions, braces, and surgery, if needed. The amount the insurance will pay depends on the coverage. For example, some insurance companies will cover 80% of the total costs of a procedure, and the athlete, parents, or guardians will be responsible for the remaining 20%. Other companies will cover 70%, with the individual paying 30%. If you have a considerable bill, you can see how this could accumulate into a large amount of money.

Insurance providers will also typically have a **copay**. A copay is a set amount of money the athlete or their family pays before the insurance will pay. For example, if you go to the doctor, you may have to pay $30 for the visit, and the insurance pays for the rest. Your copay is $30. Specialists usually have a higher copay than general practitioners do. Athletes often have dental insurance as well, and this is coordinated with the dental office in situations where oral injuries occur. All organizations also carry catastrophic insurance in the event of a life-altering injury or the death of an athlete. This is secured by the school district or organization and provides protection in the tragic event of catastrophic injury or loss.

Athletic trainers are also permitted to bill for their services. Just like doctors use codes to bill the insurance companies for the services they provide, which provides payment for services, the AT can do so as well.

> *The Current Procedural Terminology (CPT) codes for athletic training services are: athletic training evaluation (97005) and reevaluation (97006). These codes are part of the Physical Medicine and Rehabilitation (PMR) CPT family of codes. The American Hospital Association established Uniform Billing (UB) codes—or revenue codes—for athletic training in 1999. The term "qualified health care professional," as found in the CPT code book, is a generic term used to define the professional performing the service described by the code. The term "therapist" is not intended to denote any specific practice or specialty field within PMR. (https://www.nata.org/about/athletic-training)*

This is still evolving in the athletic training profession and can help prove the worth of the AT and bring revenue into the program. NATA has valuable resources on athletic training reimbursement at www.nata.org, found in the online resources.

Summary

Fiscal management is an important task that the AT completes. Depending on the program, the AT will have various levels of responsibility for determining the needs and securing the equipment and supplies for the athletes. Although the process is time intensive and often tedious, it is critical to properly plan for and distribute supplies equitably and fairly. Fiscal management is an ongoing process and should be prioritized as such. Constant attention to the changing needs of the program will help ensure appropriate supplies and resources are available for all. Athletic trainers are becoming more involved in insurance processes and must be familiar with the procedures associated with insurance coverage and billing. Additionally, major initiatives are taking place to secure reimbursement for athletic training services across the country. This helps athletic trainers bring money into their programs to help support their athletes.

Key Terms

Define the following terms found in this chapter:

- budgeting
- catastrophic policy
- copay
- fixed budget
- line-item budget
- lump-sum budget
- needs assessment
- purchase order
- reimbursement
- SWOT analysis
- variable budget
- zero-based budget

As an AT at a high school, you are on a very limited budget. You find that you need a piece of rehabilitation equipment that costs $400. You can easily justify it based on data on injury prevalence, rehabilitation protocols, and evidence-based outcomes. Your budget cannot allow the additional $400 for this equipment, and you cannot remove any other items (all are essential) from the existing budget. What ways could you use the community to help you secure this important piece of equipment?

To access supplementary material for this chapter, including the Understanding Check worksheet, vocabulary quizzes, extension activities, and chapter-specific resources and forms, visit the web resource: http://ancillaries.humankinetics.com/FundamentalsOfAthleticTrainingAndSportsMedicine5E

chapter 6

The Preparticipation Physical Exam

Objectives

After completing this chapter, the student will be able to do the following:

- Describe the typical organization of a preparticipation physical exam.
- Understand the role of a mental health exam as part of the preparticipation exam.
- Explain who should help run each station of the preparticipation physical exam.
- Understand the function and purpose of each station.
- Appreciate and use culturally competent communication in the preparticipation examination.
- Understand the unique needs of and considerations for LGBTQ+ and transgender athletes during the preparticipation examination.

A **preparticipation physical examination** is performed by a medical doctor to determine if an athlete is able to participate in a sport without extra risk of injury or illness. This exam is an essential part of ensuring that each athlete is healthy enough for physical exertion. The examination occurs before participation so that if an athlete has health issues that may exclude them from participation, the exam can prevent injury or even death. After the test, the physician reviews the findings and determines whether the athlete is able to fully participate or has limitations. This chapter explains each step of the preparticipation physical along with the staffing of each station. Professional considerations for culturally competent care will also be presented to ensure all athletes feel safe to address unique concerns based on gender, sexual orientation, ethnicity, and race.

Additionally, preparticipation physical examinations give baseline information from which to make comparisons if an injury or illness does arise. For example, if the AT is examining an athlete who is complaining of dizziness and their blood pressure seems a bit low, the AT can compare the value with the measurement recorded from a previous physical examination. In addition to a comprehensive medical history that includes medications, the preparticipation physical examination should document an athlete's height and weight, blood pressure, and pulse. Also, the ears, nose, throat, heart, lungs, abdomen, flexibility, joint stability, and posture should be examined. If a previous injury or surgery has taken place, a more comprehensive examination including special tests for stability may be performed on that specific area.

The preparticipation physical should be administered no sooner than six weeks before athletic participation (Conley et al. 2014). The timing is important because it provides the best window of opportunity to collect information since the last time the athlete participated. For athletes who require additional medical testing for clearance, six weeks will be enough time without the feeling of being rushed. The NATA position statement, *Preparticipation Physical Examination and Disqualifying Conditions* (NATA n.d.), and the American Association of Pediatrics (AAP n.d.) provide outstanding information regarding the preparticipation physical examination and its role in maintaining the health and safety of athletes and can be found in the online resources.

PREPARTICIPATION FORMAT AND PARTS

In many high schools and universities, the AT and the team physician organize a large-scale physical examination for their athletes. These physical examinations often include a set of stations with medical professionals, such as nurses, athletic trainers, doctors, and physical therapists, and the athletes move from one station to the next until they have visited each station. The athletes could progress through the stations listed in table 6.1. When the athlete first enters the exam area, they register for

Table 6.1 Personnel for Preparticipation Physical Stations

Station	Personnel
Registration	Student assistant, coach, volunteer
Height, weight, and skinfold measurements	AT, student assistant
Blood pressure, pulse rate, respiration rate, and body temperature	AT, student assistant
Vision	AT, student assistant
Joint range of motion and stability	AT
Fitness testing	AT, strength and conditioning coach
Posture	AT
Ears, nose, and throat	Physician
Heart, lungs, and abdomen	Physician
Checkout with team physician in charge who addresses mental health considerations from the intake form	Physician
Postregistration	Student assistant, coach, volunteer

the physical and receive their paperwork. Physical form requirements usually vary by state and can be found at the state athletic association websites or individual school websites. The athlete gives their name, address, and past medical history, including all medications, surgeries, and injuries, since the last exam. Often, the medical history forms are completed in advance so that the parent or guardian can help provide information. It is important for the AT to recognize and use the preferred pronouns listed by the athlete to provide sensitive, compassionate care to all athletes. The athlete then progresses through the height, weight, skinfold, and blood pressure stations.

Go online to the Resources and Forms section in the web resource to find a printable physical form.

High school physicals must be signed by the physician, and the physician does the actual physical (heart sounds, lungs, abdomen, neurological, and ears, nose, and throat). Many states specify which type of physician is able to complete the examination; this may include chiropractors, MDs, and DOs. Everything else can be done by the AT or other trained personnel. In some instances, physicals are done off-site by a physician, which is adequate in some states.

When an AT reviews an athlete's medical history, it may become apparent that an athlete has a history that should be considered. Many history forms now include mental health screening features. These inventories may include depression screenings, which are common for high school students. Figure 6.1 assists the AT in determining the significance of this issue at the time of a physical examination.

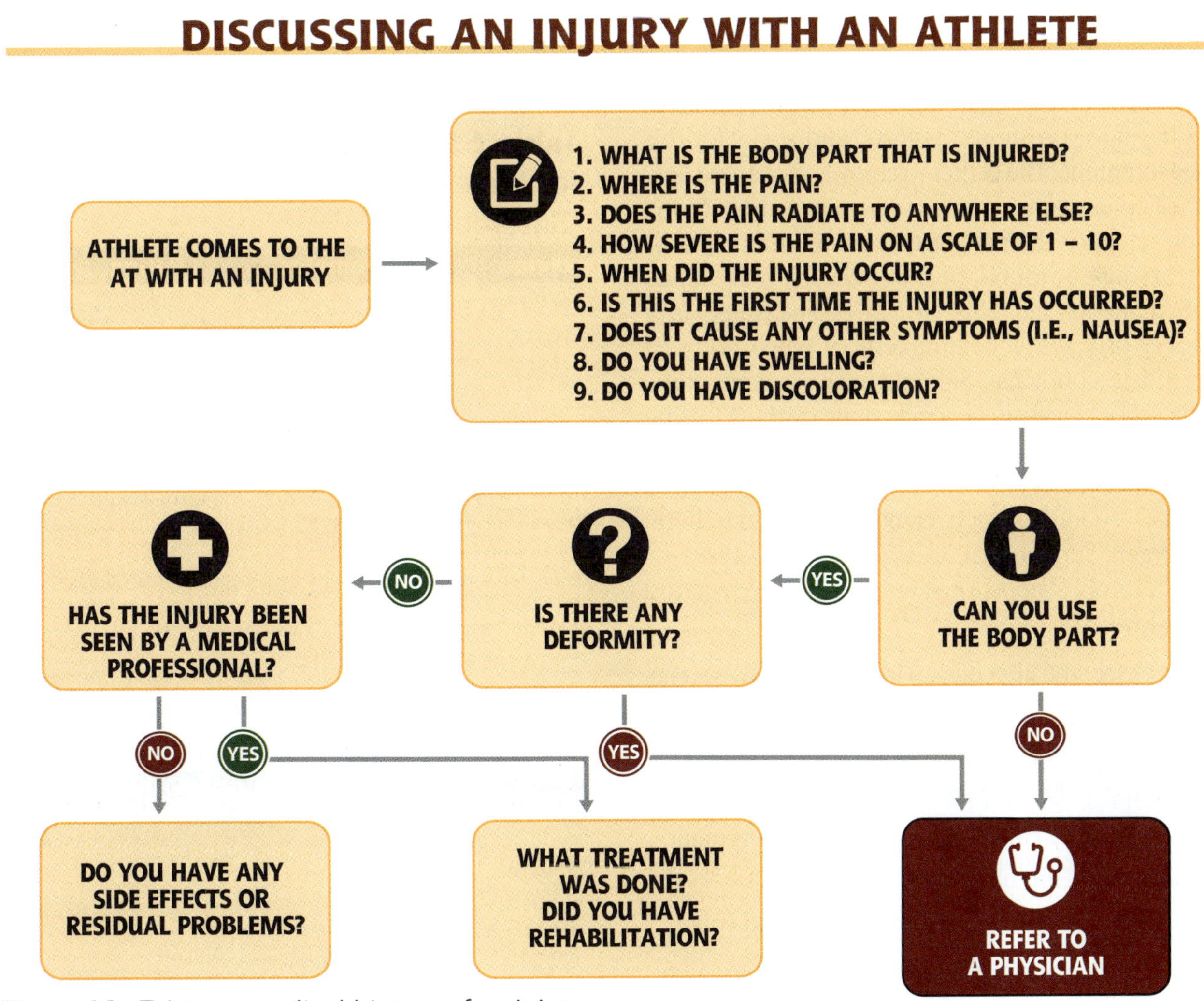

Figure 6.1 Taking a medical history of an injury.

Height, Weight, Skinfold Measurements, and Body Mass Index

Height, weight, and **skinfold measurements** are important to determine the **body composition** of the athlete. Body composition is the amount of muscle, fat, bone, and water within the body. These elements will give an indication of weight classes for such sports as wrestling or can determine if an athlete can safely lose or gain weight.

When taking the measurement for height, make sure the athlete is not wearing shoes and stands tall. The measurement should be completed to the nearest quarter of an inch, with the measurement at the top of the head while compressing the hair to the skull. This station can have a measuring tape attached to the wall.

Weight measurement must use a scale that has been certified annually to ensure the correct weight is being measured. Weight should be measured to the nearest quarter pound. This station should be shielded from other athletes since there can be some sensitivity regarding body image. Athletes should have on shorts, T-shirts, and socks for this measurement. Have them remove shoes and any other items in their pockets or on lanyards around their neck for the most accurate measurements.

Fat that is found beneath the skin is called subcutaneous fat. This fat can be measured in a variety of ways to determine how much body fat an athlete's body has. Skinfold measurements at the high school level are generally done by the AT using skinfold calipers. The calipers measure the distance from one side of a skinfold to the other. Five areas can be used to test fat content, including the thigh, abdomen, subscapular, triceps, and iliac crest.

The proper steps for skinfold measurement are as follows:

1. Select the area of skin in one of the five areas.
2. Grasp a fold of skin between the index finger and thumb.
3. Apply the calipers to the fold of the skin.
4. Read the caliper dial for the measurement.
5. Record the measurement.
6. Repeat two more times at the same spot.

Using the information from each measurement, the AT can determine the amount of body fat. The average body fat percentage varies by gender, age, and sport (tables 6.2 and 6.3). This measurement can assist the AT in making recommendations for weight gain or loss.

The body mass index (BMI) is an alternative to skinfold measurements. The calculation of an athlete's BMI is based on height in meters and weight in kilograms. Although commonly used, this measurement does not consider the lean mass and fat mass of the individual and can be interpreted incorrectly as such. The BMI for a person who is 5′9″ (1.75 m) and weighs 180 pounds (82 kg) is calculated in the following way (George 2017):

1. Multiply weight in pounds by the metric conversion of .45.
2. Multiply height in inches (69 in this case) by the metric conversion of .025.
3. Square the answer to step 2.
4. Divide the answer from step 1 by the answer from step 3.
5. Compare the BMI to table 6.4.

Table 6.2 Body Fat Percentages for Males and Females and Their Classification

Males	Females	Rating
5-10	8-15	Athletic
11-14	16-23	Good
15-20	24-30	Acceptable
21-24	31-36	Overweight
>24	>36	Obese

Note: These are rough estimates. The term *athletic* in this context refers to sports in which low body fat is an advantage.

Reprinted by permission from A. Jeukendrup and M. Gleeson, *Sport Nutrition: An Introduction to Energy Production and Performance*, 2nd ed. (Champaign, IL: Human Kinetics, 2010), 316.

Table 6.3 Body Fat Percentages for the Average Population

	<30 yr	30-50 yr	>50 yr
Females	14%-21%	15%-23%	16%-25%
Males	9%-15%	11%-17%	12%-19%

Reprinted by permission from A. Jeukendrup and M. Gleeson, Sport Nutrition: An Introduction to Energy Production and Performance, 2nd ed. (Champaign, IL: Human Kinetics, 2010), 316.

Table 6.4 BMI Categories

Category	BMI
Underweight	Less than 18.5
Normal	18.5-24.9
Overweight	25-29.9
Obese	30 or above

Source: National Heart, Lung, and Blood Institute (n.d.a.).

Our sample athlete has a BMI of

$$81 / 2.9756 = 27.22$$

Another way to classify the body composition is through predominant body type by looking at the overall build of the athlete. This is a rather subjective determination. There are three types of body composition: **endomorph**, **mesomorph**, and **ectomorph** (see figure 6.2).

- ***Endomorph:*** high fat body with a stocky body build
- ***Mesomorph:*** low fat body with a muscular build
- ***Ectomorph:*** low fat body with a slight body build

Blood Pressure, Pulse Rate, Respiration Rate, and Body Temperature

Blood pressure is the amount of pressure found in the blood vessels. A blood pressure measurement has two elements: **systolic pressure** and **diastolic pressure**. The systolic element measures the amount of pressure in the blood vessels when the heart beats, while diastolic measures the amount of pressure when the heart is at rest.

A blood pressure cuff or a **sphygmomanometer** measures blood pressure. The cuff has to fit snugly around the upper portion of the arm or the humerus. The AT needs to read the meter that determines the blood pressure, so it must face the AT. The athlete will rest their relaxed arm on the table while the AT places a stethoscope over the brachial artery at the medial aspect of the elbow joint.

To properly take a blood pressure measurement, follow the following sequence (Cleary and Flanagan 2020):

1. Apply the deflated blood pressure cuff above the elbow.

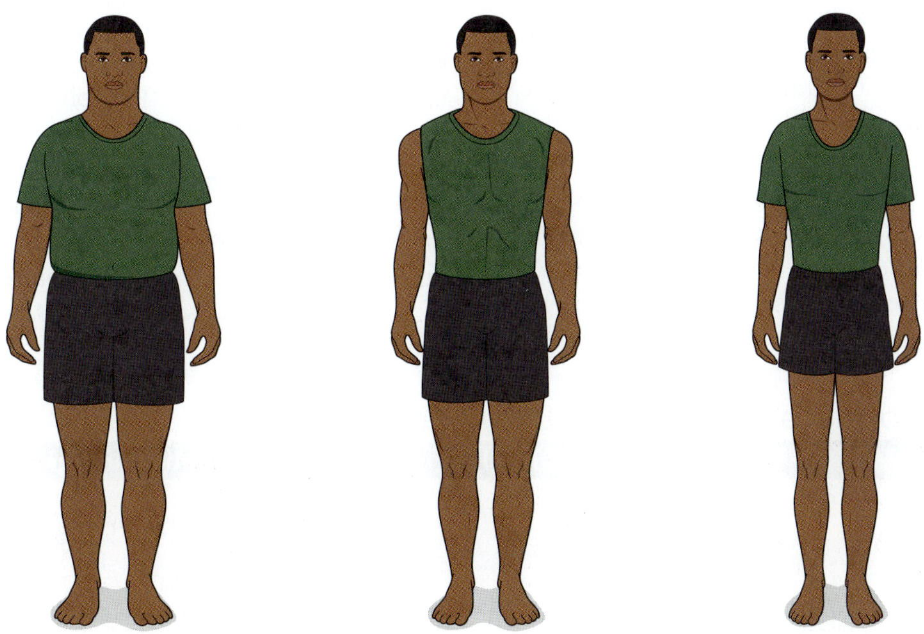

a *b* *c*

Figure 6.2 Body composition types: *(a)* endomorph, *(b)* mesomorph, and *(c)* ectomorph.

Reprinted by permission from NSCA, "Age- and Sex-Related Differences and Their Implications for Resistance Exercise," by A.D. Falgenbaum, in *Essentials of Strength Training and Conditioning*, 3rd ed., edited by T.R. Baechle and R.W. Earle (Champaign, IL: Human Kinetics 2009), 145.

2. Place the stethoscope over the brachial artery at the medial aspect of the anterior elbow.
3. Inflate the cuff to 200 mmHg.
4. Deflate the cuff at a rate of 3 mmHg per second.
5. Listen for the first audible beat sound—this will be the systolic portion.
6. Note when the sound disappears—this will be the diastolic portion.
7. Record the blood pressure as systolic over diastolic.
8. Remove the blood pressure cuff.

A typical blood pressure measurement is recorded with the systolic over the diastolic. For an adult athlete, normal blood pressure is 120/80. When an athlete's blood pressure drops 20 mmHg below their normal measurement, it is considered low blood pressure. Blood pressure is considered high when it is 140/90. Blood pressure ranges are listed in table 6.5.

High blood pressure is a concern because it can damage the heart, lungs, and blood vessels. The AT will highlight high blood pressure for the physician to follow up on during the preparticipation examination. Because managing blood pressure is important at all ages, it is essential to understand ways in which our choices affect our blood pressure.

Pulse rate tells the AT how often the heart is beating. An average resting adult pulse rate or heart rate is 60 to 80 beats per minute. An athlete will have a lower resting heart rate, and young children typically have higher resting heart rates. An athlete's pulse rate will be slower at rest than it is while physically active. The more physically active a person is, the higher the pulse rate. Often, athletes will know their target heart rate, which is calculated by subtracting their age from 220 and multiplying the result by a number within the range of 70 to 90 percent (220 − age × 70-90%). Athletes will strive to exercise for maximal aerobic benefits, and this calculation can help determine that number. The places where a pulse is taken are referred to as *pulse points*. The common pulse points assessed in an athlete are the carotid, brachial, radial, femoral, and dorsal pedis. Many fitness devices such as smartwatches can monitor heart rate throughout the day to give the athlete a record of their heart rate patterns. These are called **biometric** or **physiometric** devices.

When assessing the pulse rate, the AT will apply pressure to the pulse point using the index and middle fingers. While applying pressure, the AT will count the number of pulses in one minute. If the AT does not feel a pulse, they will recheck finger placement. No pulse indicates that the heart has stopped or blood is not flowing to that area. A normal pulse for an athlete is 60 to 80 beats per minute. When an athlete is injured, pulse rate may increase or decrease, depending on the type of injury.

The AT should record the athlete's respiration rate. Normal respiration rate is 12 to 20 breaths per minute. This is measured by physically observing the chest rise and fall for one minute. Respiration rates increase during physical activity and decrease with rest. During injury, respiration rates can increase or decrease, depending on the condition or illness. A pulse oxygen tool (pulse oximeter) is sometimes used to determine the amount of oxygen getting through the system. This small device is

Table 6.5 Normal and Abnormal Blood Pressure

Classification	Systolic (mmHg)	Diastolic (mmHg)
Child (6-11 yr)	97-120	57-80
Adolescent (12-15 yr)	102-120	61-80
Adult	<120	<80
Hypotension*	<90	<60
Hypertension	>130	>80
Hypertensive crisis	>180	>120

*Only abnormal when combined with symptoms of shock or other signs of distress.

Reprinted by permission from M.A. Cleary and K.W. Flanagan, *Acute and Emergency Care in Athletic Training* (Champaign, IL: Human Kinetics, 2020), 97. Data from Pollack and Beck (2012); Bickley and Szilagyi (2013); Marx and Rosen (2017); Pickering et al. (2005); Whelton et al. (2017).

RED FLAGS

Refer the athlete to a physician for the following conditions:

- High blood pressure 140/90 (National Heart, Lung, and Blood Institute n.d.b; Cleary and Flanagan 2020)
- Low blood pressure 90/60 (National Heart, Lung, and Blood Institute n.d.c)
- Slow heart rate (less than 60 beats per minute; Mayo Clinic 2017b)
- Rapid heart rate (100 beats or more per minute; Mayo Clinic 2018d)
- Wheezing or a crackling when breathing
- Body temperature of 100 °F (38 °C)

clipped onto your finger and uses a laser to detect oxygen levels. Any measurement above 97% is considered normal.

Measuring body temperature is called **thermometry.** Body temperature is normally 98.6 °F (37 °C). A thermometer is used to detect temperature. Types of thermometers include oral, rectal, ear, and forehead. Each type of thermometer is used differently, so ATs should follow the instructions to ensure accuracy. The most accurate temperature is rectal temperature. This is recommended in conditions of illness, especially heat illness in athletes.

Vision

Being able to see is critical in sport, so vision testing is a necessity. The AT tests vision using a Snellen eye chart. The athlete will stand 20 feet (6 m) away from the chart and read the letters on the chart in a distraction-free environment. The athlete will be asked to cover one eye and read the lowest line he can see on the chart. Then he will cover the other eye and read the lowest line. If the athlete wears glasses or contacts, an eye check is necessary. This test uses the same process but with lenses.

A typical vision is expressed as 20/20. The first number indicates which line on the chart the athlete can read and the second relates to the 20-foot line from the chart. A 20/20 means the person can read the letters that the most people can read from a 20-foot distance. When vision is expressed as 20/30 (worse than 20/20), it means that the person can see at a 20-foot distance what someone with normal sight would see at a 30-foot (9 m) distance. When the vision is expressed as 20/10 (better than 20/20), the athlete can read from a 20-foot distance what a normal-sighted person would see from 10 feet (3 m).

Joint Range of Motion and Stability

Joint range-of-motion testing is performed to determine any limitations, pain, or extra range of motion at each joint. When range of motion increases or decreases, the AT will want to determine the cause and whether it can be improved. Range of motion is tested using a special instrument called a **goniometer**. The goniometer is aligned with bony landmarks at the joint being tested. The AT reads the goniometer and records the range of motion. Other tools used for measuring range of motion are the tape measure (figure 6.3) and **inclinometer** (figure 6.4).

Table 6.6 lists the joints and normal range of motion for each (Houglum, Boyle-Walker, and Houglum 2023, Houglum 2016). Joint range-of-motion tests will be done on both the left and right sides of the athlete's body. The AT will compare both sides to determine if the range of motion is equal and normal for that person (see figure 6.5).

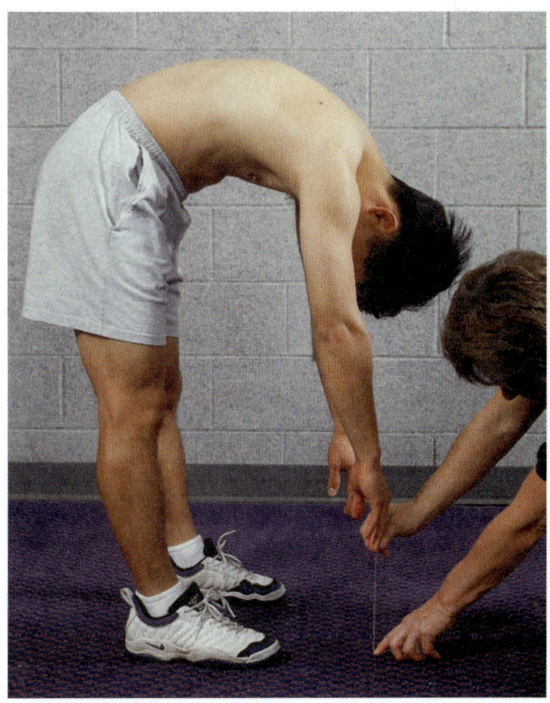

Figure 6.3 Tape measure.

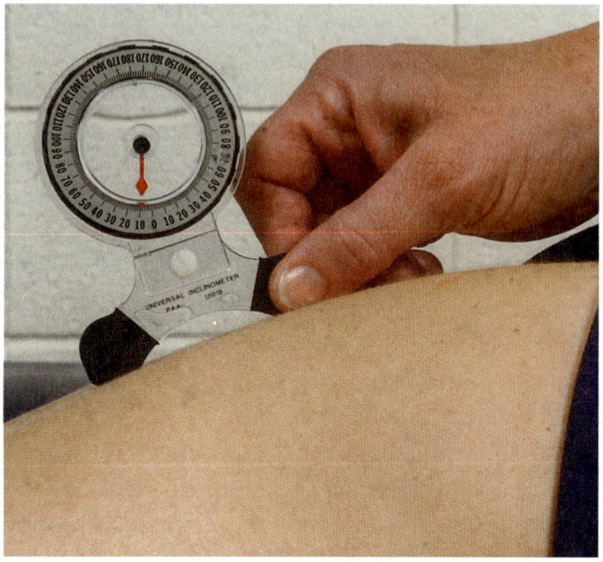

Figure 6.4 Inclinometer.

Each athlete should have their main joints tested for stability. This is especially true for athletes who had an injury that compromised the joint. Joint stability can be compromised by bony structure, ligaments, and tendons. When a joint is tested, the stability can be noted and compared in the event of injury. Joint stability tests can be found in each chapter pertaining to that body part. Unstable joints will have to be reconditioned to prevent further injury. Table 6.7 shows stress tests used for various joints.

Fitness Testing

Before physical activity, the **physical fitness** level can be determined to assist the coach with knowledge of the intensity of a workout. The baseline data can be used to help the athlete improve off-season

Table 6.6 Joint Range of Motion

Joint	Movement	Normal range of motion	Variable range of motion
Shoulder	Flexion	0°-180°	0°-170°
Shoulder	Extension	0°-60°	0°-45°
Elbow	Flexion/extension	0°-150°	0°-145°
Wrist	Flexion	0°-80°	0°-90°
Wrist	Extension	0°-70°	0°-60°
Hip	Flexion	0°-120°	0°-125°
Hip	Extension	0°-30°	10°-15°
Hip	Abduction	0°-40°	0°-45°
Hip	Adduction	0°-30°	10°-20°
Knee	Flexion	0°-135°	0°-140°
Knee	Extension	0°-15°	0°-10°
Ankle	Plantar flexion	0°-50°	0°-45°
Ankle	Dorsiflexion	0°-20°	0°-15°

- ❑ Explain the technique to the patient.
- ❑ Position the patient comfortably.
- ❑ Position the segment to be measured at the beginning of its motion.
- ❑ Stabilize the proximal portion of the segment.
- ❑ Palpate bony landmarks.
- ❑ Move to eye level.
- ❑ Position the stationary arm.
- ❑ Position the moveable arm.
- ❑ Assure alignment of the fulcrum with the joint's axis.
- ❑ Observe for substitution.
- ❑ Recheck stationary and moveable arm positions.
- ❑ Record measurement.
- ❑ Stabilize proximal segment.
- ❑ Move joint to end motion position.
- ❑ Locate bony landmarks.
- ❑ Realign stationary and moveable arms.
- ❑ Observe for substitutions.
- ❑ Recheck alignment of both arms and fulcrum.
- ❑ Record measurement.

Figure 6.5 Range-of-motion measurement technique.

Table 6.7 Stress Testing

Joints	Stress tests
Shoulder	Apprehension anterior and posterior
Elbow	Varus and valgus
Wrist	Varus and valgus
Fingers	Varus and valgus
Knee	Varus, valgus, posterior drawer, and Lachman
Ankle	Anterior drawer and talar tilt

workouts and areas of their fitness deficits. Haff and Triplett (2016) indicate that the tests described in table 6.8 can be used to test current fitness level.

Postural Alignment

The postural alignment station simply has a plumb line (a weighted string) hung from the ceiling. For correct use, the plumb line must be straight and still. The athlete should stand next to the wall so the AT can view her posture using bony markers. Ideally, the bony markers should be in alignment for proper posture.

Postural alignments are performed in the anterior, posterior, and lateral planes. Table 6.9 defines each plane and the ideal postural alignment (Houglum 2016).

When viewing the bony markers, the AT will determine whether each side of the body is level in the anterior and posterior planes. In the lateral plane, the AT will determine if the bony markers

Table 6.8 Fitness Testing

Test	What is being tested
Bench press: 1 repetition at maximum	Low-speed muscular strength
Back squat: 1 repetition at maximum	Low-speed muscular strength
Power clean: 1 repetition at maximum	High-speed muscular strength
Standing long jump	High-speed muscular strength
Vertical jump	High-speed muscular strength
300-yard shuttle run	Anaerobic capacity
Partial curl-up	Muscular strength
Push-up	Muscular strength
12-minute run	Aerobic capacity
20-yard shuttle run	Agility
40-yard sprint	Speed

Table 6.9 Postural Alignment Planes

	Anterior	Posterior	Lateral
Head	Nose	Midline of skull	Ear hole
Shoulder	Bisecting the sternum	Bisecting cervical and thoracic spines	Just anterior of shoulder
Hip	Pubic symphysis	Bisecting lumbar spine	Head of femur
Knee	Equal distance between medial aspects	Equal distance between medial aspects	Just anterior of middle of knee
Ankle	Equal distance between medial malleolus	Equal distance between medial malleolus	Just anterior of lateral malleolus

are anterior or posterior of the line. Figure 6.6 demonstrates these alignments.

Another tool used for posture assessment is the **posture grid**. This see-through plastic grid has horizontal and vertical lines on it so the AT can see symmetry of the posture. The athlete will stand behind the posture grid, and the AT will look at them at a front-facing, side-facing and rear-facing view to check for alignment based on specific bony landmarks such as the tip of the shoulder, shoulder blades (scapulae), hip bones (iliac crest), knee folds (popliteal crease), and others.

When the athlete's posture is out of alignment, their body has to compensate in another area to keep them balanced. A compensation that can occur is a contraction or fatigue of muscles or something more significant, such as scoliosis. The issue with postural imbalances is that over time, joints can degrade and muscle and ligament injuries can occur.

Physical exertion places additional pressure on the athlete's body. The AT will need to determine what conditioning or therapy is needed to create the best postural alignment.

Ears, Nose, and Throat

The physician present is responsible for assessing the ears, nose, and throat. When assessing the ears using an **otoscope,** which is a lighted tool with a magnifying feature, the physician is looking for signs or symptoms of the following:

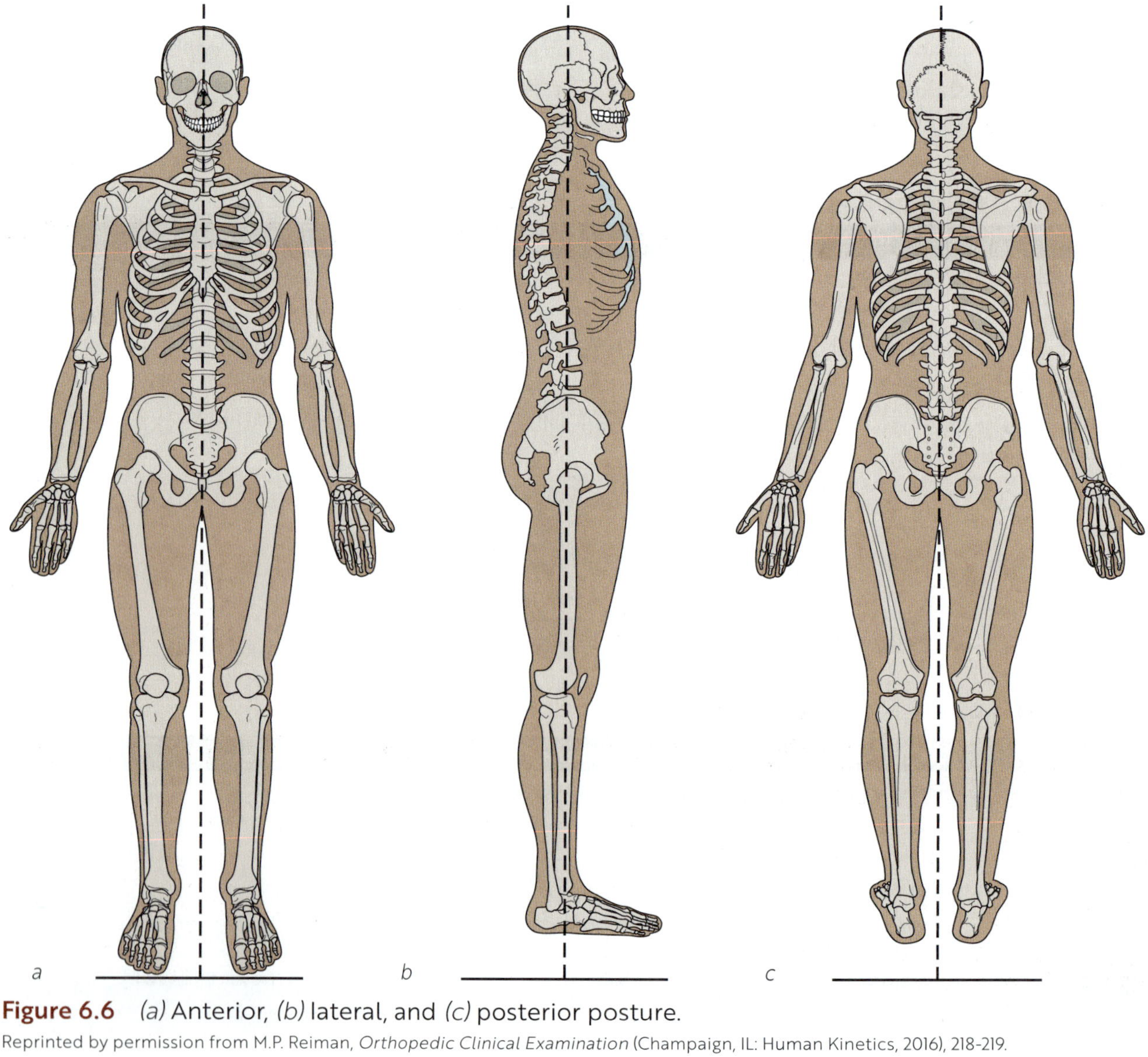

Figure 6.6 *(a)* Anterior, *(b)* lateral, and *(c)* posterior posture.

Reprinted by permission from M.P. Reiman, *Orthopedic Clinical Examination* (Champaign, IL: Human Kinetics, 2016), 218-219.

- Obstructions, such as earwax
- Infections
- Hematoma
- Decreased ability to hear

He may take this time to also use an **ophthalmoscope** to check the structure and integrity of the eye itself. This tool is like an otoscope but designed specifically for evaluating the eye (figure 6.7). Figure 6.8 shows an image of the otoscope. Can you identify the unique characteristics of each tool?

In the examination of the nose, the physician will look for the ability to breathe through both nasal passages and for alignment of the septum in the nose.

When assessing the throat, the physician will be looking for the following:

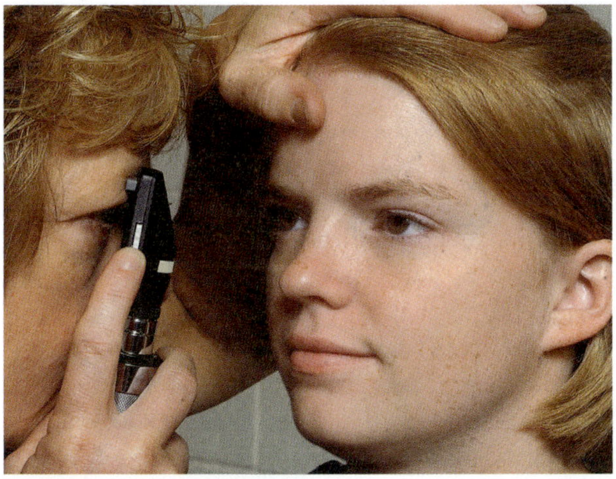

Figure 6.7 Ophthalmoscope.

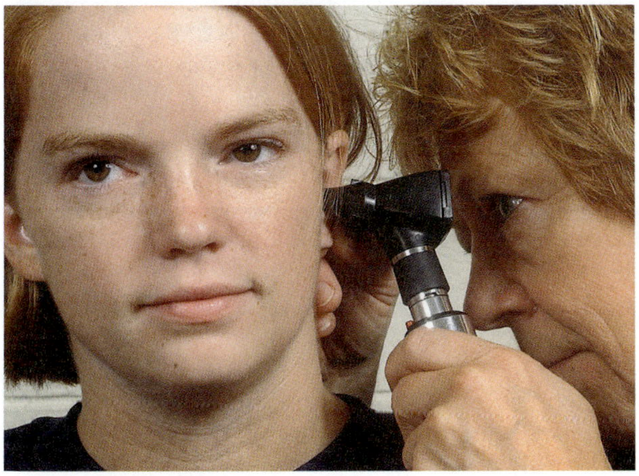

Figure 6.8 Otoscope.

- Size of the thyroid
- Ability to swallow
- Cavities or loose teeth
- Gum disease
- Swollen glands
- Signs of infection
- Discoloration in the mouth or throat

Heart, Lungs, and Abdomen

The physician will examine the athlete to determine heart, lungs, and abdominal health using a stethoscope, palpation, and **percussion**. A standard examination of the athlete's heart consists of listening for heart sounds using a stethoscope. Specifically, the physician will listen for abnormal sounds such as a prolonged swoosh sound, which is an indication of a murmur. A high-pitched sound indicates a narrowing of the blood vessels of the heart.

The stethoscope can also be used to listen to the athlete's lungs. The physician will listen for crackling, wheezing, and any other sound that is abnormal. Since the lungs are large, the physician will have to move the stethoscope to various spots. Lung sounds are compared on each side. Abnormal breath sounds can indicate asthma, bronchitis, fluid in the lungs, or an infection. A physician may have an athlete with suspected or reported asthma perform a **peak flow meter** test (see figure 6.9) to

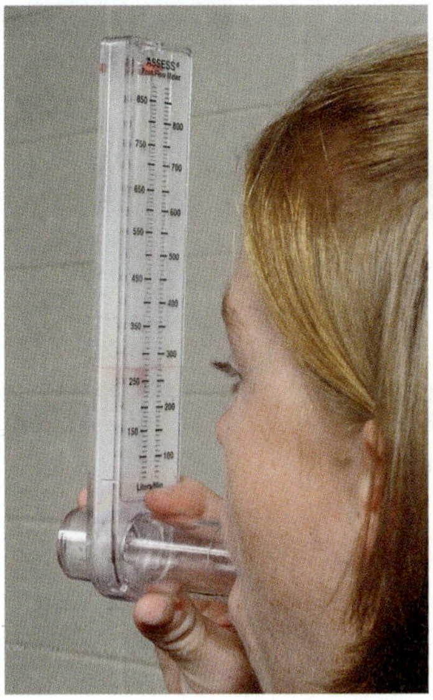

Figure 6.9 Peak flow meter.

determine the amount of air the athlete can move on expiration.

The abdomen is divided into four quadrants: upper right, upper left, lower right, and lower left. Located in each quadrant are organs involved in digestion, elimination, and reproduction. Chapter 12 covers each quadrant in more depth. During the examination of the abdomen, the physician will use their hands to palpate each quadrant. Abnormalities can include enlargement on an organ, pain, or bulging of an organ through the abdominal wall. The physician may use the stethoscope to listen for bowel sounds and pulses. Figure 6.10 shows the proper techniques for abdominal auscultations.

Percussion (tapping) is also used to listen for the sounds produced by each hollow and solid organ. This can tell the physician if there is a problem that might require additional testing.

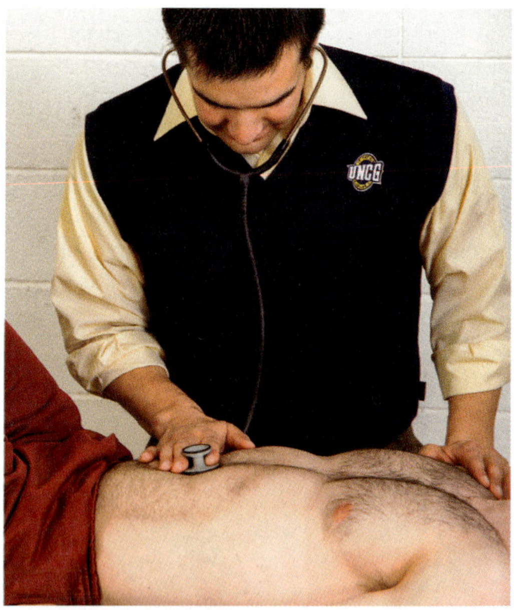

Figure 6.10 Abdominal auscultations.

Neurological

Athletic trainers are responsible for determining the function of the nervous system. The body has a central and **peripheral nervous system**. The **central nervous system** consists of the brain and spine, while the peripheral has the nerves that go throughout the rest of the body.

The nerves of the peripheral nervous system may be involved with sensation or muscular movements. The peripheral nervous system will be tested for the sensations of pain and touch. Nerves will have sensory (**dermatome**) or motor (**myotome**) functions. Each nerve has its own function, and each is assessed individually. In general, a sensory nerve will be tested by using a soft touch (cotton-tipped applicator) and sharp touch (pinwheel) along the area of innervation for that specific nerve. Motor nerves are tested by having the athlete perform specific motions associated with those innervations and can be moving the eyes to the side or raising the leg into full extension. Each nerve has its own function and is part of the advanced skill set for the AT.

Another way to assess nerves is through reflex testing. A rubber mallet tapped on tendons with intact nerves will elicit a reflex. The biceps, triceps, and patellar and Achilles tendons are the usual **reflexes** tested in this type of examination. Reflexes are graded on a scale of 0 to 4, with zero meaning no response, 1 a delayed response, 2 a normal response, and 3 a hyperresponse (table 6.10). A grade of 4 is a spasmodic response and often indicates a medical issue.

The brain has 12 fixed major nerves, called the cranial nerves, that control the senses and movements of the head and face. A physician will

Table 6.10 Reflex Grading

Reflex response	Grade	Definition
Absence of reflex	0	Areflexia
Diminished reflex	1	Hyporeflexia
Average reflex	2	Normal or average
Exaggerated reflex	3	Hyperreflexia
Clonus	4	Spasmodic alteration of muscle contraction or relaxation indicating a nerve irritation

Reprinted by permission from M.P. Reiman, *Orthopedic Clinical Examination* (Champaign, IL: Human Kinetics, 2016), 121.

examine the athlete and test each of the 12 nerves (table 6.11). The testing will involve eye movements, sensations of taste and smell, swallowing, hearing, pupil constriction, and movement of the tongue, face, and shoulders. This is important in evaluating head and neck injuries.

The central nervous system, especially the brain, needs to be tested if there is a concussion. This type of testing is referred to as a baseline. The purpose of the testing is to evaluate reaction time, memory, and decision making when the athlete is not injured. In some cases, the athlete goes through computerized testing in each area, and the responses are stored. The most commonly used computerized test is called the ImPACT test. The baseline test will be recalled in the event of a concussion as a part of a comprehensive physician evaluation to determine the significance of the injury. Each athlete will be given a baseline brain test, either face to face or with a computer. This baseline brain test will give the AT critical information about how the athlete's brain functions under normal circumstances. When the athlete is injured, the AT will compare the baseline test with a test taken after the injury.

Mental health examinations are becoming more prevalent in preparticipation screening. As an important component of overall health, a physician or other health care professional typically performs mental health examinations. Often, inventories or surveys ask the athlete to rate themselves on areas of anxiety, stress, depression, and other mental health issues. Further, any medications should be included in the health intake form to ensure that any mental health medication issues can be addressed if needed. Some athletes have a fear of disclosing they have mental health issues, but it is important to get baseline information so that the physician can monitor or refer the athlete whenever needed.

Checkout With the Team Physician in Charge

The team physician is the last person that the athlete sees during the preparticipation physical examination. At this point, the team physician checks any noted conditions or mental health concerns from the previous stations to determine whether the athlete can play or if additional testing is needed. The physician decides the athlete's status for playing.

Table 6.11 Cranial Nerves

Number	Name	Composition	Function
I	Olfactory	Sensory	Smell
II	Optic	Sensory	Vision
III	Oculomotor	Motor	Pupil reaction and size Elevation of upper eyelid Eye adduction and downward rolling
IV	Trochlear	Motor	Upward eye rolling
V	Trigeminal	Mixed	Motor: mastication Sensory: areas of the face, including the forehead, temple, nose, lips, tongue, and jaw
VI	Abducens	Motor	Lateral eye movement
VII	Facial	Mixed	Motor: facial muscles Sensory: taste
VIII	Vestibulocochlear	Sensory	Hearing and equilibrium
IX	Glossopharyngeal	Mixed	Motor: pharyngeal muscles (swallowing) Sensory: taste
X	Vagus	Mixed	Motor: muscles of the pharynx and larynx; parasympathetic control of the heart, lungs, and digestive tract Sensory: gag reflex, internal organs
XI	Accessory	Motor	Trapezius and sternocleidomastoid muscles
XII	Hypoglossal	Motor	Tongue movement

Reprinted by permission from L. Kahanov and E.K. Payne, *Athletic Training and Therapy: Foundation of Behavior and Practice* (Champaign, IL: Human Kinetics, 2022), 301.

If any restrictions are noted, a plan is discussed to remedy those conditions through either further diagnostic testing or rehabilitation.

Sometimes, the doctor may require blood work or urine tests to detect medical conditions. Common blood tests will include a **complete blood count (CBC)** and a **basic metabolic panel (BMP)**. These will detect the amount of each blood cell in the body and will also give information regarding the function of the major systems in the body such as the kidneys and liver (table 6.12). A urinalysis can also give the physician information regarding the levels of sugar, protein, or blood being excreted (table 6.13). Each test will provide valuable information to the physician if any medical conditions are suspected during the preparticipation physical examination.

After the athlete completes these additional steps, the physician will again review the data to make the final decision regarding participation.

Table 6.12 Normal Values for CBC Test

Blood contents	Normal	Function
Red blood cells (RBC)	Males: 25-35 mL/kg body weight Females: 20-30 mL/kg body weight	Carry oxygen from lungs to the rest of the body
White blood cells	4.5-11 × 10^3 cells/mcL	Fight infections and diseases Abnormal levels are signs of infection, blood cancer, or immune system dysfunction.
Platelets	150-350 × 10^3 cells/mcL	Blood cells that assist in clotting Abnormal levels may be a sign of bleeding or thrombotic disorder.
Hemoglobin	Males: 14-17 g/dL Females: 12-16 g/dL	Iron-rich protein in RBCs that carries oxygen Abnormal levels may be a sign of anemia, thalassemia, or other blood disorders.
Hematocrit	Males: 41%-51% Females: 36%-47%	Measure of how much space RBCs take up in blood Abnormal levels may be a sign of blood or bone marrow disorders.

Reprinted by permission from L. Kahanov and E.K. Payne, *Athletic Training and Therapy: Foundation of Behavior and Practice* (Champaign, IL: Human Kinetics, 2022), 329.

Table 6.13 Urinalysis Readings

Specific gravity	1.003-1.030	Low reading: diabetes mellitus, excessive hydration, renal failure High reading: dehydration, diarrhea, urinary tract infection, or renal failure
pH	5.0-9.0	Low reading: COPD, diabetic ketoacidosis High reading: renal failure, urinary tract infections
Glucose	<0.5	Diabetes mellitus, stress
Ketones	0	Diabetes mellitus, alcoholism, anorexia nervosa
Protein	0	Renal disease or injury, hypertension, fever, rhabdomyolysis
Hemoglobin	0	Urinary tract infection, sickle cell anemia, kidney disease or trauma
RBC	0	Kidney stones, vigorous activity, urinary tract infections

Reprinted by permission from L. Kahanov and E.K. Payne, *Athletic Training and Therapy: Foundation of Behavior and Practice* (Champaign, IL: Human Kinetics, 2022), 329.

Postregistration

The athlete then progresses to the postregistration booth. Here, they can pick up information regarding the findings. For example, suppose an AT found that an athlete had much less strength in one leg than in the other. Knowing that this lack of strength could create problems and increase the athlete's risk of injury, the AT would give the athlete an instruction sheet for a lower-body strengthening program to improve this condition.

MEDICAL INFORMATION FORMS

The **preparticipation physical examination** is a good time for parents to fill out a medical information card along with the athlete's medical history. It is prudent for an AT to always keep informed consent forms (permission to treat) and the athletes' insurance information and medical information with them. It is impossible to remember every condition that each athlete has. Keeping each athlete's medical information card in the medical kit allows the AT or coach to obtain crucial information at a moment's notice. For example, if a coach takes the tennis team to an away meet and one of the athletes is stung by a bee and suddenly begins to act ill, the coach can look at the medical data form to see if the athlete is allergic to bee stings. If an athlete needs advanced care at a hospital and the parent is not around, the medical data form can provide necessary information for giving proper treatment. Many high schools keep the permission

GOALS AND OUTCOMES OF PREPARTICIPATION EXAMINATIONS

The goals of the preparticipation exams are as follows:

1. To build a relationship between the student-athlete and the athletic training staff and the team physician
2. To build a relationship between the student-athlete's parents and the athletic training staff and the team physician
3. To make the AT aware of any conditions, illnesses, or injuries that may require attention when the athlete participates
4. To provide an opportunity to strengthen physical deficiencies
5. To allow students with conditions that require further medical care the opportunity to get such care before the season begins
6. To comply with association rules on participation

The outcomes of preparticipation exams are as follows:

1. Passed—This athlete can participate without any restrictions.
2. Passed with conditions—This athlete can participate in some sports but requires additional follow-up. If a physician clears the athlete of the condition, then full participation without restriction can occur.
3. Passed with reservations—The athlete will not be able to participate in contact or collision sports.
4. Failed with reservations—The athlete cannot participate in the sport requested. The physician may allow participation in less intensive sports.
5. Failed with conditions—The athlete has to return to peak health before participating. The athlete must be reevaluated to ensure health.
6. Failed—The athlete cannot participate in any sport at any time.

Adapted from Prentice (2021).

to treat and medical information on the same card. The medical information form gives information such as preferred hospital, name of primary care physician, name of dentist, insurance information, and permission to treat. However, remember that medical information is protected by law, so proper precautions must be taken to ensure that only the appropriate persons can access the medical information and forms.

Go online to the Resources and Forms section in the web resource to find a printable permission-to-treat form.

CLEARANCE FOR PARTICIPATION IN SPORT

In some instances, an athlete will need additional specialized testing to determine if they can participate. Further testing can result in several outcomes, including disqualifying an athlete from participation. In most instances, the athlete is able to participate with a little intervention, such as medication, physical therapy, bracing, or monitoring of the situation. Whenever additional specialized testing is done, the physician will have to provide the clearance for participation.

Summary

The preparticipation physical is the most crucial element in ensuring the health of athletes. The AT should assemble highly qualified people to oversee each part of the examination. In some instances, an athlete will have a previous injury or illness that will need to be evaluated more thoroughly to determine if participation can occur. The team physician will ultimately be responsible for approving the athlete's participation in sport.

Key Terms

Define the following terms found in this chapter:

- basic metabolic panel (BMP)
- biometric
- body composition
- central nervous system
- complete blood count (CBC)
- dermatome
- diastolic pressure
- ectomorph
- endomorph
- goniometer
- inclinometer
- mesomorph
- myotome
- peripheral nervous system
- physical fitness
- physiometric
- preparticipation physical examination
- reflexes
- skinfold measurement
- sphygmomanometer
- systolic pressure
- thermometry

As an AT, you will need to organize athletic training services for all athletes. You have 50 high school cross country teams come in for preparticipation screenings at the same time at your facility. How would you best address the unique needs of each athlete and respect their privacy when determining mental health issues and medications?

To access supplementary material for this chapter, including the Understanding Check worksheet, vocabulary quizzes, extension activities, and chapter-specific resources and forms, visit the web resource: http://ancillaries.humankinetics.com/FundamentalsOfAthleticTrainingAndSportsMedicine5E

Unit II

Basics of Human Anatomy and Physiology

chapter 7

Introduction to Anatomy

Objectives

After completing this chapter, the student will be able to do the following:

- Define anatomical planes and describe anatomical position.
- Label general muscular and bony anatomy.
- Understand the origin, insertion, and innervation of specific muscles.
- Describe the functions of skin, bone, muscle, ligament, tendon, and cartilage.
- Describe the types of bones and give examples.
- Describe the classification of joints and explain the types of motion produced.

An understanding of human **anatomy** is the foundation of many health care professions, including that of the certified AT. An AT must determine which structures have been injured, and they must understand what normal movements are to design appropriate rehabilitation and strength and conditioning programs. This requires understanding the structure (anatomy) and function (physiology) of the anatomical structures.

ANATOMICAL POSITION

To improve communication between health care professionals and facilitate a better understanding of human movement, medical professionals have accepted a particular alignment of the body as standard—the **anatomical position**. This position refers to an erect stance with arms at the sides and palms facing forward. The body moves in relation to three planes: the **frontal plane**, the **sagittal plane**, and the **transverse plane**. These can be seen in figure 7.1.

Health care providers use common medical terms to explain to one another where an injury is located on the body. There are many terms, and it is beyond the scope of this text to explain them all. Instead, we will present the most common terms that an AT would use in the athletic training room. For instance, you will hear the terms *anterior*, *pos-*

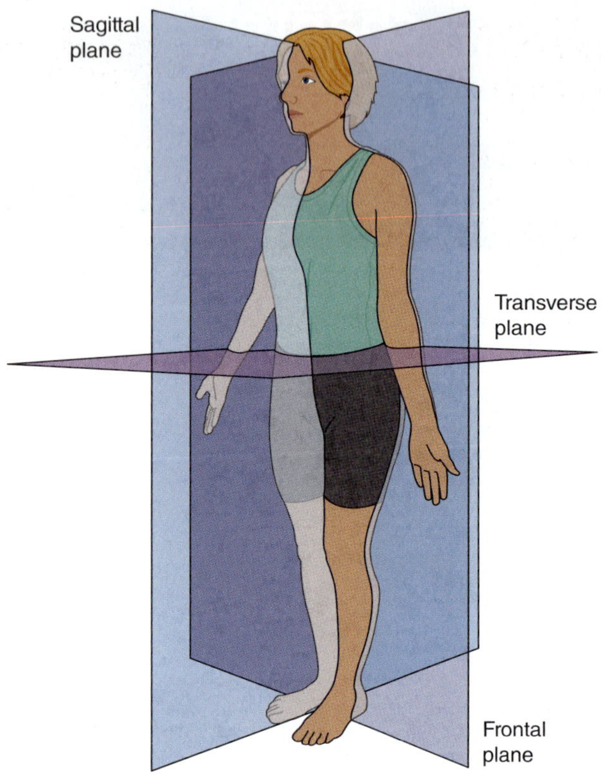

Figure 7.1 Anatomical planes. The anatomical position refers to a standing alignment with the arms at the sides and the palms of the hands facing forward. Note the planes that slice through the body. The frontal plane divides the body into front and back halves while the sagittal plane divides the body into left and right halves. The transverse plane divides the body into top and bottom halves.

Reprinted by permission from NSCA, "Biomechanics of Resistance Exercise," by E. Harman, in *Essentials of Strength Training and Conditioning*, 4th ed., edited by T. Baechle and R. Earle (Champaign, IL: Human Kinetics, 2016), 25.

terior, medial, lateral, proximal, distal, superior, inferior, dorsal, and *ventral.* These terms are all used in reference to the anatomical position. Other common terms include *superficial* and *deep.*

- ***Anterior*** refers to the front of the body. When you face an athlete, you are looking at the athlete's anterior aspect. If you were to read an injury report stating that an athlete was hit at the anterior aspect of the lower leg, you would know that the front of the leg was injured.
- ***Posterior*** refers to the back of the body. When you watch an athlete walk away from you, you are looking at the athlete's posterior aspect. If an athlete indicates that the back of the knee hurts, the AT would report that the posterior aspect of the knee is injured.
- ***Medial*** and ***lateral*** are defined in relation to the sagittal plane shown in figure 7.1. This imaginary line divides the body into left and right halves and is also called the *midline* of the body. If a body part faces the midline, it is medial, and if it is closer to the midline than another body part is, it is more medial than the other part. Thus, when you look at the side of an athlete's calf that faces the other leg, you are looking at the medial aspect. On the other hand, if a body part is located away from the midline, it is lateral, and if it is farther from the midline than another part is, it is more lateral than the other part. Thus, when you look at the outside of the calf, which faces out, you are looking at the lateral aspect. As another example, your left ear is lateral to your left eye.
- ***Proximal*** means toward an attachment or core of the body, such as where a limb attaches to the trunk of the body. Thus, the shoulder is proximal to the elbow, and the hip is proximal to the knee.
- ***Distal*** means away from an attachment or core of the body. The knee is distal to the hip. A fingertip joint is distal; one at the base is proximal.
- ***Superior*** refers to one point, or structure, being higher than another. For example, the knee is superior to the ankle. The term **cephalic** means toward the head and is synonymous with *superior.*
- ***Inferior*** refers to one point, or structure, being lower than another. For example, the pelvis is inferior to the ribs. The term **caudal** is synonymous with *inferior.*
- ***Dorsal*** and ***ventral*** are synonymous with *posterior* and *anterior,* respectively, but are often used in reference to the hand and foot. *Ventral* refers to the anterior aspect of a structure. *Dorsal* refers to the posterior aspect of a structure. An easy way to remember this is to think of the dorsal fin of a shark, which is on its back.
- ***Superficial*** means close to the body's surface; **deep** means away from the body's surface. So, your skin is superficial, while your organs are considered deep.

BODY TISSUES

Athletic-related injuries typically involve injuries to the skin, bones, cartilage, muscles, tendons, and ligaments. Before we can understand the specific injuries that occur to these tissues, we must first understand the basic function of these structures.

Skin

Skin is the outermost surface of the body. It provides the first line of defense against external forces such as insects, air, dirt, bacteria, and blows. The skin keeps bodily fluids in, picks up sensations, and secretes an oily substance. The skin is made of several layers (see figure 7.2). The most superficial layer is called the **epidermis**. The epidermis is thin and connects to the thicker **dermis** layer that is just below it. Below the dermis is the hypodermis. The hypodermis is not technically considered part of the skin, but it helps hold the skin to underlying bone and muscle tissue. The hypodermis is sometimes called the *subcutaneous layer*, which is the layer where fat is stored. The thickness of the fat layer is determined by the number of cells and the size of those cells (MedlinePlus 2017). A break in the skin is a wound.

During examination, the AT is concerned with several features of the skin. Temperature, edema (swelling), tissue mobility, hydration, and trophic changes (shiny skin, excessive hair, or hair loss). These components of the skin can help the AT understand potential problems with the skin and other regions of the body because the skin sometimes reflects physiological changes (Masaracchio and Frommer 2022).

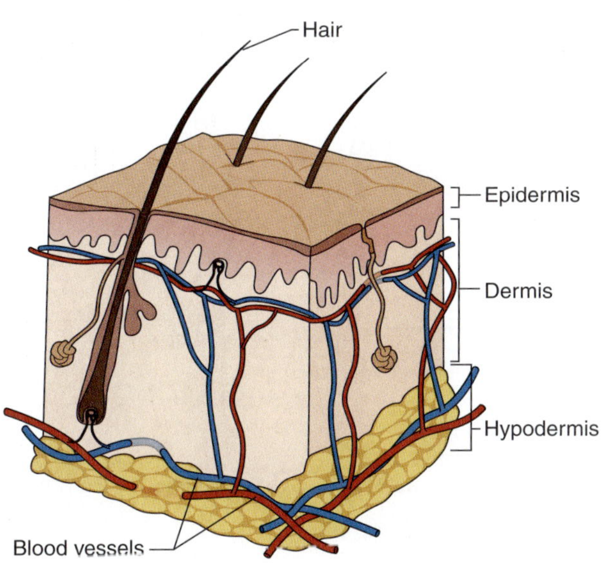

Figure 7.2 Cross-section of skin tissue.

Understanding Diversity

Vitiligo, a skin condition where pigmentation is absent, is more common in African Americans (Flanagan and Cuppett 2017). Also, skin cancer resulting from overexposure to the sun is more often found in fair-skinned people (Flanagan and Cuppett 2017).

Skin has the ability to expand; for example, it expands to accommodate an increase in muscle **girth** (the distance around a body part) from weightlifting or increased body weight. Stretch marks are lines on the skin where the dermis was stretched excessively until the elastic fibers ruptured. If the athlete loses girth, the skin will recover to a small extent.

Bones

Bones have three primary functions.

1. They protect vital organs and structures from trauma. Consider the brain. It is packaged in a hard shell (the skull) filled with fluid (cerebrospinal fluid), which helps to absorb shock and protect the brain. Similarly, the lungs and heart are surrounded by the rib cage, which supports and protects them.
2. Bones are the stiff structures that are acted on by muscles to create movement.
3. Bones are metabolically active; that is, they produce blood cells and store minerals such as calcium and phosphorus. They provide the skeleton or frame upon which the body is able to create movement.

Bones also protect the nerves and blood vessels that travel alongside them. Major vessels and nerves travel close to the bones of the body, allowing these vulnerable, fragile structures to have protection against trauma during normal activities.

The human body has approximately 206 bones and an astounding number of muscles. The skeleton is categorized into the **axial skeleton**, which includes the bones of the spine, thorax, and skull, and the **appendicular skeleton**, which includes the bones of the extremities. Although we discuss specific bones in more detail in later chapters, here we present a general discussion of bony anatomy, bone types, and joint classification. See figure 7.3 for a look at the bones of the body.

Bones come in several shapes and sizes, including long (e.g., femur), short (e.g., metacarpal), flat (e.g., scapula) and irregular (e.g., vertebra). Long bones possess an interesting feature. At the end of each long bone is an area where growth primarily takes place; this area is called an **epiphysis (growth plate)**. The area is somewhat spongy during adolescence and can be problematic for the adolescent athlete. The AT working in a high school setting should know that these growth plates are vulnerable to injury—a bone will often fracture at the growth plate. It is important to identify these injuries early because damage to an epiphyseal plate can cause long-term growth issues in that region.

Bony Prominences

When a portion of the bone is close to the surface of the skin, it is referred to as a *prominence*. This prominence act as a landmark so the AT knows where they are palpating. Typical bony prominences are the medial and lateral malleoli of the

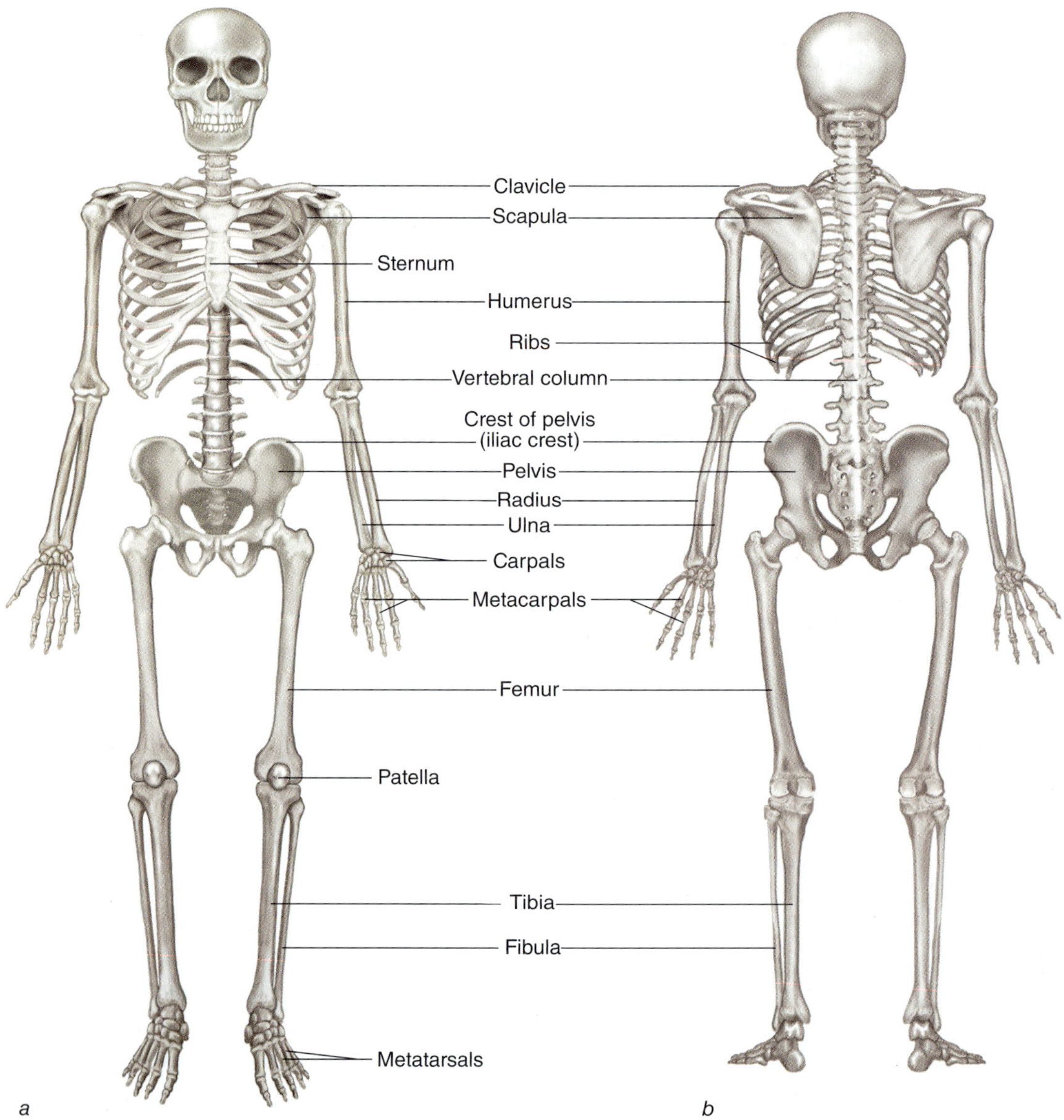

Figure 7.3 General bony anatomy: *(a)* anterior view and *(b)* posterior view.

ankle, patella, anterior superior iliac spine of the hip, olecranon process and medial epicondyle of the elbow, medial end of the clavicle, medial border of the scapula, seventh cervical vertebra, occiput of the back of the head, and the zygomatic arch of the face (see figure 7.4).

Cartilage

Cartilage covers the ends of long bones and can be found between bones. Although cartilage comes in various forms, it typically functions to join structures (for example, the ribs and sternum), absorb shock, and permit smooth bone movement.

Muscles, Tendons, and Ligaments

Muscle contractions allow the body to accelerate, decelerate, stop movement, and maintain normal postural alignment. Moreover, they produce heat. Ligaments and tendons are both composed of connective tissue. **Tendons** attach muscle to bone and transmit the force that a muscle exerts. **Ligaments** connect bones and help to form joints. Athletic trainers are responsible for knowing the tendons and the ligaments of the body as well.

Skeletal muscles are made of fibers. Each fiber can contract when a nerve impulse tells it to move.

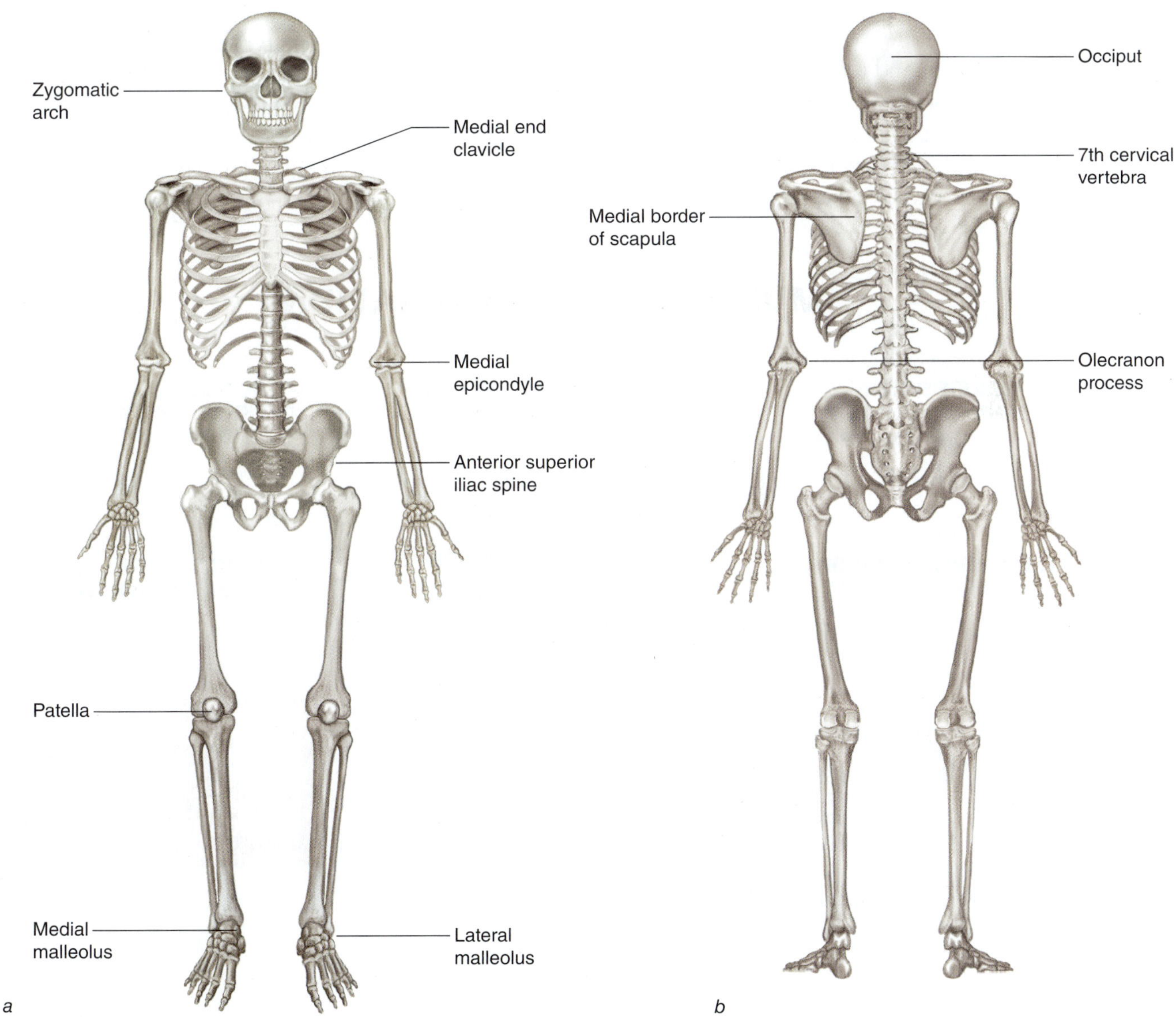

Figure 7.4 The bony prominences on the *(a)* anterior and *(b)* posterior aspects of the body.

FYI

Connective Tissue

Connective tissue is made of spindle-shaped cells that support and bind other tissues together.

These fibers have to have the correct chemical balance to move properly. Skeletal muscles are attached to bones to create movement. A tendon is a strong fibrous cord that attaches the muscle to the bone. As a person ages, the skeletal muscle degenerates and is replaced by fibrous connective tissue, which limits range of motion. See figure 7.5 for steps to consider when an athlete suffers a suspected muscle injury.

Sphincter muscles reduce the size of an opening in the body. There are sphincter muscles in the eyes, stomach, bladder, and rectum.

Cardiac muscle is found in the walls of the heart. It is muscle that contracts on its own. Smooth muscle is found in hollow organs such as the stomach, intestines, and blood vessels.

CLASSIFICATION OF JOINTS

Joints have three classifications:

- Diarthrodial
- Amphiarthrodial
- Synarthrodial

Diarthrodial joints are also known as *synovial joints*. They have fantastic mobility and consist of a **joint capsule** (a sleevelike ligament that surrounds the entire joint), a **synovial membrane** (a slick lining on the inside of the capsule), **hyaline cartilage** (a thin layer of cushioning at the ends of the bones), and ligaments. Diarthrodial joints are divided into several types, including hinge and multiaxial joints. An example of a **hinge joint** is the elbow or knee, which moves back and forth like a hinge on a door. An example of a **multiaxial joint** is the hip or shoulder. These joints can be moved in multiple directions (along many axes). The

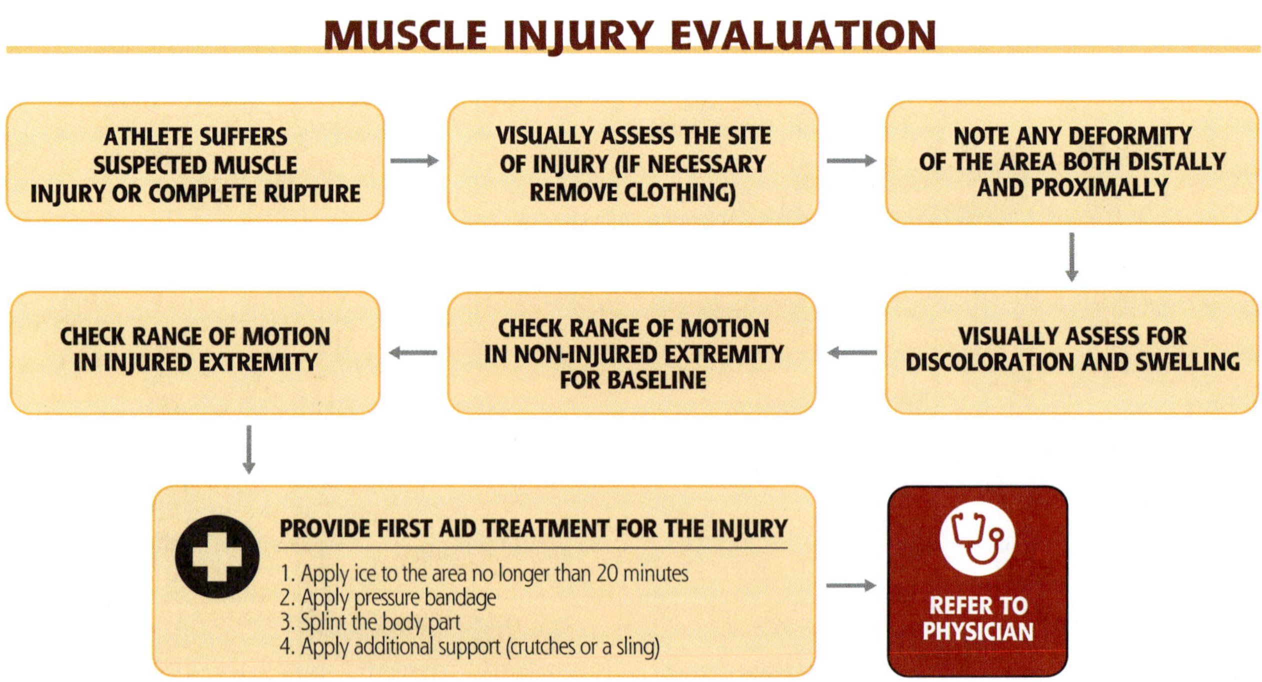

Figure 7.5 Muscle injury evaluation algorithm.

RED FLAGS

Refer an athlete who experiences any of the following symptoms to a physician:

- Sharp pain and sound of tearing
- Inability to move a body part
- A depression where a muscle should attach
- A bulge or deformity where it was smooth before injury

What Would You Do If . . .

You are in the athletic training room and the AT has stepped out to speak with a coach. You notice an athlete reading their medical report, and they ask you to explain what the report means when it states, "Limited forearm pronation and supination as well as swelling at the distal end of the radius."

shoulder and hip joints are also commonly referred to as a **ball-and-socket joint**; that is, the end of the long bone is rounded like a ball and is set into a cuplike socket of the other bone. Generally, these joints have a great deal of mobility compared with other joints.

An **amphiarthrodial joint** has cartilage attaching two bones together. They are also known as *cartilaginous joints*. An example of an amphiarthrodial joint is found where the ribs join the sternum. A **synarthrodial joint** is also called a **fibrous joint**. These joints are held together by tough connective tissue, and the joints are basically immovable. This type of joint joins the bones of the skull and the tibia and fibula in the lower leg.

MUSCLE MOVEMENT

Without muscles, the body would not be able to move. An understanding of general muscular anatomy is essential for assessment of an athletic injury and rehabilitation following an injury. Therefore, an AT must learn where muscles are located and what actions they perform. Figure 7.6 illustrates the muscles located just underneath the skin. We talk more about specific muscles in later chapters.

FYI

Axis

An axis is an imaginary line around which a segment such as an arm or leg rotates. For example, if you flex your hip (bring your knee toward your chest), you can say that the axis of motion is where the thigh (femur) joins the hip (pelvis).

Muscle tissue is divided into two categories, voluntary and involuntary. The person controls the movement of voluntary muscles, whereas the movement of involuntary muscles is automatic. Involuntary muscles include the heart, intestines, and blood vessels.

Skeletal muscles generally attach at two points and are classified by their **origin** (where they begin), **insertion** (where they end), action (what movement they do), and innervation (which nerve makes them work). The origin is the attachment to a joint that is usually at the proximal end of a bone, and the insertion is at the distal end of a joint. The bulk of a muscle (belly) lies proximal to the joint it moves. As part of the evaluation process, ATs need to understand the anatomy, including the origin, insertion, action, and innervation of the major muscles in the body. Please refer to the interactive resources to find an excellent resource for the major muscles of the body.

The muscle most responsible for a movement is called a *prime mover*. The muscle that relaxes to allow the prime mover to cause movement is called the *agonist*. If both muscles become part of the primary movement, they are commonly called *synergists*. Muscle that works against the movement is called **antagonist**. For example, in elbow flexion, the **agonist** is the biceps, synergists are the brachioradialis and brachialis, and the antagonist is the triceps. If the antagonist is tight or in spasm, it can affect the overall primary movement of a joint.

As muscles contract and produce movement, bony segments are moved in specific directions. Movement results from the angle at which the muscle pulls on the segment and the type of joint that joins the bones. Directional terms ATs and

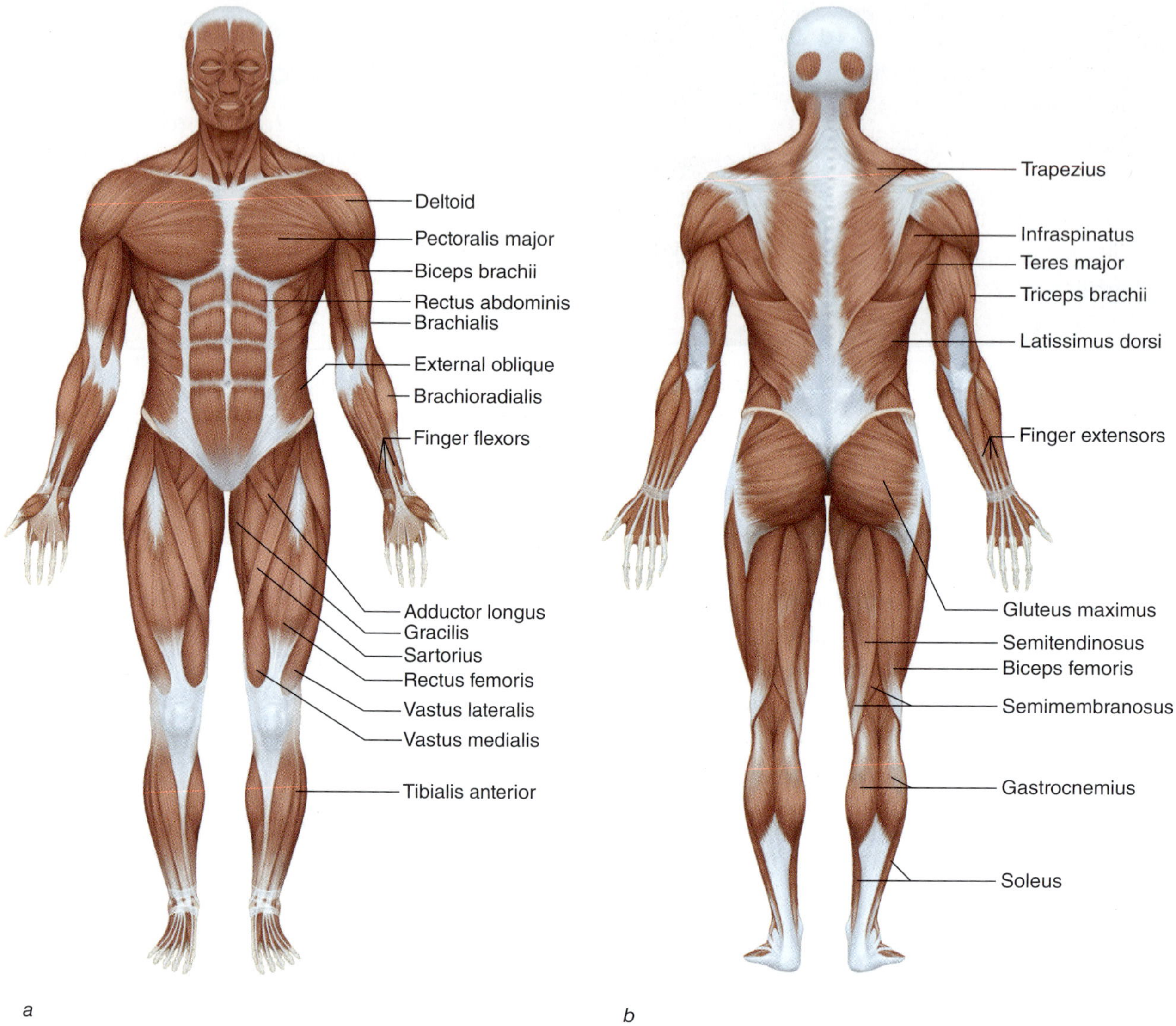

Figure 7.6 *(a)* Anterior and *(b)* posterior view of general superficial muscular anatomy.

other medical professionals use are *flexion* and *extension*, *abduction* and *adduction*, *pronation* and *supination*, *inversion* and *eversion*, *protraction* and *retraction*, *rotation*, *elevation*, *opposition*, and *circumduction* (figure 7.7 illustrates some of these movements). They are discussed in the following text.

- ***Flexion*** of a hinge joint is the bending of the joint. The anatomical position (elbows and knees straight) shows those joints in **extension**. However, hinge joints such as the knees, elbows, fingers, and toes are not the only ones capable of flexing and extending. The shoulders, neck, trunk, hip, and wrists also flex and extend.
- ***Abduction*** is movement of a body segment away from the midline (the line of the sagittal plane). For example, moving one leg outward from the anatomical position is abduction of the hip. Subsequently returning it toward the midline is termed **adduction**.
- ***Pronation*** and **supination** occur at the wrist and ankle. At the wrist, for example, if you turned your palm toward the sky as though you were going to hold a bowl of soup, you would be supinating your wrist. Conversely, if you turned your wrist so the palm faced the ground as if you were pouring out the soup, you would be pronating your wrist. In the anatomical position, the wrist is supinated.

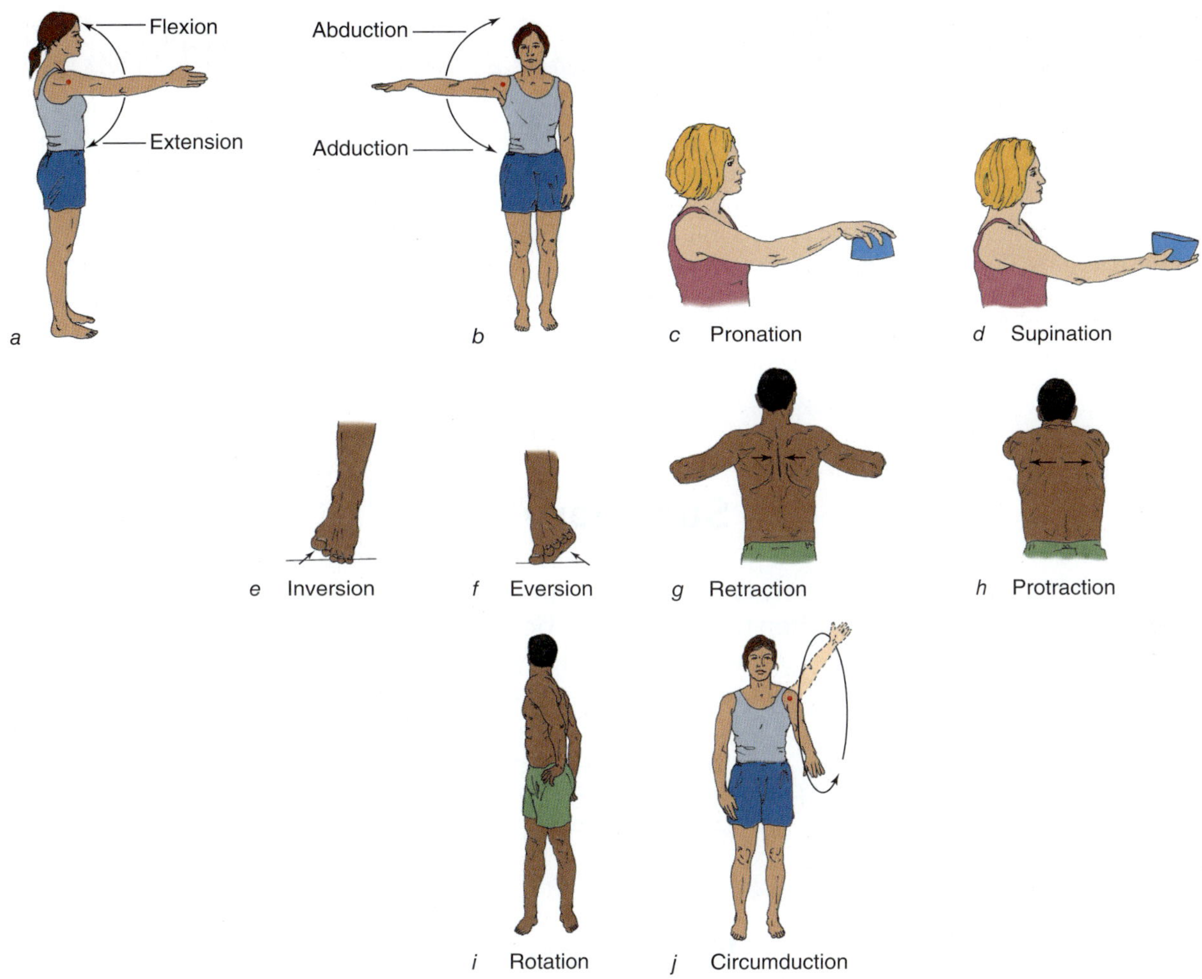

Figure 7.7 Illustrations of directional terms ATs use most often.

a, b, e, f, i, and j: Adapted by permission from J. Griffin, *Client-Centered Exercise Prescription*, 3rd ed. (Champaign, IL: Human Kinetics, 2015), 138.

- ***Inversion*** and **eversion** of the ankle can be seen in figure 7.7, *e* and *f*. Inversion occurs when the sole of the foot is turned inward, and eversion is when the sole of the foot is turned outward.
- ***Protraction*** occurs when a segment glides forward, as when the lower jaw pushes outward until the chin sticks out. **Retraction** is gliding a segment backward, as when the scapulas squeeze together.
- ***Rotation*** occurs when a bony segment (or series of segments) spins or turns on an axis. An example of rotation is turning your head to look over your shoulder. Rotation can also occur either internally (toward the midline of the body) or externally (away from the midline of the body). For example, if you rotate your humerus with the elbow bent so that your hands move away from your body, you are performing external rotation.
- ***Circumduction*** occurs when a ball-and-socket joint, such as the shoulder or hip, encompasses several directions with one movement. In so doing, the joint is moved in a circular fashion around its axis.
- ***Elevation*** occurs when a bony segment is moved in a superior direction. When you shrug your shoulders, you are elevating them. **Depression (anatomical)** occurs when a bony segment is moved in an inferior direction. When you lower your shoulders after shrugging, you are depressing them.
- ***Opposition*** occurs when you move your thumb across your hand to meet your smallest finger, or fifth digit.
- ***Reposition*** means simply returning your thumb and fifth digit to their starting positions.

The Real World

As an AT, I have had the opportunity to work with many physicians who come regularly to our school to evaluate injured athletes. I typically examine the athlete before the physician arrives to give the doctor information about how the athlete was injured and to brief the doctor on the problem. One afternoon, I told our team physician that an athlete was having pain at the fourth lumbar vertebra in his low back. After his examination, the team physician felt we should get an X-ray of the spine to make sure there wasn't a fracture. The physician thought, however, that the pain was at the third lumbar vertebra. I found it odd that we disagreed about which vertebra was injured. After receiving the X-rays, we found two interesting facts—the athlete did not have a fracture, but he did have a rare extra vertebra in his spine. Given the circumstances, we agreed that we were both right about which vertebra was involved!

Anonymous

Summary

Understanding basic human anatomy is essential for understanding athletic injuries. The AT will use precise medical terminology when talking about a body area, and the student assistant should be familiar with this terminology to understand exactly what the AT is discussing. The body is made of several tissue types: skin, cartilage, bone, ligaments, tendons, and muscle. Bones come in a variety of shapes and sizes. A joint is a point of contact between bones, and joint structure determines the type of movement possible. Muscles move the bones through the planes of the body. The ligaments, cartilage, and tendons help hold the joints together and produce smooth movement. Understanding the origin, insertion, and action of a muscle shows the potential musculoskeletal injuries.

Key Terms

Define the following terms found in this chapter:

abduction
adduction
agonist
amphiarthrodial joint
anatomical position
anatomy
antagonist
anterior
appendicular skeleton
axial skeleton
ball-and-socket joint
caudal
cephalic
circumduction
deep
depression (anatomical)
dermis
diarthrodial joint
distal
dorsal
elevation
epidermis
epiphysis (growth plate)
eversion
extension
fibrous joint
flexion
frontal plane
girth
hinge joint
hyaline cartilage
inferior
insertion
inversion
joint capsule
lateral
ligaments
medial
multiaxial joint
opposition
origin
posterior
pronation
protraction
proximal

reposition
retraction
rotation
sagittal plane
superficial
superior
supination
synarthrodial joint
synovial membrane
tendons
transverse plane
ventral

You are designing a rehabilitation program that emphasizes the major muscle groups in the shoulder region. You will need to determine which are the primary movements of the shoulder and which muscles are essential to moving in those directions. Establish a plan by identifying at least five actions of the shoulder with a primary mover as well as one exercise that could train that muscle group.

To access supplementary material for this chapter, including the Understanding Check worksheet, vocabulary quizzes, extension activities, and chapter-specific resources and forms, visit the web resource: http://ancillaries.humankinetics.com/FundamentalsOfAthleticTrainingAndSportsMedicine5E

chapter 8

Basics of Tissue Injuries

Objectives

After completing this chapter, the student will be able to do the following:

- Explain the types of soft-tissue injuries.
- Explain the processes of tissue repair and healing.
- Explain the various bone injuries.
- Explain the mechanisms of bone repair and healing.
- Understand the various medical imaging tests available for tissue injuries.

The body is made up of various tissues, each with unique characteristics and functions. In this chapter, we discuss the soft and bony tissues in both healthy and injured states. We will also discuss modern diagnostic tests to help appropriately identify injured structures and the degree to which they are damaged.

SOFT-TISSUE INJURIES

Soft-tissue injuries are often called *wounds*, *sprains*, *strains*, and *contusions*. These types of injuries are common in athletics. When a soft tissue is injured, it may bleed, become inflamed, or produce extra fluid. These injuries are often classified as acute because they occur suddenly from a high amount of force applied to the tissue over a short time. Soft-tissue injuries can have long-term complications, and when they do, they are called chronic soft-tissue injuries.

Wounds are injuries to the skin. Figure 8.1 describes the different types of soft-tissue injuries.

A **sprain** is an injury to a ligament—the strong pieces of tissue that hold adjoining bones together. A **strain** is an injury to a muscle or tendon. A tendon attaches a muscle to a bone and transmits the force that a muscle exerts. Both bleed internally, which may cause fluid to build up.

Sprains and strains are categorized in order of severity as first-, second-, or third-degree injuries. If the tissue is overstretched and there is no loss of

Incision

An incision is an open wound made by a cutting object such as a scalpel. It produces clean, smooth edges that can be of varying depths and lengths. It is rarely seen in athletics unless created through a surgical intervention or medical procedure.

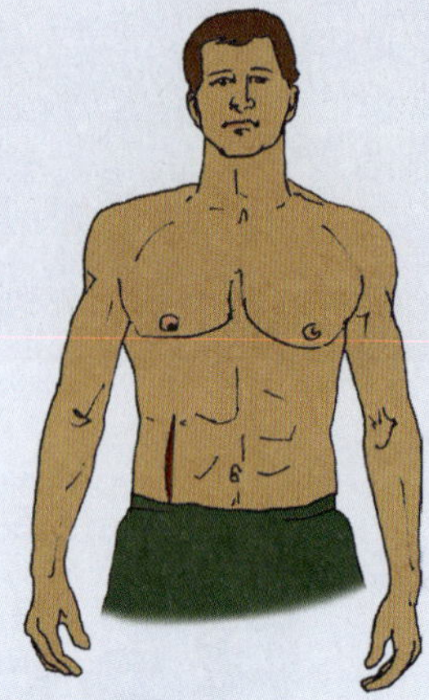

Abrasion

An abrasion results from scraping off a layer of skin. It may bleed, depending on its depth. A base runner in softball or baseball may acquire an abrasion when sliding into a base. These are often called "strawberries" or "turf burns" by athletes, but professionals in the field should use proper terminology. It is important to clean an abrasion thoroughly to prevent infection.

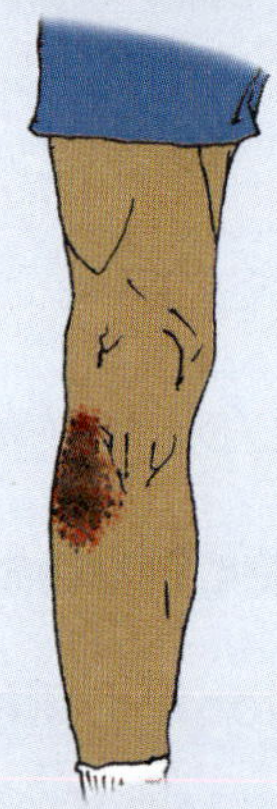

Contusion

A contusion is a closed wound and is commonly called a bruise. It bleeds under the skin, which can cause swelling, pain, and discoloration. An athlete receives a contusion from running into something, such as another person's elbow. Contusions can range in size from small to large and will change colors during the different stages of injury healing. It is common for them to go from black and blue to more yellowish as they heal. Contusions may have a hard knot in the middle of the healed area. This is a collection of blood that has calcified and is usually harmless.

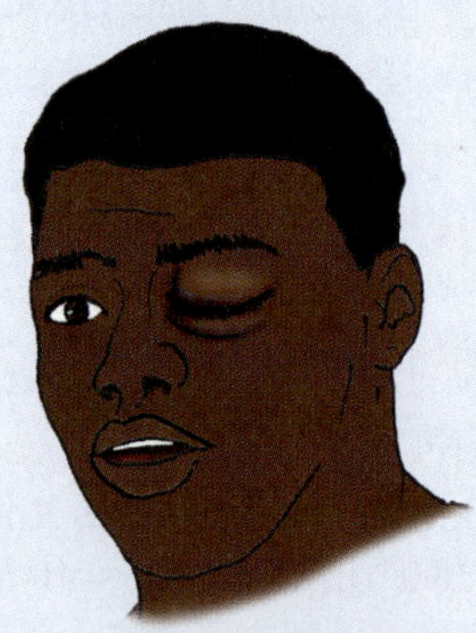

Laceration

A laceration is a jagged, irregular open wound created by a noncutting object such as a steel pole or a wall. These injuries will often bleed profusely and are difficult to close due to the uneven sides of the wounds. For example, a lacrosse player who runs into the goalpost may receive a laceration.

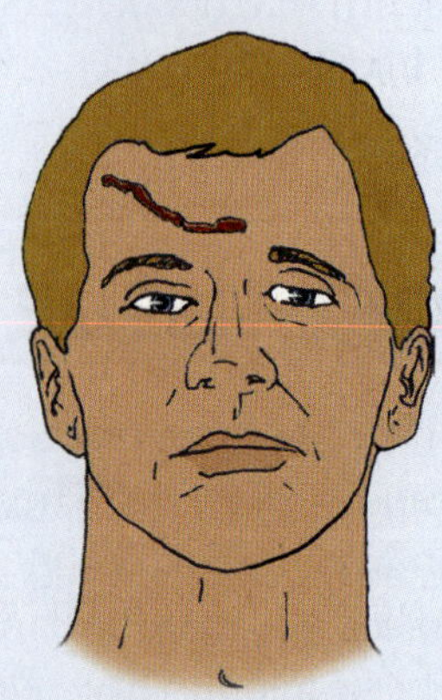

Figure 8.1 Soft-tissue injuries.

Avulsion

An avulsion is a partial tearing away of a body part. These injuries are often quite extensive and can be disturbing to see. An avulsion of a finger may occur if one catches a ring on the basketball hoop when dunking a basketball.

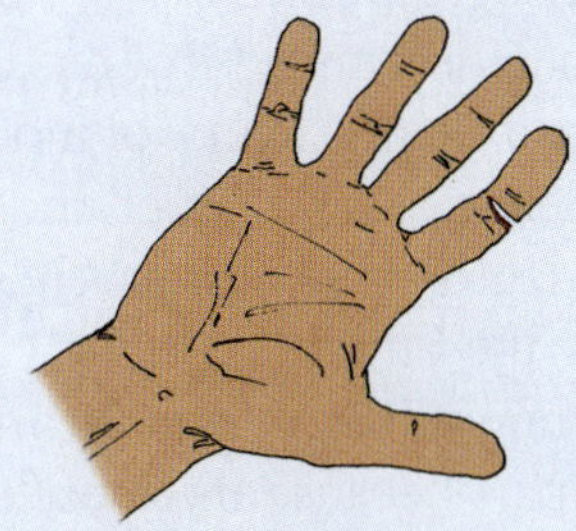

Amputation

An amputation is an open wound in which a body part is completely cut away from the body. These injuries can cause excessive bleeding and the athlete should be treated for shock immediately. Amputations are a medical emergency. Cutting off a finger with an ice skate is an example of an amputation.

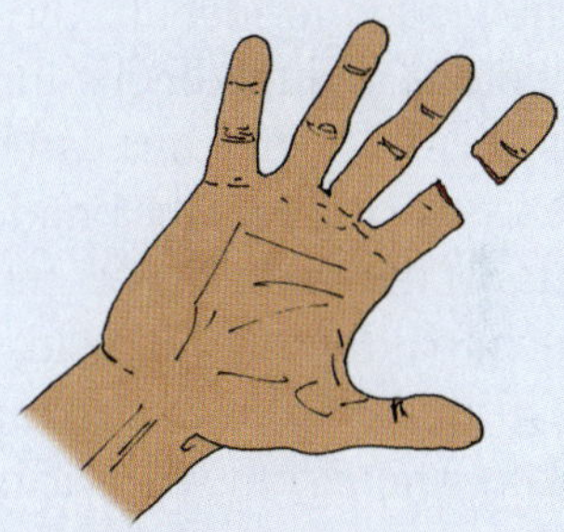

Puncture

A puncture wound occurs when a pointed object enters the body, such as if an athlete steps on a nail. Puncture wounds do not bleed much, so they are more likely to become infected than freely bleeding wounds. Using petroleum-based ointments on puncture wounds is contraindicated because it provides a plug or seal to trap the infection in the wound.

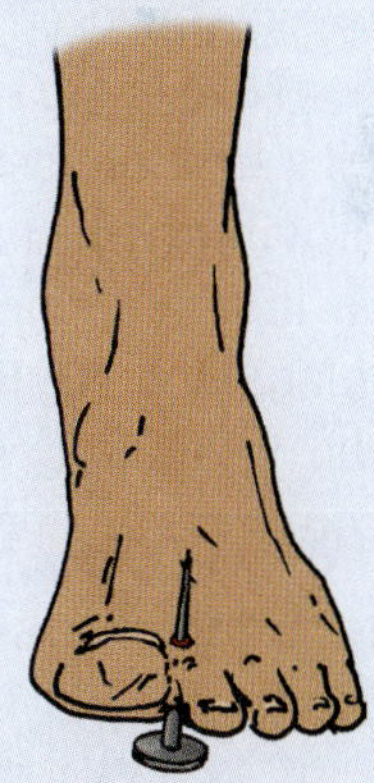

Contrecoup

A contrecoup injury occurs on the opposite side of the initial injury. This usually occurs in the brain when the head hits an unyielding object or surface. An impact to the back of the head, for example, forces the brain against the anterior part of the skull, resulting in a contrecoup injury.

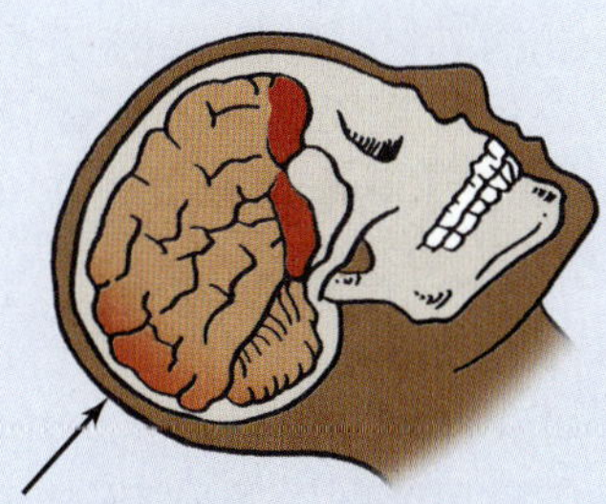

motion in the injured body part, the sprain or strain is first degree, or mild. If the tissue is partially torn and there is some loss of motion and swelling, it is a second-degree injury, or moderate. If the tissue is completely or nearly ruptured (pulled apart), it is a third-degree injury, or severe. With a third-degree injury, the athlete typically cannot function well. For strains, this means an inability to move the body part because the muscle cannot pull on the bony levers. For sprains, this means an inability to bear weight and move a joint because of pain and looseness of the joint. Sprains and strains are often painful, and it is important to rely on your anatomical knowledge to identify the difference between ligamentous and tendinous injuries.

Another soft tissue that can be injured is a nerve. Nerve tissue connects the brain and spinal cord with all parts of the body. Nerves transmit the sensations of touch, pain, heat, and cold, and they relay messages from the brain to signal a muscle to contract or relax. Therefore, when a nerve is injured, the athlete may experience a lack of sensation and even of movement. Nerves are often injured in two ways: **compression** or **traction**. A stretched nerve (traction) can send a message of extreme pain. A nerve being squeezed between two structures (compression) can cause similar symptoms. A nerve injury takes a long time to heal, and if the damage is severe, it will not heal.

One specific nerve injury is a neuroma. A neuroma is enlarged nerve tissue that develops most often in the foot. The enlargement is caused by constant compression and irritation of the nerve.

Chronic Soft-Tissue Injuries

Soft-tissue injuries can also be chronic. Chronic injuries are the result of lesser forces being applied to the body over a long time. For example, a distance runner who trains extensively every day for several months without getting enough rest may load the soft tissues enough to cause damage.

There are several types of chronic soft-tissue injuries, including synovitis, bursitis, myositis, and fasciitis.

- **Synovitis** is a chronic injury to the synovial lining of a joint. The cause can be an acute injury that is never treated properly or rested; more often, the injury is chronic and the result of repeated joint injury. When the synovium is chronically irritated, it will continue to have cellular responses to the injury. This provides a poor environment for healing in the area and results in ongoing problems at the injury site.
- **Bursitis** is the chronic inflammation of a bursa sac. Bursa sacs are located near joints where soft-tissue structures may rub near a bone. When a bursa becomes irritated, it tends to swell and can create a pocket of swelling at the joint. We have many bursas in our body, especially near our extremities. We have bursa sacs at the tips of our elbows and over 15 bursa sacs surrounding the knee region (see figure 8.2).
- **Myositis** is chronic inflammation of muscle tissue. The condition is characterized by soreness, tenderness, and mild swelling in the muscle. The injury is particularly sore when trying to contract the muscle. It can be created from overworking the muscle, from small microtears in the muscle, or from the buildup of lactic acid or other waste products. The fascia is a thick, tough connective tissue that surrounds the muscles and helps to loosely bind the skin to the underlying fat and muscle tissue. When fascia becomes strained due to overuse, it can become thickened, swollen, and painful. Chronic inflammation is called **fasciitis**.

FYI

The Suffix *-itis*

The suffix *-itis* denotes an inflammatory reaction. In chronic conditions, the inflammatory response does not resolve, preventing the body from moving on to the next stages of healing.

Corticosteroids

Corticosteroids are chemicals made in the body that help reduce inflammation. When an injury occurs, a synthetic corticosteroid may be used as a medication to help reduce inflammation, but it can also increase the healing time. These medications also have some side effects on the tissue, so it is up to the physician to use them as warranted.

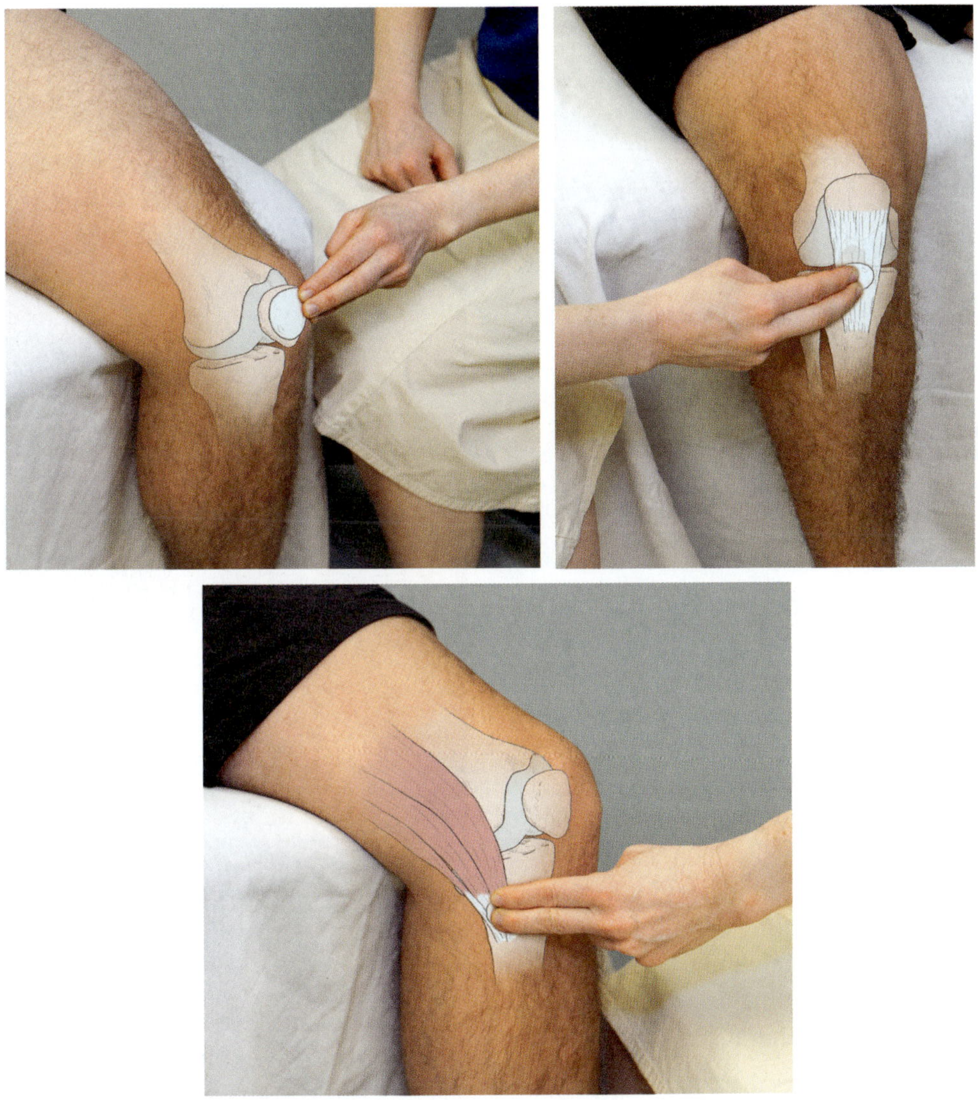

Figure 8.2 Bursas of the knee.

Reprinted by permission from M. Masaracchio and C. Frommer, *A Clinical Guide to Surface Palpation: The Art and Science of the Perfect Touch*, 2nd ed. (Champaign, IL: Human Kinetics, 2022), 377-378.

Stages of Soft-Tissue Healing

When soft tissue is injured, it progresses through three stages of healing: acute inflammatory, repair, and **remodeling**. We describe each stage in the following text and in table 8.1.

- ***Stage I: Acute inflammatory.*** When a body part is injured, cells in the area die, both from being ripped apart and from being cut off from their food and oxygen supply. In the acute inflammatory stage, an increased flow of blood to the injured area brings cells and chemicals to begin the healing process. **Phagocytes** are specialized cells that engulf and eat the dead cells. **Leukocytes** are infection-fighting white blood cells. **Platelets** carry blood-clotting materials. The acute stage lasts for about two days after the initial injury.
- ***Stage II: Repair.*** The injured area has now been filled with blood, cells, and chemicals to rebuild the area. The **fibroblasts** (fiber-building cells) begin building fibers across the area of injury. Fibroblasts form a scar. This process takes from six weeks to as long as three months, depending on the extent of the injury.
- ***Stage III: Remodeling.*** Remodeling takes up to a year or more. It is the body's way of building tissue strength in the tendons, ligaments, and muscles to withstand the stress applied to the body during activity.

Table 8.1 Tissue Healing

Inflammatory response phase	Pain, swelling, and redness Decreased collagen synthesis Increased number of inflammatory cells
Fibroblastic repair phase	Collagen fiber production Decreased collagen fiber organization Decreased number of inflammatory cells
Maturation–remodeling phase	Proper collagen fiber alignment Increased tissue strength

Reprinted by permission from NSCA, *Strength Training and Conditioning*, 4th ed., edited by G.G. Haff and N.T. Triplett (Champaign, IL: Human Kinetics, 2016), 610.

In general, the greater the injury to the tissue, the longer the healing time, although it depends on the degree of the injury, the location of the injury, the blood supply to the injury, and the age of the athlete. If blood supply to an area is poor, such as in the eyeball, the healing process will take longer. Other factors that significantly slow the healing process are poor nutrition, illnesses such as diabetes, medications such as corticosteroids, and infections. Some athletes believe that eating certain foods will hasten healing, but no research supports this.

One complication of healing is excessive scar tissue (keloid or adhesions) that results when more tissue is laid down than is necessary to repair the wound. Excessive scar tissue can delay healing, restrict the joint, and interfere with function, especially if it forms deep in joints. In some instances, scar tissue must be surgically removed so that proper movement can occur.

Tissue adhesives and adhesive strips (Steri-Strips) are used for less-serious wounds that do not require stitches. Tissue adhesive is best used when the wound edges are in close proximity and the wound is free from infection. The wound and the surrounding area must be clean and debrided. Once the area is clean and dry, the adhesive can be applied. The AT will gently squeeze the wound edges together and apply the adhesive, starting at one end and moving to the other. ATs should apply three or four layers of adhesive, allowing them to dry for at least one minute between applications. The adhesive is impenetrable to outside fluids and organisms, allowing the wound to heal (see figure 8.3).

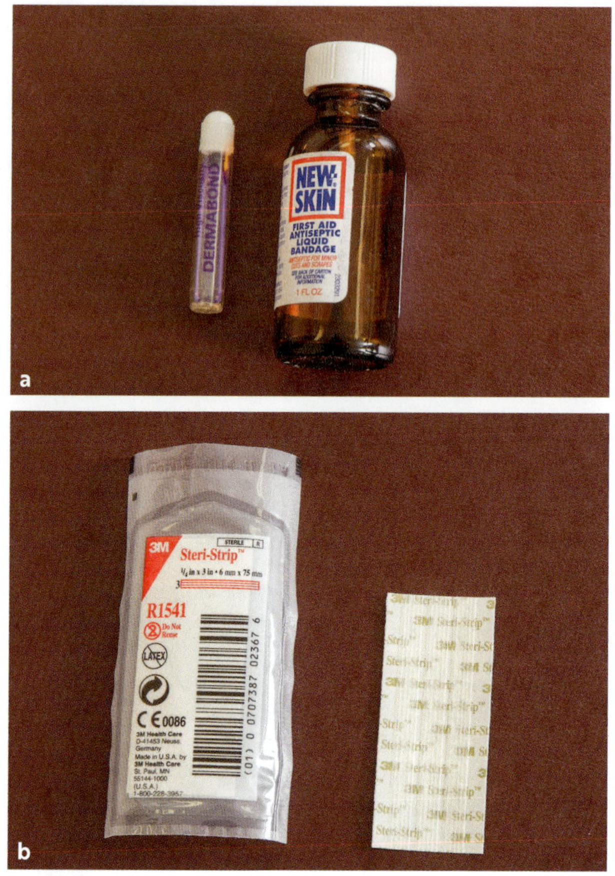

Figure 8.3 *(a)* Tissue adhesive and *(b)* adhesive strips.

Large wounds whose edges are far apart take longer to heal. Keeping the wounds closed with stitches, skin closures, or tissue adhesives will help the healing. A **suture** is made of synthetic materials, some of which are dissolvable. Dissolvable sutures are used internally and are not intended to be removed. Typically, sutures are applied one stitch at a time with a curved needle and tied with a knot off to the side. Most stitches will need to be removed after 7 to 10 days with special scissors. One of the blades of suture removal scissors is curved, which allows it to slide under the suture and easily clip the stitch. Once cut, the suture can be pulled out with forceps, usually on the side where the knot was placed. Athletic trainers should receive specific advanced training before giving stitches because there are many specialized techniques. Athletic trainers are now allowed in some states to administer sutures under the supervision of a physician (see figure 8.4).

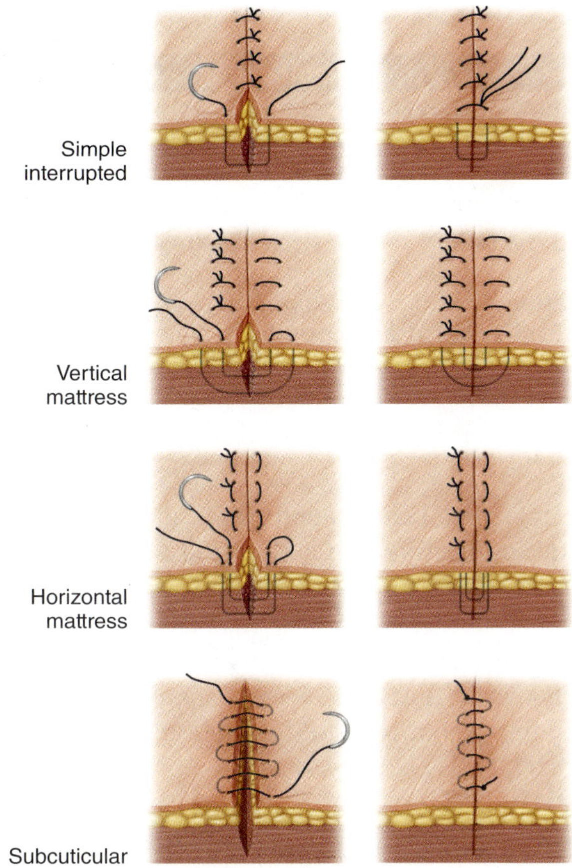

Figure 8.4 Types of sutures.

Reprinted by permission from M.A. Cleary and K.W. Flanagan, *Acute and Emergency Care in Athletic Training* (Champaign, IL: Human Kinetics, 2020), 151.

FYI

Skin Closures

A skin closure strip is a thin, tough piece of material that can bring together the edges of a wound and close a minor wound effectively. A skin closure may also be called a *butterfly bandage, butterfly stitches*, or Steri-Strips. They are tape-like materials that keep the wound edges together.

Stitches

Stitches (sutures) are used when a wound is deep or long and when fatty tissue, bone, or muscle can be seen. Stitches are done in a row, closing the edges of the wound. The length and depth of the wound will determine whether an internal layer of sutures is needed.

Tissue Adhesives

Tissue adhesives are glues used to hold the skin together for wounds that are not severe enough to require stitches.

Understanding Diversity

African Americans have a higher incidence of keloid scar formation (Mayo Clinic 2024) and are more likely to have excessive scar formation. The American Academy of Dermatology recommends diligent injury treatment to prevent scarring, including keeping the wound clean and moist with sterile petrolatum gauze, protecting the wound from the sun, and applying silicone sheets after the wound heals.

If activity is resumed too soon after an injury, healing time will be longer because the early activity can cause more cellular injury. Although athletes are always eager to get back to competition, the AT must use good judgment early in the healing process to ensure proper healing.

BONE INJURIES

ATs must be familiar with the types of bone injuries and their stages of healing. Bones go through specific healing stages just as soft tissues do. See table 8.2.

Dislocations and fractures (breaks) are common athletic injuries. Why do bones break? How much force must be applied before a bone will break? The answers to these questions vary depending on the athlete, the location where the force is applied, the bone type, the body position, and so forth.

Dislocation

When bones come together at a joint, they are said to **articulate**. A **dislocation** occurs when a significant force displaces bone so that the two bone ends in the same joint no longer line up. These are common at the shoulder, fingers, and foot and ankle but can occur anywhere there is a joint. A dislocation can also cause avulsion fractures (see figure 8.5), strains, sprains, disruption of blood flow, and disruption of nerve conduction. Dislocations present with deformity and pain and are not easily moved. Dislocations are cared for by the team physician and are not put back in place by the AT.

Table 8.2 Stages of Secondary Healing

	Reaction phase	Repair phase	Remodeling
Description	Inflammation occurs and granulation tissue formation begins.	Cartilage callus formation occurs and lamellar bone deposition takes place.	Original bone contour is regained through remodeling of the fracture site, based on Wolff's law.
Timing	It occurs immediately after fracture and requires approximately seven days to complete.	It occurs during days 7 to 14 after fracture, with callus formation peaking approximately 14 days after fracture.	It occurs during week three after fracture and may require up to five years to complete.

Reprinted by permission from L. Kahanov and E.K. Payne, *Athletic Training and Therapy: Foundations of Behavior and Practice* (Champaign, IL: Human Kinetics, 2022), 284.

Understanding Diversity

Native Alaskans are deeply rooted in holistic medicine, including spiritual aspects of healing. Integrating a holistic approach of mind, body, and spirit is essential to addressing the health care needs of this culture (Cartwright and Shingles 2011).

Fracture

Energy is required to cause a **fracture** or a broken bone. The point at which the bone breaks is called the **failure point**. Failure points vary with the athlete, age, and bone structure. For example, an athlete with a bone-deteriorating condition such as osteoporosis will have a lower failure point than an athlete with healthy bones. The epiphyseal plates (growth plates) of a young athlete are also common failure points in youth sports.

Fractures are named according to how failure of the bone occurs; for example, we say a bone has been *broken*, *cracked*, or *chipped*, or we may say it has a *hairline fracture*. These terms mean that the bone has been compromised and weakened. With any fracture, the athlete will be in a splint or cast for six to eight weeks, which is the time required for healing. However, some fractures can be splinted, and the athlete can resume participation immediately. A student assistant should be familiar with the various types of fractures (see figure 8.5).

Splinting

After a thorough assessment of the sprain, strain, dislocation, or fracture, the AT will make a decision about how to immobilize the area while the body part goes through the healing process (see figure 8.6). **Splinting** is one option for immobilizing the area and is used for the duration of the healing process. The advantages of a splint are that it is easily applied, allows for swelling, and can be removed to inspect the site of injury (Boyd et al. 2009). An athlete may be splinted while the injured area is swollen; once the swelling has gone down, casting may be the best option. A disadvantage is that it is easy for a patient to remove the splint (Boyd et al. 2009). Splinting should not be used if a site is unstable.

RED FLAGS

Call 911 for the following:

- A deformity or open fracture
- Decreased distal pulses with a dislocation
- Decreased sensation with a dislocation or fracture

Avulsion

An avulsion occurs when a ligament or tendon pulls so hard at its bony attachment that a portion of the bone is torn away. Avulsion fractures are common with sprains, strains, and dislocations.

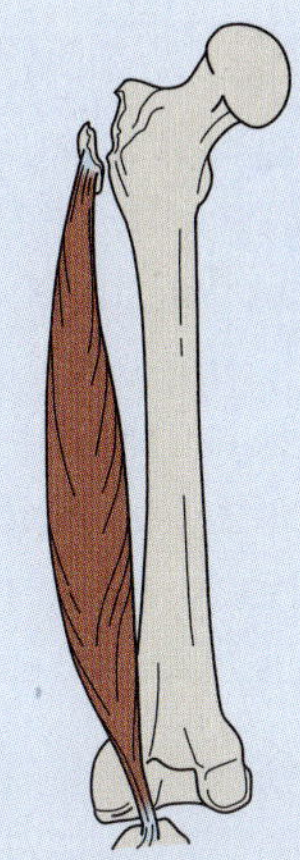

Stress

A stress fracture, also known as a fatigue or march fracture, occurs in a bone that has been subjected to a repetitive stress. That athlete will complain of a persistent sore spot over the bone. Stress fractures are microscopic and cannot be viewed on an X-ray.

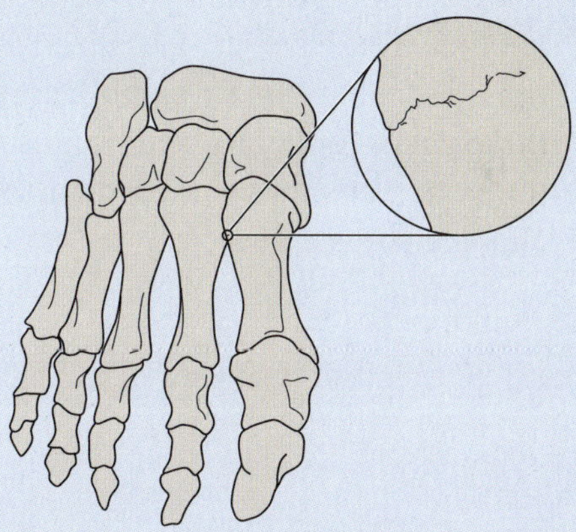

Spiral

A torsional force along the length of a bone causes a spiral fracture. Imagine that you are in-line skating and you are not very good. If your foot moves to the right while the rest of your body goes to the left, the stress may cause a spiral fracture. On an X-ray, the spiral fracture looks like the stripe on a candy cane.

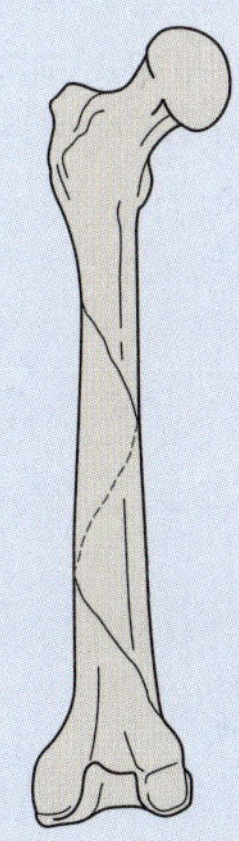

Longitudinal

A longitudinal fracture runs the length of a bone and is usually caused by an impact. A pole-vaulter who misses the mat and lands on their feet is likely to suffer a longitudinal fracture.

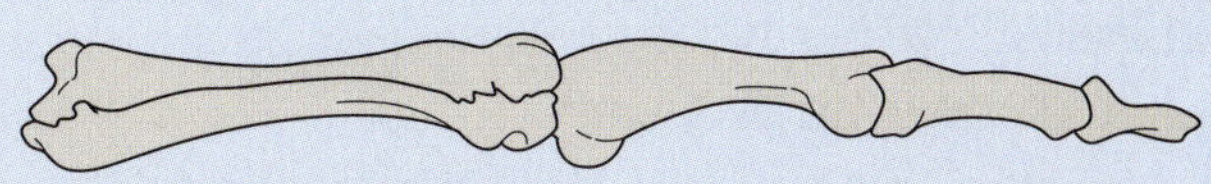

(continued)

Figure 8.5 Types of fractures.

Compression

A compression fracture occurs when opposing forces are applied to a bone from both ends at the same time. Compression fractures often occur in the spine. For example, a compression fracture may result when an athlete lands on their feet or buttocks from a height. The impact from the ground is one force, and the weight of the falling body is the other. The opposing forces cause a compression fracture in the vertebrae.

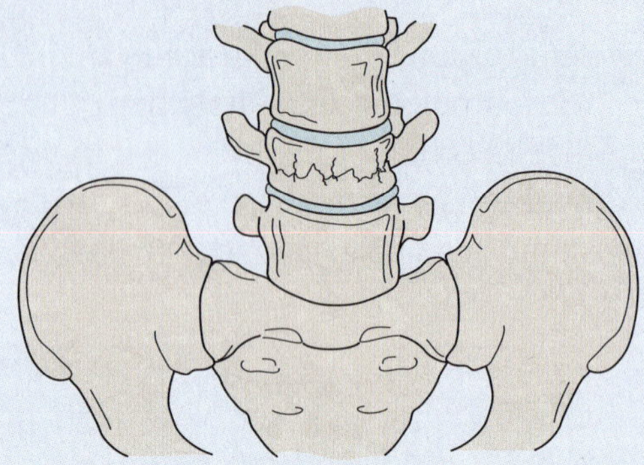

Oblique

Imagine a diagonal line across a bone from one side to another. You have just visualized an oblique fracture. An oblique fracture in a weight-bearing bone, such as a leg bone, takes longer to heal because the diagonal angle of the bone ends makes it easy for the bone to move out of alignment, even in a cast.

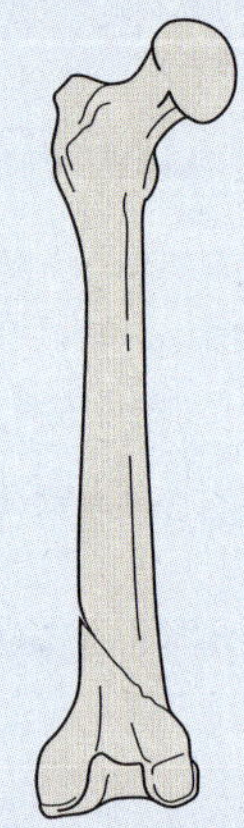

Transverse

A fracture that travels across and perpendicular to a bone is transverse. Transverse fractures occur from impacts perpendicular to the bone. A lacrosse player who brings their stick down across another player's forearms can cause a transverse fracture.

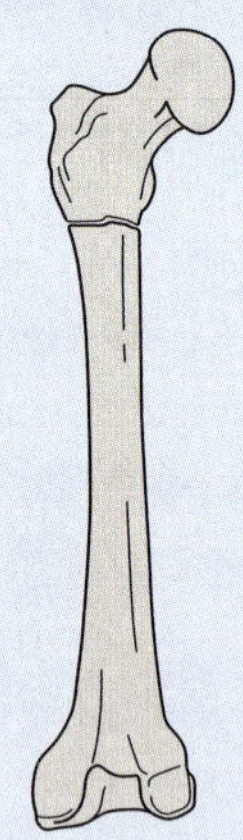

Comminuted

When a bone is crushed into smaller pieces, it is comminuted—think of a baseball catcher whose bare hand is hit by a bat.

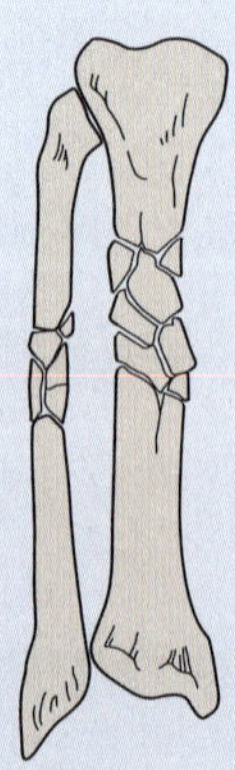

Greenstick

Adolescents' and children's bones are soft; that is, their bones still have some of the properties of cartilage. These bones tend to bend and fracture only partway through, and this is known as a greenstick fracture.

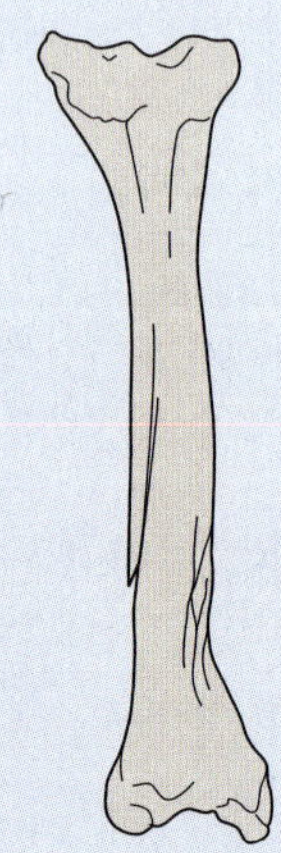

Figure 8.5 Types of fractures. *(continued)*

Depressed

A depressed fracture usually occurs from a direct blow to the skull, which indents it. This indentation is called a depression.

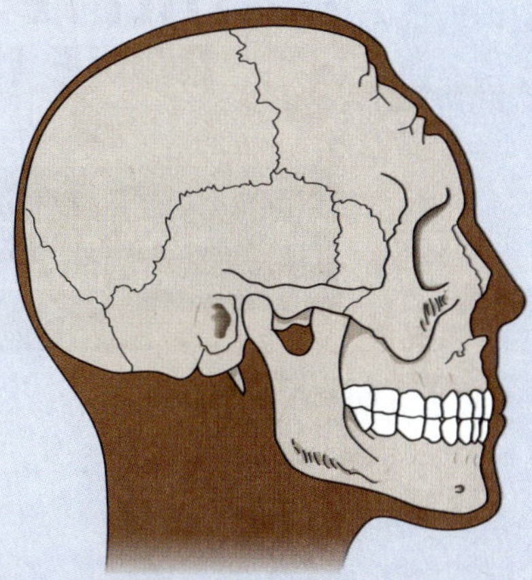

Blowout

A blowout fracture occurs when an eye is pushed hard backward and down into the eye socket. The small bones under the eye are crushed and embedded into the muscles of the eye. A blowout can occur when a hard object such as a baseball strikes the eye.

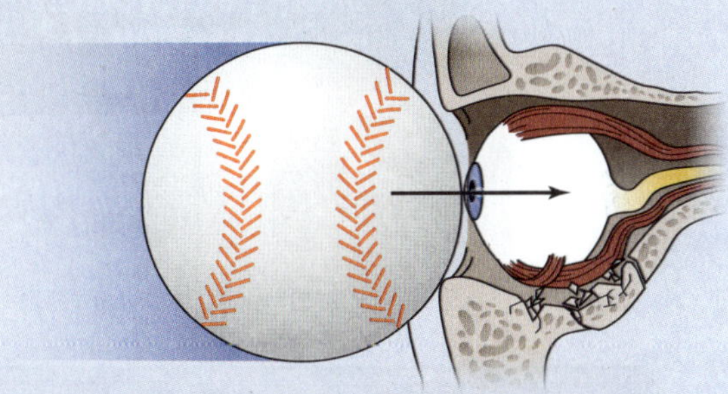

Pathologic

A disease process such as a bone tumor can weaken the bones so that a little stress will cause a fracture. Improper nutrition and eating disorders are the most common causes of pathologic fractures among teenage athletes. The bones weaken because minerals are taken from them to support vital functions.

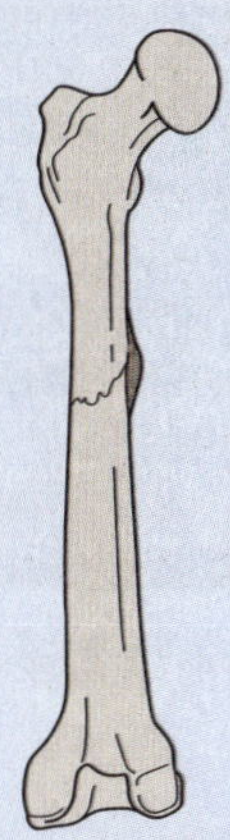

Epiphyseal

The area of a bone where bone growth occurs, the epiphysis, is susceptible to fracture because the bony tissue is stronger than the epiphysis. In adolescents and children, many epiphyseal fractures occur, especially in the long bones. Adults do not get epiphyseal fractures because their growth areas are closed; that is, they do not have active growth centers. An X-ray will not reveal a fracture of the epiphysis because epiphyses are clear on film.

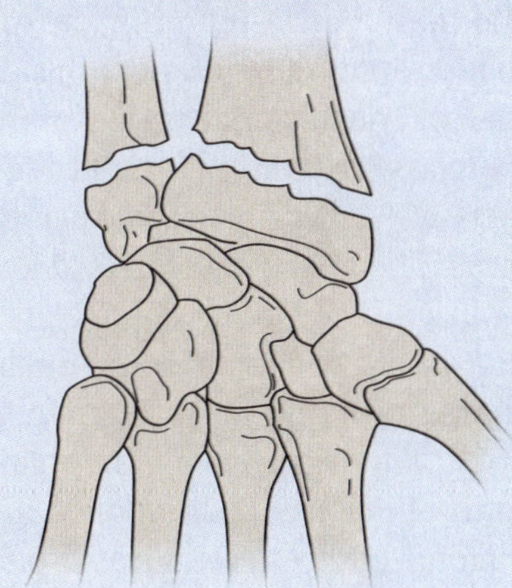

Figure 8.5 Types of fractures. *(continued)*

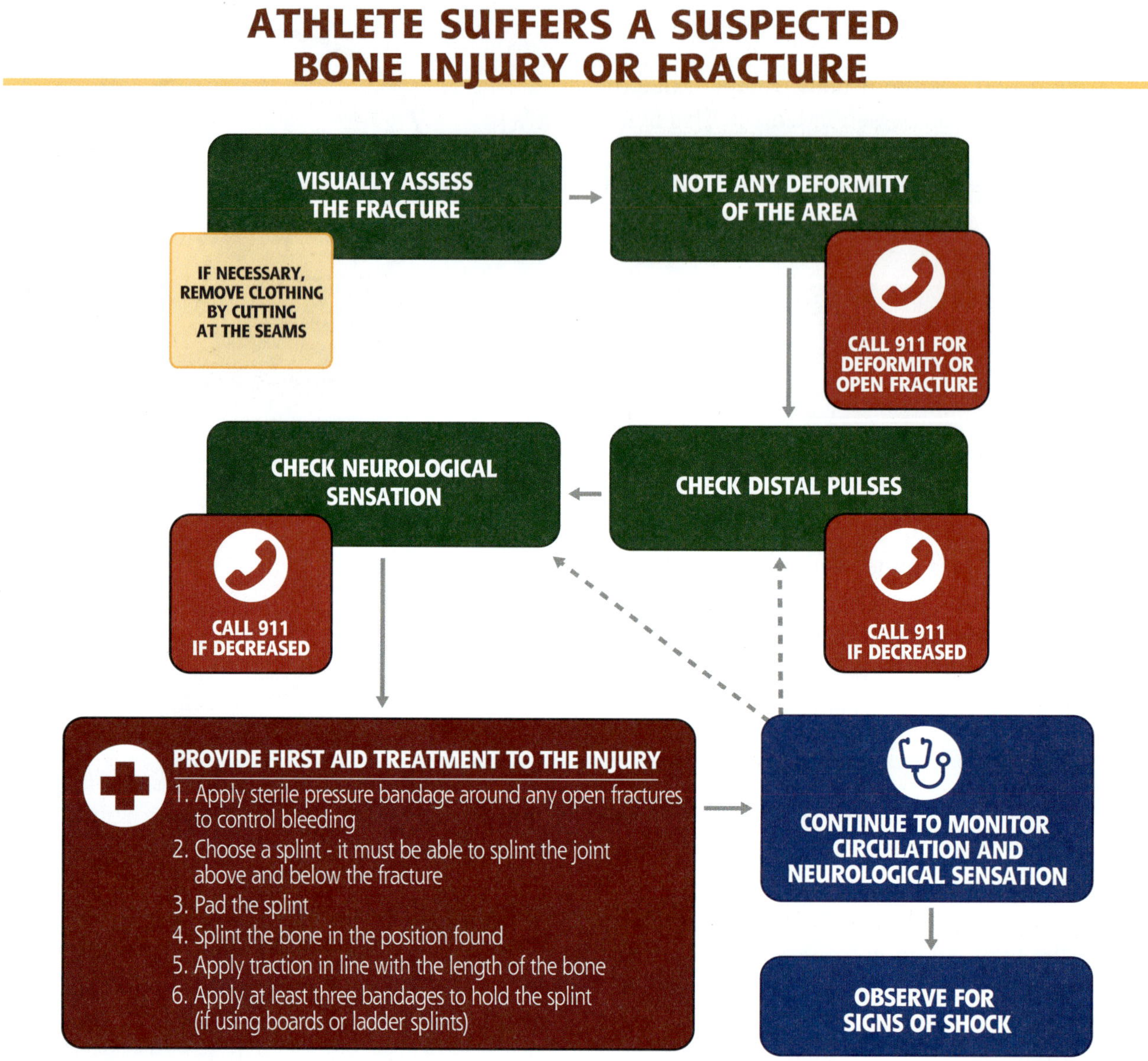

Figure 8.6 Bone fracture evaluation algorithm.

Splints can be custom made or purchased for a specific body part. Custom-made splints are best when there is swelling or a deformity resulting from the injury. The material used for the splint may be fiberglass, plaster, or a moldable plastic. New products are emerging each year as technology advances. The goal of a splint is to keep the region immobilized while being lightweight and durable.

The application of a splint includes placing stockinette over the area, padding the length of the body part, then applying the splinting material. Once the splint has been applied and molded to the contours of the area, an elastic bandage is used to hold it in place.

Casting

Casting is used when the body part involved is unstable, such as with a displaced fracture. Casting can be done once the physician has set a fracture. The advantage of casting is that it provides complete immobilization and protection. Complications include infections, skin abrasions, pain, and numbness (Prentice 2021; Cleary and Flanagan 2020).

The casting material is either plaster or fiberglass. Fiberglass comes in a variety of colors, and an athlete may select a cast color to show school pride. Although stylish, the goal is to keep the area immobilized and protected. The advantages

What Would You Do If . . .

An athlete who has had a contusion under his toenail notices that the nail is pulling away from the nail bed. He says the nail is getting stuck on his sock. He has heard that pulling the nail off will make the new nail grow faster. He hands you a pair of pliers and asks you to pull it off.

of fiberglass are that it is lighter and does not deteriorate in water.

The preparation for casting is similar to that for splinting a body part. First, the area is prepared with stockinette and padded, with more padding placed over bony prominences. Casting is applied by wrapping the material around the injured area and overlapping the previous layer by 50% with each wrap, similar to wrapping an elastic bandage (Prentice 2021; Cleary and Flanagan 2020).

Stages of Bone Fracture Healing

Like soft-tissue injuries, bone fractures go through the acute, repair, and remodeling stages of healing.

- ***Stage I: Acute.*** An injury to the bone causes the bone to break, and bleeding occurs in the area. Osteoclasts begin to eat the debris or resorb it into the body. Osteoblasts begin to add new layers to the outside of the bone tissue. This continues for about four days.
- ***Stage II: Repair.*** During the repair stage, osteoclasts and osteoblasts continue to regenerate the bone. A bony splint, or fibrous **callus**, forms (see figure 8.7). The fibrous callus, which extends both internally and externally to hold the bone ends together, is transformed into a sleeve of hard callus (i.e., bone). The process of transforming callus to bone begins at about week three and continues for three months. In most cases, after six weeks in a cast, the fracture is strong enough to allow participation with protection, and the athlete can return to competition. However, the athlete must remember that the healing process is far from complete.

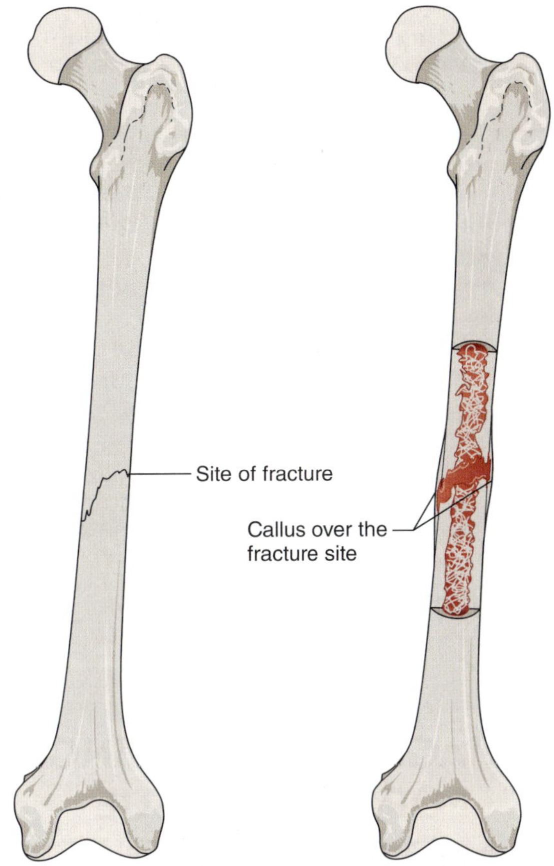

Figure 8.7 When the bone heals, a callus forms.

- ***Stage III: Remodeling.*** Stage III takes several years to complete. During this phase, the callus is reabsorbed and replaced with a fibrous cord of bone that is formed around the fracture site. Growth of this fibrous cord of bone can be stimulated through surgically implanted electrodes when the bones are not healing. Bones contain minerals that have an electrical charge, and adding electrical stimulation increases the layering of the bone. If a bone never heals, the fracture is referred to as a **nonunion** fracture. A nonunion fracture in a weight-bearing bone, such as a leg, means that the athlete will not walk. A common nonunion fracture of the wrist occurs in the scaphoid bone. Such fractures are painful and may lead to arthritis and the inability to move the wrist.

The Real World

While working in a physician's clinic, I had an opportunity to work with patients with diabetes. A common symptom exhibited by diabetics is that it takes longer for wounds to heal than it does for people without diabetes. One physician with whom I worked found that applying low amounts of electrical current to diabetics' wounds helped them heal faster. For example, one of his patients had an open wound (an ulcer) on her foot. He ran a controlled amount of current into the patient's foot and took a picture after each session to document the healing process. He found that the healing time was much faster when he used the electrical current than when he used more traditional forms of treatment.

John Robinson, ATC

DIAGNOSTIC TESTING FOR SOFT-TISSUE AND BONE INJURIES

A variety of diagnostic tests help the physician diagnose an injury and its extent. Although there are many specialized tests, this chapter will cover the basic procedures used in athletic training. These will be discussed in greater detail with imaging examples in chapter 30.

X-ray

An X-ray is a radiographic exam that will show the bones as well as other tissue. These are usually the first test ordered to rule out any fracture to the bones. It is a good test to see the alignment of the bones and detect any avulsions that may have occurred in the case of a sprain or strain.

Bone Scan

A bone scan involves injecting a radioactive isotope into a vein to illuminate the linings and more subtle parts of the bone. Bone scans are used to detect stress fractures that might not be visible on a plain film X-ray.

Computerized Tomography Scan (CT Scan)

A **computerized tomography (CT) scan** is used to look at internal structures such as the organs but will also look closely at the alignment of bony structures, especially when evaluating the spine. It is sensitive and can pick up changes to the bone surfaces, alignment of the discs, and other defects in the body. It is commonly used to detect soft-tissue injuries but can also be used for detecting tumors or bleeding in the body.

Magnetic Resonance Imaging (MRI)

An MRI is used to look at the ligaments in the body. It is often used to detect ACL tears in the knee and meniscal lesions but can be used for a range of diagnoses, including degeneration of joint surfaces, nerve injuries, and disc pathologies. It uses a magnet to create images, so this test is closely monitored before being performed to ensure the patient does not have any metal implants, pacemakers, or other medical devices that could be pulled out of the body by the magnet.

DEXA

The DEXA scan is used to determine the density of bones. It is commonly used in postmenopausal women who experience bone loss. However, many athletes can be affected by low bone density and are prescribed this test. Ongoing use of corticosteroids or inhalers, or conditions such as anorexia, amenorrhea, and nutritional deficiencies, can also cause low bone density. This test is a simple, quick way to get an accurate picture of whether the athlete has low bone density (osteoporosis and **osteopenia**).

Other advanced medical tests exist for diagnostic purposes, but these are the most common you will likely encounter as an athletic trainer. It is your role to stay abreast of new testing and diagnostic procedures as they emerge in clinical practice.

Summary

The body can get injured and, being a miraculous thing, repair itself. Indications of an injury to soft or bony tissue most commonly include pain, swelling, and bleeding. A soft-tissue injury may keep an athlete sidelined for longer than it takes a broken bone to heal. A fractured bone requires making new bone and fibers and reabsorbing the injured bone tissue. Healing time depends on the athlete's health at the time of injury and the care given during the healing process. Diagnostic tests are often used to help properly identify the location and extent of injury. Technological advances allow the AT and the physician to work together to properly identify injured structures so that appropriate treatment and rehabilitation programs can be implemented.

Key Terms

Define the following terms found in this chapter:

- articulate
- bone scan
- bursitis
- callus
- casting
- compression
- computerized tomography (CT) scan
- dislocation
- failure point
- fasciitis
- fibroblasts
- fracture
- leukocytes
- myositis
- nonunion
- osteopenia
- osteoporosis
- phagocytes
- platelets
- remodeling
- splinting
- sprain
- strain
- suture
- synovitis
- traction

As an AT in a high school setting, you encounter an athlete who has a tibial-fibular fracture that is open and displaced. You must stabilize the fracture and care for the patient until the ambulance arrives. What will you manage first? What type of splint is best when dealing with this type of injury?

To access supplementary material for this chapter, including the Understanding Check worksheet, vocabulary quizzes, extension activities, and chapter-specific resources and forms, visit the web resource: http://ancillaries.humankinetics.com/FundamentalsOfAthleticTrainingAndSportsMedicine5E

Unit III

Athletic-Related Injuries to the Head, Spine, and Axial Region

chapter 9

Head Injuries

Objectives

After completing this chapter, the student will be able to do the following:

- Describe the anatomy of the head.
- Understand that head injuries can be prevented.
- Understand common types of headaches.
- Understand the urgency involved with evaluating and caring for brain injuries.
- Describe the types of head injuries.
- Understand the long-term effects of head injuries.
- Describe and understand return-to-play criteria for head injuries.

When an athlete has a head injury, the AT must act quickly to reduce the chance of death and permanent injury. This chapter provides information to assist the student in understanding head injury and its prevention. We also address education and return-to-play criteria for athletes who have suffered head injuries.

ANATOMY OF THE HEAD

The skull is composed of 28 bones that protect the brain (see figure 9.1). A suture line is the area where two bones in the skull come together. The single moveable bone in the skull is the mandible, or lower jaw.

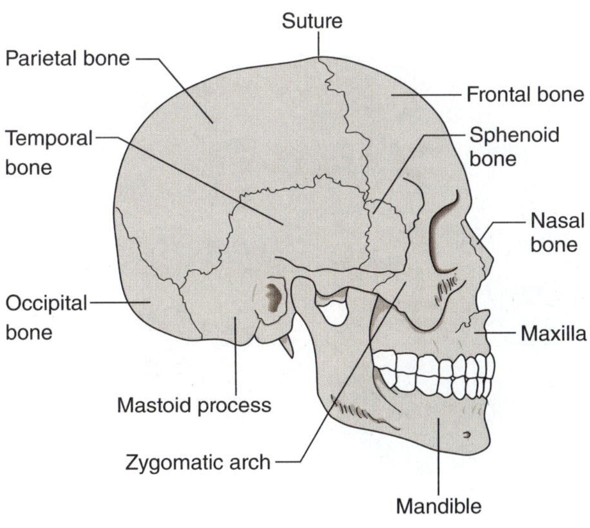

Figure 9.1 Bones of the skull.

The Brain

The brain is made of billions of cells. It weighs only about 3 pounds (1.4 kg), but it requires 20% of the body's total oxygen and 15% of the blood supply. Brain cells grow and develop until age 18. After that, brain cells can be destroyed but not reproduced. Depriving the brain of oxygen will cause unconsciousness and then death—the pupils of the eyes will dilate in 60 seconds (dilation is an indication of the inability to control the muscle of the iris of the eye). After 4 to 6 minutes without oxygen, biological brain death occurs, which means that large numbers of cells are dead.

The brain is divided into lobes, each named after the bony structure of the skull that covers it: occipital lobe, temporal lobe, parietal lobe, and frontal lobe (see figure 9.2). Each lobe is responsible for specific body functions. The brain attaches to the spinal cord at the brain stem via a crossover, so the right side of the brain controls the left side of the body and vice versa. Preserving brain function is of the utmost importance to injured athletes. Their quality of life—that is, their degree of recovery—depends on how the brain injury is evaluated and properly handled.

Cerebrospinal fluid bathes the brain and spinal cord in chemicals for proper functioning, helps maintain regular pressure around the brain and spinal cord, and protects the brain from injury. The fluid is clear amber in color. In instances of severe head injury, cerebrospinal fluid may drain from an opening in the skull, the nose, or an ear, and it should be allowed to do so. Differentiating cerebrospinal fluid from other fluids is a common field technique. Using the corner of a gauze pad, touch the fluid. If a straw-colored ring appears, it is a halo sign and indicative of cerebrospinal fluid drainage. Stopping the drainage will only increase the pressure in the skull and cause more brain damage.

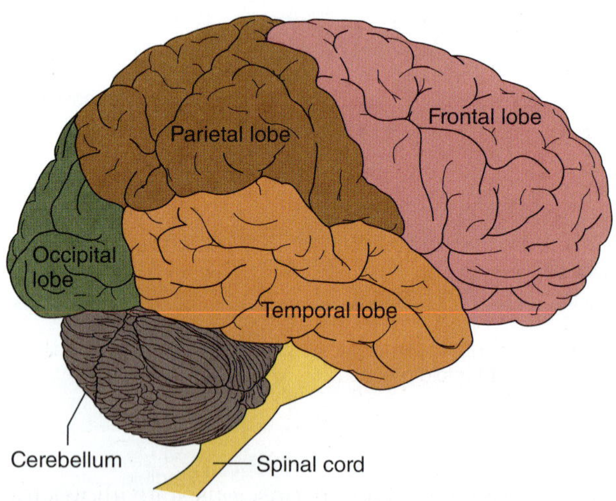

Figure 9.2 Brain areas.

Understanding Diversity

In many parts of Asia and in the Buddhist religion, the head is considered the most important part of the body (Fuller 2018). The soul of the person is said to live in the head, and touching the person's head may cause the soul to leave the body, resulting in illness. If the AT has to examine a patient's head, the AT should first explain the reason and obtain permission.

FYI

The functions of the brain are based on location.

- **Frontal lobe:** Voluntary muscle movement, emotion, and eye movement
- **Parietal lobe:** Sensation
- **Occipital lobe:** Vision
- **Temporal lobe:** Hearing, speech
- **Cerebellum:** Equilibrium, muscle actions, and some reflexes

The Scalp

The scalp is the skin that covers the skull, and it has many blood vessels, muscles, and hair. Skin protects against infections while hair protects the skin from the sun and keeps dirt and sweat away from the eyes. Blood vessels are so numerous in the scalp that even a small laceration will bleed profusely. Cartoonists draw a large lump when a character is hit in the head. This can also happen to athletes; a blow to the head may cause the many blood vessels to break open and bleed under the skin, causing a lump, or **hematoma**.

The scalp can decrease the force of an impact to the skull due to the additional padding it provides and the increased elasticity created by the tension of the connective tissue between the scalp and the skull. It is believed that without the scalp, the skull could be fractured with as little as 40 pounds (18 kg) of pressure. With the scalp, it may take 425 pounds (193 kg) of pressure before a fracture will occur. An athlete can sustain a serious head injury without a break in the scalp, however, so the AT should not be fooled by a lack of external bleeding. Bleeding inside the head is a dangerous condition that requires prompt medical attention.

PREVENTING HEAD INJURIES

Head injuries are prevented by helmets, mouth guards, rules, and common sense. A commonly forgotten piece of equipment in the battle to prevent head injuries is the mouth guard, which can prevent not only dental injuries but also concussions. If an athlete is not wearing a mouth guard, an impact to the chin can drive the mandible into the maxilla and cause the brain stem to twist slightly, resulting in loss of consciousness. A mouth guard provides spacing and shock absorption between the mandible and maxilla so that the force of the impact will not be transmitted to the brain stem. For a mouth guard to be effective, however, the athlete must be wearing one, and it must be in good condition. A mouth guard that has been chewed up or cut off will not prevent knockout. Special mouth guards for athletes with braces are available commercially or by prescription from an orthodontist or dentist.

Wearing a helmet and face mask is also important in preventing head injuries. In the early years of football, players did not wear helmets. Today, a properly fitted helmet helps protect a player's head from direct hits. The helmet prevents head injuries but not injuries of the face; thus, the face mask was introduced. Having such good equipment was an advantage but also created new concerns for sports medicine professionals.

With the head and face protected, athletes began to use the helmet as a weapon to punish opposing players. Using the head to make contact with another player is referred to as *spearing*. As spearing continued as a form of tackling, a progressive increase in the number of neck injuries resulting in permanent injury or death occurred—the helmet and face mask protected the head from direct impact but resulted in other forms of injury. Spearing has since been deemed a penalty, an offense severe enough to get a player ejected from the game. Many efforts have been launched to help educate athletes, coaches, and parents about the dangers of spearing. NATA position statements and CDC statements provide valuable information regarding head injury prevention. Links can be found in the online resources.

Athletes should be taught the proper skills so that injury can be prevented. Coaches and ATs must teach athletes that they cannot lead with the head when trying to stop an opponent; this is crucial in preventing head injuries. At the beginning of each season, a film outlining sport safety should be shown. The AT should document attendance at this safety film; recording the date and an outline of the discussion should provide legal protection if an athlete does sustain a serious head injury. The AT should also document days when safety skills are taught at practice and take attendance. They should explain the signs and symptoms of head injuries and proper care of helmets. Further, they should intervene to stop dangerous practice techniques or skills should they happen during practice sessions.

HEAD INJURY MECHANISMS

Injury to the brain can be caused by rotation of the head, but the most common mechanism is impact. The region most susceptible in the skull is the temporal region because the bone is thinnest there. **Contrecoup** injuries occur when the head is moving and receives a blow. On impact, the brain sloshes to the side opposite the blow, where it is stopped by the skull, and that is where the injury occurs. An athlete may complain of a headache opposite the impact, which is evidence of a contrecoup injury. Rotation of the head after an initial impact can cause the brain stem to stop functioning normally. The nerve receptors are overloaded with information to the brain, and brain overload causes unconsciousness. The unconscious state allows for a sorting of the impulses before the athlete returns

What Would You Do If . . .

You have been instructed to walk an athlete with a first-degree concussion into the locker room. Another athlete insists you can cure a concussion by cracking his neck. The athlete with the concussion says, "Yes, please make me better."

to consciousness. However, sometimes the athlete does not regain consciousness, and this is indicative of a critical condition.

TREATING HEAD INJURIES

Potentially life-threatening head injuries include lacerations, skull fractures, intracranial hematomas, concussions, and chronic traumatic encephalopathy. This section discusses the evaluation of each of these types of injuries.

Laceration

A laceration to the scalp will bleed profusely because of the large number of blood vessels in the scalp. Direct pressure applied to the wound will eventually stop the bleeding, but application of multiple gauze pads is usually necessary. Other blood-clotting materials are available and include clotting sprays and powders (QuickClot, HemCon Strip First Aid, WoundSeal), but direct pressure is the best first aid procedure for stopping bleeding. Lacerations of the scalp may require suturing or other wound care techniques depending on the size, depth, and severity of the laceration.

Skull Fracture

Skull fractures occur when there is significant force against the head. Types of skull fractures are depressed, linear, diastatic, and basilar. A depressed fracture pushes a portion of the skull inside toward the brain. There will be bleeding under the skin or even a laceration requiring bleeding control. A linear fracture goes across the skull. Although no bones are moved out of place, there are tears in the blood vessels on the inside of the skull. A diastatic fracture occurs along the suture lines of the skull and is seen in infants and small children. A basilar fracture involves the bones at the base of the skull. Some skull fractures, specifically the basilar skull fracture, will discolor the area behind the ear; this discoloration is called a **battle sign**. Any skull fracture is significant and requires the immediate attention of a physician.

Intracranial Hematoma

An **intracranial hematoma** is severe bleeding in the brain caused by a blow to the head, particularly over the temporal or parietal regions. The hematoma causes a significant increase in pressure on the brain, and rapid death can occur. There are two types of hematomas: subdural and epidural. The **subdural hematoma** is a leading cause of athletic-related head injury deaths. It results from bleeding between the inner layer of the dura mater (covering) and the brain. These are rapidly evolving conditions and warrant immediate care. The **epidural hematoma** is a swelling between the skull and the dura mater. The patient may be responsive initially but then deteriorates. This, too, is a medical emergency.

Sometimes an athlete is thought to have a concussion and is allowed to go home. If the athlete has a hematoma, they may die during the night. If an athlete is found in a coma, the chances of survival are only 40%. Survival depends on early examination by a physician and prompt surgical care. Physicians usually drill a hole in the skull to allow drainage of the blood and attempt to repair the bleeding vessel. If the athlete is not in a coma, the physician must give medication to put them into a coma. The comatose state keeps the athlete calm and allows the brain to heal without movement.

Symptoms of an intracranial hematoma include headaches, nausea, vomiting, loss of consciousness, paralysis of extremities on the opposite side of the injury, and battle sign. If an intracranial hematoma is suspected, EMS should be contacted for immediate transportation to the hospital. The onset of these symptoms may be gradual, so the athlete must be continually monitored. With the first indication of a condition that is worsening, the athlete must be taken immediately to the hospital. An athlete with a possible head injury should be monitored for at least 24 hours, and it is recommended they be awakened every couple of hours to check their status.

RED FLAGS

Call 911 for any of the following:

- Rise in blood pressure and drop in pulse rate
- Pupil on same side of head injury is enlarged
- Athlete is unconscious
- Athlete has difficulty speaking
- Difficulty using extremities
- Balance issues

The signs of a hematoma are a rise in blood pressure with a drop in pulse rate. The pupil on the same side as the head injury will be enlarged or dilated. The athlete may have difficulty speaking, difficulty using the extremities on the side opposite the hematoma, stiffening of posture, rapid eye movements, and lack of coordination. They may also be unconscious or in a coma. Depending on the severity of the hematoma, the athlete may fully recover or suffer permanent brain impairment or death.

Concussion

A **concussion** is the temporary impairment of brain function caused by impact to the head or by a rotation force. A rotation of the head during the impact will send a massive number of impulses to the brain all at once. The brain, not knowing what to do with all the impulses, is overwhelmed, and the athlete may be confused or dazed or may even lose consciousness. Other symptoms of a concussion include nausea, dizziness, headache, vomiting, difficulty speaking, ringing in the ears (**tinnitus**), loss of balance, unconsciousness, difficulty remembering things before or after the impact (**amnesia**), possible battle sign, and disorientation.

The potential problems related to concussions in sport prompted NATA to create a position statement on the management of sport-related concussions (Swartz et al. 2022). The position statement provides guidelines for ATs, including that ATs must be sensitive to both the causes of concussions and how concussions are presented when an athlete is injured. Also, ATs must recognize not only the common signs of a concussion (balance problems, loss of memory, and difficulty concentrating) but also the symptoms (headache, tinnitus, and nausea).

The NATA position statement also recommends that ATs collect baseline measures of mental function. This preinjury testing often involves using computers to assess an athlete's attention, reaction time, information-processing speed, concentration, and memory. Using computer programs allows an AT to identify even subtle deficiencies in brain function after an injury occurs. Such information can also help determine when an athlete can safely return to play following a concussion. Other tests commonly used to help determine if an athlete is ready to return to play are subjective self-report of symptoms and motor control tests for balance and coordination such as the following:

- Heel-to-toe tandem gait testing
- Balance Error Scoring System (BESS)
- Finger-to-nose coordination test
- Five object recall test
- Digit span test
- Serial sevens test
- Standardized Assessment of Concussion (SAC)

Each of these tests have their practical uses. Some are more appropriate for a sideline examination while others are best suited for an in-facility examination. Much research is emerging regarding the effectiveness of these tests, and athletic trainers should be familiar with the reliability, administration, and interpretation of the various concussion tests.

Predisposing Risk Factors for Concussion

During the preparticipation physical, the AT can assess the risk factors each athlete may have in conjunction with concussions. Athletes are at a higher risk of concussion if they have a history of concussions or migraines, are under age 24, are female, or play collision team sports (Swartz et al. 2022). Once the AT has background knowledge of those who are more susceptible, they should conduct a concussion assessment after a trauma, even if it is not associated with the head.

Baseline Testing

A noncomputerized cognitive test that ATs often use is the Standardized Assessment of Concussion (SAC;

Cleary and Flanagan 2020). The SAC requires an AT to obtain information from the athlete that relates to orientation (e.g., do they know what day of the week it is?), immediate memory (e.g., remembering five words), concentration (e.g., can they reverse the order of a string of numbers?), and delayed recall (e.g., can they remember the initial five words given during the immediate memory test?). The SAC test also has a neurological screening section whereby the AT examines loss of consciousness, memory loss, strength, sensation, and coordination. An athlete is given 1 point for a correct response and no points for an incorrect response. The SAC score has 30 possible points. The SAC form creates a record of an athlete's cognitive function and can be used as a pretest so the post-traumatic score can be compared. A score of 25 on the SAC is also used as one criterion for returning an athlete to play.

The SCAT-6 (https://bjsm.bmj.com/content/57/11/622) and Child SCAT-6 (https://bjsm.bmj.com/content/57/11/636) for children under 13 can be performed in approximately 10 minutes. They involve a combination of signs and symptoms; memory assessment; Glasgow Coma Scale score; cervical spine assessment; cognitive screening; concentration; decision making, and other features into a reliable, widely used test.

Along with noncomputerized cognitive testing, computerized assessment is done before participation in sport. The most commonly used program is the ImPACT. The test takes about 30 minutes to complete. The assessment has memory questions, problem-solving, response time, and attention span. The same test is administered if there is a concussion. The pre- and postconcussion tests are compared. The computerized test is one element used to determine the significance of the injury. The assessment may be administered several times to determine when the athlete has returned to the pretest level.

Every athlete must receive baseline testing, since one never knows when or how a concussion will occur. Typically, baseline tests take place at the preparticipation physical examination (see chapter 6).

Grading Concussions

Although recent literature indicates that concussions are no longer graded because it is a clinical diagnosis, many ATs and physicians still use a scale to identify the signs and symptomology of the injury. The concussion severity is usually graded in the same way as sprains and strains: mild, moderate, or severe. According to the guidelines established by the American Academy of Neurology (2020), the signs and symptoms of a mild, or first-degree, concussion include no loss of consciousness and the athlete's symptoms (e.g., dizziness) or abnormalities (e.g., loss of balance) being resolved in less than 15 minutes. A moderate, or second-degree, concussion will cause no loss of consciousness, but the athlete's symptoms and abnormalities last longer than 15 minutes. If the athlete is unconscious for any length of time, they have sustained a severe, or third-degree, concussion. The unconscious athlete may experience rapid eye movements that look like fluttering, and their pupils may be unequal in size. The pupil on the side of the head injury will be enlarged if the head injury is serious. The athlete may be in a coma, but they can hear what is being said, and it is important that someone talk to them while the AT is working. The AT will detect increased blood pressure, decreased pulse rate, and signs of shock. A severe concussion can lead to death or paralysis. The AT must be cautious when dealing with a concussion because other injuries may have occurred during the impact. They should also consider the possibility of a neck injury and keep the athlete's head still.

Other grading systems exist for concussions. The Cantu grading system, similar to that of the American Academy of Neurology, uses a grading system. Grade 1 means no loss of consciousness occurs, loss of memory lasts less than 30 minutes, and postconcussion signs and symptoms last less than 24 hours. A grade 2 concussion involves loss of consciousness for less than a minute or post-traumatic loss of memory between 30 minutes and 24 hours and postconcussion signs and symptoms lasting one to seven days. A grade 3 concussion will show loss of consciousness of over a minute, memory loss longer than 24 hours, or postconcussion signs and symptoms lasting longer than seven days (AAN 2020). Remember, new guidelines are moving away from grading concussions and gauging their affect by symptomology; however, this information is still important as you begin to understand the severity and injury characteristics of this complex condition.

HEAD INJURY CLASSIFICATION

- Severe head injury—GCS score of 8 or less
- Moderate head injury—GCS score of 9 to 12
- Mild head injury—GCS score of 13 to 15

Adapted from: American Academy of Orthopedic Surgeons (2011).

Any athlete with a suspected head injury should be removed from play. When the athlete is removed from the playing field, it is not uncommon for teammates to hit the player on the head and say, "Hang in there." Although they are trying to be supportive, they're actually contributing to the concussion. Athletes must be instructed ahead of time to keep their hands off so that only the AT touches the injured athlete. This is part of the preseason education all participants and parents are required to have.

Assessing the consciousness level should be done using the Glasgow Coma Scale, or GCS (see table 9.1). The scale is used to determine the severity of the brain injury. The scale assesses AVPU, which stands for **a**lert, **v**erbal, **p**ain, and **u**nresponsiveness. The scale is broken into three areas: motor response, verbal response, and eye opening. Each category has a grading scale, and the final score is determined by adding all the scales together. The final score is assessed against the chart to determine the athlete's prognosis. The higher the number on the grading scale, the greater the chance of returning to normal.

Regardless of whether the athlete loses consciousness, a concussion should make the AT wonder about other injuries that may have occurred. It is best to use a backboard for any athlete with a moderate or severe concussion. An old saying goes: "If there is a head injury, suspect a neck injury too." If an athlete has lost consciousness, they must

Table 9.1 Glasgow Coma Scale

Response	Grading scale	Score
Eye opening		
Spontaneous eye opening	4	
Eyes open to speech	3	
Eyes open to pain	2	
No eye opening	1	
Verbal		
Oriented	5	
Confused conversation, able to answer questions	4	
Inappropriate words	3	
Incomprehensible speech	2	
No response	1	
Motor		
Obeys commands for movement	6	
Purposeful movement to painful stimulus	5	
Withdraws in response to pain	4	
Flexion in response to pain (decorticate posturing)	3	
Extension in response to pain (decerebrate posturing)	2	
No response	1	

From the Centers for Disease Control and Prevention.

be referred to a physician the day of the injury or transported by EMS to the closest emergency room.

An athlete who has suffered a concussion will need to be monitored by a physician to determine when it is safe to reenter competition (see figure 9.3). The NATA position statement on concussion management states that an athlete should be monitored every 5 minutes after the concussion until the condition clears or the athlete is referred for advanced care. In general, an athlete will not be allowed back into competition after the first concussion until there are no remaining signs or symptoms. Specifi-

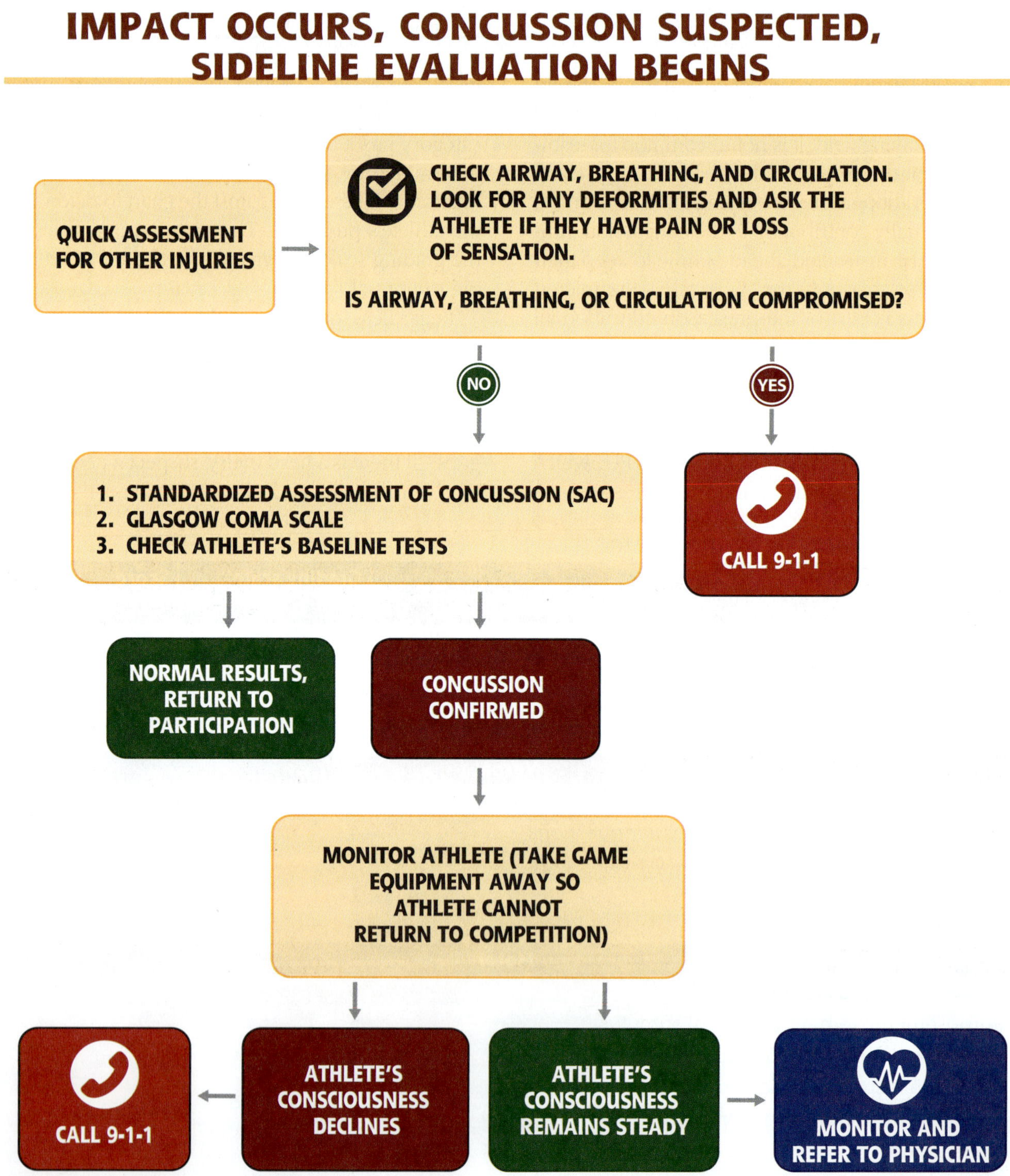

Figure 9.3 Sideline concussion evaluation and process.

cally, the athlete will have no headache, nausea, dizziness, or amnesia and will have regained full coordination and normal blood pressure. After a second concussion in a year, the athlete must have at least 1 month free of all signs and symptoms before returning. A third concussion in 1 year puts the athlete out of competition for a year, starting the day of the third concussion. An athlete who has suffered a concussion should be told about the signs and symptoms of concussions and the implications of repeated impacts. This condition has gotten much press and can result in second-impact syndrome. Athletes may have postconcussion syndrome, where their signs and symptoms persist months after the injury, so careful evaluation and restrictions should be in place for all who have suffered a concussion. An athlete who has suffered one concussion is four times more likely to suffer another.

The AT and team physician should make the decision about an athlete returning to participation. In general, athletes who have suffered a concussion should not return to participation until completing a progression of physical activity and follow-up assessments that begin only after they are free of all concussion symptoms (see table 9.2). Assessments should be compared with previous SAC tests (if performed). The progression of activity involves engaging in exercises such as stationary biking, push-ups, sit-ups, and low-level running. The AT must reassess the athlete to determine if the concussion symptoms reoccur during activity. If symptoms occur at this time, the athlete is not ready to progress to other activities, and more rest is required. If the athlete is symptom-free, they can then participate in sport-specific activities that do not pose a risk of further injury, such as noncontact activities. These activities should be done for several days, with the AT reassessing. At this point, the athlete can have **neurocognitive testing** to make sure they are back to normal. Once this is the case, the athlete can return to full sport activity, assuming a physician has cleared the athlete for play. The minimum guideline is for an athlete to be symptom-free for at least seven days before returning to contact activities.

Table 9.2 AT Concussion Assessment and Exertion Progression Log

Original assessment		
Return-to-play decisions	**Criteria for return to play**	
Return to play	☐	If athlete had no signs and symptoms of a concussion
Sit out for 15-30 min	☐	If signs and symptoms lasted fewer than 5 min and athlete had no more signs or symptoms and had completed exertional testing
Sit out for rest of game	☐	If athlete had all the signs of a concussion and had any episode of blacking out, can wait to refer but must see physician before return to play
Do not return to play	☐	If athlete was unconscious, call 911 for help

Exertional testing			
Activity	**Pass**	**Fail**	**Comments**
Run	☐	☐	
Jog	☐	☐	
Sprint	☐	☐	
3 broad jumps	☐	☐	
3 sets of 10 vertical jumps	☐	☐	
Figure 8	☐	☐	
Box drills	☐	☐	
Balance drills	☐	☐	
Sport-specific activity, treadmill, elliptical	☐	☐	

Based on McCrea (2001).

What Would You Do If . . .

The AT has instructed you to take the blood pressure of an athlete with a head injury every five minutes and let them know about any changes. The first blood pressure is 160/92. The athlete is responsive but talks about a headache. The next blood pressure is 126/84. The athlete then vomits.

Postconcussion Syndrome

Postconcussion syndrome is the persistence of symptoms after a concussion. Symptoms may include headache, ringing in the ears, dizziness, and confusion. The athlete should be seen by a physician for a follow-up evaluation. Returning to play too soon following a concussion increases the chance of developing this condition. Postconcussion syndrome usually does not last more than a week or two but can extend for months.

Return Protocols for Academics

The concussed athlete's brain may require rest or alternative learning experiences. The AT will need to engage teaching staff and administrators in postconcussion care. Athletes may have many difficulties when returning to the classroom, experiencing reductions in the ability to concentrate and understand concepts, attention span, memory, and reaction time (McGrath 2010). Athletes may also be light sensitive (photophobic), requiring them to wear sunglasses or minimize screen time. The physician may indicate that the athlete may be limited in their capacity to fully return to the classroom.

It has been found that the concussed athlete's brain needs rest to repair the damage (Centers for Disease Control and Prevention 2024). An athlete who returns to the learning environment taxes the injured brain, thus slowing the repair. It is important to follow a progression to allow the healing process to occur.

The Centers for Disease Control and Prevention (2024a) has a HEADSUP training program that is accessible to students, parents, teachers, nurses, and other health care professionals involved in the care of the concussed student. It uses a five-stage approach for returning the cognitively impaired athlete to school.

1. No school
2. Half day of school with accommodations
3. Full day of school with accommodations
4. Full day of school without accommodations
5. Full day of school and physical activity

The progression through each of these stages depends on how the athlete is improving and functioning. Athletes who have learning disabilities, migraines, or some mental health issues before the concussion may find that it takes longer to recover and thus may progress more slowly through the stages (Centers for Disease Control and Prevention 2023). The physician will determine how quickly the athlete can progress through the five stages. The CDC HEADSUP has guidelines for recovering after a concussion (see figure 9.4).

Second-Impact Syndrome

It is thought that damage from concussions and brain injury is cumulative. Therefore, if an athlete is allowed to return to participation before the symptoms of the first concussion have completely subsided and they receive another blow to the head, the athlete can quickly lose brain function and go into a coma. **Second-impact syndrome** can occur when an athlete receives more than one concussion or blow to the head in a relatively short time. Such trauma may disturb the blood supply to the brain and present signs of a minor concussion, followed quickly by a semicomatose state. Athletes who have suffered brain injuries must not be allowed to return to participation until they are symptom-free and have obtained written permission from a doctor. Second-impact syndrome can be deadly, and caution should be exercised with each concussion to ensure the athlete is not returned too soon.

Chronic Traumatic Encephalopathy

Repeated trauma to the head can lead to degeneration of the brain, which is called **chronic traumatic encephalopathy (CTE)**. CTE is a condition that most often occurs in athletes who participate in contact or collision sports, such as lacrosse,

Talk to your health care provider if symptoms don't go away within two to three weeks or get worse after you return to your regular activities. Taking these steps may help speed your recovery:

- Avoid activities that can put you at risk for another injury to your head and brain.
- Stay connected to friends and loved ones and talk with them about how you are feeling. Support from family and friends can help with your recovery.
- Ask your health care provider about medications that are safe to take during recovery to help with symptoms.
- Limit screen time and loud music before bed, sleep in a dark room, and keep to a fixed bedtime and wake-up schedule.

The First Few Days

- Rest is good the first few days after a mild TBI or concussion because this is when symptoms are more severe.
- You may need to take a short time off from work or school, although usually no more than one or two days.
- Find relaxing activities like reading and taking a short walk with a friend.

Start Light Physical Activity

- After one or two days of rest, ease back into your regular activities even if you still have some mild symptoms. If your symptoms get worse, you should cut back on that activity.
- Ask your health care provider for written instructions about when you can safely return to work, school, or other activities, such as driving a car.

When Your Symptoms Are Nearly Gone

- When your symptoms are mild and nearly gone, you can return to most of your regular activities.
- Recovery from a mild TBI or concussion means you can do your regular activities without experiencing symptoms.
- Recovery may be slower among older adults, young children, and people who have had a concussion or other TBI in the past.

Figure 9.4 Steps to take to feel better after a mild traumatic brain injury or concussion.
Adapted from CDC. Available: www.cdc.gov/traumatic-brain-injury/response/.

mixed martial arts, boxing, football, rodeo, rugby, and ice hockey.

CTE is sometimes suspected while the athlete is alive when known normal behaviors change. However, it is not formally diagnosed until an autopsy is performed postmortem. Suicidal thoughts, balance issues, speech difficulty, aggressiveness, memory loss, dementia, and depression are signs and symptoms that may occur (Mayo Clinic 2017). It is imperative that the AT follow strict guidelines to prevent CTE when returning athletes to competition.

Headaches

In addition to brain trauma or concussions, athletes often suffer from headaches. Headaches can range from minor to debilitating and should be evaluated carefully by the AT. Headaches are often defined by their symptoms or location. Common types of headaches are sinus, tension, cluster, and migraine. The location of zones of pain are featured in figure 9.5.

- Sinus headaches often occur in a butterfly shape around the top of the eyes, down the nose, and under the eyes. This is the location of some of the major sinuses in the face. When irritants, allergies, or infections strike, the buildup of pressure in the sinuses will cause headaches in these regions.
- The tension headache is usually a result of stress. In addition to the headache, which goes around the head from the temples to the back of the head to the forehead, athletes may experience fatigue in their shoulder muscles as a related

The Real World

One afternoon, at 2:35 p.m., our high school dismissed students. My student trainers and I went to work in the training room. It was a fairly busy Monday. My students were preparing athletes for football, soccer, and volleyball, while I was checking a few of the injured athletes. At approximately 2:50 p.m., the athletic director announced over the PA system that I was needed in the parking lot—there had been an accident. By the sound of his voice, I could tell we had a big problem.

I ran out of my training room at full speed. When I hit the doors just outside the athletic office, the athletic director met me, and we ran on together. The accident had occurred at the far end of the parking lot. I surveyed the scene as we approached. Several students were standing around, looking at something on the ground. On the right, next to a car, a distraught female student was talking with one of the teachers. I started asking questions as I made my way through the gathering of students. Someone said that a girl had fallen off the hood of the car while it was moving.

The next thing I saw took my breath away. Lying on the ground was a student who had been in my office earlier in the day to arrange for a tutor. She was pale, sweaty, and bleeding from her ears, nose, and mouth. I saw a patch of bloody hair on the pavement about 2 feet (.5 m) from us and 8 to 10 feet (2.5-3.0 m) from the car. All I had to do was look at the athletic director, and he got on his radio to his secretary to call an ambulance.

Because I suspected both head and neck injuries, I stabilized the student's head and neck. I immediately used the jaw thrust maneuver to open the airway with minimal head movement. When her airway opened, she made a gurgling noise, and a bloody froth bubbled from the corners of her mouth. As I continued to stabilize her head and neck, I asked a health teacher, who was at my side, to check the girl's pulse. Her pulse was faint, and her breathing was irregular. She was nonresponsive, and her face was covered with blood. An assistant principal was there with gloves and paper towels, and I had him gently clean her face so I could determine the major source of bleeding. I told the athletic director to keep bystanders back, and I sent the head custodian to the school entrance to direct the ambulance to us. While I was stabilizing the girl's head and neck and maintaining her airway, I was also trying to get a response from her. As we waited for the ambulance, I realized that I did not have gloves on, but it was too late to worry about that. We seemed to wait forever. The girl started to choke, and we had to logroll her just as the ambulance made its way into the parking lot.

I continued to maintain the girl's head and neck while the paramedic checked her vitals. While he was doing this, she became combative. The paramedic got a collar on her, and I fought to maintain her head and neck stability while we put her on the backboard and then the stretcher. The paramedic asked me to ride in the ambulance to continue to maintain her head and neck. I held her head between my forearms while a second paramedic tried to get an IV going. Despite her restraints, it took several attempts; she was a lot stronger than I ever could have imagined. We were about a block from the hospital when she started to vomit, and she aspirated. Now, clearing her airway became the priority. The paramedic yelled at me to grab the suction line as he turned it on. As he was suctioning the bloody vomit from her mouth, I was trying not to vomit on both of them.

We arrived at the emergency room, and I was still maintaining her head and neck. They did a cross-table X-ray, which was negative for cervical spine fracture, and I was allowed to discontinue stabilization. I stayed with the girl in the ER until her parents got there. The doctor told me it was too early to tell how she would be. When I walked out of the ER, I met the athletic director, who was waiting to give me a ride back to school. It was like coming back to the real world. I hadn't even thought about getting back to school or about practice.

The young woman spent two weeks in the ICU being treated for a subdural hematoma. She later returned to school, showing few effects of the injury. I, however, learned that my job extends far beyond the training room—and I always grab a pair of gloves on my way out the door.

Becky Clifton, ATC

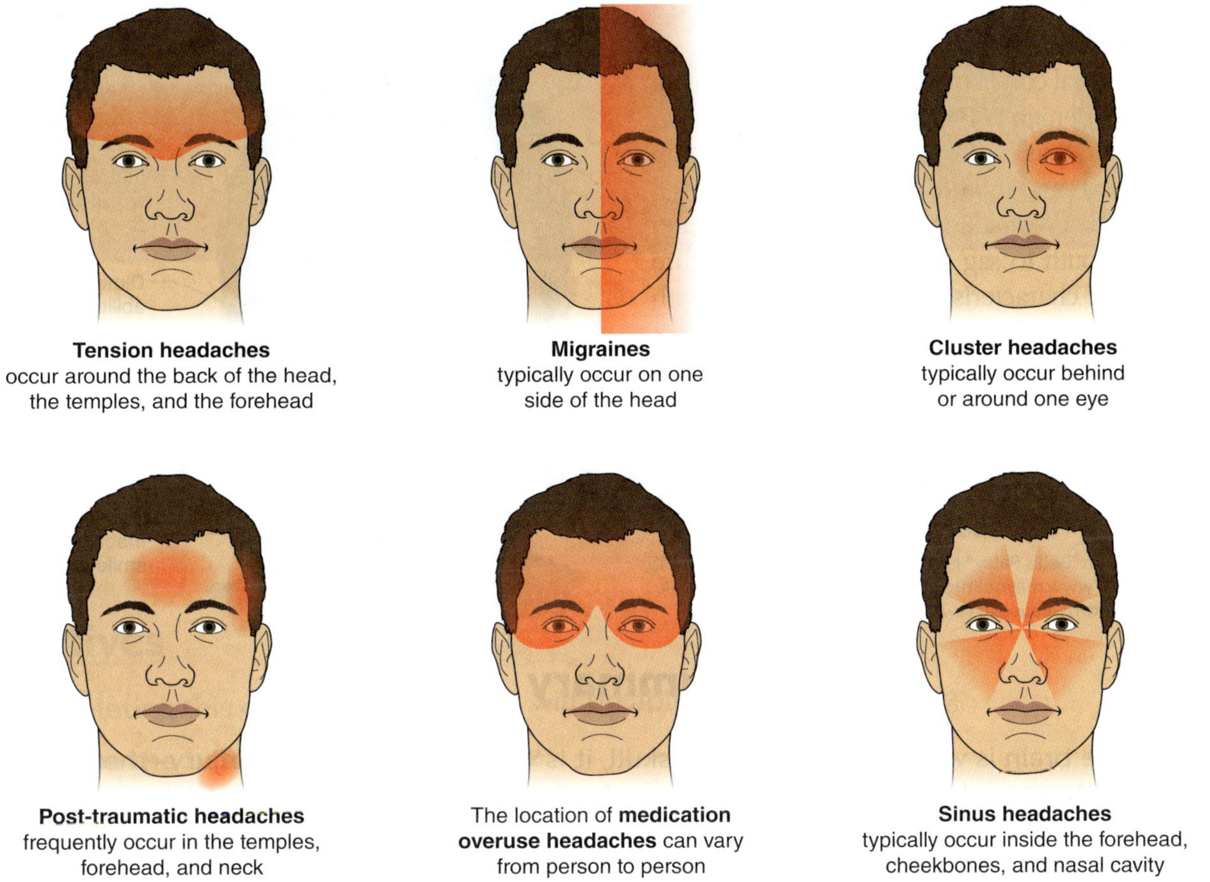

Figure 9.5 Zones of headaches.

Adapted from "Types of Headache by Location and Symptoms," Medical News Today, last modified August 9, 2024, https://www.medicalnewstoday.com/articles/headache-chart.

response. Tension headaches can be caused by any stressor.

- Cluster headaches are less well understood but form with pain behind one of the eyes. They can also be associated with eye redness, watering, or drooping. The causes of cluster headaches can be variable and have been hard to identify, although smokers seem to get cluster headaches more often than nonsmokers.
- Migraine headaches are the last type. These headaches are often severe and debilitating when they strike. The pain is usually limited to one side of the face and is often associated with visual and auditory defects, numbness and tingling, nausea, vomiting, and insomnia. Migraines can be attributed to many different causes but generally are associated with illness, stress, dietary patterns, and hormonal changes.

Headaches are often treated with over-the-counter pain medications such as acetaminophen, ibuprofen, or aspirin. People with medical conditions should check with their physician to see which over-the-counter medication is best for their medical problems. When severe, persistent headaches are treated by a physician with prescription medication.

Weightlifter's Cephalgia

Cephalgia is common with experienced weightlifters. When an athlete lifts a heavy load, they perform a Valsalva maneuver, where they bear down and increase the pressure inside their body, including the head. As a result, weightlifters often experience headaches from the repeated blood flow restrictions occurring throughout their multiple lifts. Although these are often not serious, they are uncomfortable and can cause the athlete to be apprehensive.

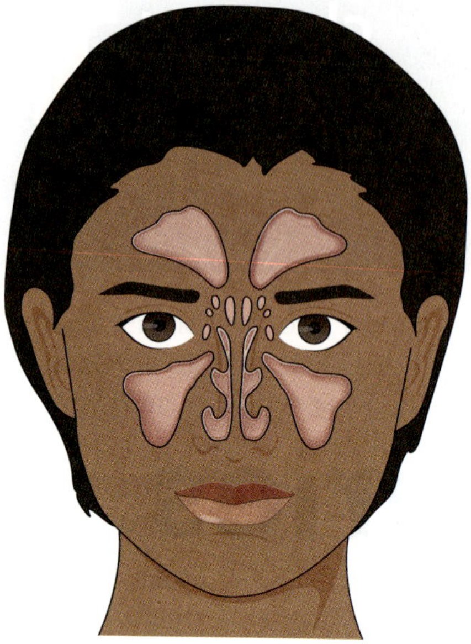

Figure 10.2 Sinuses.

The Eye

The eye sits in a socket known as the *orbital foramen*, or *orbit*. Most of the eye is hidden inside the orbital foramen, which protects the eye on three sides and serves as an attachment point for the muscles that move the eye. Lack of eye movement can indicate either a head injury or a serious eye injury (figure 10.3 shows the anatomy of the eye).

The eye itself has anterior and posterior chambers. The two chambers are filled with fluid, which gives the eye its rounded shape. An injury that causes fluid to drain from the eye is likely to cause permanent damage, even blindness.

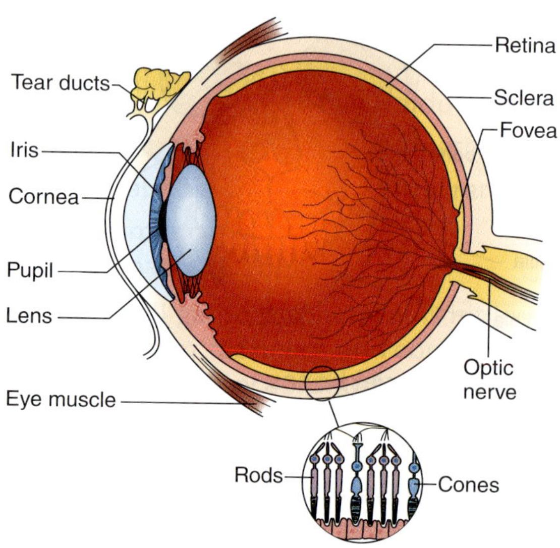

Figure 10.3 Anatomy of the eye.

Understanding Diversity

Color blindness is the inability to be able to distinguish between certain colors (Colorblind Guide n.d.). According to Colorblindguide.com, 3.7% of the United States population is color blind. Most of those who are colorblind are male. The most common form of color blindness is red-green. With red-green color blindness, the green looks more red, while another form of red-green blindness makes the red look more green and less bright (National Institute of Health 2019).

The covering of the eye has a white area and a clear center. The white outer covering of the eye is the sclera. A change in sclera color indicates that the athlete has a problem or an illness, such as liver disease, lack of oxygen, or poisoning. The clear center portion of the eyeball covering is the cornea. The cornea protects other important structures from injury. It covers the iris and pupil and admits light to the interior. The cornea is made up of thousands of tiny cells that can be injured by wearing contact lenses too long or by something that scratches the eye.

The iris is the contractile, colored portion of the eye, and in its center is the pupil, which is the opening in the iris. The iris responds to light, changing the size of the pupil. In bright light, the pupil gets smaller, thus limiting the light entering the eye. In a dark room, the pupil gets larger, allowing all available light into the eye. Also located in the anterior portion of the eye is the lens, which focuses the entering light rays on the retina. A poke in the eye may dislodge the lens, blurring or changing an athlete's vision. Finally, the **conjunctiva** lines the inner surface of the eyelid and continues over the forepart of the eyeball.

The main structures at the posterior aspect of the eye are the retina and the optic nerve. The retina lines the back of the eye and contains rods and cones. Rods provide vision in black and white, and cones provide color vision. The retina receives the image the lens forms and converts it into chemical and nerve signals that the optic nerve sends to the brain, where vision occurs. Damage to the optic nerve can cause blindness. Injury to the optic nerve that has resulted in blindness will also prevent the pupil from functioning.

In the upper outside (that is, superior lateral) edge of each eye is a gland that makes tears. Tears wash diagonally across to the nose and drain into it through a duct. In the rims of each eyelid are small glands that secrete lubricating fluid, allowing the eyelid to open and close smoothly.

Vision is measured by an arbitrary standard. Originally, the test consisted of reading letters on a chart from a distance of 20 feet (6 m). A person who could read the smallest letters was said to have 20/20 vision. Today's vision tests relate to that standard. A person who can see near objects more clearly than distant ones is nearsighted, and a person who can see distant objects better than near ones is farsighted. These common vision problems are treated with corrective lenses or eye exercises.

Muscles of the eye are divided into two categories: extrinsic and intrinsic. Table 10.1 provides muscle locations and functions.

What Would You Do If . . .

An athlete comes running into the athletic training room. They are in tears, cannot see, and have pain in their eyes. The athlete reveals that they are wearing a friend's contact lenses because they wanted to try them out.

The Ear

The ear has three distinct areas: the external ear, middle ear, and inner ear (see figure 10.4). The external ear is composed of the pinna, ear canal, and tympanic membrane. The pinna, which is the projecting portion of the external ear, is cartilage covered by skin. Its purpose is to catch sound and funnel it into the auditory canal.

Table 10.1 Muscles of the Eye

Extrinsic muscles	Attachments	Functions
Lateral rectus Medial rectus Superior rectus Inferior rectus Superior oblique Inferior oblique	Bones of the orbit and the eyeball	Movement of the eye superiorly and inferiorly, externally and internally, and obliquely
Intrinsic muscles	**Attachments**	**Functions**
Iris Ciliary	Interior layer of the eye	Size of the pupil and shape of the lens

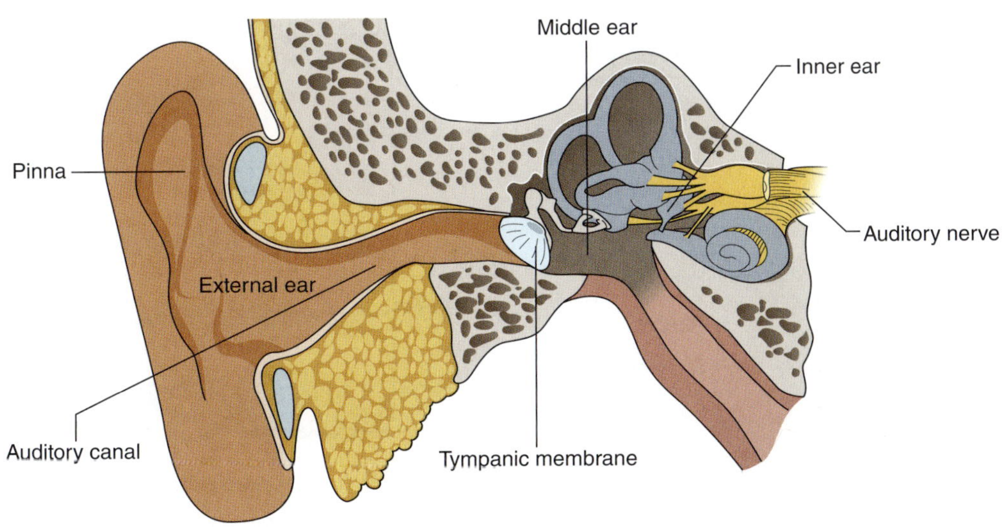

Figure 10.4 Anatomy of the ear.

The auditory canal carries sound from the pinna to the tympanic membrane, or eardrum. Earwax, which is designed to keep dirt away from the sensitive eardrum, is found in the auditory canal. Too much wax in the ear prevents or delays sound from reaching the middle ear.

The Nose

Two small bones, called the *nasal bones*, attach to the frontal bone of the skull. About an inch (2.5 cm) in length, the nasal bones make up the bridge of the nose. The rest of the nose is cartilage.

Inside the nose is the septum, which is a piece of cartilage that separates the left and right sides of the nose. Hairs inside the nose filter impurities from the air. The palate, which is the roof of the mouth, separates the mouth from the bottom of the nose.

Air that is inhaled through the nose is warmed, moisturized, and cleansed before reaching the lungs. In winter, breathing through the nose will decrease lung pain caused by inhaling cold air through the mouth. Athletes with asthma and upper-respiratory infections should breathe moist air.

The Mouth

The mouth is made up of the mandible (lower jaw), maxillae (upper jaw), temporomandibular joint, tongue, palate (roof of the mouth), and teeth. There are three primary glands in the mouth: **submandibular**, **sublingual**, and **parotid** (see figure 10.5).

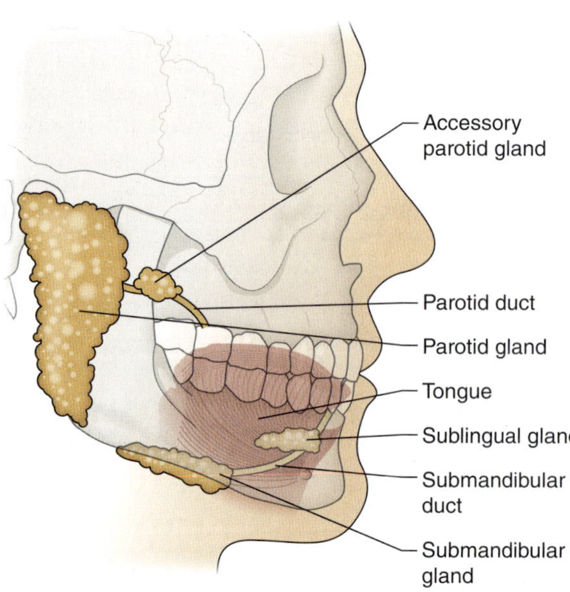

Figure 10.5 Glands of the mouth.

Reprinted by permission from K.W. Flanagan and M. Cuppett, *Medical Conditions in the Athlete*, 3rd ed. (Champaign, IL: Human Kinetics, 2017), 308.

The submandibular, sublingual, and parotid glands all secrete saliva but to different parts of the mouth and oral cavity.

The mandible attaches to the skull at the temporomandibular joint and is the only moveable bone in the face. The mandible moves during speaking and eating. The teeth give the face shape and are used to chew food; they are attached to both the mandible and the maxillae. An adult has 32 permanent teeth.

A tooth is composed of the crown, which is the visible portion above the gumline, and the root, which is below the gumline (see figure 10.6). The crown is capped with a thin layer of enamel, which protects against tooth decay. The root contains pulp and dentin. Dentin is the hard, bony portion of the tooth. The pulp is the soft portion of the tooth containing the nerve and blood supply. The nerve is sensitive to pain, pressure, and temperature, and the blood supply brings oxygen and nutrients to the tooth to keep it alive. A live tooth is white in color, whereas a dead tooth is dark gray. The teeth have a specific arrangement in the mouth and are referenced by their number. Figure 10.7 shows the numbering system for teeth.

The teeth, tongue, and saliva work together to prepare food to be swallowed. The salivary glands under the tongue and in the back of the mouth provide saliva to begin digestion. The saliva makes it easier for the teeth to break down food, and it binds the food together before the food is sent to the stomach.

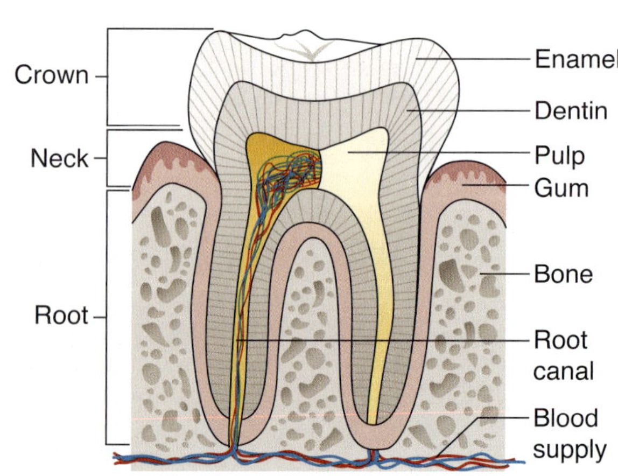

Figure 10.6 Cross-section of a tooth.

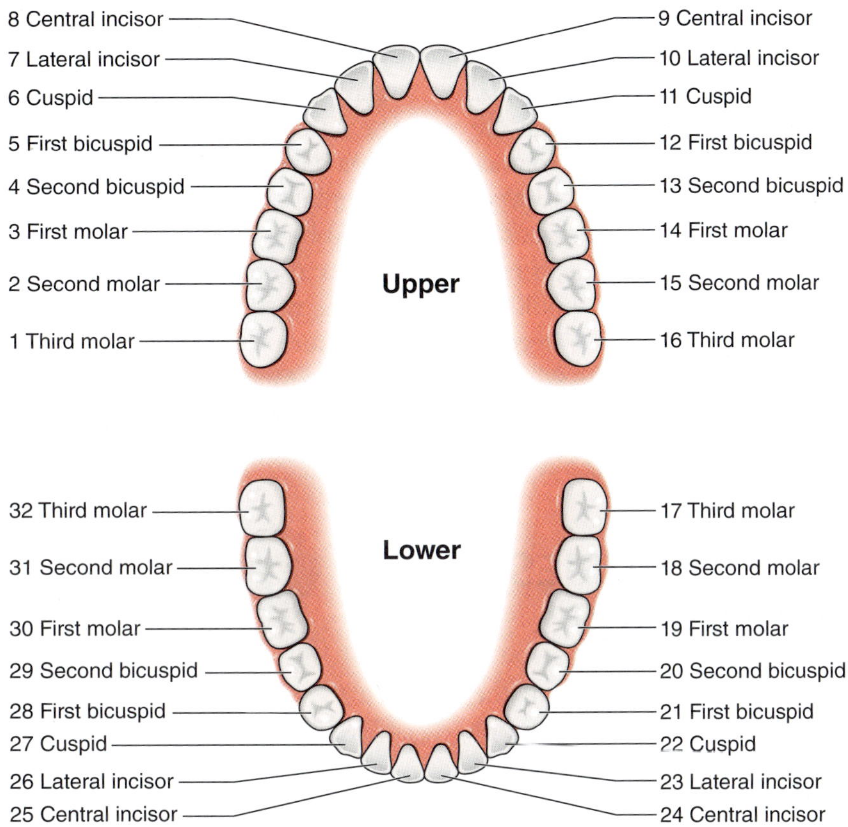

Figure 10.7 Diagram of teeth by number.

Data from News Medical Life Sciences. Available: https://www.news-medical.net/health/Universal-Numbering-System-for-Teeth.aspx.

The muscles used for chewing include the masseter, temporal, and pterygoid. Table 10.2 lists the muscles involved in chewing, including attachments and functions.

PREVENTING FACIAL INJURIES

Preventing facial injuries requires common sense. Athletes who fail to wear the proper equipment can easily become injured—a prime example is a catcher who does not wear a face mask when warming up a pitcher. Equipment is available in all sports to prevent facial injury; it includes helmets, mouth guards, face masks, goggles, protective eyewear, and headgear. Mouth guards are relatively inexpensive, but repairing injuries to the teeth and jaw is expensive. A properly fitted athletic face mask decreases the number of eye, nose, face, and mouth injuries. The face mask should be spaced a minimum of 1 inch (2.5 cm) from the nose; if it is closer, an impact to the mask can cause it to distort inward, resulting in injury to the face or nose. When selecting a face mask, make sure that no game equipment, such as a hockey puck or stick

Table 10.2 Muscles of the Mandible

Muscle	Attachments	Functions
Masseter	Zygomatic arch and the mandible	Closing the mouth
Temporal	Temporal bone and mandible	Closing the mouth
Pterygoids	Inferior surface of skull and mandible	Grinding the teeth

blade, can get through the openings in the mask and hit the face. Protective eyewear is crucial in preventing blindness. All sports have the potential for eye injuries; balls, sticks, elbows, and fingers are common items that injure eyes. Because eye injuries are unpredictable, it is best for all athletes to wear eye protection designed for their sport. Eye guards, which are similar to glasses and generally consist of plastic frames and lenses, or goggles should be worn if face masks are not worn (see the Recommended Eye Protectors for Selected Sports sidebar). Athletes with fractures of the nasal bones, skull, or jaw should wear special padding, masks, or helmets to prevent additional injuries.

TREATING EYE INJURIES AND CONDITIONS

Eyes are precious, and it is better to err on the side of caution and send the athlete to a doctor or **ophthalmologist**, even if the eye injury does not seem serious. Have a trained physician or specialist evaluate the injury to determine the seriousness and treatment to prevent permanent injury or vision loss. The AT should also think about other injuries that might have occurred along with the eye injury. For example, a head injury is a definite possibility that should be assessed.

Eyes move in coordination. Even if an eye is injured, it still tends to move with the uninjured eye. If an eye must be patched or shielded, the AT should cover both eyes. This will reduce the movement of both eyes and help protect the injured eye from further irritation.

? What Would You Do If . . .

You find the lost contact lens of a soccer player. It is covered with dirt and grass.

RECOMMENDED EYE PROTECTORS FOR SELECTED SPORTS

These are the specific types of eye protectors recommended for these sports; all other sports wear custom eyewear or polycarbonate eye protection.

- ASTM F803
  - Baseball or softball fielder
  - Basketball
  - Soccer
  - Track and field
- ASTM F3077
  - Lacrosse
  - Field hockey (also ASTM F27130)
- NOCSAE DOC.24: Baseball or softball catcher
- BS 5883: Water polo or swimming
- ASTM F513: Ice hockey forwards and defenders
- ASTM F1587: Ice hockey goalies

ASTM = American Society for Testing and Materials; BS = British Standard; NOCSAE = National Operating Committee on Standards for Athletic Equipment.

Data from American Academy of Ophthalmology (2013); S.J. Dain, "Sports Eyewear Protective Standards," Clinical Experimental Optometry 99 (2016): 4-23; U.S. Lacrosse (2017), "Approved Eyewear List," www.uslacrosse.rg/safety/equipment/approved-eyewear-list.

Chemical Burns

Chemical burns can be disastrous. Although seen in labs or work facilities, these can happen if an athlete comes in contact with any chemical agent such as caustic cleaning agents. If an athlete experiences a chemical burn, it is important to flush it out with water. Remove all clothing that has the chemical on it so that the chemical does not burn through to the athlete's skin. If only one eye is affected, be sure to flush the eye so the water flows away from the uninjured eye. Immediately refer the athlete to a physician or call EMS.

Conjunctivitis

Conjunctivitis is more commonly known as *pink eye*. The conjunctiva turns red, and the eye appears to be irritated. Conjunctivitis has a variety of causes, including bacteria, allergies, eye irritants (e.g., soap), viruses, and diseases (Flanagan and Cuppett 2017). Symptoms of conjunctivitis include redness, irritation, crusting matter along the corners and lid of the eye, blurred vision, and itching.

A physician needs to examine the eye to determine the cause. Pink eye is usually caused by a highly contagious virus, so to prevent others from getting it, the athlete should stay at home until effectively treated and no longer contagious. Eye drops will be necessary for effective treatment.

For those who have the allergic form of conjunctivitis, an antihistamine or separating the athlete from the allergen will work. An athlete who has a bacterial infection will need antibiotics.

Foreign Body

A foreign body in the eye causes tears, which attempt to wash the foreign body toward the nose. In some instances, tears will not clear the eye. In these cases, rinsing with water from the nose outward can flush the particle out of the eye or over to one side where it can be removed.

If the object is stuck under the eyelid, the AT or athlete should lift the lid outward over the bottom lashes. The bottom lashes can brush the object out. If this process does not remove the object, it will be necessary to invert the upper eyelid. To invert the eyelid, grasp the lid and pull it outward; place a cotton-tipped applicator in the fold of the lid, and lay the lid over the applicator. This exposes the underside of the lid so that the object can be removed. If the inversion technique fails, the athlete should be referred to a physician for care. Both eyes must be patched to decrease eye movement and prevent scratching of the cornea. Figure 10.8 shows the process for removing a foreign object from the eye.

Embedded Object

An embedded object is stuck in the eye; it may have been blown into the eye, for example, or a blow from a ball may have shattered a contact lens. No matter how the object entered the eye, the care received will determine the quality of the athlete's vision in the future. The athlete will know the object is in the eye. They will reach for the eye and tears will occur, resulting in pain, visual impairment, and anxiety.

The best treatment is to place an eye shield over both eyes and send the athlete to a physician. If the object is sticking out of the eye, the AT will not remove the object but will stabilize it with bulky dressings. The physician will determine the severity of the injury, surgically remove the object, and stop

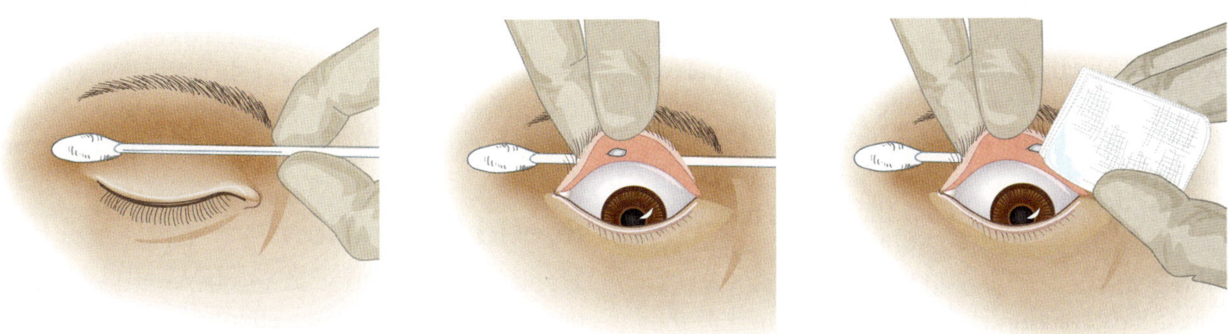

a b c

Figure 10.8 Removing foreign object.

Reprinted by permission from M.A. Cleary and K.W. Flanagan, *Acute and Emergency Care in Athletic Training* (Champaign, IL: Human Kinetics, 2020), 239.

> **? What Would You Do If . . .**
>
> A golfer comes into the training room assisted by several others. They tell you that someone yelled, "Fore," and when the golfer turned to look, the ball hit her in the eye. The athlete is in extreme pain and wants you to remove her contact lens. You can see several pieces of her contact lens sticking into her eye.

any fluid release. The physician will prescribe antibiotics, and the eye will remain patched for about a week. A vision test will be necessary to determine visual acuity. Eye guards and goggles will help the athlete protect the eye from reinjury.

Dislodged Contact Lens

Contact lenses come in two types: hard and soft. A hard contact lens covers the pupil of the eye, whereas a soft lens covers the entire cornea. A displaced hard contact lens feels like a rock in the eye. The athlete's vision will be impaired, and the displaced lens will irritate the eye. Usually, the athlete knows where the lens is in the eye because of the initial pain. When the eye is examined, the lens can be seen because of its color in contrast to the sclera. Some people believe that the lens can be lost behind the eye, but that is impossible. The lens will be in the eye—the AT just has to keep looking. The hard lens can be moved back over the pupil, and usually the athlete can do this if the AT provides a mirror. If the athlete cannot remove it, the AT can remove it using a small suction cup device that is placed over the lens. The athlete should then clean the lens before placing it back in the eye.

The displacement of a soft lens is less uncomfortable. The athlete will know the lens is out of place because they will not be able to see. A soft lens is more difficult to put back in place because it tends to curl up. The athlete should wash their hands and then gently grab the lens. They must use caution, because roughly handling a soft lens will tear it. The lens should be cleaned with sterile contact lens solution before being returned to the eye. Sometimes an athlete believes that putting the lens in their mouth to rinse it is acceptable. The practice of placing a hard or soft contact lens in the mouth is like dipping it in garbage before reinserting it. This practice must be discouraged!

REMOVING A CONTACT LENS

1. Wash and dry your hands before removing any lenses.
2. Pull down your lower lid.
3. For soft lenses: Look up or to the side, and gently move your lens to the white of your eye. Using your thumb and index finger, gently pinch the lens and lift it off your eye.
4. For gas-permeable lenses, open your eyes wide and pull the skin near the corner of your eye toward your ear. Bend over your open palm and blink. The lens should pop out into your palm.

Adapted from WebMD. Available: www.webmd.com/eye-health/ss/slideshow-contact-lens-tips.

Corneal Abrasion

A **corneal abrasion** or laceration is caused by being poked in the eye with a foreign object or by wearing contact lenses too long. An abrasion is superficial, whereas a laceration is deeper and more severe. The athlete will experience pain and feel as if something is lodged in the eye. They will have tears and sensitivity to bright light. If the injury is not treated, the eye may become infected, or the athlete may have permanent vision problems. The physician treats the abrasion by patching the injured eye for 24 hours and applying antibiotic ointment. The athlete will need help getting to the hospital because of limited vision. If wearing a contact lens too long caused the injury, a restriction will be placed on the athlete to keep this from recurring. Sunglasses may be worn while recovering. Corrective lenses may be necessary if the cornea becomes distorted. The athlete may have difficulty returning to competition for fear of reinjuring the eye, but using eye guards or goggles will help overcome this fear.

Eyelid Laceration

Think of an athlete who reaches out to grab the head of the opposing wrestler to gain control for a takedown. The opponent jerks his head away from the grasp but gets poked in the eye and experiences immediate eye pain. The eye is bleeding, and the athlete refuses to pull his hand away so the AT can determine the extent of the injury. Once the athlete relaxes, the AT can see that the eyelid is lacerated, maybe all the way through to the margin of the eyelash.

The immediate procedure is to control the bleeding with direct pressure. The AT will question the athlete about their ability to see clearly to determine the extent of other possible consequences of the poke. An eyelid laceration is similar to most lacerations except the tear duct may also be injured, possibly resulting in permanent damage. Once the bleeding is controlled, the athlete must be referred to a physician, ophthalmologist, or plastic surgeon to repair the lid.

A plastic surgeon should repair a laceration of the eyelid to prevent scarring or permanent deformity of the lid. The ophthalmologist will want to check the eye for proper vision and to ensure that there are no other complications.

Athletes should keep their fingernails short to prevent eyelid lacerations (this is a rule in wrestling). Goggles can also prevent this type of injury.

Black Eye or Periorbital Contusion

A hard blow to the eye may cause a black eye or periorbital contusion. As with any contusion, a black eye is caused by bleeding and discoloration just under the skin, which affects the tissue surrounding the eye but not the eye itself. Therefore, the athlete will not complain of visual impairment, but there will be swelling and pain. If the athlete complains of any other difficulty, a referral to a physician is necessary. Ice application over a black eye is an accepted treatment.

Hemorrhage Into the Anterior Chamber (Hyphema)

A blow to the eye can cause bleeding in the eye. A **hyphema** is blood pooling in the anterior portion of the eye. The athlete will complain of both the inability to see and of pain. They should have both eyes covered with a protective shield, but the AT should not apply an ice pack. The physician needs to determine the severity of the injury. The athlete with a hyphema may suffer permanent damage, blindness, or cataracts.

Detached Retina and Retinal Tears

A blow to the eye or even a hard sneeze can cause the retina to detach. The athlete will experience pain, but the surest sign of a **detached retina** is that the athlete sees sparks, lights, and flashes that nobody else can see. The athlete may indicate that they are having difficulty seeing or that things look foggy. The athlete should be referred to a physician who can do laser surgery to repair the detached retina. Sometimes, the retina will tear as well. Any injury to the retina requires prompt attention to ensure proper care and preserve vision. When the athlete returns to activity, they must wear protective goggles to prevent reinjury. If a physician does not repair the damage promptly, blindness could result.

Subconjunctival Hemorrhage

Athletes who have a terrible cough from an upper-respiratory infection are prone to **subconjunctival hemorrhage**. The constant coughing may cause the small vessels in the eye to rupture, turning the conjunctiva red. An athlete may also get poked in the conjunctiva or hit by a ball, which causes the same result.

Although the eye looks painful, the athlete experiences minimal or no pain and no visual impairment. It is best to refer the athlete to a physician for an eye exam to be sure no other structures are injured. The treatment for this hemorrhage is to do nothing. The athlete is allowed to participate without restriction. Their biggest problem will be the funny looks they get from others concerned about the appearance of their eye.

Orbital Roof Fracture

A blow to the eye or the area just above the eye can cause a fracture in the roof of the orbit. When this happens, the athlete will experience pain, a headache, signs and symptoms of a concussion, and a hematoma over the area. The nose may bleed, and cerebrospinal fluid may drain from the nose. This injury requires immediate care by a physician. Hospitalization for observation and care of the fracture and rest will most likely be required. The athlete will not be able to return to competition for about a year.

Sinus Fracture

A sinus fracture can occur from a sharp blow to the face—for example, from a baseball taking a bad hop or from a stick across the face. A headache, dizziness, and unsteadiness may occur. The athlete's nose may bleed on the same side as the injury. He will experience pain, but once the bleeding has stopped, the AT should do a quick assessment of the injury. With this fracture, air seeps into the skin and tissues around the eye and nose, resulting in a crackling sensation when the area is touched. The AT should apply ice and immediately refer the athlete to a physician. The physician will order special X-rays to determine the exact location of the fracture.

A complication of this injury is a concussion, which could diminish the athlete's ability to give a history. In the case of a blow to the face, it is always prudent to recommend a physician's evaluation and manage the acute situation with caution.

Blowout Fracture

A blow to the eye can force the eyeball backward into the socket. The thin bones beneath the eye absorb the sudden increase in pressure and fracture. This type of fracture is referred to as a **blowout**.

The athlete may experience double vision and may not be able to feel much pain because surrounding nerve endings are damaged. The athlete may also experience numbing of the lip and upper jaw on the same side as the injury. The muscles of the eye often get caught in the fractured bones. Therefore, the AT may notice that the athlete cannot control the injured eye—it will be looking in a different direction than the uninjured eye. The eye may appear to be sunken in the socket. There will be immediate swelling, and the conjunctiva will begin to discolor. The athlete may have a bloody nose on the same side as the injury, and the bleeding may fill the sinus, making it difficult to breathe. The eye may bulge when the athlete attempts to blow their nose.

The AT should call 911 and help control any bleeding. The athlete should be monitored in case their condition worsens. A physician may have to surgically repair the fracture and release the muscles. The athlete may suffer permanent vision problems, including glaucoma and cataracts. They will remain out of competition for several months.

Boxers wear headgear to prevent such eye injuries. Although blowout fractures are rarely seen in wrestling, basketball, and racquetball, athletes in these sports should wear eye protection to prevent them.

Ruptured Globe

The globe—the eyeball itself—can be ruptured by any object small enough to hit the eye, such as a squash ball or racquetball. When examining the eye, the AT will notice a lack of roundness of the globe and a hemorrhage of the eye. Associated injuries may include an eyelid laceration, blood in the front of the eye, the interior contents of the eye spilling out, or the pupil being out of round (see figure 10.9). Any sign that the globe has been ruptured requires that the AT cover both eyes with protective eye shields that will not allow external pressure. The athlete must be taken to the emergency room immediately and referred to an ophthalmologist if their eyesight is going to be saved. The athlete will not be able to return to competition for months.

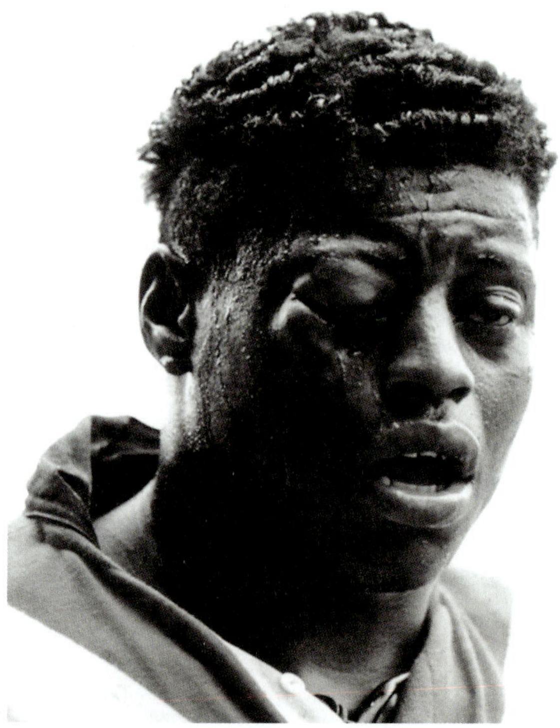

Figure 10.9 Any time there is excessive swelling with possible leakage of fluid, a ruptured globe should be suspected. In this case, both eyes should be patched and the athlete sent to the emergency room immediately.

Photo courtesy of Active Images.

! RED FLAGS

Call 911 for any of the following:

- The globe of the eye is leaking fluid.
- The globe of the eye is outside the socket.
- The athlete can no longer move his eye after injury.
- A glass lens has been embedded in the eye.

TREATING EAR INJURIES

The external ear helps to funnel sound to the inner ear, and the inner ear plays a role in equilibrium. With its placement on the side of the head, the ear does not have a high incidence of injury. In high school athletics, earrings are barred from competition because of the potential for ear injury.

Swimmer's Ear (Otitis Externa)

Proper ear care requires that the ear and the canal be dried after swimming. A swimmer cannot always remove water from their ear, such as when they are hurrying to get home or water is stuck in the ear. If water remains in the ear, the canal can become inflamed, which is referred to as *otitis externa*, more commonly called **swimmer's ear**. The athlete will experience pain, itching, hearing loss, and possibly a smelly discharge from the ear. It will be easy to notice the discharge and the swollen, red canal. If the infection is not controlled, it can spread deeper into the canal. The athlete should be sent to a physician for ear drops and antibiotics. Prevention of swimmer's ear can be as simple as drying the ear after swimming by using a hair dryer on a low setting. Rubber or wax plugs are sometimes used to reduce the flow of water into the ear, but these can increase the risk of infection because they irritate the ear canal. Also, when using plugs, hearing is impaired, making it difficult to hear coaches. Some athletes prefer to use alcohol-based ear drops, which dry the ear canal.

Many athletes clean their ears regularly to prevent infection, but this, too, can become problematic. Cerumen, or earwax, is an important barrier to infection, and regular cleaning that forces wax out of the canal may not only irritate the canal but also increase the risk of infection (American Academy of Otolaryngology 2020).

Otitis Media

Unlike otitis externa, which affects the external ear, otitis media is an infection in the middle ear. It is common with a cold, sore throat, or even an upper-respiratory infection. Although most common in children, adults can get this infection. They will have pain in the ear, fever, loss of balance, and sometimes hearing problems. Any athlete suspected of having a middle ear infection should be referred to the physician for antibiotic treatment.

Foreign Body

In athletics, foreign bodies in the ear are rare, but bugs have been known to be in an athlete's ear. The athlete will have the sensation that something is in the ear and may experience pain.

Probing the ear with a cotton-tipped applicator may push the object farther into the ear and should be avoided. The AT could also rupture the eardrum while trying to get the object out. A physician can remove an object using mineral oil or special tweezers.

Cauliflower Ear (Hematoma Auris)

Wrestlers are the athletes who suffer the most from **cauliflower ear**. The wrestler involved usually is not wearing headgear and gets hit hard in the ear, or their head is pushed hard into the wrestling mat.

The Real World

One night while I was covering a high school football game, an athlete whose nickname was Cowboy came over to the sidelines as the defense came off the field. The team physician and I were there when the athlete stated that he was experiencing ear pain. After removing his helmet, I examined his ear and saw a fly at the entrance to the ear canal. I must have startled the poor insect because it retreated back into the ear. The physician asked if I had a penlight. I produced one, she aimed it at the ear, and the fly immediately came forward—drawn to the light and buzzed away, solving Cowboy's dilemma.

Todd Keasling, ATC

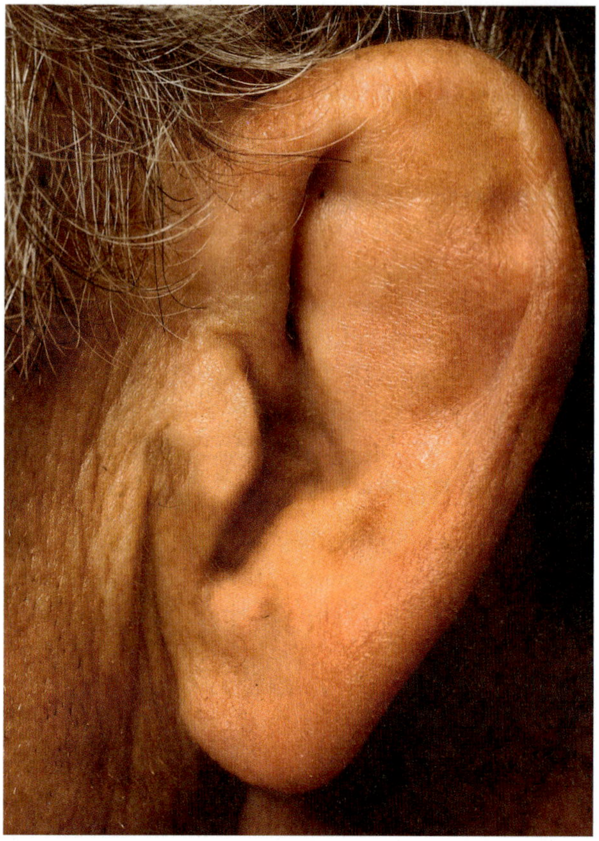

Figure 10.10 Cauliflower ear.

The pinna of the ear begins to bleed internally, causing swelling, redness, and pain. As the ear heals, there is an excessive growth of reparative tissue, which distorts the pinna, causing it to look like a piece of cauliflower (see figure 10.10).

Treatment of cauliflower ear starts with ice and compression with moldable material, performed by the team physician. The team physician may lance, or drain, the ear to reduce the swelling and use steroid medication to keep the hemorrhage under control. In more complicated cases, the physician may remove the tissue through surgery. Some athletes opt for plastic surgery to fix the ear if it is permanently distorted. Wearing headgear and applying petroleum jelly to reduce friction can prevent cauliflower ear.

Pinna Laceration

Ears stick out from the head enough that they may get in the way. Athletes should never wear earrings in practices or competitions because they increase the vulnerability of an already exposed body part. An earring can be caught by another athlete's finger, tearing the earlobe. Even in sports in which the ears are protected by a helmet, earrings may be jammed against the wearer's head if the head is struck, causing serious discomfort and even injury. A laceration of the pinna is treated the same as any other wound—by controlling the bleeding with direct pressure, which can be applied on both sides for rapid control.

When a portion of the pinna is no longer attached, the missing piece must be found so that it may be reattached. The detached part should be wrapped in sterile gauze, put in a plastic bag, and placed in a container full of ice. (It is appropriate to place it on ice as long as the ear is not directly touching the ice.) In the case of a laceration, the athlete should be referred to a physician for stitches and a tetanus shot. The athlete can prevent lacerations and other wounds of the pinna by wearing proper protection and removing earrings.

Ruptured Eardrum

A tear of the tympanic membrane, or **ruptured eardrum**, can occur from an ear infection, a blow to the side of the head, loud noises, and atmospheric pressure. The athlete may experience loss of hearing, buzzing in the ear, and drainage from the ear. A physician will have to examine the ear using an otoscope and do a hearing test to determine the extent of the injury. In some cases, no treatment is necessary, and the membrane will heal on its own. In other cases, antibiotics will be necessary to deal with the ear infection, if that was the cause. For severe ruptures or ruptures that do not heal, surgery may be necessary. An athlete will need to wear headgear to protect the membrane and must not put anything in the ear, such as a cotton swab.

TREATING NOSE INJURIES

For some athletes, the nose is always in the way. In boxing, it is constantly being smashed by a fist. Wrestlers can find their noses rubbed into the mat and even used as a carrying handle by opponents. And basketball players' noses seem to be attracted to the elbows of opposing players. The nose is vital: It warms incoming air and acts as a filter to catch particles.

Nosebleed (Epistaxis)

When an athlete goes up to head a soccer ball and it lands on their nose, the impact can cause an **epistaxis**, or bloody nose. An athlete may get a nosebleed from constantly blowing their nose during a cold. Athletes taking certain medications, as well as those who have had a recent nosebleed, are prone to epistaxis.

The nose will bleed from one or both nostrils, and if the nosebleed is from a blow, it will be painful. The AT should instruct the athlete to lean forward while pinching the nose. Applying ice and packing the nose with gauze that has been soaked with an astringent (medication that slows bleeding) are helpful. Leaning the head backward forces the blood into the throat, obstructing the airway, and should be avoided. The athlete should lean forward to allow blood to discharge from the nose and should spit out any blood draining into the throat—swallowing blood will cause vomiting. Discourage any attempt to blow the nose, because this will start the bleeding process again. If there is excessive bleeding (gushing like a faucet) from the nose, the athlete should be treated for shock and sent to the hospital for evaluation. The physician may cauterize the bleeding vessel.

Deviated Septum

The septum is the piece of cartilage that separates the left and right sides of the nose. A deviated septum has moved to one side, causing decreased airflow through the nasal passageway. Any form of direct impact to the nose can cause a deviation.

The blow to the nose will have caused a nosebleed, so follow the instructions for epistaxis first. Then wait a day or two to test the athlete for a deviated septum by blocking off one nostril and having the athlete force air out of the nose and then repeating the procedure on the other side. If one nostril forces more air through than the other does, the septum may be deviated. If the athlete has a deviated septum, the nose may also be broken. To evaluate the septum, shine a flashlight or penlight up each nostril. The septum should be in the middle of the nose. If either side looks smaller, the septum is likely deviated to that side. The athlete should be referred to a physician to determine if surgery is necessary. Many athletes with a deviated septum choose not to have surgery. Wearing a face mask will prevent further injury to the nose.

Nasal Fracture

A direct blow to the nose can fracture one or both nasal bones. There will be a severe nosebleed, often similar to water running from a faucet. The AT will treat the athlete by having them lean forward. Pinching the nose may not be possible. The AT uses gauze to catch the blood as it comes out of the nose and applies ice. Gauze should not be forced into the nostril to slow bleeding.

The athlete may indicate that they heard a snap and may have pain and difficulty breathing. The AT should observe deformity (flat on one side) and swelling. They may hear **crepitus**, or crunchiness, during palpation and observe a deviated septum. The athlete should be referred to a physician for care. The physician may proceed with surgery to put the bones back into place. Some athletes who opt to avoid surgery suffer from a permanently deformed nose. In the days after a nasal fracture, the athlete will have black eyes from internal bleeding that pools underneath the orbits of the eyes. See figure 10.11 for more on assessment and care of an injury to the nose.

Sinusitis and Rhinitis

Sinusitis is a medical condition indicating inflammation in the sinuses. The frontal sinus is located above the eyebrows; the ethmoid is located along the sides of the nasal cavity; the sphenoid is located below the eyes; and the maxillary is in the cheek region. Sinuses can get infected and cause pain in these regions as they swell and create pressure. Sinuses can fill with fluid and cause drainage along with the pressure. Athletes with sinus pain and pressure should be referred to a physician for treatment. **Rhinitis** is inflammation of the nasal tissues where the blood vessels in the nose expand. This creates an environment similar to sinusitis: inflammation, pain, and pressure. Rhinitis can be in response to an allergen such as smoke, pollen, or other substance; it can be nonallergic, which is caused from weather or infection. Rhinitis can be treated with saline flushes, over-the-counter antihistamines and anti-inflammatories, or medical treatments by a physician. Chronic rhinitis can lead to sinusitis and the infection of the sinuses if not treated properly.

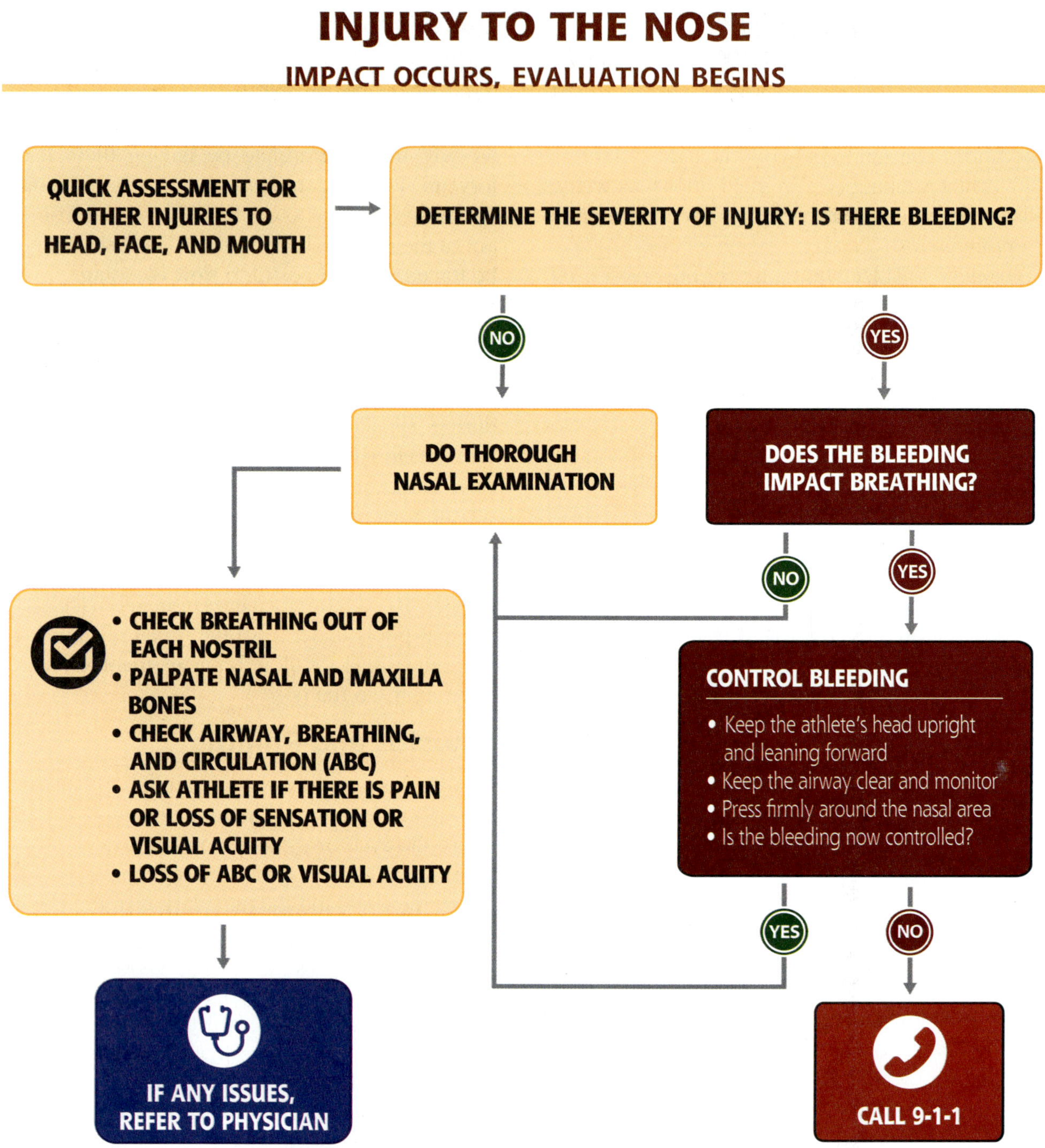

Figure 10.11 Care of an injury to the nose.

TREATING MOUTH INJURIES

Although some believe that losing teeth is no big deal because they can always get false teeth, they are wrong. False teeth are not nearly as good as real teeth at biting and chewing, making it difficult to get the nutrition the body needs. The AT should use caution when treating the mouth—some athletes may bite because of a seizure or because they are gagging. It is also the responsibility of the athletic trainer to prevent sports-related orofacial injuries by

> **What Would You Do If . . .**
>
> A couple of volleyball players are horsing around in the locker room. One slips and hits their mouth on the edge of the sink. They bring two fractured front teeth into the training room and hand them to you.

educating their athletes about protective devices and proper equipment (American Academy of Pediatric Dentistry 2023).

Tongue or Cheek Laceration

The mouth has a significant blood supply, so a lot of blood flows if the mouth is injured. This can be scary. Lacerations can occur in a variety of ways, including accidentally biting oneself. Bleeding can be controlled by applying direct pressure in most cases. If the cheek is pierced through to the inside of the mouth, direct pressure should be applied, both internally and externally. The cheek and tongue do not usually require stitches unless the laceration is large and deep.

Examination of the tongue is a unique practice. Most athletes do not like to have their tongues touched. But it is important to properly evaluate the tongue for lesions, wounds, or other issues. First, put on a pair of gloves after cleaning your hands properly. Next, have the athlete sit in front of you on a chair. Take a clean piece of gauze and grab the end of the tongue as the athlete protrudes it from his mouth. Rotate the tongue to the left, right, and up so that you can check the surfaces, including the undersurface of the tongue. Any lesions, growths, or other problems should be referred to a dentist or physician.

Tooth Fracture

Direct impact to the lower jaw or the teeth can result in a tooth fracture. The athlete will experience pain and difficulty closing their mouth. A fracture can be seen if the tooth is examined closely. In some instances, a portion of the tooth will be gone. If a portion has broken off, it should be sent with the athlete to the dentist. Although the portion cannot be put back on, the dentist may find it helpful when reconstructing the tooth. The broken tooth may die and have to be removed.

Tooth Dislocation

Direct impact to a tooth can knock it out of the jaw. The athlete will experience severe pain, bleeding, and swelling. The dislodged tooth needs to be handled carefully. Caring for a lost or dislocated tooth is important to ensure the viability of the tooth. After putting on gloves, the AT should pick up the tooth with a sterile gauze pad. It must be kept moist and should be placed in a designated saline tooth container or a glass of milk. The athlete must be seen by a dentist so that the tooth can be put back in place, assuming it is not too severely injured to be reinserted. The AT should treat the bleeding socket, placing a piece of sterile gauze where the tooth was located and having the athlete gently bite down to keep it in place with direct pressure. In addition to caring for the tooth, be sure to evaluate the surrounding areas of the face for injuries and consider a potential head injury as a result of the blow.

Dental Caries

Dental caries or cavities are weaknesses in the tooth enamel caused by poor dental hygiene, poor nutritional habits, or sometimes medical conditions. Dentists often find dental caries during an exam, but an athlete may come to you with tooth pain and sensitivity to air and temperatures (cold or hot fluids). Pain with pressure on the tooth is often a sign of an emerging or developed cavity. Dentists will have to put a filling in the tooth if it can be saved and will always recommend good dental hygiene such as brushing, flossing, and mouthwash to protect the enamel on the teeth.

Jaw Fracture

Imagine getting hit in the face by a sharply hit baseball, a scenario that is not uncommon in athletics. A direct blow to the jaw, either upper or lower, can result in a fracture. The athlete will experience pain that increases with movement. When the AT observes the area of impact, they will be able to see swelling. If the lower jaw has been fractured, they may be able to observe a space between teeth that was not there previously. The athlete will have discoloration under the tongue, and their teeth may not line up. Palpation will reveal crepitus, and the athlete will be cautious about moving the jaw. The AT should make sure all the teeth are in place and the airway is clear.

Ice should be applied to the area, as tolerated by the athlete, who should be referred immediately to a physician for care. The physician will realign the jaw for proper closure and wire the mouth shut. The athlete will eat through a straw for four to six weeks. Some athletes are allowed to return to activity as long as a special face mask protects the jaw.

Improper care or neglect of a jaw fracture can result in permanent deformity. The jaw may not be able to open wide enough to allow for eating a hamburger, for example, and malalignment of the teeth can lead to further mouth problems.

What Would You Do If . . .

One of your friends shows you his ice hockey helmet, which has a crack in the back portion that he has glued together. He says there is no rule that prevents him from playing in a game with his repaired helmet.

Temporomandibular Dislocation

A blow to the chin or a violent, forced opening of the mouth can cause a dislocation. The athlete will immediately grab and hold their mouth to keep it from moving. The jaw will lock itself in place when the local muscles spasm, and the athlete will be in extreme pain. The jaw will look deformed, locked open, or to one side. The AT can feel that the condyles are out of normal position. The AT should never try to put the jaw back in place because the area around the jaw is filled with nerves and cartilage that can be permanently damaged. The team physician should relocate the jaw, which must be kept shut for several weeks. Some physicians wire the jaw shut to ensure this rest.

Temporomandibular Joint Dysfunction

Temporomandibular joint (TMJ) dysfunction is a condition in which the muscles surrounding the joint spasm. The spasms can be caused by stress, a blow to the mandible, or an injury to the muscles. The dysfunction can cause misalignment of the teeth, an inability to open the mouth fully, clicking of the jaw, earache, pain in the musculature of the mouth, and headaches.

The Real World

I was covering a girls' soccer match. With two minutes left in the first half, the opposing team was inside the scoring circle. From where I was standing, I could see a lot of bodies kicking and flailing around as our team was defending. Then our goalie was on the ground with the ball in her hands, and I knew something was wrong by the reaction of our players. The official summoned me onto the field. Our goalie had been kicked in the mouth, and there was blood everywhere. Unfortunately, she had not been wearing a mouth guard. She was conscious and spitting out blood. I did a head and neck evaluation and found no other problems. When examining her mouth, I saw blood coming up from her gums in the molar region. She was able to move her mouth to talk, but her jaw was painful in the front. I packed sterile gauze between her gums and teeth all the way around her mandible. I had her put ice on the jaw where she had pain. Her father wanted to drive her to the emergency room because that was quicker than calling an ambulance. I felt she was stable enough and agreed he should take her. I gave her a pan to hold on her lap because she was still spitting blood.

The textbooks say to use a wrap around the patient's jaw and apply ice if there is a suspected jaw fracture. However, in this case, I chose not to follow that protocol. The athlete was spitting blood that would have gone into her stomach if I had strapped her jaw the way the books say. Blood is an irritant to the stomach, and chances are she would have started vomiting, thus complicating matters. The emergency room physician said I did the right thing. The mandible was fractured in two places in the front of the jaw. On the X-ray, it looked as if a triangle had been cut into the mandible. This player's soccer season was over. However, the athlete was back in goal next year, wearing a mouth guard.

Suzy Heinzman, ATC

During examination, the AT may find a lack of range of motion, holding of the jaw, poor alignment when opening or closing, or crepitus. Treatment of TMJ dysfunction includes relaxing the jaw muscles, such as from massage or trigger-point techniques. In some instances, the athlete may require muscle relaxants or pain medication. A dentist may choose to make a bite splint to prevent TMJ dysfunction from reoccurring.

Medical Conditions of the Mouth

Oral Candidiasis

Oral candidiasis is a fungal condition in the mouth that results in a white coating over the tongue and cheeks. This is commonly called thrush and is sometimes caused by antibiotics. This condition is treated by rinsing the mouth with antiseptic mouthwash but sometimes will require antifungal medications prescribed by a physician.

Leukoplasia

Leukoplasia is another oral condition that presents as thickened white areas in the mouth. It can be caused by repeated irritation to an area but may also be a sign of precancerous growths in the oral cavity. A dentist will treat these lesions by removing them and evaluating them. Prompt attention to any oral lesions is prudent care.

Squamous Cell Carcinoma and Kaposi's Sarcoma

Squamous cell carcinoma and Kaposi's sarcoma are both oral cancers, although they can also be found in other areas of the body. Squamous cell carcinoma is identified as lesions in the mouth that do not heal, while Kaposi's sarcoma are more purplish in nature and may appear as nodules or patches. Kaposi's is associated with the human papilloma virus (HPV). Proper and prompt referral for any oral lesions is the proper course of treatment.

Piercing Issues

Some athletes opt to have their body parts pierced, commonly the ears but also the tongue, lips, or nose. This can be problematic because some body parts, such as the mouth, are not sterile. Other complications for piercing include infections, broken teeth, irritation of the soft tissue, allergic reactions to metal, and nerve damage (California Dental Association 2017). Adding to the complication is the fact that people who do the piercings do not have to be licensed or use sterile equipment. Some piercers lack the knowledge of anatomy to understand where blood supply and nerves are located.

> **What Would You Do If . . .**
>
> You observe a basketball player chewing the end off his mouth guard.

An athlete who suffers an infection or nerve damage should be referred to a physician for care. An athlete with an allergic response can remove the jewelry and replace it with a plastic piece or remove it all together. An irritation is generally caused by the post of the jewelry. It may be dealt with by removing the piercing or using dental wax over the area.

Orthodontic Concerns

Braces are common among athletes; therefore, the AT will need to be prepared for emergencies that may result. It can be alarming when athletes experience discomfort from their braces being tightened or protruding wires. Athletes could even swallow a piece of their braces. The most common issues associated with braces are as follows:

- ***Irritation of lip or cheek.*** Braces can rub against the inside of the mouth, causing irritation. This can be resolved by using a dental wax that is applied to the brace. The wax can be made pliable by rolling it between the fingers.
- ***Embedded braces.*** An impact to the mouth can cause braces to be stuck to the soft tissue of the cheek. This can be painful and cause a lot of bleeding. The first step for the AT is to control the bleeding with direct pressure so they can examine the area. Next, the AT will have to carefully remove the tissue from the brace. Once the tissue is removed from the braces, the AT will control the bleeding that may result. To prevent future incidents of this kind, the AT will recommend a mouth guard.
- ***Wire protrusion.*** Sometimes a wire from the braces will come off and stick outward, causing irritation. It is best to use a cotton-tipped applicator

and press the wire so that it lies flat against the teeth (American Association of Orthodontists n.d.). If the protruding wire cannot be pushed into a position of comfort, apply dental wax to the wire. The athlete needs to see a dentist so the brace can be properly repaired.

- ***Soreness after tightening.*** When braces are adjusted, it is normal for the athlete to experience soreness for about a week. When this happens, the AT can offer solace that this pain is only temporary. The AT may recommend soft food or a liquid diet during this time.
- ***Ligature comes off.*** A ligature is a rubber band that attaches to the braces. These rubber bands are very small but easy to reattach. The AT can use a pair of tweezers to put the ligature back in its original placement (American Association of Orthodontists n.d.). If the ligature breaks off, it is best to have the athlete go to a dentist.
- ***Swallowing a piece of the bracing.*** In rare cases, an athlete may swallow a piece of the brace. First, make sure the athlete does not have an obstruction of the airway. If there is an obstruction, follow the instructions in chapter 25 for care. If the airway is not obstructed, have the athlete go to a physician to determine next steps.

Summary

Any impact to the face could injure the eyes, nose, ears, or jaw and could result in permanent disfigurement. Impairment of the facial organs can be devastating to the injured athlete. To prevent facial injuries, an AT should work with the equipment staff to make sure proper equipment is provided and with coaches to make sure the athletes wear the equipment. Facial injuries should be treated conservatively and evaluated by the team physician and dentist. Many disease pathologies can manifest in the anatomical structures of the face. Identifying the signs and symptoms and initiating proper referral will help your athletes get the care they need in a prompt, professional manner.

Key Terms

Define the following terms found in this chapter:

- blowout
- cauliflower ear
- conjunctiva
- conjunctivitis
- corneal abrasion
- crepitus
- dental caries
- detached retina
- epistaxis
- hyphema
- ophthalmologist
- parotid
- rhinitis
- ruptured eardrum
- sinusitis
- subconjunctival hemorrhage
- sublingual
- submandibular
- swimmer's ear
- temporomandibular joint (TMJ) dysfunction

An athlete walks into the athletic training facility. They have been hit in the nose with a field hockey stick. The nose is bleeding profusely and appears to be bent to one side. What are your actions to immediately control the bleeding? What do you do after you stop the bleeding?

To access supplementary material for this chapter, including the Understanding Check worksheet, vocabulary quizzes, extension activities, and chapter-specific resources and forms, visit the web resource: http://ancillaries.humankinetics.com/FundamentalsOfAthleticTrainingAndSportsMedicine5E

chapter 11

Throat and Thorax Injuries

Objectives

After completing this chapter, the student will be able to do the following:

- Understand the basic anatomy of the throat and thorax.
- Understand how to prevent injuries of the throat and thorax.
- Know the care necessary to treat an injury to the throat or thorax.
- Understand the implications of illness or injury related to specific organs in the thorax.
- Understand the fundamentals of monitoring devices and diagnostic testing for selected conditions.

The thorax is between the neck and abdomen. The organs in the thorax are protected by the rib cage and other bony structures. Compromise of the organs and passageways in the throat and thorax is life-threatening. Prompt care can save an athlete's life.

ANATOMY OF THE THROAT

The throat contains the carotid arteries, jugular veins, larynx, trachea, and esophagus. Because these structures are so sensitive and vital to life, the AT must understand their purpose and location (see figure 11.1).

The **esophagus** is the passageway for food going from the mouth to the stomach. It lies in front of the cervical vertebrae and behind the trachea and larynx. The **trachea** is made up of circular rings of cartilage; it is the main trunk of the system of tubes through which air passes to and from the lungs for the exchange of oxygen and carbon dioxide. The **larynx** is the modified upper part of the trachea and contains the vocal cords.

One **carotid artery** and one **jugular vein** pass on each side of the trachea. The carotid arteries carry oxygenated blood to the brain while the jugular veins carry unoxygenated blood away from the brain. Severing one of these vessels can cause death in a short time, so neck protection is vital in

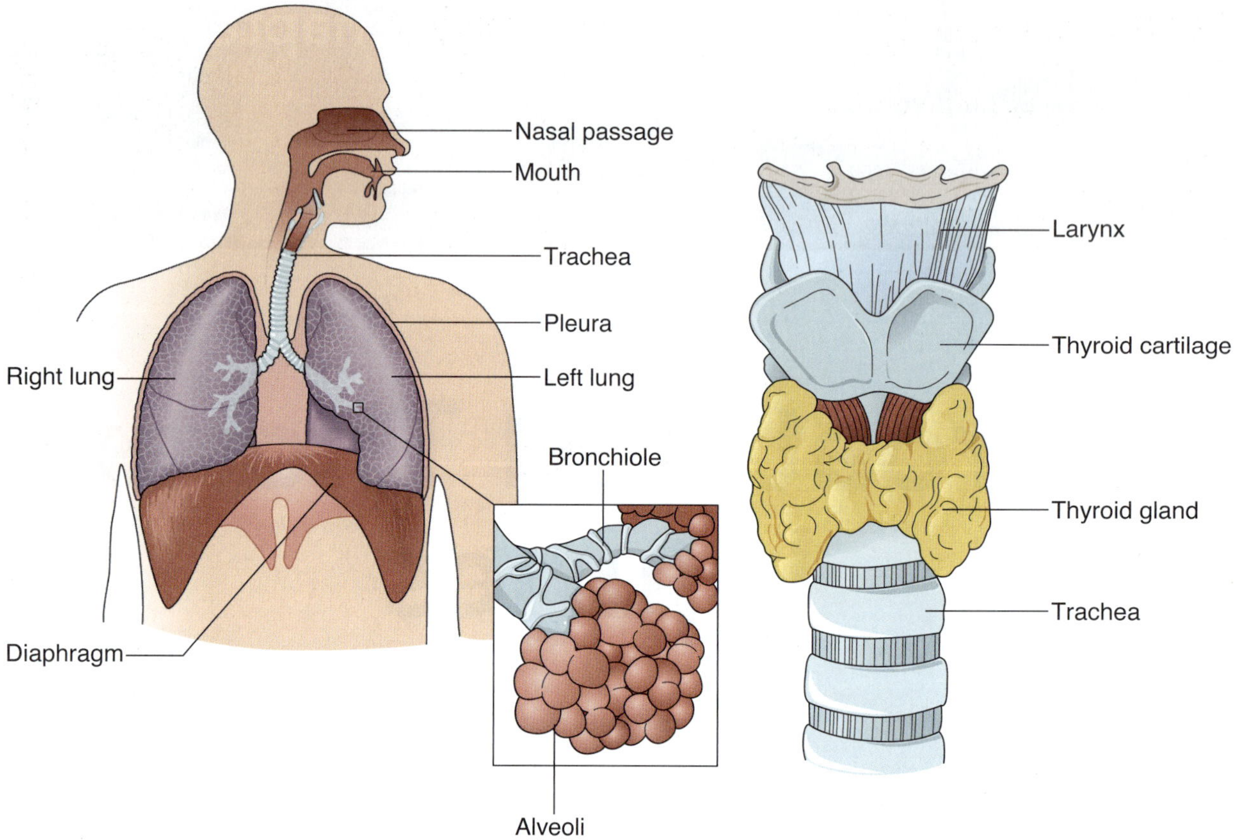

Figure 11.1 Anatomy of the thorax and throat.

sports such as ice hockey and field hockey (Behnke and Plant 2022).

ANATOMY OF THE THORAX

The bony structure of the thorax is made up of the thoracic vertebrae posteriorly, 12 ribs on each side, and the sternum anteriorly (see figure 7.3). These bones protect the sensitive organs in the thorax. The two lowest ribs do not attach to the sternum and are called *floating ribs.*

Heart and Lungs

The heart is about the size of a fist and is responsible for pumping blood to all parts of the body. The blood carries nutrients and oxygen to cells and carbon dioxide and waste products away from cells. The heart is divided into four chambers: the upper chambers, which include the left and right atria, and the lower chambers, which include the left and right **ventricles** (see figure 11.2). The ventricles are generally larger and have thicker walls than the atria because they pump the blood throughout the body.

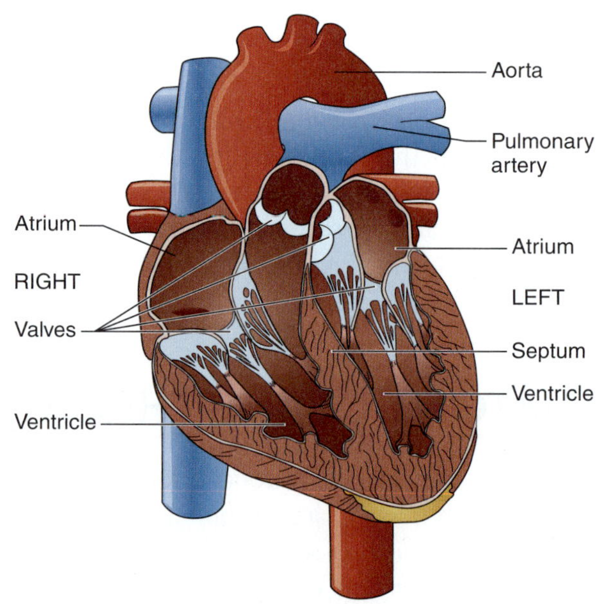

Figure 11.2 Interior of the heart.

Understanding Diversity

Situs Inversus

Situs inversus is a genetic condition in which the organs of the chest and abdomen develop on the reverse side of the body. So, organs found on the right side develop on the left side. This condition occurs in 1 of 10,000 births and is more common among males (Cleveland Clinic 2022).

Exercising the heart muscle makes it larger and more efficient at pumping. However, an enlarged heart can also be a sign of heart disease.

The heart pumps blood to the lungs and around the body (see figure 11.3). The right **atrium** fills with blood from a vein, which is carrying waste products and carbon dioxide. The right ventricle receives blood from the right atrium and pumps it to the lungs to get rid of carbon dioxide and pick up oxygen. The left atrium fills with the oxygenated blood from the lungs. The left ventricle, which is the largest chamber of the heart, receives the oxygenated blood from the left atrium and pumps it throughout the body. The main artery leaving the heart is known as the aorta. The aorta travels downward through the chest and abdomen, and other large arteries branch off to the head (carotid arteries), arms (brachial arteries), and legs (femoral arteries) (see figure 11.4). After the oxygen-rich blood has been delivered to and used by the tissues, the deoxygenated blood returns to the heart through major veins (see figure 11.5).

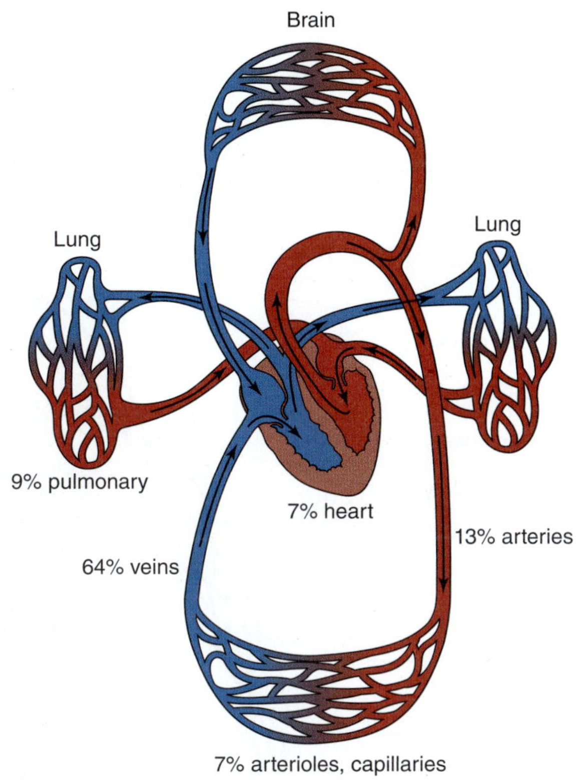

Figure 11.3 Circulation of blood through the heart and distribution to the body.

The sinoatrial (SA) node and **atrioventricular (AV) node** in the right atrium begin a contraction. The SA node is called the pacemaker of the heart. A slight delay in impulses conducted from the nodes through the heart allows blood to be squeezed from one chamber to another. Injured or diseased electrical nodes cause the heart to stop or to beat ineffectively. Irregular heart activity is called an **arrhythmia**.

The lungs, which are located on each side of the heart, exchange oxygen and carbon dioxide and dissipate body heat. The trachea divides into two bronchi, the bronchi further subdivide into bronchioles, and each bronchiole ends in an alveolus, an air-containing cell of the lungs (see figure 11.1). In the **alveoli**, the exchange of oxygen and carbon dioxide occurs. The lung tissue is divided into sections, or lobes. There are three lobes in the right lung and two lobes in the left lung. Lung capacity

FYI

Veins

Veins carry waste products and carbon dioxide back to the heart (except for the pulmonary vein, which carries oxygenated blood to the left atrium).

Arteries

Arteries carry nutrients and oxygenated blood away from the heart and throughout the body. Arteries are elastic vessels that can expand and contract with changes in blood pressure.

Oxygen Rich

As blood passes through the lungs, it picks up oxygen and becomes oxygenated, or oxygen rich. Oxygen is important to feed the cells of the body so they can perform their individual duties. All cells in the body rely on oxygen to remain viable.

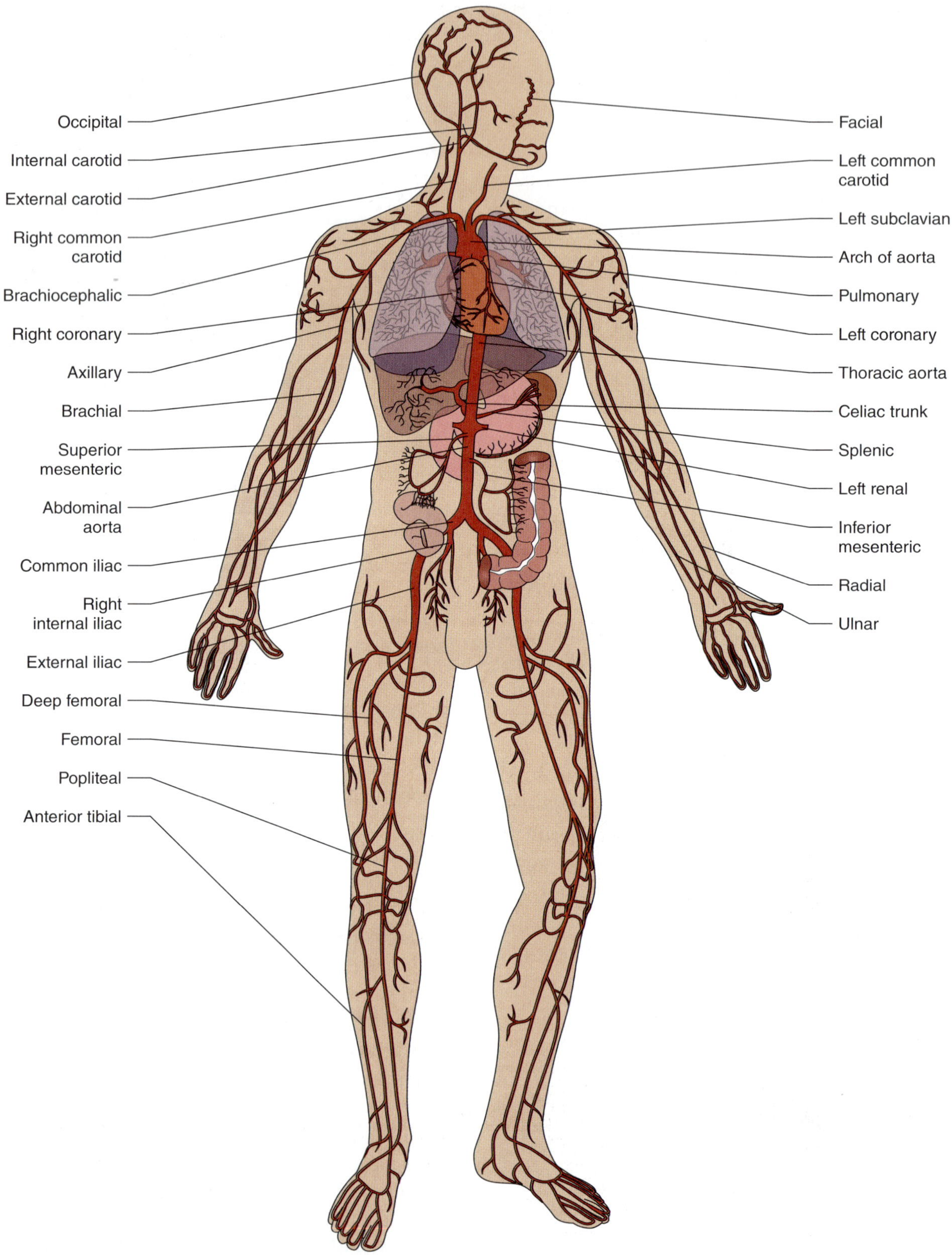

Figure 11.4 Major arteries.

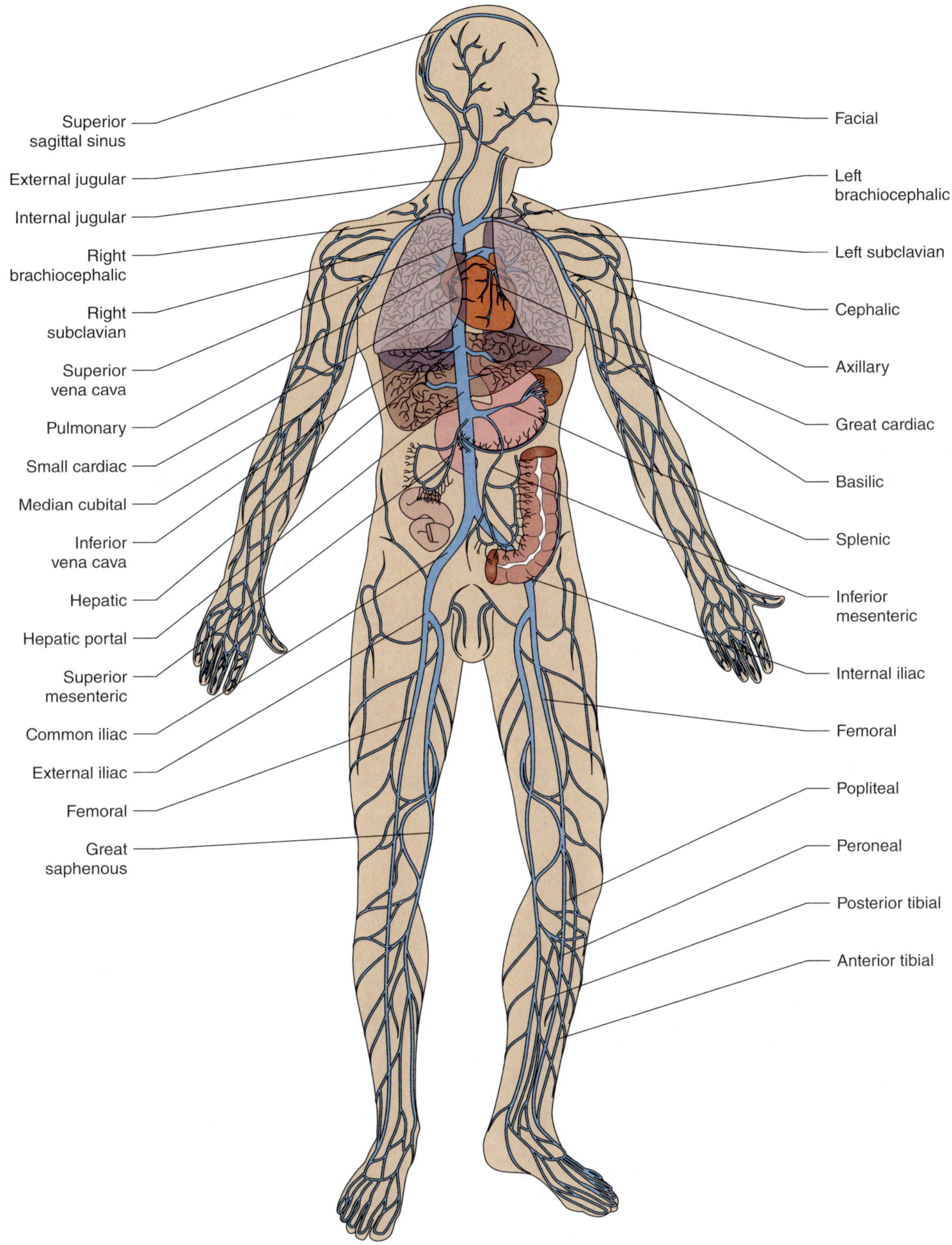

Figure 11.5 Major veins.

is hampered by smoking, pollution, and lung disease. The bronchi are filled with cilia, which are small hairlike projections that help remove foreign substances such as dust and pollen. Coughing and sneezing help to keep the trachea and bronchi clear and remove phlegm and allergy-causing agents.

Lung function and breathing rate are controlled by carbon dioxide receptors. When receptors register the presence of too much carbon dioxide, inhalation occurs. Exercise increases cell metabolism and causes cells to need more oxygen and eliminate more carbon dioxide. This increased cellular need increases the number of breaths per minute. Over time, the ability of the lungs to exchange air effectively increases as the athlete exercises, and the athlete's breaths become deeper and more forceful. Moreover, a conditioned athlete will return to a normal breathing rate more quickly after exercising compared with someone who is out of shape. This return to normal breathing rate is called the recovery rate.

A thin, lubricated tissue called the pleura lines each half of the thorax and is folded back over the surface of the lung on the same side. The pleurae allow smooth movement of the lungs as they encounter the wall of ribs during inhalation and exhalation. There is a small space between the pleura and the lung.

Diaphragm

The **diaphragm** muscle separates the thorax and the abdominal cavity. The diaphragm contracts and pulls down to assist in inhalation and moves upward to push air out of the lungs on exhalation (see figure 11.6). The diaphragm has three openings to allow passage of the esophagus, abdominal aorta (artery), and inferior vena cava (vein). It is supplied by the phrenic nerve. Breathing patterns are also important to understand as an athletic trainer. Figure 11.7 shows the specific breathing patterns you might see in your athletes.

Breathing Patterns

Breathing patterns are anchored in exhalation and inhalation patterns. Regular breathing patterns bring oxygen to the tissues and release carbon dioxide as a waste product. Learning to manage breathing patterns is important in injury management to facilitate the relaxation and control of the diaphragm. Breathing in through the nose and out through the mouth for a count of 5 seconds each helps the athlete focus on breathing and slowing down respirations to allow for better oxygenation. Further, positioning the athlete in an upright position when medically indicated will help open the thoracic region to allow for better lung expansion. Bending

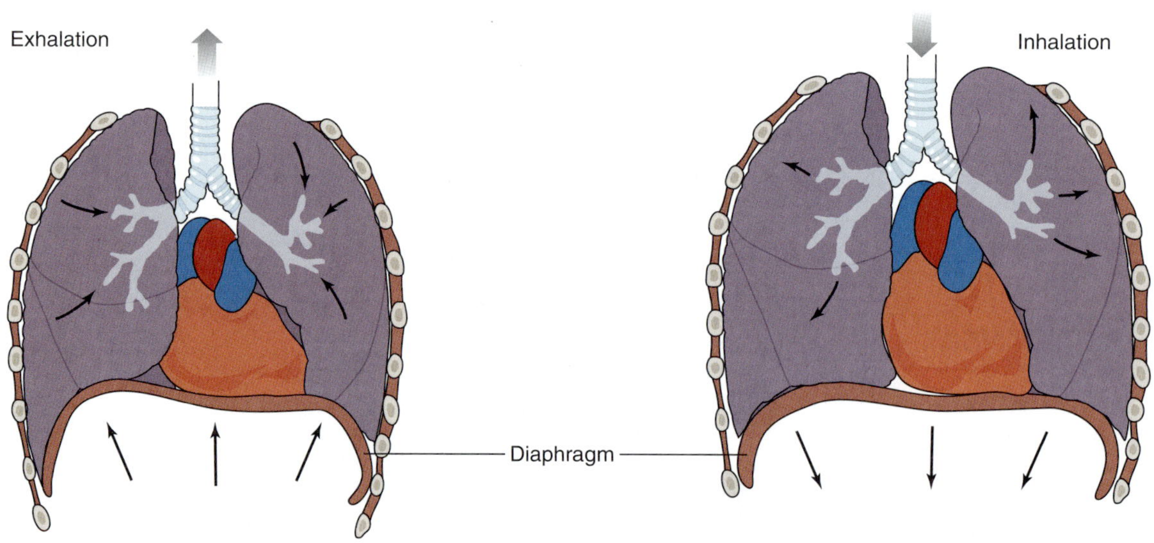

Figure 11.6 Breathing. The diaphragm moves upward during exhalation and downward during inhalation.

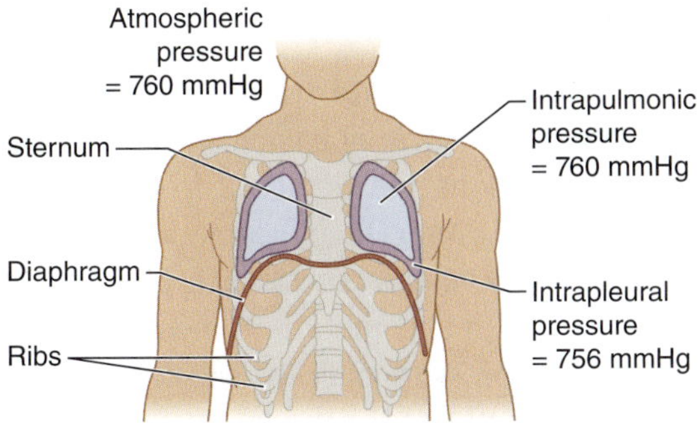

a Resting positions of the diaphragm and the thoracic cage, or thorax. Note the size of the rib cage at rest.

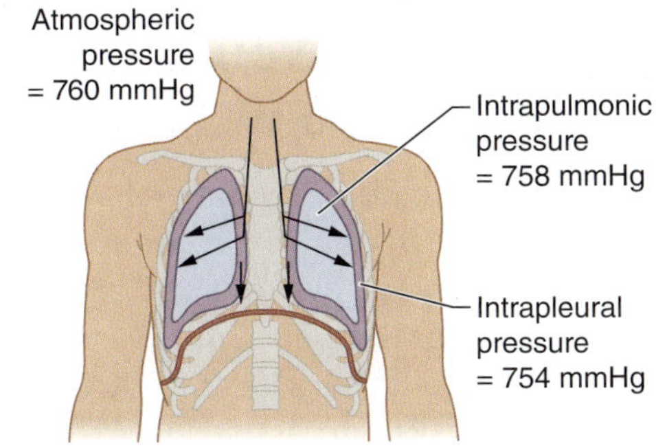

b The dimensions of the lungs and the thoracic cage increase during inspiration, forming a negative pressure that draws air into lungs.

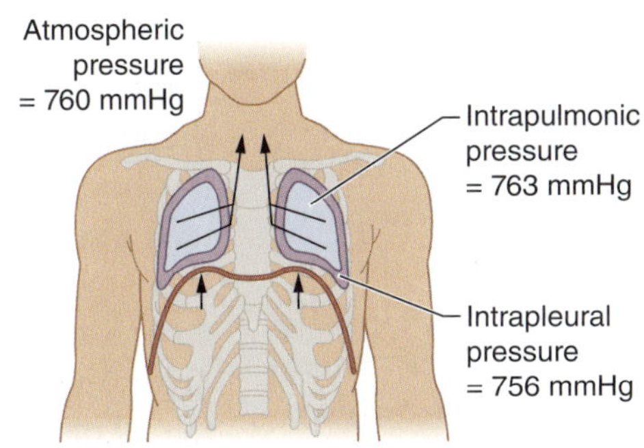

c During expiration, the lungs' volume decrease, thereby forcing air out of the lungs.

Figure 11.7 Breathing patterns.

Reprinted by permission from W.L. Kenney, J.H. Wilmore, and D.L. Costill, *Physiology of Sport and Exercise*, 8th ed. (Champaign, IL: Human Kinetics, 2022), 194.

over will not allow the lungs to fully expand and should not be recommended.

PREVENTING THROAT AND THORAX INJURIES

Protective equipment and rules in athletic contests are designed to prevent injuries to the throat and thorax because these areas contain organs that are vital to life. Thus, athletes wear throat protectors in softball, baseball, lacrosse, field hockey, and ice hockey. In field hockey, lacrosse, football, ice hockey, softball, and baseball, protective equipment—shoulder pads, chest protectors, and sternal pads—is provided for the thorax, especially for goalies. A safe distance between the boundary of a playing surface and objects such as bleachers, fences, scorers' tables, and spectators is 15 feet (4.5 m). In addition, walls, tables, and fences are often padded to prevent injury to athletes who may collide with these objects. Even with these precautions, injuries to the throat and thorax can occur, requiring the AT to react efficiently and effectively to help the athlete.

Many Little League softball and baseball players are required to wear chest protectors when batting because of the danger of being struck in the chest with a ball. If a ball strikes the chest just before a heartbeat is initiated, it can cause the heart to beat irregularly or even stop, which could result in death. Although Little League organizations do not typically have ATs on staff, as an AT you can work with youth organizations to provide educational materials and seminars for parents and coaches to inform them of the importance of protective equipment.

When buying equipment to protect an athlete in a potential life-and-death situation, get the best

> **? What Would You Do If . . .**
>
> You are proudly wearing your new student assistant's uniform of a white sweater. This is the first sweater you have received after working with the AT for two years. At the ice hockey game, the goalie suffers a lacerated vein in the neck. You are asked to assist the AT in stopping the bleeding. Blood is everywhere—it is definitely going to get on your new sweater.

available. Make sure the equipment is certified and will do what it claims. When a baseball hits the chest of a Little Leaguer, the chest protector is supposed to absorb the force and reduce the impact on the heart. However, some of the chest protectors Little Leaguers use are not certified and may increase the chance of irregular heartbeat if a ball hits the chest because they focus the impact over the heart. Protective equipment is not an area where buying used is a good idea. It should be properly fit to the athlete and designed for the individual sport for which it is being used. For example, you do not want to wear a lacrosse chest protector for baseball. The composition of the ball and the force at which it can affect the body are different in most sports.

TREATING THROAT INJURIES AND CONDITIONS

Throat injuries can be simple or devastating. Most of the injuries that occur to the throat are contusions caused by blows from sticks, feet, or arms. Contusions can be treated by applying ice. In any type of throat injury, the athlete will experience coughing, spitting, difficulty breathing, and pain. If the airway is compromised or the athlete has difficulty breathing, it is prudent to refer the athlete for immediate care. Swelling that evolves over time can further restrict the airway after the initial injury. Err on the side of caution in these injuries (Cleary and Walsh Flanagan 2020).

Throat Laceration

A throat laceration could occur, for example, when one player's ice skate goes across another player's throat. Lacerations that are not deep can be handled with direct pressure. Deep lacerations or those that affect a jugular vein or carotid artery are true medical emergencies and require immediate treatment. Apply direct pressure over the site of the laceration and treat the athlete for shock. The athlete will be placed on their side with their feet elevated. The injured side must be placed closest to the ground. Throat lacerations can allow oxygen into the circulatory system, which can cause an **air embolism** and sudden death. If air enters the vein or artery, it can block blood flow. Reduced blood flow causes tissue death. The air embolism gravitates toward the body part that is elevated—in this case, the feet. The vessels in the neck are large, and a massive amount of blood will be lost rapidly, so the AT must respond quickly to save the athlete's life. To review procedures for treating hemorrhages, see the Hemorrhage section in chapter 25.

Cartilage Fracture

A severe blow to the throat can result in a fracture of the circular cartilaginous rings of the trachea, which can be life-threatening. This can happen with a direct blow from another player or from a piece of equipment striking the throat region. The athlete will have difficulty breathing and talking, gasp for air, spit up blood, complain of pain, and be very anxious. Their skin may turn a bluish color due to lack of oxygen. The AT must exercise caution when treating a cartilage fracture because the trauma also may have caused a cervical spine fracture. This is a medical emergency. The AT will place the athlete on a backboard for transport to the hospital and apply ice to the area to reduce swelling. Those treating the athlete must remain calm to keep the athlete calm. Keep the airway free of blood and make sure medical care is on the way. Prepare for emergency medical intervention while waiting for EMS by having an AED ready on-site.

Medical Conditions of the Throat

Athletes often come to the AT complaining of a sore throat. Although this is not the result of an injury,

The Real World

At an ice hockey game, a young man was trying to stop a shot on goal with a diving headfirst slide. The slap shot hit him square in the throat. It was immediately apparent that he was in a life-threatening condition. The team physician and AT jumped onto the ice before play was stopped. They quickly assessed him and found he had difficulty breathing, a blue skin tone, an inability to speak, and rapid swelling over the throat. They iced his throat and put him on a backboard. His breathing was constantly monitored, and the physician was ready to make an emergency airway. Paramedics arrived and took the young man to the hospital. He recovered—with a deeper voice and partial loss of the use of his vocal cords. He now wears a throat protector, and he slides feetfirst to stop slap shots!

Lorin Cartwright, MS, ATC

it is the AT's responsibility to identify the signs and symptoms of common conditions. **Tonsilitis** is an inflammation of the tonsils and results in a sore throat, fever, and hoarse voice. Athletes will have visibly swollen tonsils (or redness in the tonsil area) when the back of the throat is inspected. **Pharyngitis** is inflammation of the pharynx. People with this condition often have pain in their throat, swollen glands, and throat irritation. **Laryngitis** is an irritation of the voice box or vocal cords from overuse or irritation. This can also cause pain, redness, and discomfort when talking. Most athletes will get better with rest, fluids, and over-the-counter pain medications; however, it is always prudent to have them check with a physician if they have a fever or do not feel better in a few days. Anytime the athlete reports a difficulty swallowing or breathing from these conditions, they should be sent immediately to the emergency room for care.

TREATING THORAX INJURIES AND CONDITIONS

Many people suffer from conditions such as asthma or experience hyperventilation. Additionally, if the thorax is not adequately protected, it is vulnerable to blunt trauma that can result in fractures of the ribs or sternum. Moreover, severe trauma may cause a lung or cardiac injury. Some medical conditions can also put an athlete at risk and the AT should identify them in order to provide proper preventive and acute care.

Hyperventilation

Hyperventilation is quick, deep breathing at a rate of more than 24 breaths per minute, which leads to abnormal loss of carbon dioxide from the blood. The condition can be caused by an athlete becoming too excited and beginning to breathe rapidly or by an underlying illness such as diabetes. If the athlete does not get breathing under control, they will experience lightheadedness; numbing of the fingers, toes, and lips; and loss of consciousness. As hyperventilation continues, muscular contractions will occur in the limbs. To treat hyperventilation, the AT should talk calmly to the athlete and encourage them to control their breathing rate.

Exercise-Induced Asthma

Asthma is a chronic inflammation of the breathing passageways to the lungs. The triggers can be many, but in this instance, exercise causes the asthma attack. The bronchi spasm and narrow the breathing passageways. This narrowing causes the athlete to wheeze and struggle with taking a full breath. The feeling has been described as if one is breathing through a straw. An athlete may also experience tightness of the chest, their lips and fingernails may turn blue, and they may cough and produce mucus.

The immediate treatment is to have the athlete stop activity, sit upright, and breathe in through the nose and out through the mouth (see figure 11.8). The athlete should take the medication that has been prescribed before the attack gets worse. This medication is typically in an aerosol form called an inhaler. Emergency or rescue inhalers are short acting and will open the airways immediately, and long-lasting inhalers are intended to prevent attacks by keeping the airway open all the time. Inhalers are prescribed for individual athletes and should not be given to anyone other than the person for whom it is prescribed.

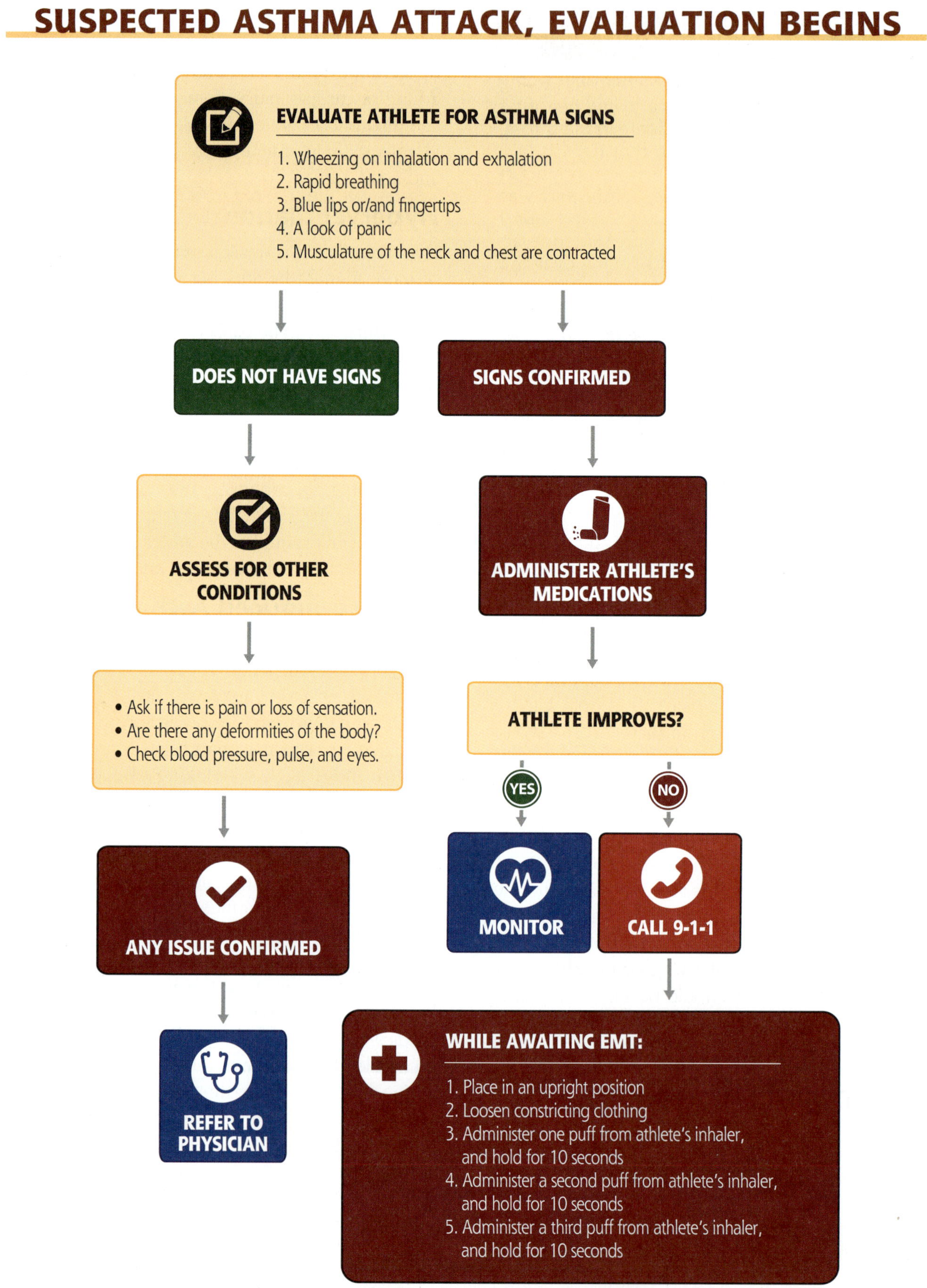

Figure 11.8 Treating an asthmatic attack.

If medications are not available or not working, breathing must be controlled, even though the person feels as if they are not getting enough air. Breathing in through the nose humidifies and cleans the air. Exhalations should last for a count of five. If mucus is coughed up, the athlete should lean forward and remove it. They should continue to control their breathing and relax as much as possible. If the athlete is unable to breathe or is progressively worsening, EMS must be called, and the AT must be prepared to perform CPR, including getting the AED.

One successful preventive method is to have athletes take their medication about 20 minutes before exercise. Athletes who have a known asthma problem should be tested during their preparticipation physical with a spirometer. A spirometer is a device that measures air volume, both in and out. The spirometer measurements are recorded on the athlete's physical form. The spirometer can be used to test air volume at the time of a suspected attack; if it is less than the preparticipation amount, an asthma attack should be the diagnosis.

Jogger's Nipple

Jogger's nipple is most commonly found among male athletes. It occurs when the shirt one is wearing rubs against the nipple repetitively. It is called *jogger's nipple* because long-distance runners suffer this condition most often. The nipple becomes irritated, sometimes to the point where application of a lubricant or bandages becomes necessary.

Prevention involves using a lubricant or applying an adhesive bandage over the nipple. Often, the athlete will find a fabric that will help to prevent this injury. Moisture-wicking clothing will help to prevent chafing. If the irritation does not subside with minimal treatment, a physician may have to evaluate the athlete to determine if an infection has occurred.

What Would You Do If . . .

An athlete comes off the playing field where you are standing and is having trouble catching their breath. You ask what happened and they say, "I just got the wind knocked out of me. I'll be fine in a minute." The minute passes, and they are still struggling to catch their breath.

Blow to the Solar Plexus

The typical cause of a solar plexus injury is a blow to the area of the diaphragm that hits the nerve in the solar plexus. When this occurs, the athlete will struggle to take a breath because the diaphragm spasms. After a short time, the diaphragm relaxes, and the person is able to breathe normally again. The AT should reassure the athlete while they recover and have the athlete practice controlled breathing patterns. Further, keeping the athlete upright will give the diaphragm and lungs more room to recover through normal movements.

Pulmonary Contusion

A pulmonary contusion is a bruise of the lung due to impact, such as from a baseball to the chest or a tackle. The contusion results in an accumulation of blood and other fluids in the lung tissue. Unfortunately, the accumulated fluid keeps the lung from exchanging oxygen and carbon dioxide, and the larger the contusion, the more serious the injury. The athlete will have difficulty breathing and may have a bluish skin color. Pulmonary contusions can also cause a tear in the lung if the rib is compressed into the lung tissue. Application of ice may be helpful, but EMS must be called immediately to ensure the proper imaging tests and treatment.

Myocardial Contusion

The heart can become bruised from an impact over the chest, such as from a ball or a shoulder into the chest. An athlete may experience chest pain, especially over the sternum, and a rapid heart rate. The athlete may become unconscious from the blow. In this instance, the injury merits calling EMS and treating the athlete for shock while preparing to administer CPR if needed.

Rib Contusion

A rib contusion is caused by the same impact or compression as a rib fracture, but the force does not cause a fracture. There is pain, and signs and symptoms may be similar to those of a rib fracture.

When the AT evaluates the athlete, there is pain over the site of the impact but not on compression away from the site.

Treatment involves ice application and rest. An athlete may participate as pain allows. The area may have to be padded to allow participation. A rib belt or pads can also be used in collision and contact sports to protect the ribs from injury. A variety of rib pads are available and specific to individual sports.

Ruptured Diaphragm

Though infrequent, the diaphragm can rupture from a blow to the general area of the diaphragm. The athlete will present with difficulty breathing with no real trauma to the chest. The athlete may have other internal injuries, most likely in the abdominal region. If the AT auscultates the chest, bowel sounds may be heard.

Treatment is to care for the presenting signs or symptoms. If the athlete is having difficulty breathing, elevating the head will be helpful. Treat the athlete for shock and call EMS while preparing for CPR. This injury is hard to diagnose, so immediate medical referral is necessary.

Sternal Fracture

Sternal fractures occur because of direct impact. Impact to the sternum that causes a fracture can be expected to also cause internal injuries, so the heart and lungs may be involved. A suspected sternum fracture is treated with application of ice and a referral to the hospital. If the sternum is only contused from the impact, the athlete could possibly return to activity with a special sternal pad.

Rib Fracture

A rib fracture is caused by direct impact or chest compression. On rare occasions, a sudden violent muscular contraction, such as throwing a baseball, will cause a rib stress fracture. Blows to the front or back of the ribs generally do not result in inward displacement of the fractured rib. Blows to the lateral aspect, however, are more likely to lead to inward penetration, causing complications such as internal bleeding or a punctured lung.

An athlete with fractured ribs experiences pain and difficulty breathing. The pain increases with inhalation, and the athlete usually holds a hand over the injured area to support the ribs, which is called splinting. The area may be deformed due to swelling. A key to determining if a rib is fractured or severely contused is to note whether the athlete experiences increased pain with inhalation but not exhalation. If there is pain during both inhalation and exhalation, the athlete more likely has a contusion.

Treatment for uncomplicated rib fractures involves applying ice and sending the athlete for X-rays. The team physician will restrict the athlete's physical activity until inhalation is not painful. If the athlete participates in a collision or contact sport, all activity should be stopped for six weeks. When the athlete returns to competition, they should wear protective padding or equipment.

Flail Chest

Flail chest occurs when several consecutive ribs are fractured in two or more places (see figure 11.9). This injury occurs from an impact directly to the ribs. The entire fractured portion moves in and out when the athlete breathes; however, the portion moves opposite to the normal breathing pattern. Normally the chest expands and the ribs move outward during inhalation, and during exhalation, the chest moves inward. With a flail chest, the fractured portion moves outward during exhalation and inward during inhalation. This movement creates

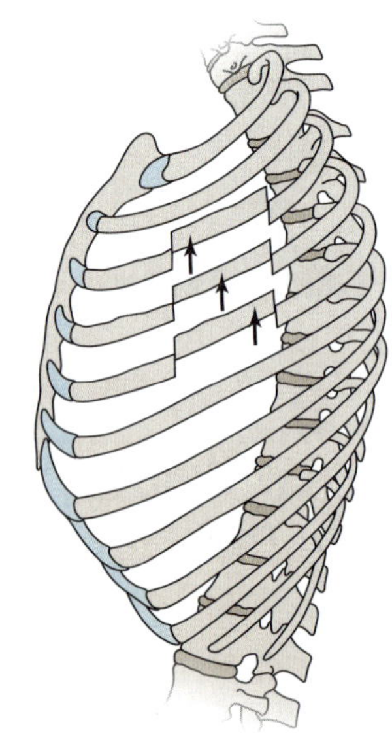

Figure 11.9 When two or more ribs are broken in two places, it makes flail chest possible—the broken section of ribs move inward toward the heart and lungs during inhalation and outward during exhalation.

extreme pain and difficulty breathing. Breathing will be painful and distressed, the athlete will be anxious, and skin tone will be bluish. The athlete should be checked for other internal injuries, especially lung contusions.

Treatment of a flail chest includes decreasing the movement of the fractured ribs. This can be accomplished by placing an object such as a light sandbag or pillow over the fractured segment to keep it from moving. The athlete can be placed on the injured side as a way of controlling the movement of the flail chest, and they also should be treated for shock. This is a medical emergency and requires rapid advanced care.

Pneumothorax

A **pneumothorax** is the presence of air in the pleural cavity, commonly known as a collapsed lung, which can occur either with or without trauma. A traumatic pneumothorax can occur from a rib puncturing the lung, a gunshot wound, or a severe laceration. A nontraumatic pneumothorax occurs due to a weakness of the lung tissue. When a pneumothorax occurs, the injured lung moves toward the center of the chest, which puts pressure on the heart and the other lung. Because only one lung is functioning, the athlete will have trouble breathing and will gasp for air. As the athlete continues to breathe, air goes through the hole in the lung and into the chest cavity, which causes the collapsed lung to compress the heart and opposite lung even further.

Spontaneous Pneumothorax

When the lung tissue has an imperfection, it can cause the lung to collapse, which is also known as a spontaneous pneumothorax. There need not be any impact or illness associated with a spontaneous pneumothorax; the athlete may have appeared healthy in the past and had no previous signs of illness. The athlete will have trouble breathing and chest pain and possibly have a bluish color of the skin if breathing is poor.

The athlete should be placed so that the side with the injured lung is closest to the ground. The AT will treat the athlete for shock and get them to a hospital. In general, a spontaneous pneumothorax will heal itself without surgical intervention but should be evaluated by a physician.

Tension Pneumothorax

An athlete with a pneumothorax may develop a more serious problem called a *tension pneumothorax*. As air leaks out of the collapsed lung and into the chest cavity, it forces the lung to press against the other lung and the heart. If the AT observes the trachea deviated to the side of the throat, they should suspect tracheal shifting. As pressure builds in the chest, the trachea moves away from the side of the pneumothorax. If the trachea moves, the athlete will experience severe respiratory distress. As more air enters the chest cavity, more pressure builds against the heart and uninjured lung. As the pressure mounts, the heart begins to labor as blood flow and breathing are impeded. Death can occur if the athlete is not treated rapidly. If the athlete has an external puncture wound, partially cover it, leaving one side unsealed. Sealing the wound entirely will prevent the inner air from escaping, worsening the tension pneumothorax.

With tension pneumothorax, the athlete will experience respiratory distress, absent breath sounds on the injured side, anxiety, and bluish skin color. Their pulse will be rapid and weak, and their blood pressure will drop. As the pneumothorax worsens, tracheal deviation and neck vein distention will occur, as will bulging of the muscles between the ribs. The AT should place the athlete so that the side with the injured lung is closest to the ground, treat them for shock, and get them to a hospital. This injury requires a physician to insert a chest tube to allow air to escape as well as possible surgical intervention.

Sucking Chest Wound

If the wall of the chest is punctured and air from the outside is drawn noisily into the cavity, the athlete has a sucking chest wound (see figure 11.10). In this injury, the lung is not punctured. However, the air that is being sucked into the chest cavity applies pressure on the lungs and heart, causing distress. The athlete will have difficulty breathing, and circulation may become impaired, resulting in a bluish skin color. The athlete is best treated by sealing the

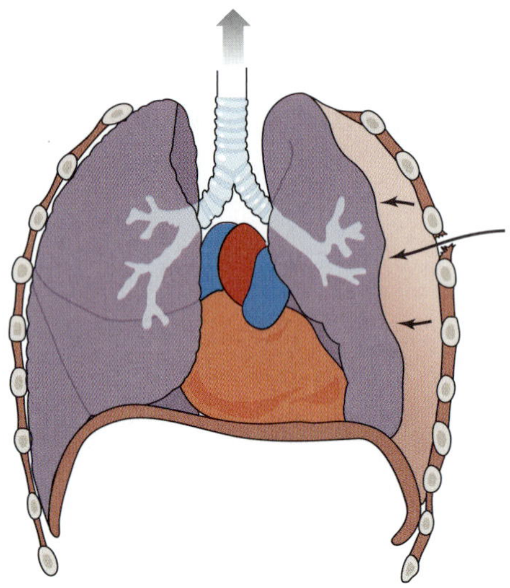

Figure 11.10 Sucking chest wound. When the chest is pierced, air can enter the chest cavity directly from the outside, which causes the lung on the same side to compress. Breathing becomes difficult.

wound with a cellophane wrap or a piece of plastic from a plastic bag. EMS must be called immediately.

Hemothorax

A **hemothorax** is blood in the chest cavity. The bleeding can occur from an internal injury, such as a ruptured lung or blood vessel. A hemothorax may also occur from an external wound that penetrates the chest, such as a javelin into the chest.

A hemothorax is similar to a pneumothorax in that the blood puts pressure on the heart and lungs, which decreases their ability to function normally. As blood fills the chest cavity, the athlete will have difficulty breathing, may turn blue from lack of oxygen, may become unconscious, will have a rapid weak pulse, will sweat, and will go into shock. Breath sounds may be absent on the side of the bleeding.

Bleeding into the chest cavity is serious and requires immediate care to prevent death. The AT must call EMS for immediate transportation to the hospital and control the bleeding as best they can. The athlete may require CPR if advanced help is delayed.

Cardiac Tamponade

Blows to the thorax can affect not only the lungs but also the heart. There is a thin pericardial sac around the heart. When fluid fills the sac, it places pressure on the heart to the point where it may stop beating. An injury to the heart increases fluid in the sac. In athletics, the most likely cause is a blow to the chest.

Cardiac tamponade is a medical emergency that will cause death if not diagnosed and treated

! RED FLAGS

Call 911 if any the following signs or symptoms exist with a throat or thorax injury:

- Difficulty breathing
- Wheezing
- Low blood pressure of 90/60 (National Heart, Lung, and Blood Institute n.d.)
- Uncontrolled severe bleeding
- Rapid breathing
- Shock
- Narrow pulse pressure
- Bluish skin color
- Extreme pain
- Hearing bowel sounds in the chest
- Deformity

quickly. The athlete will be in shock, with all the signs and symptoms. The defining sign of cardiac tamponade is a narrowing pulse pressure, meaning the systolic and diastolic pressures come closer together after each repetitive taking of the blood pressure. EMS must be called and oxygen administered. On arrival at the emergency room, a needle will be inserted into the chest to remove the fluid.

Dorsal Aortic Rupture

The aorta can be ruptured with a severe deceleration force to the chest over the dorsal aorta. This is often seen in car accidents when the strap of the seat belt tightens rapidly during a sudden deceleration. In sport, the most common deceleration is a severe blow to the chest, such as a hit in football.

In dorsal aortic rupture, the aorta commonly tears away from the heart, and the athlete most often bleeds to death in seconds. Those who do not die may have a partial tear and can bleed to death more slowly. They will show signs of shock and will be anxious. The deceleration, or severe blow, may be the most revealing determination of this injury. If this happens, EMS must be called, and the athlete must not be moved. Movement can cause the aorta to shift, resulting in immediate death.

Medical Conditions to the Thorax

Pneumonia

Pneumonia involves an infection in the lungs. Pneumonia can be either viral or bacterial. Pneumonia makes it hard for the athlete to breathe and is commonly associated with a fever, cough, and fatigue. Proper care involves referral to a physician for a chest X-ray and prescription medication. A pneumonia vaccine is now widely available but is often used for persons older than 40.

Pleurisy

Pleurisy is created by an inflammation between the lining of the lung and the chest wall. Pleurisy causes pain with breathing and is typically caused by another infection, such as bacterial pneumonia or viral flu. Although this is painful, the treatment for pleurisy is rest and anti-inflammatory medications. Athletes will likely be referred for an X-ray.

Emphysema and Chronic Obstructive Pulmonary Disease

Emphysema and **chronic obstructive pulmonary disease (COPD)** are respiratory conditions commonly associated with smoking. Emphysema results when the air sacs in the lungs get clogged with mucus, making it difficult to breathe. People with emphysema will be short of breath, fatigued due to lack of oxygen, and typically have a bad cough. COPD is a chronic condition of the lungs that results from scarring of the lung tissue. It creates obstructions in the lungs, making air exchange difficult. People with COPD will have lower than normal oxygen saturation (as measured by a pulse oximeter) and will often breathe more rapidly but shallower. Emphysema and COPD are managed through medical care teams that are usually led by a pulmonologist.

Bronchitis

Bronchitis is an infection in the bronchi of the lungs. This is commonly seen in the wintertime and is associated with the common cold. It is also associated with smoking and worksite inhalants or chemicals that cause damage and inflammation to the bronchi. Bronchitis can cause more severe symptoms and is characterized by a hoarse cough and thick mucus. Bronchitis should be treated by a physician.

Tuberculosis

Tuberculosis is a serious bacterial infection that affects the lungs. Although most people are vaccinated against tuberculosis in the United States, it is still a medical condition that might evolve in the athletic training setting. People with tuberculosis will report with a cough, night sweats, and weight loss. Any athlete reporting these symptoms should be referred immediately because tuberculosis is spread through air droplets when coughing and could create a potentially contagious environment in the athletic training facility if not managed promptly.

Lung Cancer

Lung cancer is characterized by lesions or tumors in the lungs. Lung cancer can affect people of all ages and is commonly associated with smoking or exposure to hazardous inhalants through work or at home. Many people who have lung cancer, however, have not smoked. As with any cancer, abnormal cells replicate to create tumors. Lungs can be the original site of the cancer or they can be a secondary site where it has metastasized. Cancers are classified by stages, with stage I being the least serious and stage IV being the most advanced. Lung cancer is diagnosed through CT and PET scans, and care is managed by an oncologist.

Cardiomyopathy and Sudden Cardiac Death

Cardiomyopathy and sudden cardiac death are conditions that you hope you never encounter as an AT. With cardiomyopathy, the heart muscle becomes weakened and is unable to pump blood through the body effectively. Cardiomyopathy can lead to heart failure, where the heart is simply unable to circulate the blood effectively, causing debilitation and eventually death. Sudden cardiac death is a loss of cardiac function that results in the death of the athlete. It occurs without warning typically, and even with prompt medical attention, the athlete may not survive. Sudden cardiac death is a difficult situation for the AT and team because it often occurs on the athletic field or court. Many organizations are available to help the AT and their team cope with these sudden losses. ATs Care is NATA's peer-to-peer support group of trained colleagues who can help you deal with a sudden loss at your school. Valuable resources regarding how to get trained for this and how to seek help should you need it are found at www.nata.org.

Aneurysms

Aneurysms occur in vessels in the body. They occur when a blood vessel has a weakened spot on the wall causing it to bulge out and rupture. Once the vessel ruptures, it is a true medical emergency. Aneurysms can occur in any vessel in the body, but aneurysms in the brain and in the abdominal aorta are common sites. Each of these carries unique dangers and should be referred immediately to EMS or the hospital for urgent care. The long-term effects of a ruptured blood vessel in a major organ such as the heart or brain can be life-altering or fatal.

Coronary Artery Blockage

Coronary arteries supply the heart muscle itself (figure 11.11). They are the plumbing system of the heart. Several key vessels are associated with blockages: left anterior descending (LAD), right coronary artery (RCA), left coronary artery (LCA), and the left circumflex (CX) artery. Vessels in the heart become blocked by plaque buildup inside the vessel. This results in decreased blood flow to that part of the heart. Blockages are diagnosed using an electrocardiogram (ECG), along with other tests (figure 11.12). If a blockage is found, the cardiologist will likely put in a stent to hold that part of the vessel open. If many are blocked, open heart surgery may be needed. Although all the vessels are important, the LAD is commonly called the widowmaker because when it is significantly blocked, the chance of survival is low.

Myocarditis

Myocarditis involves an inflammation of the heart muscle itself. Commonly caused by an infection, myocarditis should be diagnosed and treated by a physician. Athletes with myocarditis will report chest pain, shortness of breath, and fatigue. Immediate referral is prudent.

Hypertension

Hypertension is another term for high blood pressure. The pressure the blood exerts against the walls of the arteries will be measured by a sphygmomanometer or blood pressure cuff, as discussed in chapter 6. If someone has a systolic pressure above 140 mm/Hg and a diastolic pressure above 90 mm/Hg, they will be diagnosed with hypertension. There are many causes of high blood pressure, but poor diet, no exercise, high stress, and genetics all play an important role in this condition. Physicians manage this condition with recommended lifestyle changes and prescription medications when needed.

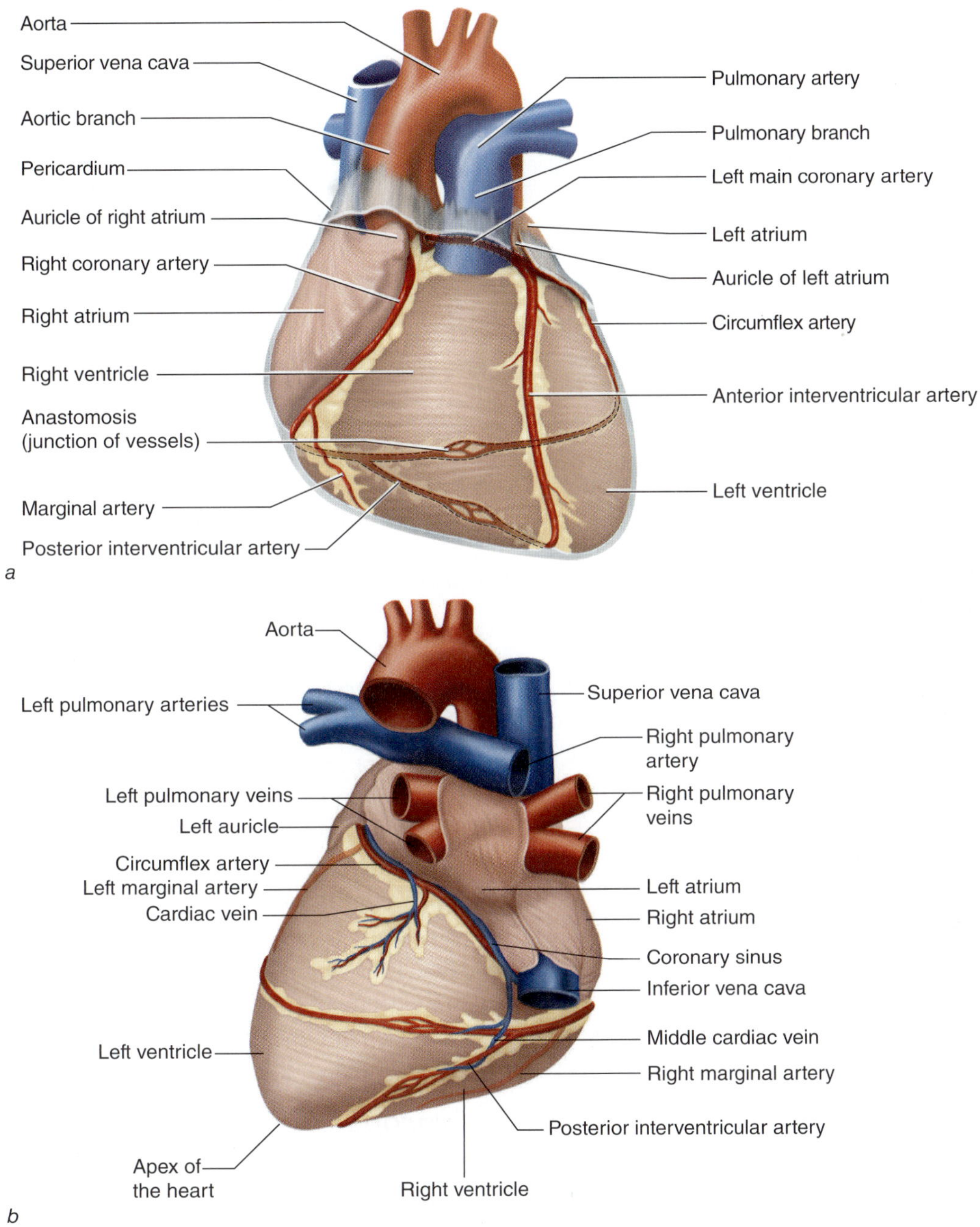

Figure 11.11 Coronary arteries: *(a)* anterior and *(b)* posterior.

Reprinted by permission from R.S. Behnke and J. Plant, *Kinetic Anatomy*, 4th ed. (Champaign, IL: Human Kinetics, 2022), 181.

Deep Vein Thrombosis

Deep vein thrombosis (DVT) is a blood clot that forms in the deep veins of the body. When a clot forms in the vein, it occludes blood flow as it returns to the heart. As a result, blood will start to build up in distal parts to thc clot, causing significant discomfort. People with DVT will experience deep pain and pressure. A DVT is a serious condition, and any suspected DVT should be referred immediately to a physician for care. These are diagnosed clinically as well as with ultrasound technology. DVTs commonly form after surgery or on long plane rides due to long periods of inactivity.

Embolism

An **embolism** is an air bubble or blood clot that moves through the circulatory system and reaches a

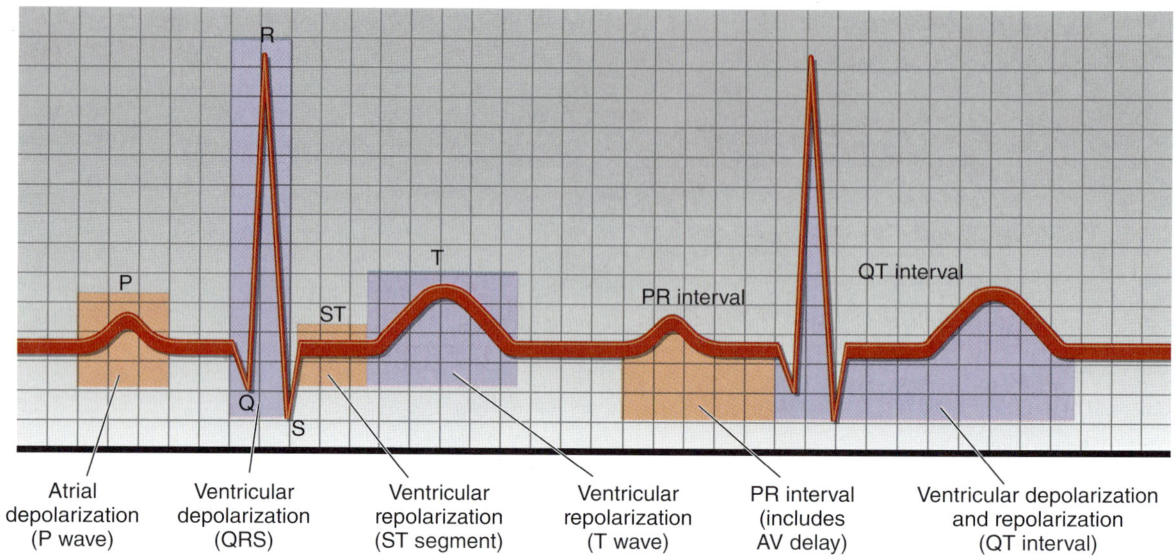

Figure 11.12 ECG.

Reprinted by permission from M.A. Cleary and K.W. Flanagan, *Acute and Emergency Care in Athletic Training* (Champaign, IL: Human Kinetics, 2020), 307.

specific part of the body. Emboli are potentially fatal when they land in the lungs (pulmonary emboli) or brain or heart. These are often sudden medical events that require prompt advanced medical interventions to ensure survival.

Anemia

Anemia is a condition that affects the blood. Since our blood is made up of different components, doctors evaluate the different cells as well as the amount of hemoglobin in our blood. Hemoglobin helps carry oxygen to our cells, so if an athlete is anemic, they will feel tired, fatigued, and dizzy. They will be advised to increase the amount of iron in their diet or may be prescribed iron tablets. These athletes are often treated by a hematologist.

Hemolysis

Hemolysis is the breakdown of the red blood cells in the body. Although our bodies normally do this to destroy older cells and replace them with more efficient ones, sometimes the body does this prematurely, resulting in a decrease in red blood cells and anemia. Hemolysis can be stimulated by certain medications, stress, toxins, and even intense exercise. Any athlete who reports fatigue and shortness of breath and has a blue tinge to the white of their eyes should be referred for evaluation.

Peripheral Artery Disease

Peripheral artery disease (PAD) affects the blood supply at the farthest parts of the circulatory system. People with PAD will have poor circulation in their feet, hands, tip of nose, ears, and other distal parts. Due to disease, the peripheral (small) vessels close down, causing discoloration (bluish tint), lack of sensation, coldness, and other problems. People with PAD often experience amputations due to the extremely poor blood flow to certain regions. Diabetic patients, the elderly, and smokers are particularly vulnerable to this disease.

Syncope

Syncope is a condition where an individual loses consciousness for a brief period. There are many causes of syncope, especially related to the thorax and throat diseases. However, syncope can occur for many different reasons, including stress, shock, or heat. Treatment for syncope involves a prompt evaluation of the cardiorespiratory function. If they have a pulse and are breathing, a secondary evaluation for the potential cause can resume.

Mitral Valve Prolapse

Mitral valve prolapse (MVP) is commonly associated with women after menopause. Hormonal changes in the body are said to weaken the valve, causing it to be less effective. However, athletes at any age, including men and women alike, can experience MVP. As a result, the valve does not close completely, causing blood from one chamber of the heart to backflow into the adjacent chamber. This is called regurgitation. A physician can typically hear this using a stethoscope, but sometimes advanced medical testing is required, such as an echocardiogram, to see the detailed anatomy of the valve (figure 11.13). A cardiologist will treat patients with MVP.

Breast Lumps and Cancers

Breast lumps and cancers are conditions that require referral if brought to the AT's attention. Athletes are encouraged to perform breast self-examinations to detect any changes in the density or surface texture of the breast. A gynecologist or physician can evaluate the mass. Sometimes, the doctor can determine if it is worrisome or not, but most often, an ultrasound imaging test or mammogram (see figure 11.14) will be ordered. These tests show the specific size, shape, and composition of the mass. Some masses are benign and will be evaluated periodically by the physician. Masses that are suspected to be cancerous will require further consultation and treatment by an oncologist (Johns Hopkins Medicine n.d.).

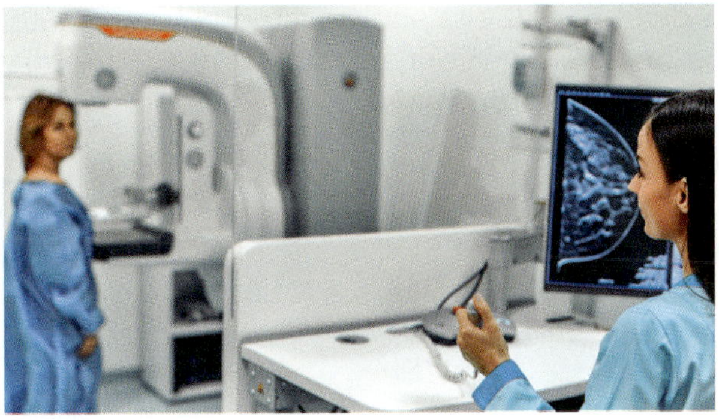

Figure 11.14 Mammogram.
Valerii Apetroaiei/iStock/Getty Images

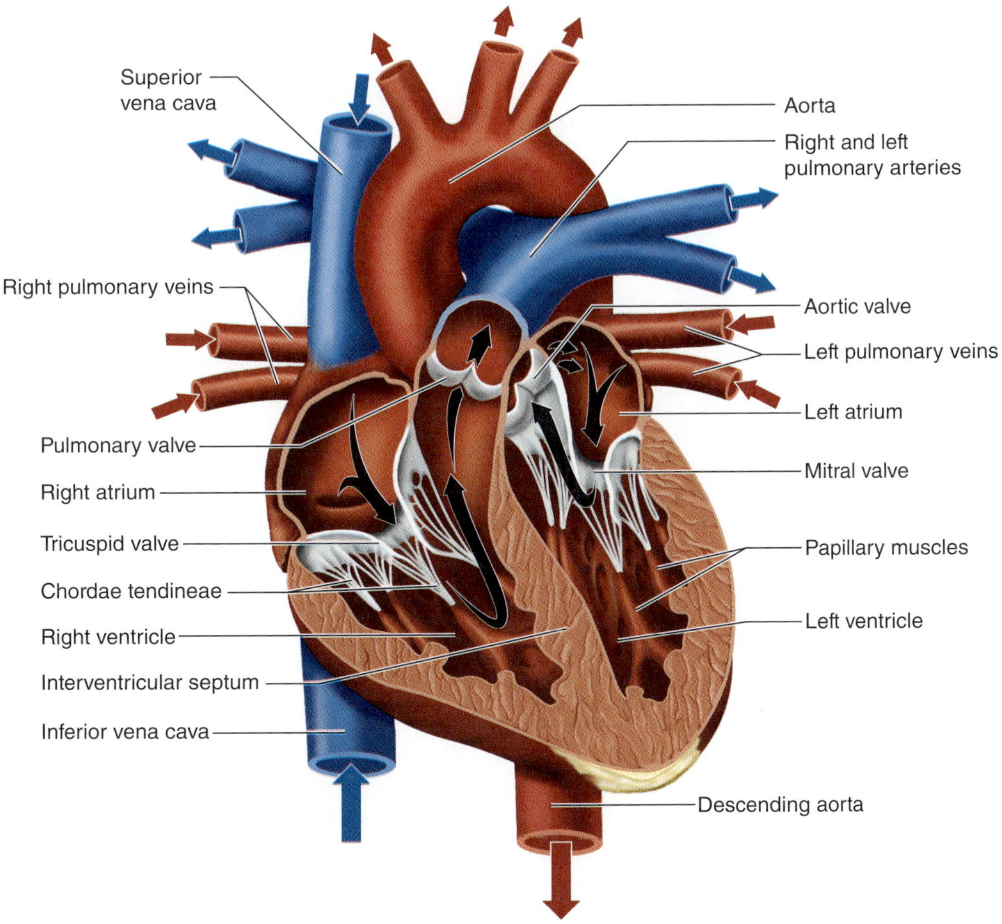

Figure 11.13 Heart valves.
Reprinted by permission from R. Behnke, *Kinetic Anatomy*, 4th ed. (Champaign, IL: Human Kinetics, 2022), 182.

Summary

Injuries to the throat and thorax can cause severe, permanent damage or even death. The AT must be able to evaluate injuries to the throat and thorax because prompt treatment is crucial to an athlete's survival. The history, signs, and symptoms will define the injury. Most injuries to these areas are preventable if the athlete is wearing the proper equipment. Luckily, few injuries occur in these areas, and when they do occur, most are not life-threatening. For serious injuries, EMS is needed immediately. As the scope of the AT expands, becoming familiar with common medical conditions and terminology associated with injuries to the throat and thorax will help you better serve your athletes. Proper identification will facilitate prompt referral for advanced care when needed.

Key Terms

Define the following terms found in this chapter:

- air embolism
- alveoli
- aneurysms
- arrythmia
- atrioventricular node (AV)
- atrium
- cardiac tamponade
- cardiomyopathy
- carotid artery
- chronic obstructive pulmonary disease (COPD)
- deep vein thrombosis (DVT)
- diaphragm
- ECG
- embolism
- emphysema
- esophagus
- flail chest
- hemothorax
- jugular vein
- laryngitis
- larynx
- mitral valve prolapse (MVP)
- myocarditis
- pharyngitis
- pleurisy
- pneumonia
- pneumothorax
- sinoatrial node (SA)
- tonsilitis
- trachea
- ventricles

As an AT, you work with the school nurse to help students get the general medical care they need. A student-athlete reports to your office with a sore throat. The school nurse is out of the building today, so you need to determine if they should go home and see a physician. How do you differentiate between tonsilitis, pharyngitis, and laryngitis? When should you refer the student to a physician?

To access supplementary material for this chapter, including the Understanding Check worksheet, vocabulary quizzes, extension activities, and chapter-specific resources and forms, visit the web resource: http://ancillaries.humankinetics.com/FundamentalsOfAthleticTrainingAndSportsMedicine5E

chapter 12

Abdominal Injuries

Objectives

After completing this chapter, the student will be able to do the following:

- Understand the anatomy of the abdomen.
- Understand that an abdominal organ may cause referral of pain.
- Understand the implications of illness or injury related to specific organs.
- Understand and be able to identify signs and symptoms for selected abdominal conditions.
- Understand how to prevent injuries of the abdomen.
- Describe the care necessary to treat an abdominal injury.

Although abdominal organs are not generally protected by padding, abdominal injuries occur infrequently. A serious abdominal injury, however, may not become apparent for days and can be life-threatening. In this chapter, we discuss function of the abdominal organs, injury prevention, and treatment.

ANATOMY OF THE ABDOMEN

The abdominal cavity is bounded by the lumbar spine posteriorly, the diaphragm superiorly, the abdominal musculature anteriorly, and the pelvis inferiorly. For purposes of discussion, the abdominal cavity is divided into four quadrants by an imaginary horizontal line running across the abdomen through the navel and an imaginary vertical line running from the sternum through the navel to the area between the legs (see figure 12.1). The upper right quadrant lies just below the ribs on the athlete's right side, and it contains the liver, a portion of the pancreas, the right kidney, the gallbladder, and the large and small intestines. The upper left quadrant lies just below the ribs on the athlete's left side, and it contains the stomach, a portion of the liver, a portion of the pancreas, the left kidney, the spleen, and the large and small intestines. The lower right quadrant contains the large and small

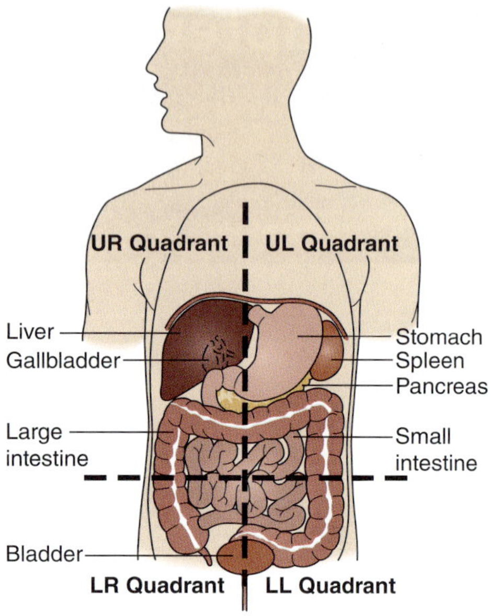

Figure 12.1 The abdominal quadrants.

intestines, the appendix, a portion of the bladder, the uterus and right ovary (in women), and the prostate (in men). The lower left quadrant contains the large and small intestines, a portion of the bladder, the uterus and left ovary (in women), and the prostate (in men).

The abdomen has both hollow and solid organs. Hollow organs are tubes that assist in transporting substances from one organ to another and are connected to one another by sheetlike membranes. Injuries to the hollow organs, such as the bladder, intestines, stomach, and appendix, rarely cause rapid death but can make the athlete quite ill. Moreover, the hollow organs tend to move and bend away if an athlete is hit in the abdomen. Solid organs such as the liver, kidneys, and spleen aid in body chemistry. They can cause rapid death if injured because they have a large blood supply.

Abdominal organs can be divided into three categories: digestive organs, urinary organs, and reproductive organs. The organs included in the digestive system are the stomach, liver, pancreas, large and small intestines, appendix, spleen, and gallbladder. The organs of the urinary system are the kidneys, ureters, and bladder. Organs of the female reproductive system include the ovaries and uterus. Organs in the male reproductive system include the prostate and seminal vesicles. Accessory abdominal organs are pictured in figure 12.2.

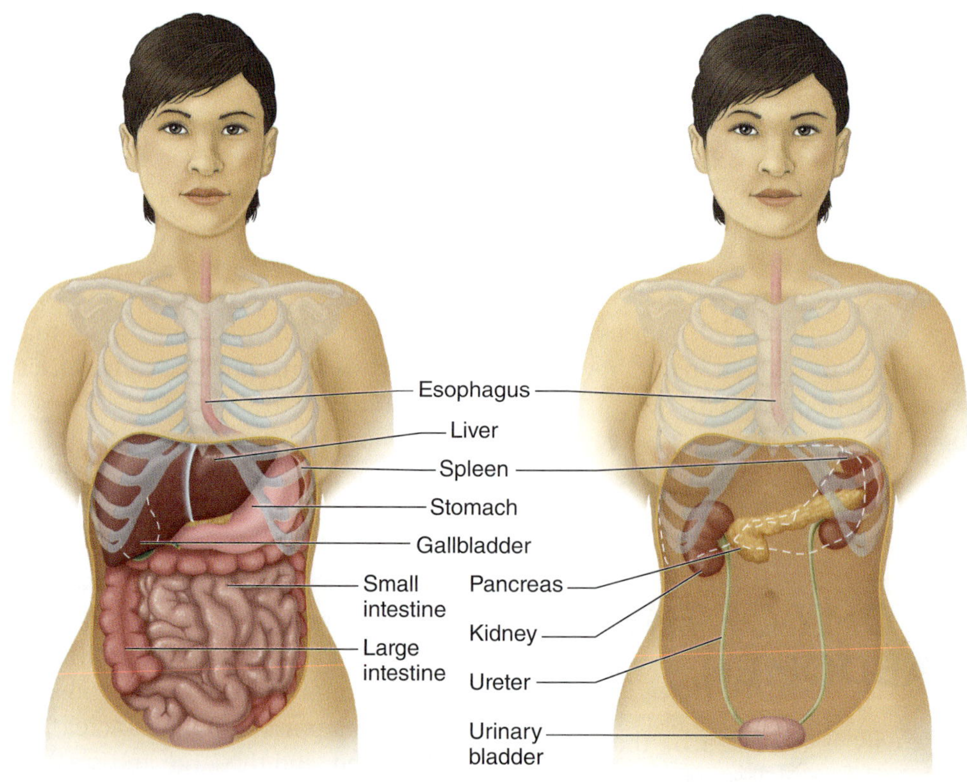

Figure 12.2 Accessory abdominal organs.

Reprinted by permission from M. Masaracchio and C. Frommer, *A Clinical Guide to Surface Palpation: The Art and Science of the Perfect Touch*, 2nd ed. (Champaign, IL: Human Kinetics, 2022), 285.

The abdominal organs, when injured or diseased, will refer pain to another part of the body. The following list indicates the abdominal organ and its **referral point** (Cleary and Flanagan 2020; Stanford Medicine 2016):

- Liver: right shoulder area and back
- Kidney: below rib cage, wrapping from back to front
- Appendix: lower right abdomen halfway between navel and anterior superior iliac spine of the hip (McBurney's point)
- Gallbladder: just below right rib cage and possible right shoulder
- Pancreas: left shoulder and midabdominal region
- Stomach: below rib cage to chest
- Bladder: over the bladder
- Small intestine: navel
- Large intestine: sacrum
- Spleen: left shoulder and over the spleen (Kehr sign)

During an evaluation, the AT can palpate each quadrant to determine if any of the organs may have been injured. It is important to have the athlete bend their knees when palpating to take the slack out of the abdominal musculature and allow for easier palpation. When palpating a quadrant, the AT will use the flat surface of their fingers (see figure 12.3). The AT will compress the abdomen and ask if the athlete experiences any pain. The pain can occur as the AT is compressing inward or when pressure is released. The AT will be determining if the abdominal muscles tighten, which is a sign of internal injury.

ATs often use the stethoscope to hear sounds in the body. It is used to listen to heart, lung, and bowel sounds. Using a stethoscope to hear a sound in the body is called auscultation. If a suspected injury to the abdomen has occurred, the AT uses a stethoscope to hear sounds in each quadrant. Figure 12.4 shows where abdominal auscultations are performed. The AT can hear abnormal bowel sounds or the lack of bowel sounds, an indication of injury. It is typical to hear gurgling in the abdominal region.

Digestive Organs

Immediately above the stomach lies the esophagus. It is a flexible tube extending about 10 inches (25 cm) to the top of the stomach. It is a transportation tube that joins the stomach at the gastroesophageal sphincter. Sphincters are openings or valve-like structures that allow the flow of materials like food from one region to another and prevent backflow into the previous region. The next organ in the gastrointestinal tract is the stomach. The stomach secretes gastric juices that assist in breaking down food before it enters the intestines. It has three main parts: the fundus, body, and pyloric regions, and it is shaped like a flask. The stomach empties into

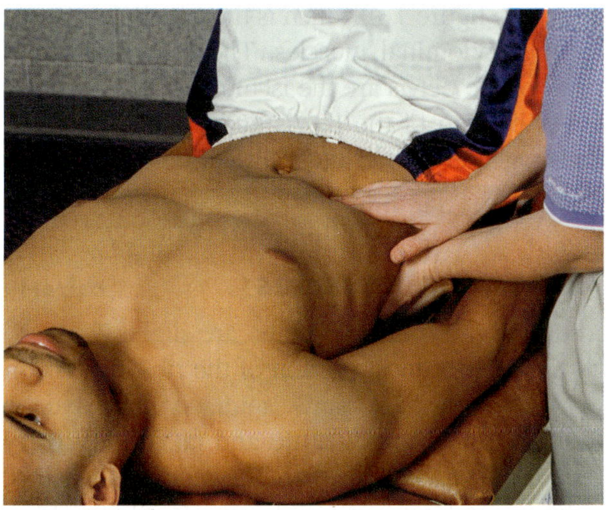

Figure 12.3 Palpating an abdominal quadrant.

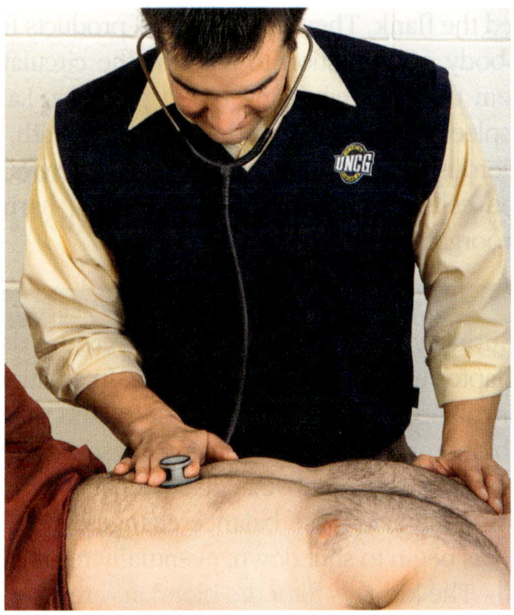

Figure 12.4 Auscultation of the abdomen.

abdominal muscles. Most sports do not allow tackling or checking (physically moving an athlete) from behind so that athletes can protect themselves. Boxing has a rule that says it is illegal to hit below the belt. Before games, all athletes should be reminded to empty their bladders because full bladders are more prone to rupture on impact than empty ones. Simple strategies and education can help athletes prevent painful and dangerous abdominal injuries.

TREATING ABDOMINAL INJURIES AND CONDITIONS

Injuries in the abdominal cavity, especially to the hollow organs, are rare. The solid organs—the liver, spleen, and kidneys—can be injured, and internal bleeding may result. The AT should assess any athlete who has received a blow to the abdominal area, especially if they have abdominal pain, signs of shock, muscle spasms, or blood in the urine. See figure 12.6.

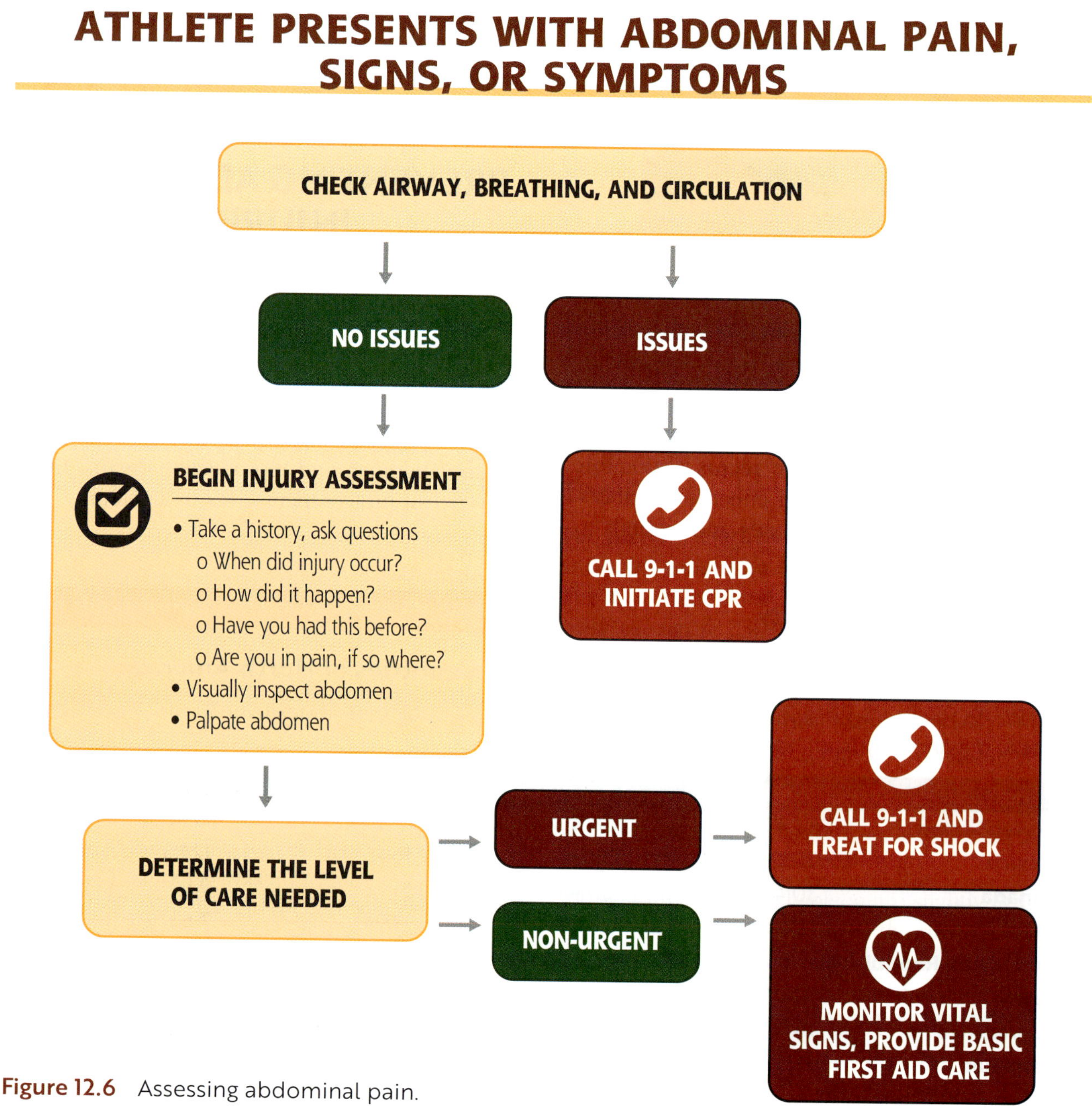

Figure 12.6 Assessing abdominal pain.

RED FLAGS

Call 911 if an athlete experiences any of the following:

- An injury that refers pain
- Spleen injury
- Liver injury
- Protrusion of abdominal organs
- An object penetrating the abdominal wall
- Blood in urine
- Pain when palpating abdominal quadrants
- Painful urination

Side Stitch

A side stitch refers to pain just below the ribs in the upper abdominal region. There are various theories about why this pain occurs—a lack of oxygen to the abdominal muscles, improper breathing technique, eating food just before exercising, air trapped in the abdominal organs, and muscle spasms are a few—but in general, less fit people tend to get more stitches. Athletes experiencing the pain of a stitch resolve it by stopping exercise or by pressing directly over the area. If an athlete believes the stitch is a result of eating, they should change their eating patterns. A muscle spasm stitch can be resolved by raising the arm on the same side as the pain and leaning away from the painful area. Pain that does not resolve needs to be referred to a physician for further evaluation.

Hernia

A **hernia** is a lump of tissue, usually the intestine, that bulges through a weakness in the abdominal wall. There are two types of hernias: femoral and inguinal (see figure 12.7). Hernias can result from increased abdominal pressure, which may occur if the athlete holds their breath while weightlifting or going to the bathroom. The lump may go away when they lie down and bulge again when they stand up or exert abdominal pressure. In men, the intestine may go through the inguinal canal and stay in the scrotal sac. The athlete may or may not have pain. A hernia must be surgically repaired, although a truss, or strap, can be used temporarily to apply pressure to keep the bulge inside the abdomen. A truss does not work for inguinal hernias and cannot be used by athletes who participate in contact sports or sports such as weightlifting that require the exertion of internal abdominal pressure. If not treated, the bulge of tissue can get stuck in the abdominal wall or inguinal canal, which is called *strangulation*. Strangulation cuts off the blood supply to the tissue, and eventually the tissue will die. If intestinal tissue is involved, a bowel obstruction will result. The obstruction prevents the passage of waste material from the body, causing pain and illness, and must be surgically repaired.

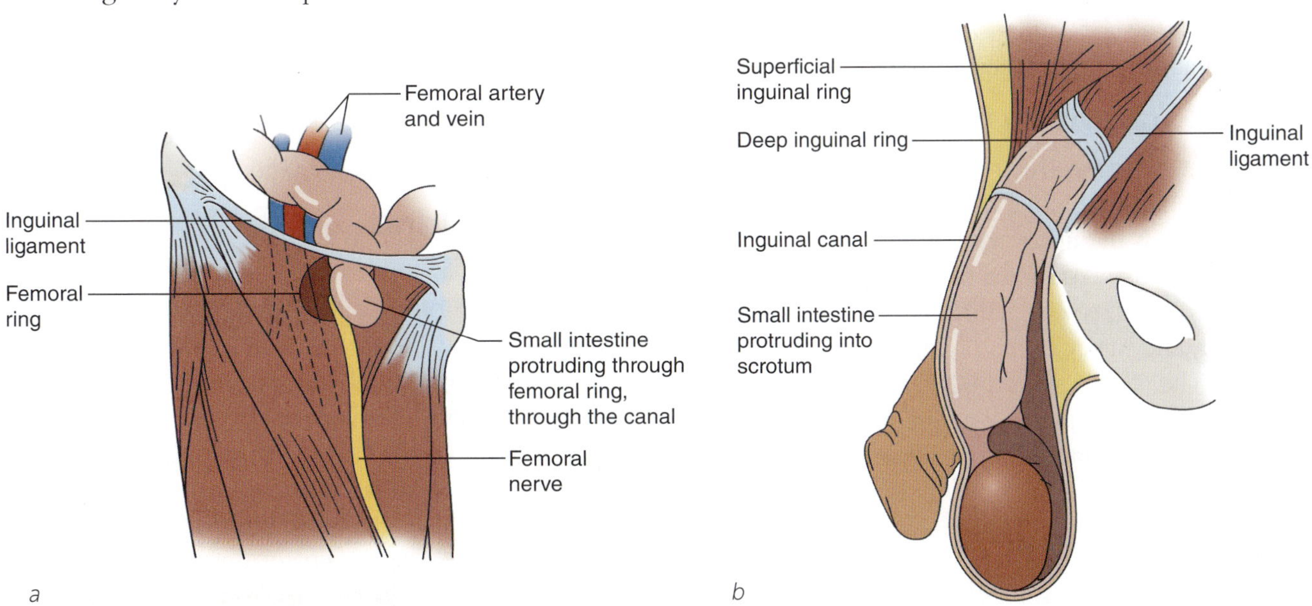

Figure 12.7 *(a)* Femoral hernia and *(b)* inguinal hernia.

Reprinted by permission from S. Shultz, P. Houglum, and D. Perrin, *Examination of Musculoskeletal Injuries*, 4th ed. (Champaign, IL: Human Kinetics, 2016), 626.

FYI

Enzymes

An enzyme is a protein that allows a biochemical reaction to take place at normal body temperature but is itself not changed in the reaction.

Inguinal Canal

The inguinal canal is a hole in the abdominal wall in the groin region.

Mechanism of Injury

The *mechanism of injury* refers to the way in which an injury occurs. The mechanism can be observed if one is paying attention during a practice or game or it can be explained by the athlete.

Appendicitis

When the appendix becomes inflamed, it causes pain between the navel and the hip, better known as **McBurney's point**. The athlete will be in more pain upon release of the pressure at McBurney's point than with the initial pressure inward. This is called rebound pain. The inflammation of the appendix increases and is called *appendicitis*.

Along with significant pain, the athlete is likely to exhibit nausea, vomiting, a fever, loss of appetite, and abdominal bloating (Mayo Clinic 2023). This athlete needs to be treated by a physician so an immediate referral is necessary. In some cases, the appendix can rupture, spewing the contents of the colon into the abdominal cavity. Surgery is urgent in this situation to prevent sepsis or systemic infection.

Blunt Trauma to the Abdomen

An athlete who receives a blow directly to the abdomen is subject to blunt force trauma. An example of blunt force is the impact of the handlebars when a bike rider crashes during a race. The blunt force can cause bruising, severe pain, difficulty standing up straight, and injury to the organs in the abdominal cavity. The athlete should be treated for shock and needs immediate medical attention. The following are specific abdominal organs that can be injured, along with their signs and symptoms.

Pancreas Injury

The pancreas lies just behind the stomach near the liver and the spinal column. It is prone to injury during deceleration—for example, when an athlete running with the ball hits a wall. The wall does not cause the injury, but as the pancreas shifts forward when the rest of the body has stopped, it tears. The athlete will have pain in the middle of the abdomen to the back as well as nausea, vomiting, and signs of shock. The athlete should be referred to the hospital for additional examination—a ruptured pancreas must be surgically repaired. Even with repair, pancreatic injuries are often long-standing and create digestive issues during the healing process.

What Would You Do If . . .

Everyone in the locker room is gathered around an athlete who is showing off a quarter-sized bulge near his navel. He pushes on the bulge and it disappears, but when he holds his breath and bears down, the bulge reappears. Everyone laughs, and he continues showing off.

Liver Injury

A blow to the upper right abdomen can result in a contusion or rupture of the liver. The athlete will experience pain over the area that may radiate to the right shoulder. As the athlete loses blood, they will go into shock, have a rapid, weak pulse, and experience a drop in blood pressure. They must be referred to a physician immediately or transported by ambulance if needed. The AT should be suspicious of a liver contusion if the athlete receives any blows to the area. The athlete may die if the liver is ruptured and it goes untreated.

Blood in Urine

Occasionally, an athlete may tell you that their urine is tinged pink or red. This means that there is blood in the urine. The AT's assessment will include determining if the athlete has been ill, experienced painful urination, received any impact to the abdominal organs, or did strenuous exercise. Dehydration can also cause blood in the urine. The athlete will likely be referred to a physician for evaluation. Cross country runners are prone to **hematuria** (blood in the urine) due to their strenuous exercise routine (Mayo Clinic 2017a).

Kidney Injury

A direct blow over the kidney can cause a contusion, laceration, or rupture. The athlete will experience pain just under the posterior ribs to the side of the spine commonly called the flank, and the pain may radiate to the bladder. Pain will increase with trunk extension and ease with knee or hip flexion. The athlete may feel nauseated and vomit. Urine may have visible blood, and the blood loss may cause the athlete to go into shock. Thus, the injury requires prompt emergency care and hospitalization. Generally, an athlete with a kidney injury is required to rest for several weeks before returning to competition. Possible complications of kidney injuries are scarring of the kidney and hypertension. Educating the athlete to monitor signs for hematuria for the next 24 hours after injury will help with early detection if delayed signs and symptoms appear. Urine strips are also commercially available to detect subtle blood in the urine (see figure 12.8).

What Would You Do If . . .

A cross country runner reports that they have blood in their urine. They do not remember being hit over their kidney.

Bladder Injury

A bladder rupture causes urine to leak into the surrounding area. The athlete may have painful urination, a contusion over the bladder, or blood in the urine. They should report any of these symptoms to the AT. In severe cases of bladder injury, athletes go into shock, causing rapid heart rate, decreased blood pressure, anxiety, and sweating. When the injury mechanism suggests a bladder injury, the athlete should be referred to a physician for immediate evaluation. The AT should instruct the athlete to look for the signs and symptoms listed previously and report problems immediately. A ruptured bladder can cause urine to be leaked into the pelvic region, causing infection.

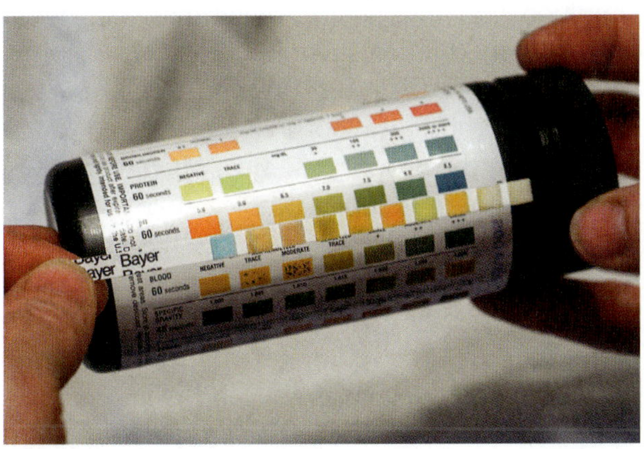

Figure 12.8 Urine strips.

Spleen Rupture

A blow to the abdomen may injure the spleen. A spleen that is enlarged from an infection is more prone to rupture, so athletes recovering from illnesses, especially mononucleosis, should not be allowed to play without a physician's permission. Athletes with a spleen injury will experience abdominal pain and perhaps pain in the left shoulder, which is referred to as **Kehr's sign**. The left shoulder pain is caused by internal bleeding that puts pressure on the diaphragm, which presses on a nerve, causing referred pain to the shoulder. The athlete will often indicate that they are nauseated, experiencing cramps, and are weak, and they may pass out. On examination, the AT may note abdominal spasms, vomiting, rapid heart rate, decreased blood pressure, and shock. The athlete must be transported by EMS to a hospital immediately—an injured spleen is a medical emergency. A ruptured spleen can bleed severely, causing rapid blood loss and a drop in blood pressure. The spleen can, however, splint itself and appear to be fine after a blow to the splenic region. Athletes must be fully evaluated and educated to watch for signs of splenic rupture. The athlete can go home and the spleen can rupture later once the splint (clot) moves, so always be sure to err on the side of caution with these injuries.

An athlete with less severe spleen injuries will be hospitalized overnight for observation. A ruptured spleen must be surgically removed. Athletes who have had their spleens removed are able to play sports after complete recovery. The spleen can be protected from injury with padding.

The Real World

While I was working a summer basketball camp, one of the athletes was accidentally kneed in the abdomen. When we got to him, he complained of high pain levels in the lower abdomen off to the left side. We determined that he could move, so we helped him walk to the sideline and finished our evaluation. He exhibited tenderness over the spleen with a positive Kehr's sign. The coach encouraged the athlete to walk it off, but because a Kehr's sign most often suggests a spleen injury, I overruled him. We removed the athlete to the training room, where he began to show signs of shock. We thought his spleen must be ruptured, and we called EMS immediately. While we waited, we monitored his vital signs and treated him for shock. He showed a decreasing level of consciousness and a significant drop in blood pressure. We recorded vital signs at 5-minute intervals before EMS arrived, and that cut down on time of transfer from our care to theirs. He was taken to the local hospital and was later airlifted to a larger hospital. He did have a ruptured spleen, and he was rushed into surgery. The athlete recovered fully, and the next summer he was back at the same camp.

Alex Embry, ATC, EMT

Penetrating Abdominal Injury

Penetrating abdominal injuries present with external bleeding and an open wound. If an object that has penetrated the abdominal wall causes a wound, the AT will not remove it. The AT will apply direct pressure around the object, stabilize it, and call 911.

Some penetrating injuries can be the result of the athlete's own anatomy, such as a fractured bone, like a rib, or from an external source, such as a limb or implement. The concern with all penetrating wounds is the possibility that the object may have injured one of the abdominal organs. Injuries to abdominal organs will require a physician's assessment, so immediate care is necessary.

COMMON MEDICAL DIAGNOSES OF THE ABDOMEN

Several abdominal conditions plague athletes throughout their careers. Some are more common than others, but the AT should consider each one with care.

Constipation and Diarrhea

Athletes often experience either **constipation** (the inability to have a regular bowel movement) or **diarrhea** (loose bowel movements). There are many causes for these, such as certain foods, dehydration or overhydration, stress, parasitic infestations, or infection. Regardless of the cause, the AT should take a careful history to find out the duration and potential source of the problem. Constipation can cause abdominal pain, discomfort, bloating, and general malaise. Diarrhea can cause fatigue, dehydration, and even shock if too much fluid is lost. Proper interventions include regulating fluid intake, monitoring the dietary makeup of fluids the athlete consumes, and nutritional interventions to support good bowel habits, such as increasing fiber. Over-the-counter medications are also available to help these situations, but if persistent, they should be evaluated by a physician to rule out more serious conditions.

Common Gastrointestinal Conditions

Gastro-esophageal reflux disease (GERD) is a condition affecting the gastrointestinal system and is commonly called reflux or acid indigestion. It is characterized by the reflux of stomach acid into the esophagus, causing a horrible taste and burning sensation in the esophagus. Most often associated with spicy foods, eating late or eating rich foods and then lying down can also make the symptoms worse. Over-the-counter medications are available to help mild cases, but athletes with persistent problems should be referred to a physician to rule out more serious conditions.

Upset stomach is a common term used by athletes to describe a range of conditions affecting the gastrointestinal tract. Gastroenteritis is an inflammation of the gastrointestinal system causing pain, diarrhea, cramping, and nausea. It is commonly called the stomach flu and is a viral infection. Although over-the-counter medications can make you more comfortable, prevention through proper hygiene habits is the best option.

Cholecystitis is a condition describing an inflamed, swollen gallbladder that can cause much pain and discomfort. Although more commonly seen in women than men and in people over the age of 40, anyone can experience this condition. It occurs when bile gets trapped in the gallbladder and causes pain, nausea, and vomiting. Gallstones (hard particles that build up in the gallbladder and get stuck in the duct) can also cause this condition. A medical referral is often needed, where advanced medical testing is performed to properly diagnose and manage this condition. Sometimes, the gallbladder will need to be removed surgically to treat the problem (Johns Hopkins Medicine n.d.).

Diverticula are outpouchings in the lining of the large intestine that trap food in them, causing inflammation, infection, and pain (see figure 12.9). **Diverticulitis** results when a person typically does not have enough fiber in their diet to keep the waste products moving through the system, appropriately causing some of these products to get stuck in these little pouches. As the waste sits in these areas, they fester and become problematic for the athlete. Nuts, seeds, and popcorn are often attributed to diverticulitis symptoms in patients. Diverticulitis is often treated by a physician with rest, diet changes, and antibiotics, but if it is severe, it may require surgical intervention. Referral to a physician is prudent (Cleveland Clinic n.d.).

Irritable bowel syndrome is characterized by fluctuations between diarrhea and constipation. It is often affected by food choices and stress and can

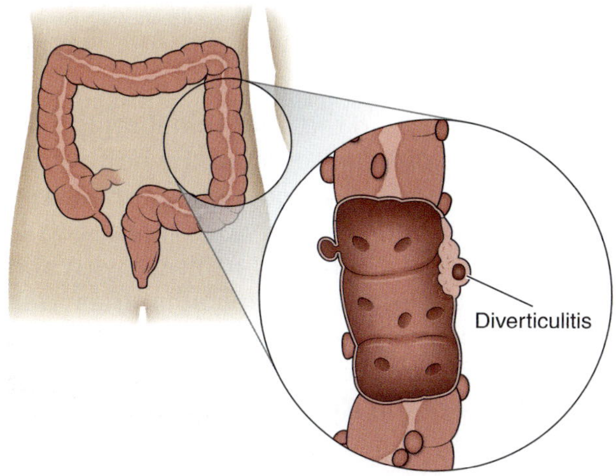

Figure 12.9 Diverticulitis.

cause discomfort for the athlete. Referral to a gastroenterologist can help the athlete as many pharmacological agents are available for this condition. Another gastrointestinal disease is called **Crohn's disease**. This is an autoimmune digestive disorder causing diarrhea, fever, rectal bleeding, weight loss, and abdominal pain and cramps. This is a serious medical condition that ranges in severity from mild to severe and requires the intervention of a physician (Parker 2017).

Parasitic infections can occur in athletes, although they are not as common as viral or bacterial infections. There are many parasites, but giardia is seen in people who drink unclean water or consume products that are not washed well. Giardia causes explosive diarrhea, cramping, and abdominal pain. Since the danger of dehydration is high with this infestation, it is best to get the athlete to a physician if a parasitic infection is suspected. Sometimes, athletes will need supplemental fluids in the form of an intravenous solution if they have these symptoms for too long.

Summary

Most of the organs in the abdominal region are involved in the digestive process and therefore are hollow. It is difficult to injure the hollow organs, but the solid organs of the abdomen can be seriously injured. The AT must know where the organs of the abdomen are located to evaluate abdominal injuries. Some serious injuries will not be immediately evident because they have delayed signs and symptoms. Athletes with abdominal injuries require immediate aid from EMS. The number of serious abdominal injuries in sport has been reduced by players following rules restricting body contact and wearing required protective equipment. Medical conditions in the gastrointestinal tract can affect athletes and their ability to perform at their full capacity. It is the responsibility of the AT to identify signs and symptoms and secure appropriate medical referral when needed.

Key Terms

Define the following terms found in this chapter:

- bile
- constipation
- Crohn's disease
- diarrhea
- diverticulitis
- gastro-esophageal reflux disease (GERD)
- hematuria
- hernia
- irritable bowel syndrome
- Kehr's sign
- McBurney's point
- referral point

An athlete comes to you reporting stomach pains. They have been eating many strawberries because they just came into season. The athlete says that they often have belly pain after eating foods with seeds and almost always after eating nuts. They are vegetarian but have diverticulitis. What would you advise relative to their current stomach pain? What recommendations would you give for food choices that do not aggravate the diverticulitis?

To access supplementary material for this chapter, including the Understanding Check worksheet, vocabulary quizzes, extension activities, and chapter-specific resources and forms, visit the web resource: http://ancillaries.humankinetics.com/FundamentalsOfAthleticTrainingAndSportsMedicine5E

chapter 13

Genitourinary and Gynecological Injuries and Conditions

Objectives

After completing this chapter, the student will be able to do the following:

- Understand the basic anatomy of the female and male genitourinary and reproductive systems.
- Identify common signs and symptoms for conditions affecting these systems.
- Understand the evaluation, treatment, and referral processes associated with common injuries and conditions.

Athletes come to the AT with a range of medical concerns. ATs must be able to identify signs and symptoms of medical conditions of the genitourinary and reproductive systems to ensure appropriate medical care and referral. Although it is not within the scope of the AT to prescribe medications, correctly identifying medical conditions and injuries can facilitate prompt medical care through referrals. A word of caution: Due to the sensitive nature of genitourinary and reproductive system evaluations, you must take a thorough medical history in a private setting to ensure confidentiality. Further, physical examination and evaluation of the genital or reproductive regions is always referred to the physician.

GENITOURINARY ANATOMY

The genitourinary anatomy of the female and male include some similar physiological features and other anatomical features that are distinctly different. The kidneys are fist-sized organs located in the mid back region called the flank. They rest under the lower posterior ribcage. Most people have two kidneys. The kidneys maintain fluid balance, remove waste products from the blood, and control blood pressure and red blood cell formation. Each **kidney** is connected to a tube called the **ureter**, which extend posteriorly where they connect to the urinary bladder. The bladder is a hollow organ that stores urine for excretion from the body. The urinary bladder is then emptied through the urethra or the tube that exits the male or female genitalia. Figure 13.1 shows the anatomy of the urinary tract.

Understanding Diversity

As an AT, it is important to understand terminology regarding a person's identity. Using the proper terminology is critical in establishing trust with your athletes and patients. As a health care provider, it is important to treat your patients with respect and consider their identity as you navigate their medical concerns.

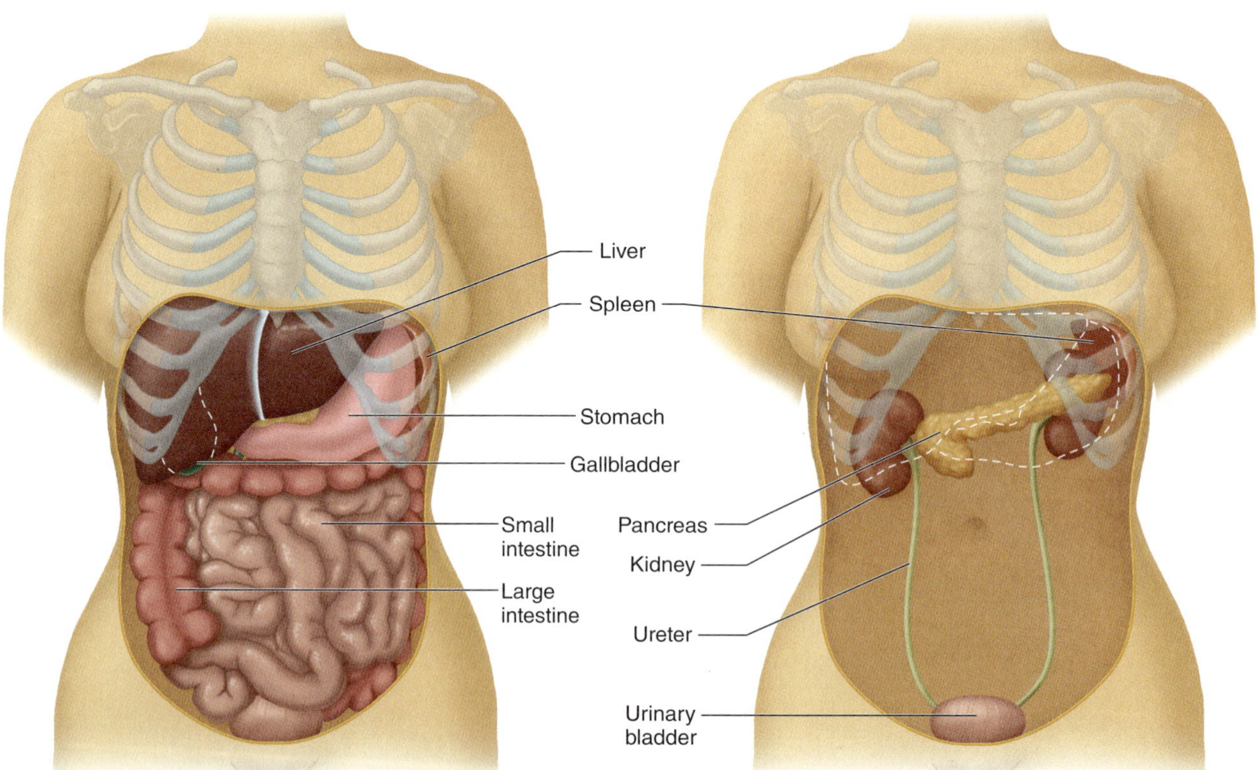

Figure 13.1 Anatomy of the urinary tract.

Reprinted by permission from M.A. Cleary and K.W. Flanagan, *Acute and Emergency Care in Athletic Training* (Champaign, IL: Human Kinetics, 2020), 330.

Female Reproductive Anatomy

The female reproductive system is comprised of several key structures (see figure 13.2). These structures are housed internally in the pelvic region and have important functions anatomically as well as hormonally. The ovaries (right and left) are on each side of the pelvis in the lower abdominal quadrant. These walnut-shaped organs are suspended from the uterus and the **fallopian tubes**. The **ovary** produces eggs and does so from menarche (the start of menses) through menopause (the end of menses). The fallopian tubes are located off the uterus and are considered tubelike projections. They carry the egg from the ovary to the uterus, where it will either be shed if not fertilized or create an embryo if fertilized. The uterus is the thick-walled, triangular organ that acts as the host for embryo development. The uterus has a distal cervical canal that ends at the cervix. The cervix then opens into the vagina.

Male Reproductive Anatomy

The male reproductive system is characterized by key anatomical structures (see figure 13.3). The testicles (2) are housed outside of the body in a scrotal sac. This helps to regulate the temperature of the testicles (also called *testes*), which is an important factor in sperm production. Typically, the testicles must be 4 to 11 °F (2-6 °C) below core body temperature for maximal sperm production (Gao et al. 2022). The epididymis sits above the testes and connects to the spermatic cords. The spermatic cord is a combination of vesicles, artery, nerve, and a duct. These structures transport sperm through the reproductive system out the urethra of the penis.

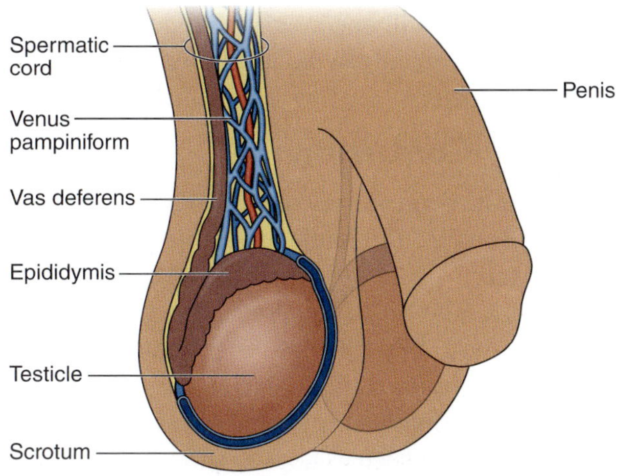

Figure 13.3 Male reproductive organs.

Reprinted by permission from M.A. Cleary and K.W. Flanagan, *Acute and Emergency Care in Athletic Training* (Champaign, IL: Human Kinetics, 2020), 332.

INJURIES AND CONDITIONS OF THE URINARY SYSTEM

The urinary system keeps the fluids and salts of the body regulated. It removes waste from the blood and keeps blood pressure and volume at optimal

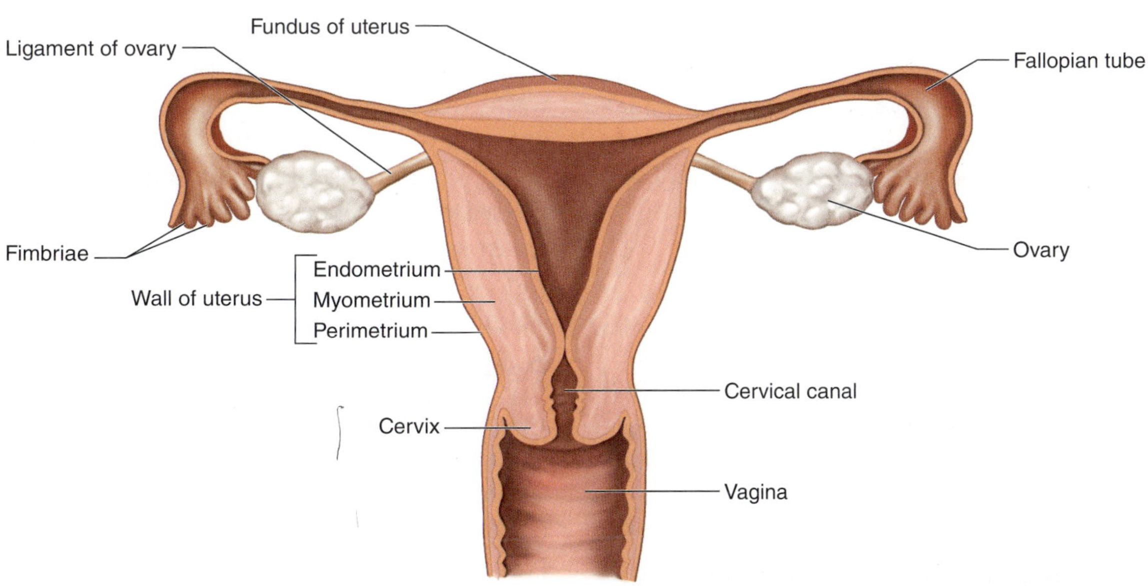

Figure 13.2 Female reproductive organs.

Reprinted by permission from M.A. Cleary and K.W. Flanagan, *Acute and Emergency Care in Athletic Training* (Champaign, IL: Human Kinetics, 2020), 331.

levels. The AT will encounter the following conditions (Kahanov and Payne 2022; Cleary and Walsh Flanagan 2020).

Kidney Contusion

As mentioned previously, the kidneys are located in an area called the flank, at the bottom region of the posterior rib cage and around the lateral side of the ribs. The kidneys are situated there so they are protected, but they are vulnerable to contusions through direct blows to the mid or low back in contact and collision sports or with direct hits from equipment such as hockey and lacrosse sticks. Further, kidneys can be contused through percussion or vibration from a hard fall onto the buttocks. An athlete with a kidney contusion will have pain in the flank. They may also report blood in their urine immediately or days after the contusion. Most athletes feel nauseated when the injury occurs and should be monitored to ensure no serious injury to the kidney has occurred. Referral is always prudent when you suspect an injury to the kidney.

Kidney Stones

Kidney stones are calcifications that get lodged somewhere in the urinary tract. Some people are prone to kidney stones, while others are not. Excessive calcification forms small stonelike masses in the genitourinary tract that must be excreted by the body if they are not dealt with medically in-clinic. As these stones move through the kidney to the ureters and out the urethra, they create a significant amount of pain and sometimes bleeding. Kidney stones can have many causes, but dehydration is an aggravating factor. If an athlete reports unbearable pain in the flank without any contusion or fall, they will need to be referred to a physician to rule out a kidney stone.

Urethritis

The **urethra** is vulnerable to inflammation due to its proximity to the end of the urinary tract. The urethra is the exit point for urine and can be irritated by bacteria or organisms caused from sweat and urination. Patients who report pain with urination, sometimes associated with blood in the urine, should be referred to the physician. As always, good personal hygiene can prevent urethritis but is not the cause of all urethral conditions.

UTI

Any inflammation in the urinary tract is generally classified as a UTI. It can involve all aspects of the urinary tract but most often affects the bladder and distal parts of the system. Patients with a UTI will experience pain with urination, urgency in urination, more frequent urination, and often pain over the bladder region. UTIs are treated with prescription medications, so referral to a physician is necessary. Encouraging your patient to drink plenty of fluids is prudent to help to flush the system of any harmful infection.

INJURIES AND CONDITIONS OF THE FEMALE REPRODUCTIVE SYSTEM

The female reproductive system includes the uterus, ovaries, fallopian tubes, cervix, and vagina. It creates hormones and is responsible for fertility, menstruation, and sexual activity.

Vaginitis

This condition results from inflammation in the vagina and can cause itching, discharge, and pain. Bacterial vaginosis, yeast infections, and trichomoniasis are common vaginitis conditions (Mayo Clinic n.d.b). Vaginosis is characterized by a grayish-yellow, odoriferous discharge, while yeast infections typically present with a thick white discharge. Trichomoniasis presents with a greenish-yellow frothy discharge. Patients reporting any of these to the AT should be referred to a physician for proper diagnosis and treatment. For an expanded description of these conditions, please visit www.mayoclinic.org/diseases-conditions/vaginitis/symptoms-causes/syc-20354707.

Pelvic Inflammatory Disease

Pelvic inflammatory disease (PID) is a chronic condition where the pelvic organs are affected by a disease pathology or condition that creates an unhealthy environment. PID can be associated with sexually transmitted infections, endometriosis, or other conditions and may result in fertility issues and chronic pain. Any athlete who reports pelvic pain should be referred to a physician or **gynecologist** for medical examination and treatment.

Amenorrhea and Dysmenorrhea

Amenorrhea is the absence of a menstrual period and is classified as primary or secondary in nature. Primary amenorrhea occurs if the patient has not yet reached menarche due to a biological abnormality. Secondary amenorrhea occurs when a woman started her period but now fails to have her period or has irregular periods for 3 to 6 months. There are many causes for amenorrhea but it warrants a referral to a physician or gynecologist for medical diagnosis and treatment. **Dysmenorrhea** is the medical term for painful menstruation. Although many women have some cramping and pain during menstruation, pain that is intense and limits activities of daily living should be referred to a gynecologist for treatment and to rule out any medical problems such as cysts, endometriosis, or other conditions.

Endometriosis

This is a condition where endometrial tissue grows inside and outside of the pelvic cavity. The athlete will present with pelvic pain, low-back pain, and abdominal pain, all of which are worse during menstruation. Adolescents with dysmenorrhea (painful menstruation) should be referred to a physician for diagnosis and care.

Ovarian and Cervical Cancer

Ovarian and cervical cancers are conditions that affect women of all ages. Any changes in menstrual function premenopausal or any pain or changes postmenopausal should be evaluated by a gynecologist. A pap smear is a clinical test that can be used to check for abnormal cells on the cervix, which may indicate cervical changes or cancer. Women are encouraged to have this examination done annually as a preventive measure for early cancer detection. Ovarian cancer is harder to detect through annual screening, but any changes or masses should be reported to the physician for further medical testing. Often, an ultrasound or CT scan will be performed to detect ovarian masses or cancer. Treatment for these conditions varies depending on the stage of the cancer. Patients with cancer are referred to an **oncologist** to help manage the treatment.

Pregnancy and Ectopic Pregnancy

Pregnancy results when a female egg and male sperm combine to create an embryo. Women can get pregnant while on birth control, especially if they do not take their birth control pills regularly or are on antibiotics, which decrease the effectiveness of the pill. Pregnancy is a well-known risk of sexual intercourse, and is often an emotional experience. Any AT who is aware of a pregnant athlete should refer them to a medical professional for prenatal care and counseling. Further, guidelines exist for participation in sports for pregnant athletes, so it is wise to work together with the medical team to ensure a safe environment for the pregnant individual. **Ectopic** pregnancies occur when the egg is fertilized in the fallopian tube. The embryo begins to grow in the fallopian tube rather than in the uterus, creating a painful, potentially dangerous situation. There will be extreme pain over the ovarian region and likely abnormal bleeding. This is an emergency because of the potential for deadly blood loss and should be referred immediately to prevent any further complications.

INJURIES AND CONDITIONS OF THE MALE REPRODUCTIVE SYSTEM

The male reproductive system includes the penis, testes, and scrotum as well as the prostate gland and urethra.

Testicular Contusion

The testicles are vulnerable to direct contact in many sports. Although protective equipment such as an athletic support and athletic cup are widely available, some athletes choose not to wear them. Testicular contusions occur with direct contact to the testes and result in pain and spasming. When injured, the testicles will ascend in spasm toward the core of the body, and the athlete can be incapacitated for a time due to the pain. Although many strategies have been used to help the athlete, having him lie on his back with his knees to his chest will help break the spasm, as will standing in a bent-over position. It is important to advise the athlete to check their urine and monitor any swelling to ensure more serious complications do not arise.

Testicular Torsion

The testicles are suspended and have the potential to twist upon themselves within the **scrotum**, creating a lack of blood flow to the testicle itself. The patient may report one-sided scrotum pain and may experience swelling. A **testicular torsion** is a true medical emergency and requires prompt referral to preserve the viability of the testicle. Blood flow will need to be restored immediately, which may require surgery.

Hydrocele and Varicocele

A water-filled cyst around the testicle in the scrotum is called a **hydrocele**. These cysts are often painful and are typically noticed by the athlete when inflammation or injury is present. A varicocele is an enlargement of the veins in the scrotum. This occurs when the blood fails to circulate out of the scrotum and stays trapped in the veins around the testicles (Mayo Clinic n.d.a). Again, medical referral is the prudent treatment for these suspected conditions. For more information, please see https://www.mayoclinic.org/diseases-conditions/varicocele/diagnosis-treatment/drc-20378772.

Testicular and Prostate Cancer

The prostate gland is a small organ located deep in the reproductive system behind the testicles. It is often a site for cancer formation in males. The prostate is checked during physical examinations by physicians in men over the age of 40. However, it is not impossible for a younger man to experience prostate problems. Often, they report difficulty urinating and pain in the region. They report having to go to the bathroom more often but not feeling like they can completely eliminate all the urine. Testicular cancer is another cancer of the male reproductive system. Men will likely find a mass in or around their testicle with or without pain. Just like with women and breast self-examination, testicular self-examination is an important step in early detection. Athletes with cancer work with a medical team, including an oncologist.

SEXUALLY TRANSMITTED INFECTIONS

Athletes trust their ATs, and the AT is often the first line of medical counsel for students having medical issues. Although sexually transmitted infections are quite personal, many athletes will reach out to the AT for guidance. Understanding the signs and symptoms communicated to you by the athlete will help you secure a prompt, proper referral for the athlete (Kahanov and Payne 2022, pp. 358-361).

Herpes Simplex Virus (HSV)

Genital herpes is a lifelong condition characterized by pain, painful urination, genital skin ulcers, fever, and swelling. This disease is contagious and can easily be spread through direct contact during times of viral shedding. A physician will treat the patient after a careful evaluation to ensure proper immediate care and education regarding the spread of the virus.

Genital Warts

Genital warts are caused by the human papillomavirus (HPV) and are typically asymptomatic. Most often, the athlete identifies the wartlike growth, which gives them concern after feeling pain and seeing redness around the anus or genitals. Athletes will be referred to a physician who will determine if medical agents, pharmacological agents, or surgical treatment is needed.

RED FLAGS

The following signs and symptoms require referral to a physician:

- Abdominal pain or pain in a specific region of the genitourinary anatomy
- Blood in the urine or bloody discharge
- Frequent urination or inability to urinate
- Abnormal discharge
- Unusual lumps, warts, lesions, or textures in the genital structures
- Fever, nausea, and vomiting after injury or spontaneous with pain

The Real World

A young male athlete reported to football camp with no medical conditions prohibiting him from participation. In a game, he went over the top of the line and was immediately struck by the defense. He landed on the field on his back with his knees pulled up and was in considerable pain. Upon arriving on the field, the AT ruled out a solar plexus injury and determined it was a testicular contusion. Within minutes, the athlete was in excruciating pain. The AT transported him to the athletic training facility, where the team physician evaluated the injury. Upon examination, they discovered that the testicles had swollen to the size of cantaloupes. The AT called the emergency squad, and the athlete was taken immediately into surgery. He had torn a blood vessel in the testicles, which resulted in a huge collection of blood in the scrotum. This was a true medical emergency, and prompt attention by the medical team resulted in a positive outcome for the athlete.

Kimberly Peer, EdD, ATC, FNATA

Chlamydia

A commonly reported infectious disease, chlamydia can lead to pelvic inflammatory disease. This condition is characterized by yellow or bloody discharge and pain with urination. Some patients report pain in the lower abdomen as well. Athletes who report this type of discharge should be referred to a physician for evaluation and treatment, which is usually antibiotics.

Gonorrhea

This is another disease that is classified by discharge and pain in the reproductive organs. Women usually show signs later than men, and the complications from this disease can result in fertility issues and reactive arthritis. This condition, like all suspected sexually transmitted infections, requires referral to the physician for proper care and treatment.

Summary

Genitourinary conditions can occur in athletes of all ages. Although most are referred to physicians for diagnosis and care, it is important for the AT to identify signs and symptoms through a careful history and appropriate examination. As the first line of communication for many athletes, the AT must be educated on and prepared to address medical conditions in all major systems of the body.

Key Terms

Define the following terms from this chapter:

amenorrhea
dysmenorrhea
ectopic
fallopian tubes
gynecologist
hydrocele
kidney
oncologist
ovary
pelvic inflammatory disease (PID)
scrotum
testicular torsion
ureter
urethra

You are approached by a student who was recently hit in the testicles while playing soccer. The pain was immediate but subsided during the next few minutes. However, it has been 24 hours and the athlete is still experiencing considerable pain in the testicular region. What are your treatment recommendations and to whom will you refer this athlete? Explain your rationale.

To access supplementary material for this chapter, including the Understanding Check worksheet, vocabulary quizzes, extension activities, and chapter-specific resources and forms, visit the web resource: http://ancillaries.humankinetics.com/FundamentalsOfAthleticTrainingAndSportsMedicine5E

chapter 14

Spinal Injuries

Objectives

After completing this chapter, the student will be able to do the following:

- Describe the basic anatomy of the spine.
- Explain common spinal injuries that occur with athletic participation.
- Identify common signs and symptoms of spinal injuries.
- Explain the treatments performed by ATs for specific spinal injuries.
- Describe common postural problems.

Like other joints in the body, the joints in the spine consist of articulated bones supported by muscles and ligaments. However, the spinal column is more complex than many joints and includes other structures such as discs and nerves. Because it protects the spinal cord, injuries to the spine can be life-threatening and need careful attention by the AT. Most spinal cord injuries are in the lumbar and cervical regions, so this chapter considers only injuries to those areas.

ANATOMY OF THE SPINE

The spine is a complex structure of bones with four segments—the **sacrum** (tailbone area), **lumbar spine** (lower spine), **thoracic spine** (middle spine), and **cervical spine** (upper spine; see figure 14.1). Normal anatomical position and muscular strength keep the spinal segments aligned properly. The spine should have curvature at each of these areas. Normal alignment is termed a **neutral spine**—this means that the spinal curves of the lumbar, thoracic, and cervical region are curved neither too much nor too little, and the spine is comfortable. Such a position is anatomically the strongest.

Bones

The bones in the spine are separated by discs and held together by ligaments. The muscles of the spine and trunk permit many movements and help to stabilize the spine.

The bones of the spine are called *vertebrae*. There are 7 cervical, 12 thoracic, 5 lumbar, and 5

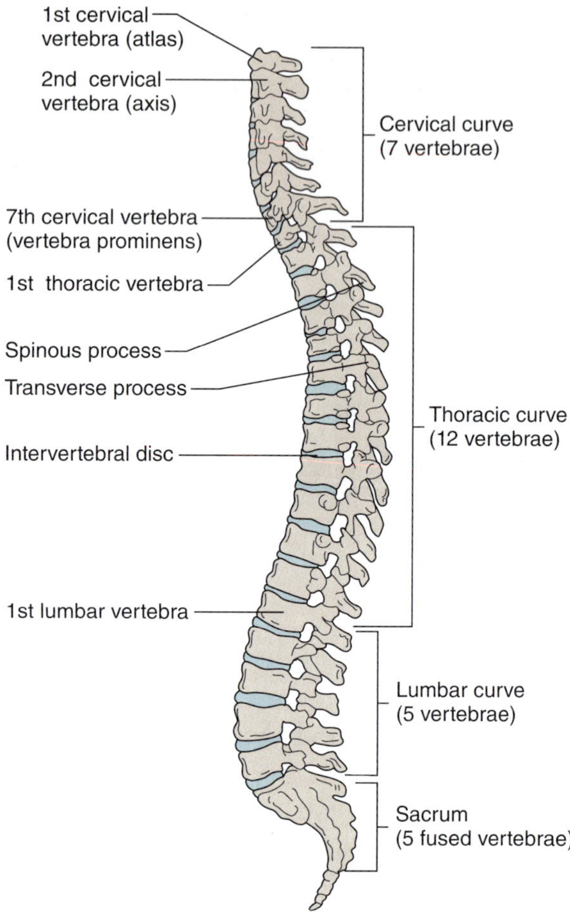

Figure 14.1 Lateral view of the spine. The natural anterior and posterior curves of the spine allow it to absorb shock. Note also the differences in size of the cervical, thoracic, and lumbar vertebrae.

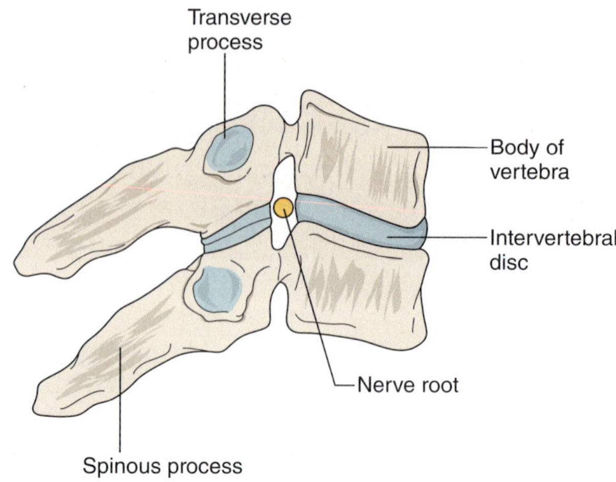

Figure 14.2 A normal vertebra. Each vertebra has a body, a transverse process, and a spinous process. An intervertebral disc lies between each pair of vertebrae to absorb shock.

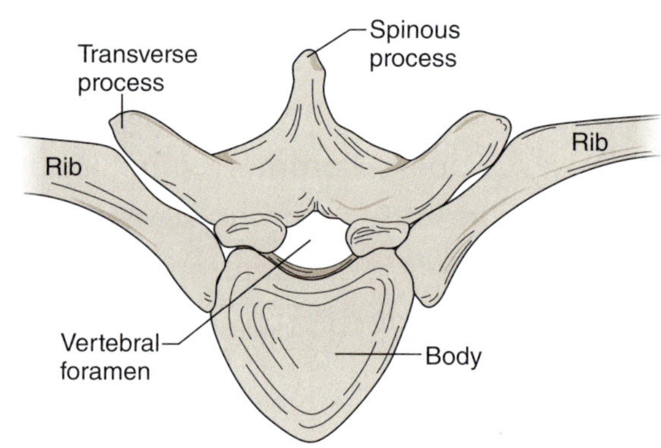

Figure 14.3 Inferior view of normal vertebra.

sacral (which are fused together) vertebrae. Though there are differences between the vertebrae of each region, they also share many similarities. For example, each vertebra has a body, a spinous process, and a canal through which the spinal cord passes (see figures 14.2 and 14.3). The bony spinal column has several functions: protecting the spinal cord, holding the body upright for walking, and serving as a site for muscular attachments.

Discs

The **intervertebral discs** that lie between the vertebrae absorb shock and resist compression during activity. They separate the vertebrae, which allows movement and flexibility, and they provide space for nerves to exit the spinal cord and enter the rest of the body. Figure 14.4 shows a disc cross-section.

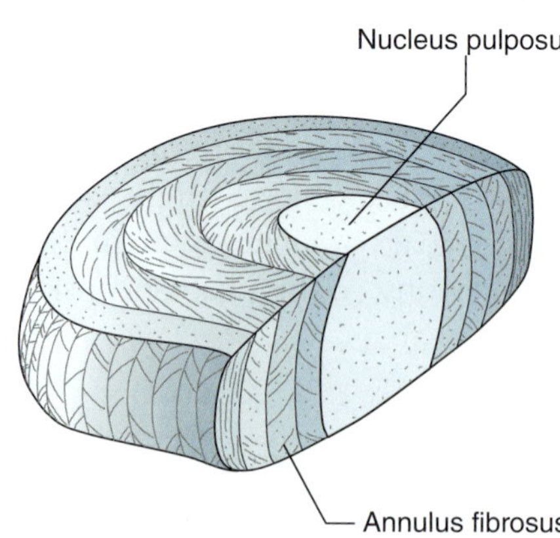

Figure 14.4 Disc cross-section. The disc lies between the vertebral bodies. The nucleus pulposus, located at the center of the disc, is a jellylike substance.

A disc has two parts: a jellylike core called the **nucleus pulposus** that is surrounded by several layers of cartilage called the **annulus fibrosus**. The discs of the spine do not receive any blood supply, so they do not have the same healing potential as other tissues of the body. The discs are compressible—a person is slightly taller first thing in the morning than later in the day, after gravity has been compressing the discs, and in old age we become shorter.

Foramen

A **foramen** is an opening, and there are several foramen in the spine of particular importance to the AT. The vertebral foramen is the opening where the large spinal cord itself passes behind all the bodies of the vertebrae. It is protected in this bony structure as long as the vertebrae remain in proper anatomical position (figure 14.5). The intervertebral foramen is where the parts of the vertebrae come together to create an opening on each side of the vertebrae. The opening is created from the junction of the bottom of the top vertebrae coming together with the upper part of the lower vertebrae (figure 14.6). These facets create a hole to allow for the nerve roots that come off the spinal cord itself to go out to the various parts of the body. As these nerve roots leave the upper spine, they are called the brachial plexus and innervate the upper part of the body (figure 14.7). Where they exit out of the

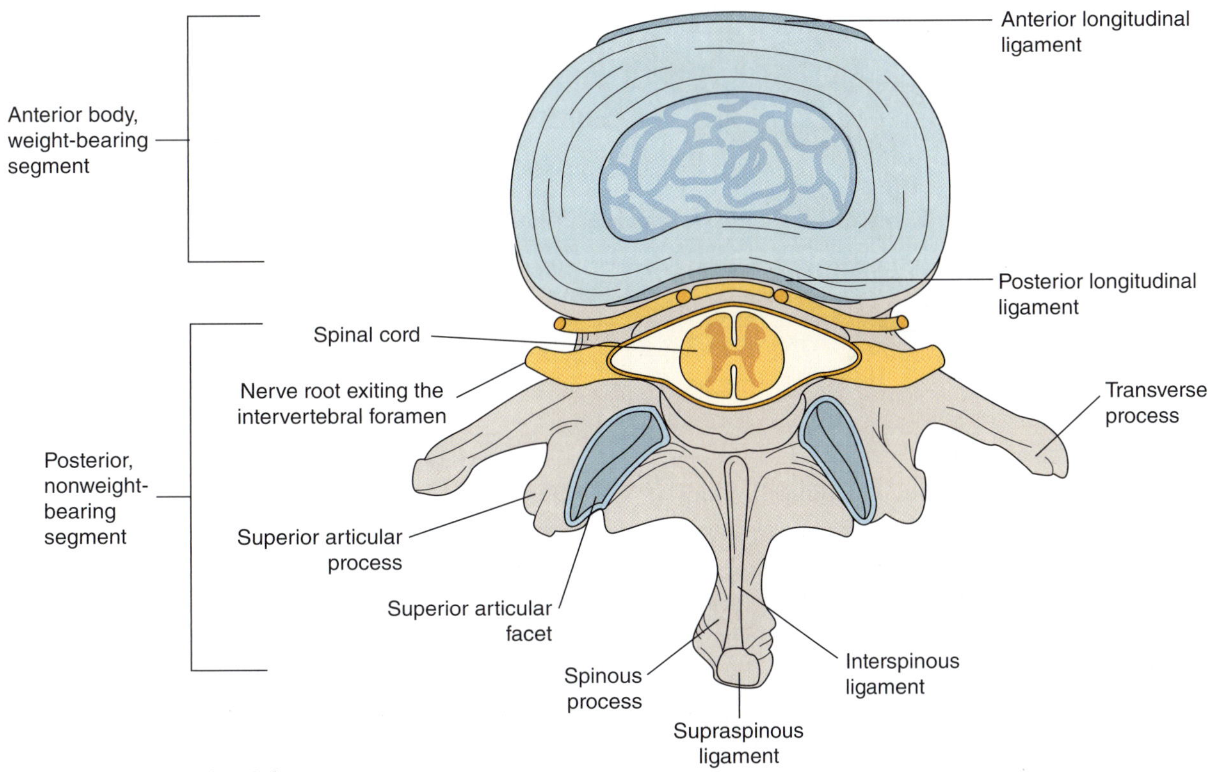

Figure 14.5 Vertebral foramen.

Reprinted by permission from S.J. Shultz, P.A. Houglum, and D.H. Perrin, *Examination of Musculoskeletal Injuries*, 4th ed. (Champaign, IL: Human Kinetics, 2016), 369.

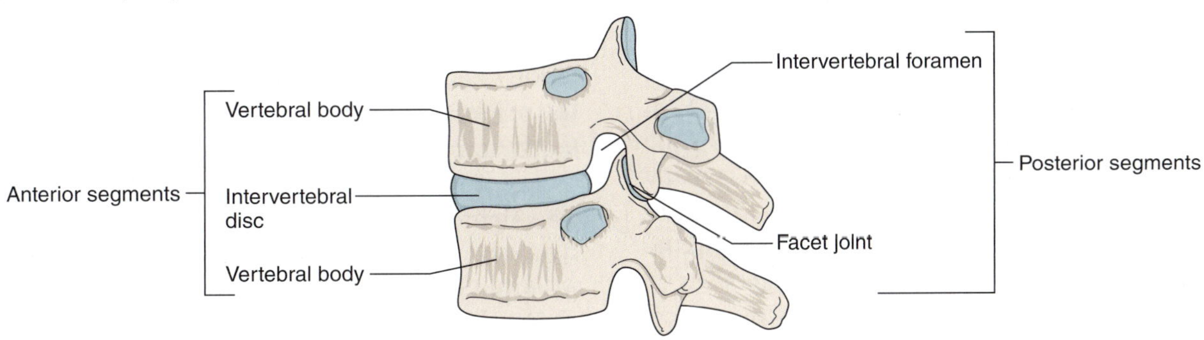

Figure 14.6 Intervertebral foramen with nerve roots.

Reprinted by permission from S.J. Shultz, P.A. Houglum, and D.H. Perrin, *Examination of Musculoskeletal Injuries*, 4th ed. (Champaign, IL: Human Kinetics, 2016), 368.

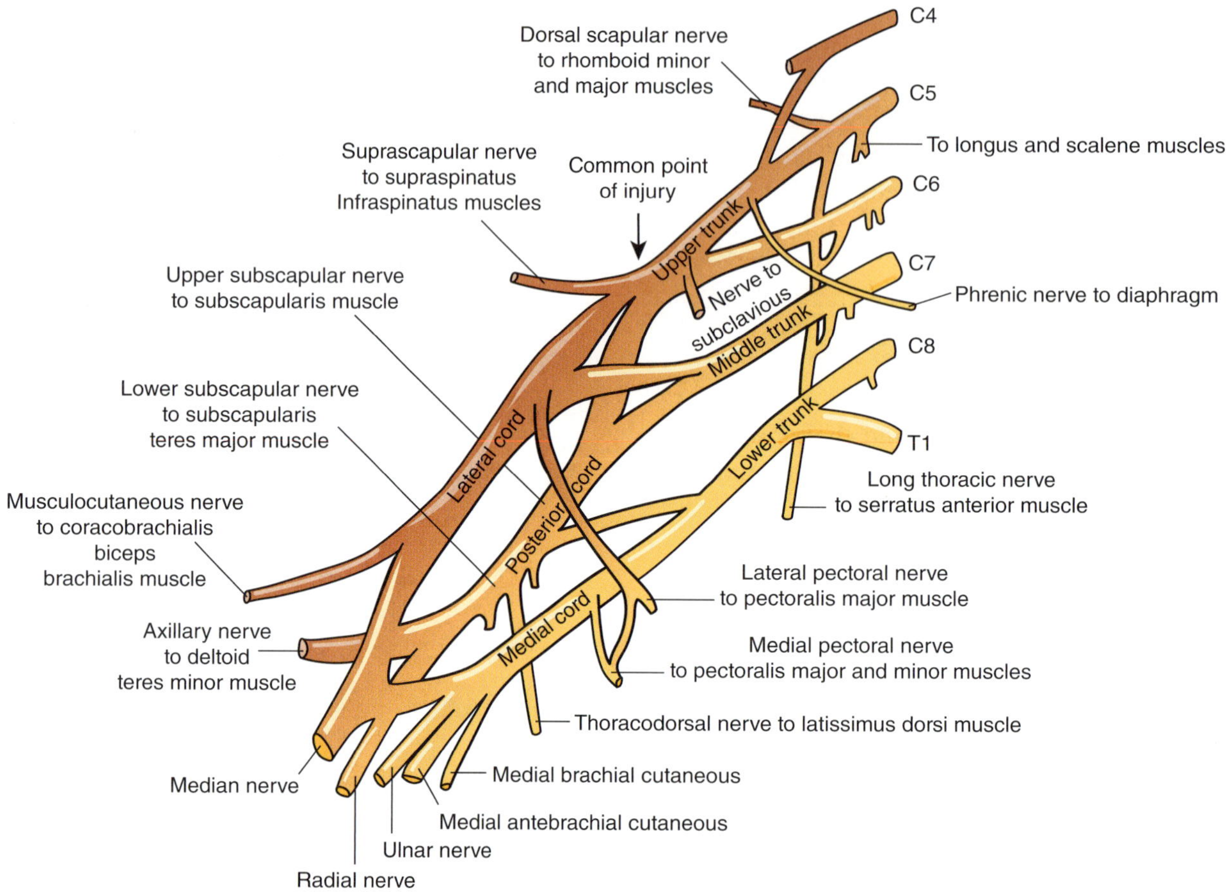

Figure 14.7 Brachial plexus.

Reprinted by permission from S.J. Shultz, P.A. Houglum, and D.H. Perrin, *Examination of Musculoskeletal Injuries*, 4th ed. (Champaign, IL: Human Kinetics, 2016), 219.

lower part of the spine, they are called the lumbar plexus. Figure 14.8 shows the dermatomes associated with the lumbar plexus. Each of these nerve roots have a specific function in the body and can be evaluated individually by an experienced AT.

Muscles and Tendons

The muscles of the trunk and neck attach to the spine via tendons and provide both a wide range of movement and much-needed stability. James Porterfield and Carl DeRosa, two highly respected physical therapists, describe the spine as a mast on a ship (1991). A mast has many cables attached to it at various points that extend to different places on the ship. These cables keep the mast stable as the wind catches its sail. Likewise, the spine has many muscles attached at various points that extend to the pelvis, legs, and arms. These muscles keep the spine stable as the body performs tasks such as throwing, catching, and kicking. If the ship has a mast that bends and folds, the sail will not catch the wind effectively. Similarly, if the body has a spine that bends and gives because of poor stability, it will not perform athletic tasks effectively. This concept is called **dynamic stabilization**, meaning that the muscles of the spine, legs, abdomen, and chest must all be strengthened and in balance to provide stability and prevent injury when a person is engaging in work or sport-related activities (figure 14.9).

The abdominal muscles are crucial for supporting trunk movement, especially the rectus abdominis and the internal and external obliques. The spinal extensors run the entire length of the spine posteriorly and attach to various structures, including the pelvis, ribs, and vertebrae. These muscles work together to keep the body upright.

The upper trapezius extends the cervical spine (see figure 7.4). It attaches to the occipital bone (back of head) and fans out to each side of the neck before attaching to the acromion process of the scapula (see figure 7.3).

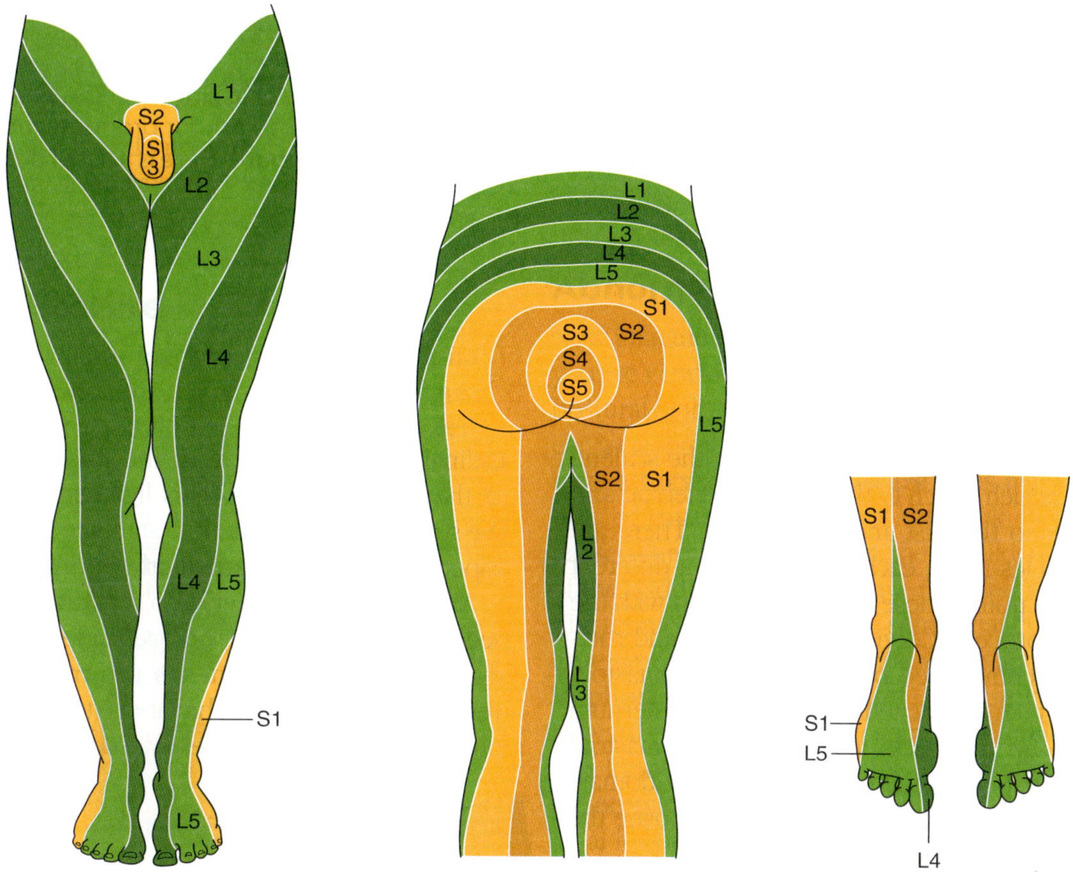

Figure 14.8 Lumbar plexus.

Reprinted by permission from S.J. Shultz, P.A. Houglum, and D.H. Perrin, *Examination of Musculoskeletal Injuries*, 4th ed. (Champaign, IL: Human Kinetics, 2016), 383.

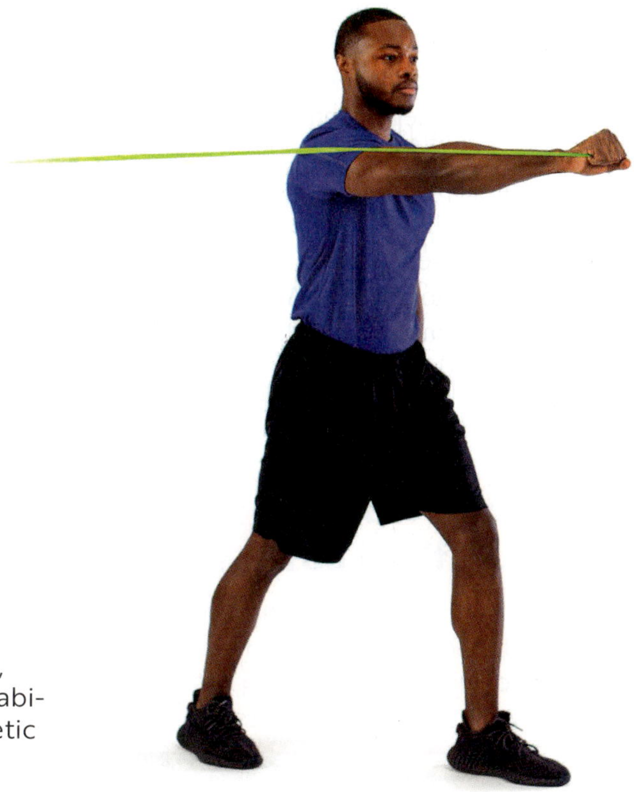

Figure 14.9 Contracting the abdominal, leg, chest, and back muscles creates dynamic stabilization of the spine to help people do athletic activities safely and more effectively.

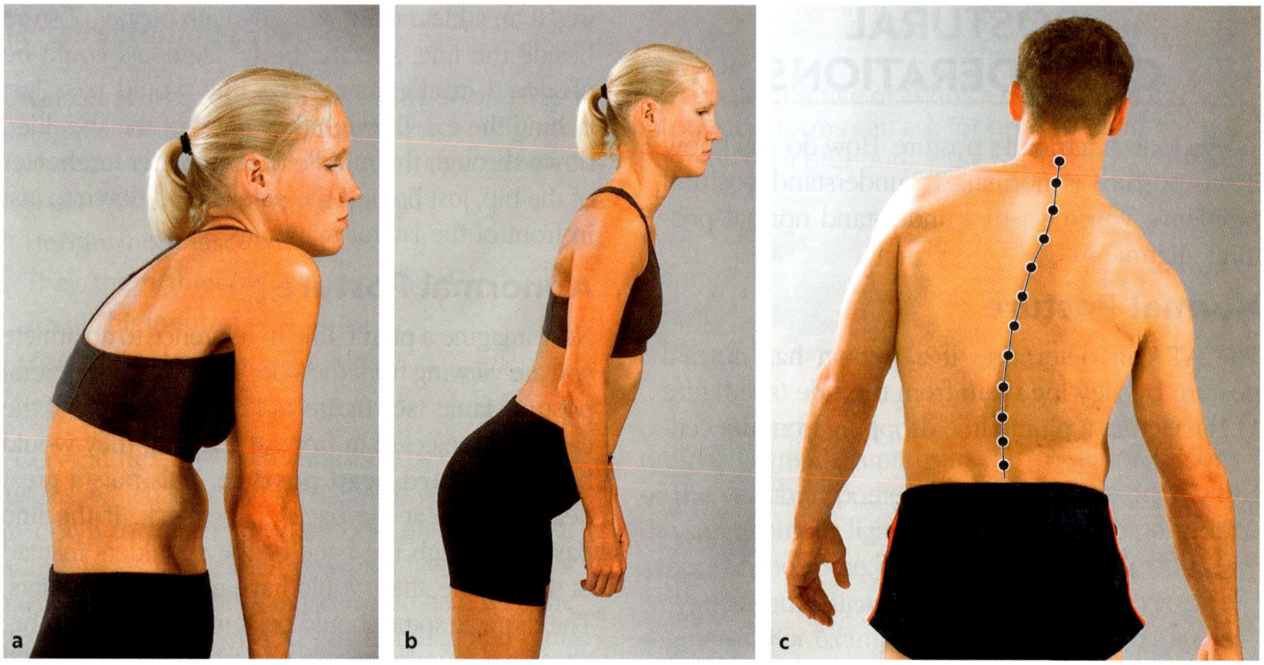

Figure 14.12 Abnormal postures: *(a)* kyphosis, *(b)* lordosis, and *(c)* scoliosis.

Spinal Stenosis

Spinal stenosis is a narrowing of the spinal canal or the intervertebral foramen. A stenosis can occur at birth or be caused by a bulging disc or a bony spur. The symptoms include pain, muscular weakness, and numbness. The cervical and lumbar spine are the most likely areas for a stenosis (Mayo Clinic n.d.).

Athletes can take steps to prevent poor postural habits, such as imagining balloons attached to their head that are pulling up straight. Athletes can also alternate carrying their book bag or gym bag on opposite shoulders. Putting a heavy book bag on the same shoulder every day throughout the high school and college career can take its toll on the spine. Athletes can stay fit and exercise regularly, too. The body is made to move, and being a slug will cause stiffness. Be kind to the spine, and use proper posture whenever possible.

PREVENTING SPINAL INJURIES

Preventing injury to the cervical and lumbar regions of the spine is an active process. Athletes should participate in exercise and flexibility programs, maintain proper posture, learn to lift properly, use proper technique (e.g., proper tackling in football), and perhaps use back support when lifting heavy objects.

Exercise and flexibility programs are necessary for the muscles surrounding and supporting the spine, especially the abdominal muscles. A strong abdomen can help decrease stress on the lumbar spine. The muscles around the hip should also be strengthened because the hip directly influences the spine. If the hip is tilted forward, the spine will move into extension, and if the hip is tilted backward, the spine will move into flexion. Therefore, the hip musculature should be both flexible and strong to allow proper movement and positioning in the lumbar region.

Proper lifting procedures reduce the risk of injury (see figure 14.13). Businesspeople understand that if an employee improperly lifts a weight, they can injure their back. To prevent such injuries, businesses have begun sending employees to training called *back school*. Back schools are short-term instructional programs that teach people proper posture and lifting techniques. Proper lifting technique is maintaining a slight curve in the lumbar spine while lifting with the knees and the hips

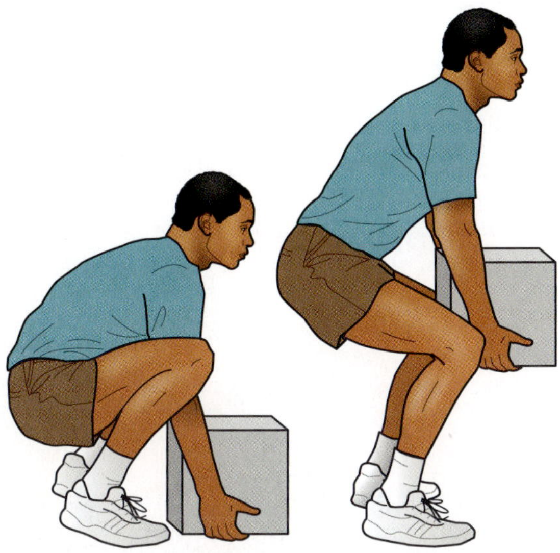

Figure 14.13 Proper lifting entails keeping the head up, the feet in a wide stance, and the spine in a neutral position. Also, keeping the load close to the body reduces stress on the back.

Adapted by permission from E.T. Howley and B.D. Franks, *Health Fitness Instructor's Handbook*, 4th ed. (Champaign, IL: Human Kinetics, 2003), 63.

rather than the spine. It also involves keeping the head up when lifting. A lifting posture in which the spine is too rounded or flexed may cause a strain or disc injury.

Back supports have become popular recently. Go to any home repair store, lumberyard, or even some grocery stores, and you will see many of the workers wearing these belts. Back supports increase the pressure around the spine and decrease the amount of stress to the vertebrae. A back support, however, should not take the place of other means of injury prevention—using the brace alone cannot prevent all injuries.

Recognizing that proper technique plays a role in preventing cervical spine injuries, NATA published a position statement regarding the head-down technique in football (Heck et al. 2004). It states that initiating contact at the top of the helmet (also known as spearing) creates an axial load. An **axial load** occurs when force is applied to the head while the head is lowered into flexion; this load straightens the cervical spine like a drinking straw. If you take a drinking straw and push on the ends hard enough, it will eventually bend. A similar event occurs at the cervical spine, causing vertebrae fractures.

According to the NATA position statement found in the online resources, axial loading is the key mechanism for catastrophic injuries in football; thus, football players should tackle with the shoulders while positioning the head in an upward position. Many coachers teach athletes to see their tackling targets. This is a cue to remind players to keep the head up while tackling.

TREATING LUMBAR SPINE INJURIES AND CONDITIONS

As with other parts of the body, the spine is susceptible to ligament, muscle, tendon, and bone injuries. In addition, the discs that lie between the bodies of the vertebrae cause unique problems.

Bone Injuries

Bone fractures are possible in the lumbar spine, especially with severe mechanisms of injury such as compression; for instance, forcefully landing on the buttocks could cause a compression fracture. Fractures of the spine are hard to determine without an X-ray. However, if an AT knows the mechanism of injury and finds a great deal of back pain, muscle spasm, and tenderness when touching the vertebrae, a fracture must be suspected. If the AT suspects a lumbar fracture, the athlete should be treated conservatively; that is, they should be put on a backboard with the help of appropriate emergency medical personnel and taken to the nearest hospital.

Two common bone injuries found among athletes are **spondylolysis** and **spondylolisthesis**. These bony problems are most commonly found in athletes such as gymnasts because they arch their backs and subject their spines to a great deal of hyperextension. Spondylolysis is often described as a stress fracture or bone degeneration of the vertebrae, specifically at a location referred to as the *pars interarticularis*. The pars interarticularis is located on a thin portion of the vertebrae between the superior and inferior facets. The location of the bone degeneration is important because if the fracture fails to heal, it can separate, causing the spine to become unstable. The resulting instability allows a vertebra to slip forward (shunt) on the vertebra below it. This is called *spondylolisthesis* (see figure 14.14). The most common location for this injury is the fifth lumbar vertebra slipping forward on the first sacral vertebra.

Spondylolysis and spondylolisthesis are serious problems, and they require examination by a physician. In many instances, the athlete is required to discontinue the aggravating activity and wear a lumbar brace to keep the vertebral segment stable. The athlete must then perform extensive rehabilitation that focuses on strengthening the trunk muscles in a neutral spine position.

Disc Injuries

One of the most common injuries of the lumbar spine is a disc bulge (see figure 14.15). This condition is not common in younger athletes, but older athletes seem to be susceptible to it. Although some people call it a *slipped disc*, that is not an appropriate term. The disc is attached to the body of the vertebra and rarely slips forward or backward. In a disc bulge, the jellylike nucleus pulposus at the center of the disc pushes through the rings of cartilage. For example, if you were to place the palms of your hands on the top and bottom of a jelly donut and squeeze, jelly would begin to ooze through the layers of dough. Similarly, when a disc is compressed, the nucleus pulposus begins to press through the layers of cartilage around it and eventually can press against the outer layer, causing it to bulge.

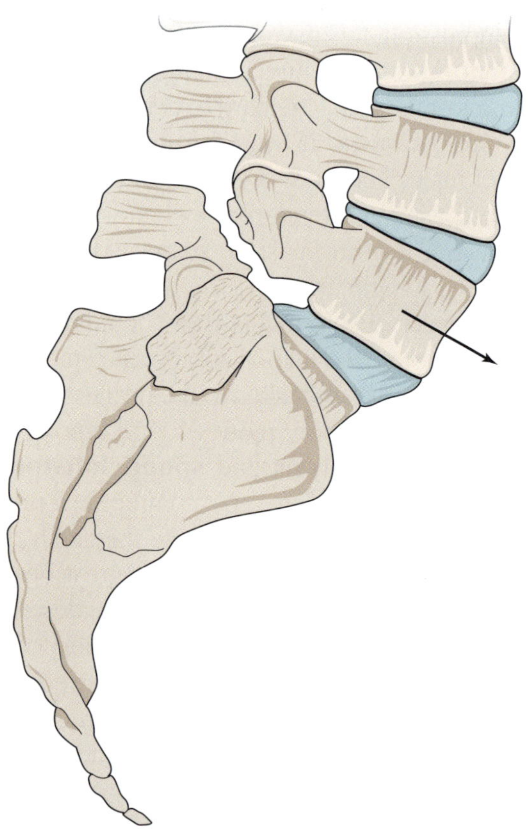

Figure 14.14 Spondylolisthesis.

RED FLAGS

The following are signs and symptoms of spinal injuries that require emergency care:

- An axial load mechanism of injury
- Difficulty breathing
- Deformity of the spine
- Loss of sensation in extremities
- Shooting pains in extremities
- Loss of motion in extremities
- Pain along the spine
- Loss of consciousness
- Low blood pressure of 90/60 mmHg (National Heart, Lung, and Blood Institute n.d.)
- Heart rate less than 60 beats per minute

Discs rarely bulge toward the front of the spine for two reasons. First, the front of the spine is covered with a thick ligament called the *anterior longitudinal ligament,* and second, most people have postures that flex the spine forward most of the time. Flexion of the spine tends to put more pressure on the front of the disc, pushing the nucleus pulposus toward the posterior. Most often discs bulge posteriorly to one side or another, which may put pressure on the nerve exiting the spinal cord at that level (see figure 14.15).

Disc bulges are aggravating and can be disabling. If the disc bulge puts pressure on a nerve, numbness, tingling, and pain can occur down the leg. Another characteristic of this condition is pain in the lower back that increases with sitting. **Sciatica** occurs from pressure on the sciatic nerve that runs from the sacrum to the posterior aspect of the legs. Sciatica occurs because of a bulging disc, a bone

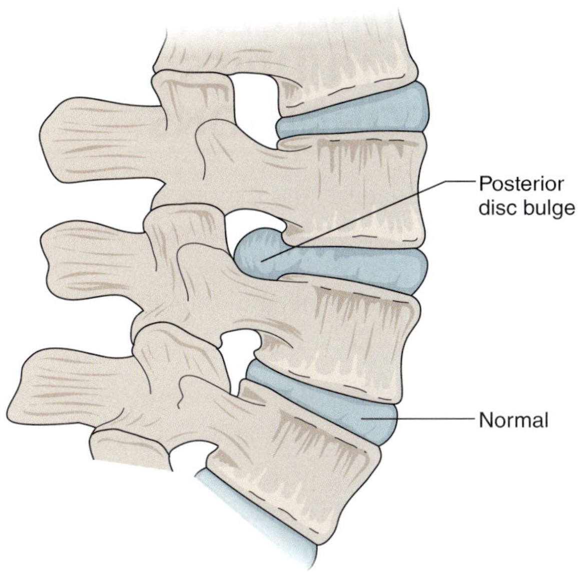

Figure 14.15 A posterior disc bulge. As the spine is flexed, pressure is put on the anterior part of the disc, which encourages the nucleus pulposus to push through layers of the annulus fibrosus.

spur, or a stenosis of the spine. Typical symptoms include shooting pain down the hip and into the leg and muscular weakness of the affected leg.

Treating an athlete with a disc bulge requires the AT to understand the causes of this condition. Most often, disc bulges are the result of poor posture and body mechanics that put the spine in a great deal of flexion over a long time. For example, a softball infielder who does not maintain a neutral posture may await a pitch with the spine flexed forward. If this same person also sits with a slouchy posture and uses poor lifting mechanics, they may eventually be at risk of a disc bulge.

Under the direction of the team physician, an AT may initially treat a disc bulge by using active rest, as with a sprain (see the section on Ligament Injuries). Also, correcting poor posture and helping the athlete move into spinal extension can be helpful. It is thought that if proper posture and body mechanics are used, the nucleus pulposus will not bulge quite as much, which will give the athlete relief. The AT should make certain that none of the exercises aggravates the leg pain or causes more numbness or tingling. As the athlete progresses, extension exercises, and sometimes traction (discussed in chapter 21), may help reduce the disc bulge. Athletes should also be taught about proper sitting, standing, and lifting postures that minimize pressure on the disc, and they should avoid prolonged sitting. Strengthening the spine with lumbar stabilization techniques is also helpful.

Muscle and Tendon Injuries

An AT rarely sees a ruptured muscle at the lumbar spine, but mild and moderate strains are common. Characteristics of lumbar strain include pain to one side of the spine, spasm, and lack of movement. Also, the athlete will often present with pain on the opposite side of the direction in which they bend. For example, if they bend to the left and the pain is on the right side of the spine, the muscle to the right of the spine may be strained. The pain associated with sprains is localized, whereas pain caused by a muscle strain usually moves up and down the length of the muscle, especially when the athlete tries to use the muscle while bending. Remember that the spine is like a mast on a ship, and the muscles are the guy wires. If the spine is bent to one side, the muscles on the opposite side will attempt to stabilize it. The AT can initially apply ice to the injury, and gentle stretching using a knees-to-chest routine often speeds healing. Once pain is decreased, flexibility and strength can be restored to normal using strengthening and stretching routines. The AT should observe the athlete for proper posture and lifting mechanics to prevent reinjury.

> **FYI**
>
> **Compressing the Spine**
>
> Sitting creates a greater compressive load on the spine than standing does.

Torticollis

Torticollis is a condition of the neck in which the head is tilted toward the shoulder where a muscle strain or sprain has occurred. The chin is turned away from the injured side of the neck. Turning or tilting the head to its normal position is painful. The AT will treat the torticollis with cryotherapy, heat therapy, gentle stretching, massage, trigger-point release, and range-of-motion exercises.

Ligament Injuries

Sprains at the lumbar joints commonly occur when athletes are forced into excessive trunk flexion or attempt to flex the spine and rotate at the same time. An example of this mechanism is when a football player is tackled and forced forward. When the trunk flexion is combined with rotation, the posterior aspect of the vertebral joints can separate and stretch over the ligaments. Characteristics of a lumbar sprain include pain to one side of the spine and limited movement because of pain and muscle spasm. An AT who takes a thorough history of the injury and performs special spinal tests can determine if the ligaments are involved, although it can be difficult to differentiate from a muscle strain. During an assessment, an AT might gently perform a stress test that pushes each vertebra anteriorly. This will usually be painful if the joint is sprained, but it should not be painful if a strain is present, unless the strain is severe. Of course, an AT will not perform such a test if signs or symptoms of a fracture are present.

When a sprain initially occurs, the AT should treat it the same as any other acute injury. As we will discuss in chapter 25, the critical treatment in this phase is PRICES, which stands for **p**rotection, **r**est, **i**ce, **c**ompression, **e**levation, and **s**upport. Many believe that heat should always be used for spine injuries. With an acute injury, however, this may do more harm than good because heat tends to increase swelling and pain. But 48 hours postinjury, it is typically all right to use heat.

Though rest is recommended, complete bed rest is no longer the accepted norm. Rather, the athlete should engage in active rest, maintaining a comfortable neutral spine position and gently performing strengthening exercises to stabilize the spine. (Strengthening exercises are discussed in chapter 22.) As the initial inflammation subsides, the AT can have the athlete begin flexibility exercises as well as advanced lumbar stabilization exercises as long as they do not aggravate the area. The spinal musculature needs to be strengthened in preparation for return to activity.

TREATING CERVICAL SPINE INJURIES AND CONDITIONS

As you might imagine, the injuries incurred at the cervical spine are similar to those at the lumbar spine. However, the cervical spine has more mobility than the lumbar spine, and thus the treatments differ.

Bone Injuries

Bone injuries to the cervical spine include fractures and dislocations, which can have devastating results, including permanent disabilities and death. Fractures to the cervical spine are often the result of an axial load, as discussed earlier in the chapter. This occurs when a force is applied to the head while it is lowered into flexion that straightens the cervical spine, resulting in vertebra fractures. A dislocation of the cervical vertebrae often results from a combination of excessive neck flexion and rotation.

Cervical spine fractures and dislocations have similar signs and symptoms. The athlete will often report pain around the cervical spine and weakness, numbness, and tingling down the arms. With a dislocation, there is often a visible deformity, but because of equipment or positioning, it is sometimes difficult to observe. A high cervical spine dislocation is especially concerning because this can place potentially fatal pressure on the nerves that serve the heart and lungs.

Most spinal cord injuries occur in the cervical and thoracic regions (Johns Hopkins Medicine n.d.). Injuries in these areas must be treated with caution because they may have caused a partial or complete tearing of the spinal cord. An injury as significant as a partial or complete tear of the spinal cord can result in quadriplegia or paraplegia, based on the level of the injury.

Quadriplegia results in the loss of use and sensation in both arms and legs. The injury occurs to the spinal cord in the cervical spine. **Paraplegia** results in the loss of function and sensation in the legs. Paraplegia occurs when the spinal cord is injured in the thoracic, lumbar, or sacral region.

Initial care for these injuries is identical. Emergency care procedures should be followed. The NATA's position statement, *Acute Management of the Cervical Spine—Injured Athlete*, provides a comprehensive perspective on all aspects of acute management. It can be found in the online resources. However, the fundamentals include ruling out life-threatening conditions and immobilizing the neck to place the athlete on a backboard. If the athlete is wearing a helmet and a cervical fracture or dislocation is suspected, the helmet should be left in place because attempting to remove it may cause excessive movement of the neck, which could lead to further damage. Although most people think of football helmets, ATs should know whether to remove other helmets as well. Baseball, softball, hockey, and lacrosse all have helmets to consider. Regardless of the helmet, the face mask should always be removed if immediate access to the airway is needed and if the patient will be transferred with equipment on (Cleary and Flanagan 2020, p. 271). Appropriate emergency medical personnel should take the athlete to the nearest hospital facility. See figure 14.16 for protocol for determining when to immobilize an athlete.

Disc Injuries

Disc injuries in the cervical spine are not nearly as common as those in the lumbar spine, but they can occur. An athlete with a cervical disc bulge often will report more neck pain while sitting and while flexing the neck forward than while standing and walking. They may also report discomfort down the back between the shoulder blades. Treatment for disc bulges of the cervical spine includes improving neck posture and then progressing to cervical extension exercises that do not aggravate the condition. Cervical traction can also be used by the AT under the direction of the team physician to help reduce the disc bulge. Full neck mobility and strength should gradually be regained. As with suspected fractures, if an athlete presents with severe symptoms, such as numbness, tingling, and burning of the arm, they should be put on a spine board and referred to a hospital. The AT should consult the team physician regarding the athlete's return to participation following this condition.

The Real World

After school, the AT was called to assist an injured female gymnast. She had been performing a back flip in the gym when she landed shoulders and neck first. She was lying face down, with her right arm under her body and her head turned to the side. The initial exam revealed point tenderness along her trapezius muscle and lower cervical spine. All neurological signs were fine. The athlete was laughing and wanted to get up. The AT felt extra caution was necessary based on how she fell, so EMS was summoned. The student became upset, but the AT reassured her that this was the best option. The AT knew that appearances and an athlete's attitude do not always represent an accurate picture.

Several hours later, the injured girl's father called the AT to thank him for being so cautious. The girl had suffered a fracture dislocation of C3 and fractures of C4 and C5. By insisting that she be backboarded and transported, the AT may have saved her from paralysis or death. The athlete was placed in a special neck brace for three months. The fractures healed, but the C3 dislocation remained out of alignment, so she had surgery to fuse the vertebrae. The young woman kept a positive attitude and was courageous throughout her ordeal. She was a definite inspiration to those around her. And although she was unable to return to gymnastics, she is now able to function normally in other aspects of her life. She even teaches gymnastics to younger athletes and has recently enrolled in a college athletic training curriculum.

Roger Kalisiak, ATC

Muscle and Tendon Injuries

A cervical muscle strain can also occur from a whiplash injury by the mechanism described in the following section. Characteristics of cervical muscle strains include muscle spasm, restricted range of motion, weakness against resistance, pain,

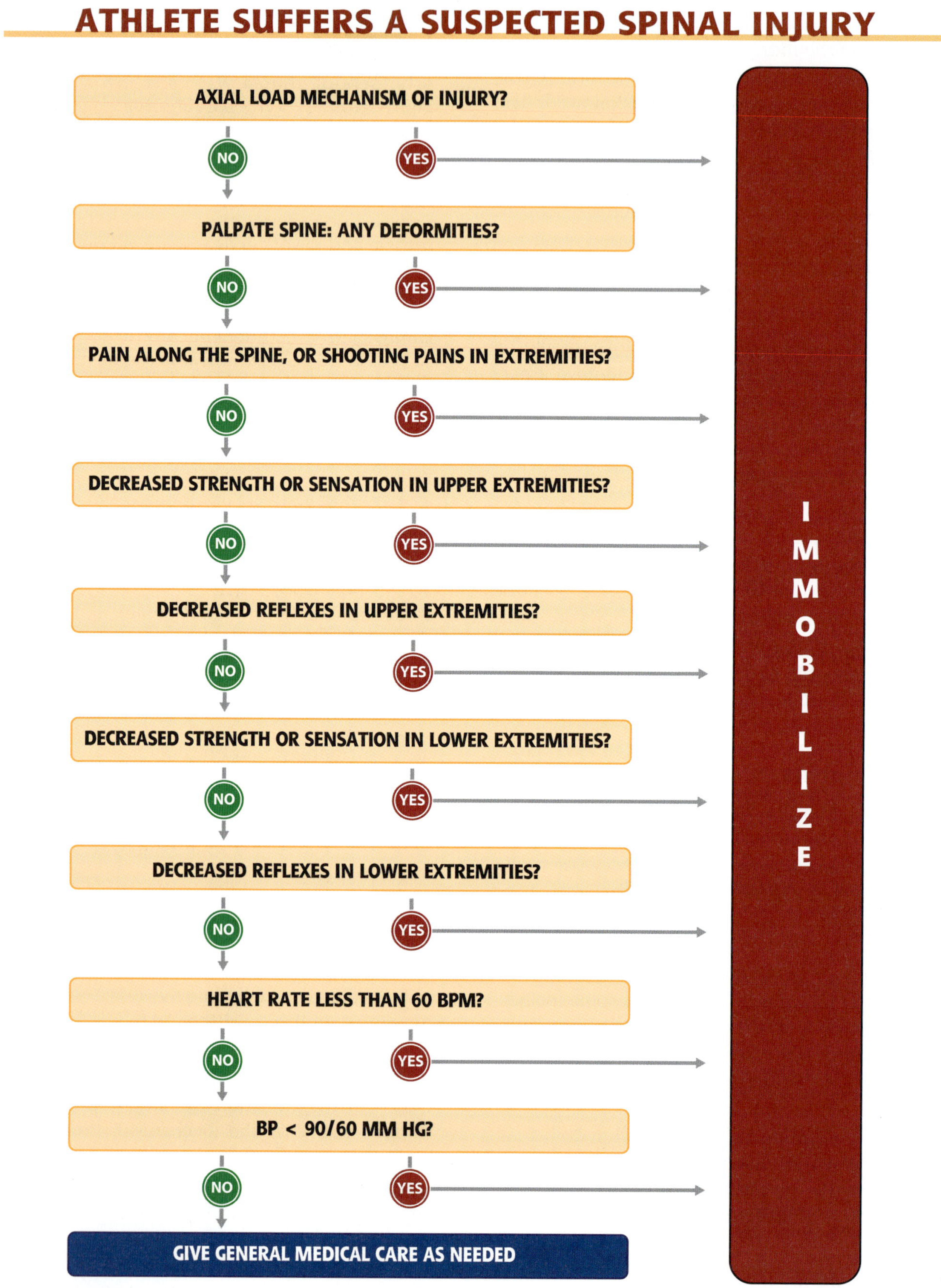

Figure 14.16 Protocol for determining when to immobilize.

and tenderness of the muscle. An AT should treat cervical strains much like cervical ligament sprains. The criteria for returning to play are the same as for cervical sprains. Manual resistance works well for strengthening the neck. Not a lot of exercise equipment is designed specifically for the neck; an alternative is performing cervical stretches while a partner provides resistance with their hand.

Ligament Injuries

Despite having an excellent range of motion, the cervical spine is subject to ligament sprains when it is forcefully moved beyond its normal range. Cervical sprains are usually the result of hyperextension or hyperflexion of the neck. Take a football receiver who stops, turns toward the quarterback to catch the ball, and then gets tackled by a defender. When hit forcefully from behind, the receiver often suffers a whiplash injury—in fact, many a receiver would say that he felt as if he were hit by a car. The body is forced forward by the blow while the head moves backward, placing the cervical spine into extension and stretching the ligaments and muscles at the front of the neck. When his body stops—because he hits the ground or is tackled from the front—his head snaps forward, stretching the posterior neck ligaments and muscles.

Cervical ligament sprains have symptoms of neck and arm pain. The athlete may even complain of pain between the scapulae. Because of the possibility of a spinal cord injury, the AT must thoroughly evaluate any neck trauma. Provided there is no sign of nerve injury, the AT can treat the neck. As with many other ligament injuries, the neck needs to be treated with protection, rest, ice, and support. No compression with an elastic bandage should be applied to the neck, however, because this may slow blood flow to the brain. A neck brace can be used to help the athlete hold the head up. A follow-up examination from the team physician is necessary to rule out any other conditions. Further treatment for the cervical spine sprain includes strengthening exercises to regain stability, and full range of motion should be reestablished. Before the athlete is allowed to return to participation, they must have the following:

- Full strength
- Full range of motion
- Full confidence
- No symptoms
- Physician clearance

Brachial Plexus Injuries

The brachial plexus is a network of nerves that exit the cervical spine and run through the shoulder and down the arm. An athlete who falls, runs into, or attempts to tackle another player can stretch the brachial plexus. Picture a linebacker tackling an opponent. As he makes the tackle, the shoulder is pressed downward and the neck is forced into a stretch in the opposite direction. This mechanism of injury often stretches the brachial plexus, resulting in burning, tingling, numbness, and stinging sensations of the arm and shoulder (see figure 14.17). For this reason, this condition is often called a **burner** or **stinger**. Depending on the severity of the injury, the burner may last for a matter of seconds or minutes. More severe cases can last much longer, even weeks. Treatment is often neck-strengthening exercises and range-of-motion stretching of the area. A football player is usually fitted with a neck roll that limits lateral flexion. Before returning to play following a burner, an athlete must have the following:

- No symptoms
- Full strength
- Full range of motion of the neck and shoulder
- A problem-free neck and shoulder evaluation by the AT and the team physician

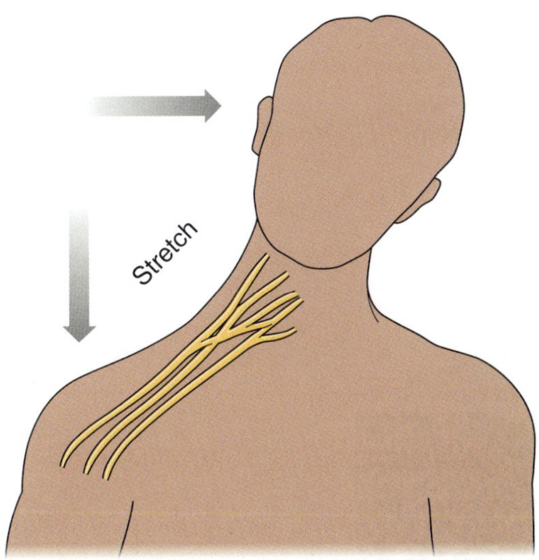

Figure 14.17 Stretching the brachial plexus causes burning, tingling, numbness, and stinging sensations of the arm and shoulder.

Summary

The spine is an articulated series of vertebrae that protect the spinal cord, and numerous muscles attach to it. A neutral spine, promoted by proper posture, is stable and absorbs shock. The spine may receive sprains and strains in the lumbar and cervical regions, but because of the spinal cord, nerve roots, and discs, other injuries to the spine may be more serious, even life-threatening. After any injury to the spinal area, an athlete must learn proper bending and lifting techniques and perform muscle-strengthening exercises to reduce the risk of further injury.

Key Terms

Define the following terms found in this chapter:

- annulus fibrosus
- axial load
- burner
- cervical spine
- dynamic stabilization
- foramen
- forward head posture
- intervertebral discs
- kyphosis
- lordosis
- lumbar spine
- neutral spine
- nucleus pulposus
- paraplegia
- quadriplegia
- sacrum
- sciatica
- scoliosis
- spinal stenosis
- spondylolisthesis
- spondylolysis
- stinger
- thoracic spine
- torticollis

An athlete comes to your clinic and indicates that the physician, an orthopedic surgeon, has diagnosed them with scoliosis. The doctor has recommended no surgery but indicates that exercises might help. In addition to stretching, the doctor says that pain can be managed with modalities. Is this a chronic or acute condition? Based on this condition, would you use ice or heat to manage the pain and why?

To access supplementary material for this chapter, including the Understanding Check worksheet, vocabulary quizzes, extension activities, and chapter-specific resources and forms, visit the web resource: http://ancillaries.humankinetics.com/FundamentalsOfAthleticTrainingAndSportsMedicine5E

Unit IV

Athletic-Related Injuries to the Upper Extremity

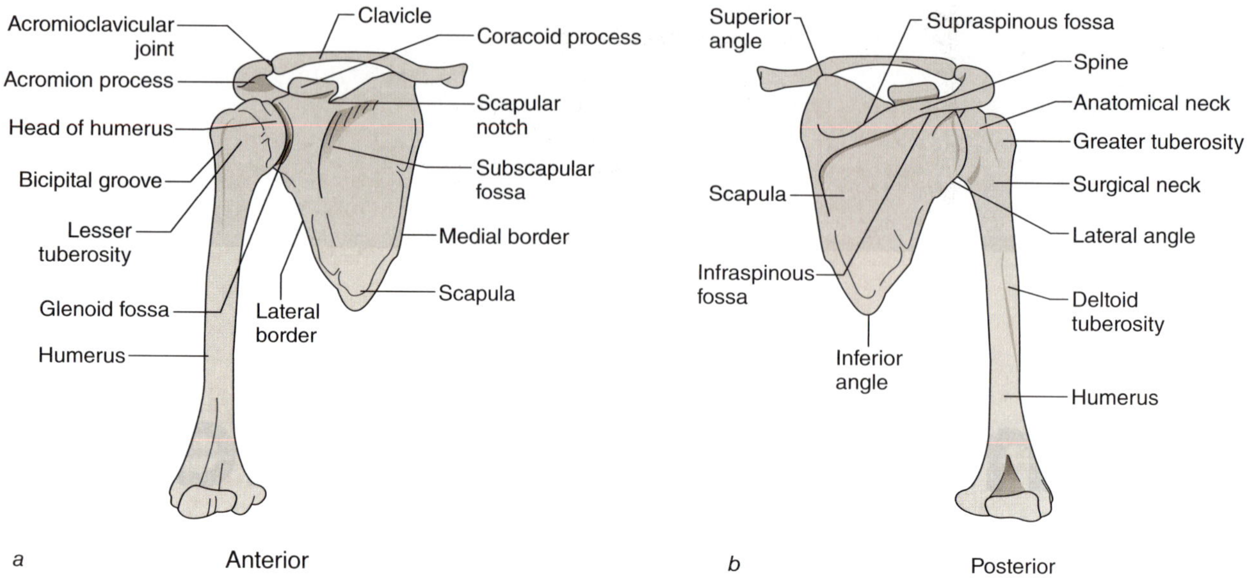

Figure 15.1 The bones of the shoulder girdle: *(a)* anterior view, *(b)* posterior view.

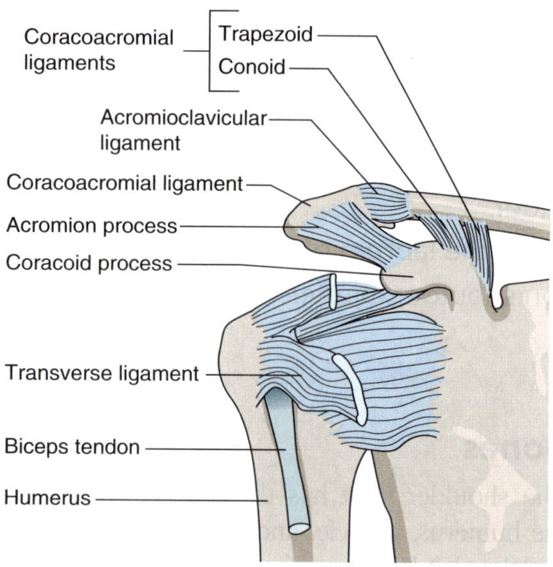

Figure 15.2 The ligaments of the shoulder.

ligaments hold the glenoid fossa and head of the humerus together, the acromioclavicular ligament creates a connection between two points on the scapula, the coracoclavicular ligament holds down the clavicle with two distinct parts (conoid and trapezoid), and the transverse ligament holds the biceps tendon in the bicipital groove. These help provide stability to an otherwise unstable anatomical joint.

Muscles and Tendons

The **rotator cuff** has four muscles—the subscapularis, infraspinatus, teres minor, and supraspinatus (see figure 15.3)—and their associated tendons that

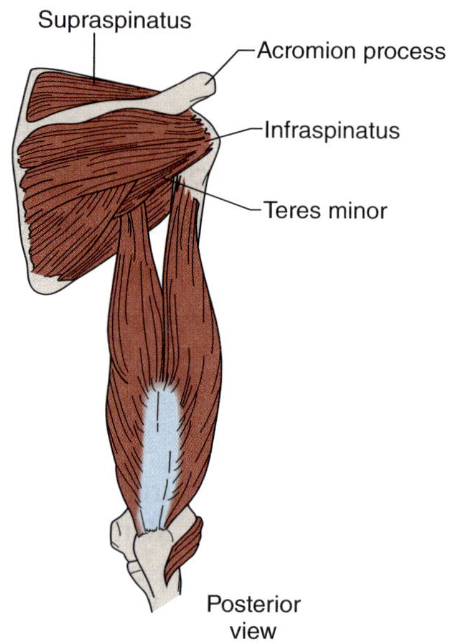

Figure 15.3 Rotator cuff muscles. The three posterior muscles are depicted. The subscapularis is found at the anterior aspect of the scapula and runs to the anterior aspect of the superior humerus.

insert into the humerus. These muscles are responsible for rotating the arm internally and externally as well as abducting the shoulder. The rotator cuff muscles are easy to remember if you use the acronym **SITS** (**s**ubscapularis, **i**nfraspinatus, **t**eres minor, and **s**upraspinatus).

The deltoid muscle lies over the head of the humerus. It attaches to the acromion process and the lateral aspect of the humerus. The deltoid abducts, flexes, and extends the shoulder.

The muscles in the anterior portion of the shoulder are the pectoralis major and minor. The pectoralis muscles attach at the sternum and the anterior portion of the humerus.

The biceps muscle flexes the elbow. It attaches to the humerus and coracoid process on one end and to the radius on the other. The biceps tendon runs through the bicipital groove and is kept in the groove by a ligament. The triceps muscles oppose the biceps. They extend the forearm and shoulder. The triceps attach to the posterior of the humeral head and scapula (see figure 7.3*b*).

Ligaments and Joints

The shoulder girdle has several joints held together by ligaments, but the most injured ones include the acromioclavicular joint and the glenohumeral joint. The acromioclavicular joint is made up of the acromion process of the scapula and the distal end of the clavicle. It is held together by the acromioclavicular ligament. The muscles that hold the scapula to the thorax allow movement in the scapulothoracic joint. This may be the most forgotten joint in the shoulder, but it is essential to its motion and strength.

The glenohumeral joint is the articulation, or point of contact, of the head of the humerus and the glenoid fossa, the saucer-like portion of the scapula. The glenoid fossa is shallow, making the joint susceptible to injury. The end of the humerus is covered with a hard articular cartilage that moves against the glenoid fossa. This is called the labrum. The glenoid labrum can be injured and is often called a **SLAP lesion**, which stands for **s**uperior **l**abrum from **a**nterior to **p**osterior lesion (see figure 15.4). These are common in swimmers, throwers, and volleyball players. A capsular ligament, also known as the glenohumeral ligament, surrounds the entire glenohumeral joint from the scapula to the humerus, maintaining the scapula and humeral head in proper relationship and giving the joint stability. Muscles hold the scapula close to the thoracic ribs.

Bursa

The shoulder has four bursas: the subacromial, subcoracoid, subdeltoid, and subscapular. Each bursa

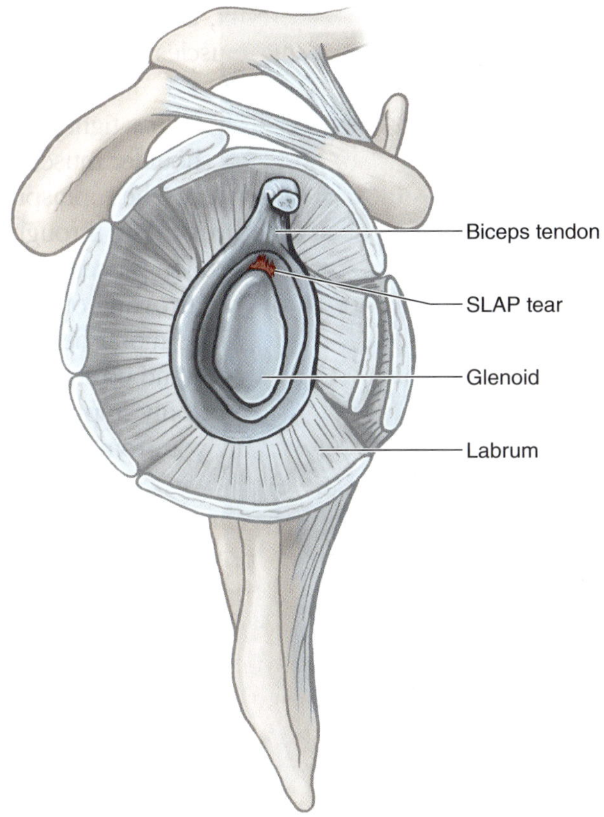

Figure 15.4 SLAP lesion.

is associated with bony prominences or muscles as its name indicates. The function of a bursa is to act as a cushion between tendons and bones. The bursa is a fluid sac that allows the muscular tendon and bone to move smoothly. In some cases, the bursa can become injured, either by overuse or direct impact.

PREVENTING SHOULDER INJURIES

The AT and the athlete must know what kinds of shoulder injuries occur and how to prevent them. Shoulder injuries are often caused by muscle weaknesses, postural problems, and the nature of the sport.

Addressing Muscular Weakness

The saying "out of sight, out of mind" applies to weight training in that people often lift weights only for those muscles they can see in the mirror the head of the humerus can cause an epiphyseal fracture. Falling on the elbow and driving the humerus into the glenoid fossa can also cause an epiphyseal fracture. Epiphyseal fractures have the same signs and symptoms as humeral fractures: pain, inability to use the arm, a desire to hold the arm still, and feeling a pop. Injuries to the epiphyses can cause permanent growth impairment. Application of ice, splinting, and a sling are the best courses of action the AT can take. The physician will determine the severity of the epiphyseal injury and the treatment.

Some epiphyseal injuries require surgery to hold the humerus head to the shaft. These cases are obviously more serious. Teenage pitchers are prone to epiphyseal injury from excessive throwing. Because of this, pitchers should be limited in the number of games they are allowed to play as well as the number of pitches they throw. With this injury, the athlete has pain around the circumference of the humerus. Pain will be exaggerated with flexion, as during the throwing motion. Caution must be exercised when dealing with this injury or the loss in range of motion could be permanent. The team physician must see the athlete, and immobilization is essential.

Avulsion Fractures

Avulsion fractures can occur in the shoulder. Avulsions may accompany a glenohumeral or acromioclavicular sprain. Recall that avulsion fractures are those in which a ligament or tendon pulls away a small portion of the bone as it is stressed during an injury. When the humerus is dislocating from the glenoid fossa, the capsular ligament is stressed and can sometimes pull on the scapula, resulting in an avulsion fracture. The athlete will experience pain associated with the dislocation and the avulsion fracture. It is difficult, if not impossible, for the AT to know if an avulsion fracture exists. An AT must assume an avulsion fracture until an X-ray reveals otherwise. Splinting and ice are appropriate care for sprains.

Glenohumeral Dislocations and Subluxations

Glenohumeral dislocation means that the head of the humerus is out of its socket (see figure 15.6). Subluxation means that the head of the humerus

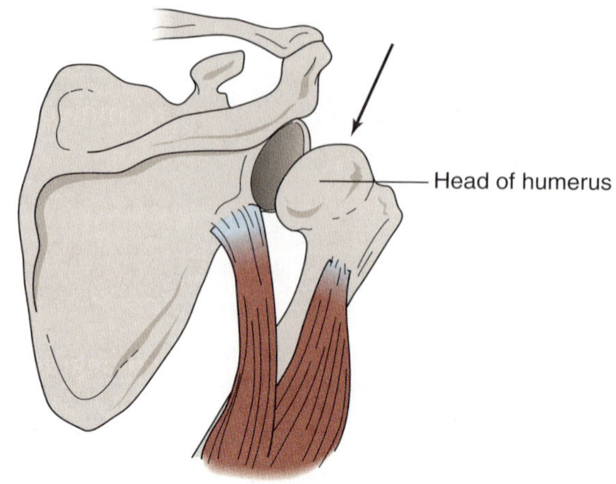

Figure 15.6 Shoulder dislocation occurs at the glenohumeral joint. The head of the humerus drops out of the socket, injuring the capsular ligament. The most common direction for a shoulder dislocation is anterior.

came out of its socket and then went back in. The cause for both injuries is usually the same—excessive abduction and external rotation—but the results are different. Dislocations and subluxations require attention by the AT and team physician.

A dislocation will sometimes cause the head of the humerus to tear the capsular ligament anteriorly. The instability of the capsular ligament allows the head of the humerus to shift forward, which is the most common type of shoulder dislocation. The athlete will experience pain and an inability to use the shoulder. When the AT looks at the dislocated shoulder, they will see a deformity at the deltoid muscle; the shoulder will not be round but flat. The team physician must put a dislocation back into place. For a subluxation, the athlete may indicate that they felt the shoulder go out of its socket but then pop back in. An X-ray is necessary to determine the extent of the dislocation or the subluxation—there may be associated fractures, a tear in the cartilage of the glenoid fossa, or nerve or blood vessel injury.

An athlete may not indicate to the AT that they have experienced a shoulder subluxation. Eventually, the athlete will notice changes as more subluxations occur. There can be permanent injury to the nerves, cartilage, and blood vessels. The athlete who has a dislocation or subluxation should strengthen the muscles of adduction and internal rotation. They may also wear a harness that restricts external rotation and abduction. An athlete who experiences recurrent subluxations or dislocations will require surgery to repair the capsular ligaments.

MUSCLE, BURSA, AND TENDON INJURIES

Most shoulder muscle and tendon injuries are caused by overuse. Athletes who throw, shoot, or repeat a swim stroke are prone to overuse injuries in the shoulder. Overuse injuries require rest, ice application, immobilization, and referrals to physicians for care. Common muscle and tendon injuries occur to the rotator cuff. Injury to the rotator cuff can also lead to impingement syndrome and bicipital tendon problems or involvement of the bursa.

Rotator Cuff Strain

Similar to other strains, a rotator cuff strain is categorized as a first-, second-, or third-degree strain. As noted in chapter 8, first-degree strains are indicated by pain with no loss of stability or range of motion. Second-degree strains will have pain with loss of stability and range of motion. Third-degree strains will have pain with partial or complete loss of stability and range of motion.

Rotator cuff strains occur from excessive motion beyond the normal range. Most often, the supraspinatus muscle is injured. The athlete will have pain with motion and sometimes when the shoulder is not moving. The pain generally occurs with abduction of the shoulder. If the athlete is unable to abduct, a complete tear, or third-degree strain, is suspected. Strains caused by repetitive movements can also result in crepitus and impingement syndrome. A complete tear must be surgically repaired, whereas a first- or second-degree tear can be treated initially with PRICES and then with gentle strengthening and flexibility exercises.

Impingement Syndrome

An athlete develops **impingement syndrome** from repetitive overhead movements. Freestyle swimmers, throwers, and tennis players are prone to impingement syndrome. The supraspinatus and biceps muscles run together through a space beneath the acromion process. If the space narrows—from swelling, tendinitis, weak posterior muscles, or poor posture—the two muscles are impinged in the space. This creates pain and discomfort with overhead movements and pressure when lying on the involved shoulder. Treatment includes modifying activity, strengthening the posterior muscles of the shoulder, and improving flexibility of tight pectoral muscles.

Bicipital Tendinitis

Bicipital tendinitis is common among athletes who are constantly raising their arms above their heads, such as tennis players. The repetitive nature of the movement will irritate the tendon in the bicipital groove. The AT may be able to palpate the tendon and feel crepitus. The athlete must stop the repetitive action causing the tendinitis. Pain is common, especially when repeating the motion that caused the tendinitis. Immobilization in a sling will make the athlete more comfortable. The team physician may prescribe ultrasound therapy and anti-inflammatory medication.

Biceps Tendon Rupture

The biceps tendon can rupture from either a direct blow or severe contractional forces. When the tendon ruptures, the athlete will be unable to flex the elbow. There will be a noticeable change in the appearance of the muscle as the tendon rolls up on itself—it will look like a golf ball under the skin (see figure 15.7). The arm must be iced and

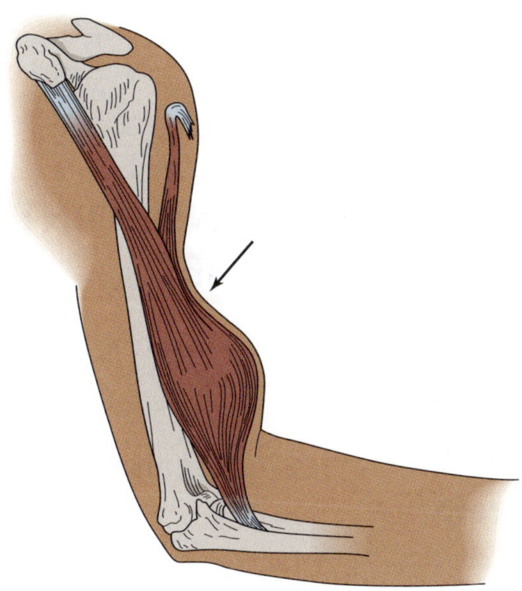

Figure 15.7 Biceps tendon rupture.

immobilized, and the athlete should be referred to a physician. The physician will surgically repair the tendon so that the muscle can return to full function.

Bursitis

Bursitis is an inflammation of the bursa, either by overuse or direct impact. There may also be involvement with other tissues in the shoulder complex. When an overuse injury occurs, the bony structure or joint can degenerate, causing a roughened surface that aggravates the bursa. Sports that involve throwing or repetitive overhead motion are the likely culprit in overuse injuries. Bursitis will present with shoulder pain during the throwing action, especially at the acromion process. The AT can treat the bursitis based on the symptoms with referral to a physician.

Thoracic Outlet Syndrome

The thoracic outlet exists between the first rib and the clavicle. Thoracic outlet syndrome occurs in several ways but results in a narrowing of the thoracic outlet when the scalene musculature contracts and lifts the first rib. Some symptoms are a dull, aching pain and sensation changes from the neck into the hand. If the vein in the area becomes compressed, the athlete will experience edema in their hand and a blue discoloration. Sports that involve overhead movements are usually to blame. Because of the loss of sensation or blood flow, this injury is considered a medical emergency. The physician will do a complete assessment of the neck and upper extremity to determine the severity of the injury. For more on how to distinguish between soft-tissue shoulder injuries, see figure 15.8.

LIGAMENT AND JOINT INJURIES

Several shoulder girdle joints are prone to sprains. The joints that are most commonly sprained include the acromioclavicular and glenohumeral joints.

Acromioclavicular Ligament Sprain

A sprain of the acromioclavicular ligament is referred to as a **shoulder separation** (see figure 15.9) so as not to confuse it with a glenohumeral ligament sprain. Although these joints are in close proximity, they involve different structures. The acromioclavicular joint can be injured by impact to the top of the shoulder or by falling on an outstretched arm. Falling on the elbow forces the humerus up and into the acromioclavicular joint. The athlete will indicate pain with movement whether it is a first-, second-, or third-degree sprain. The more serious sprains cause the clavicle to move superiorly. In a third-degree separation, there will be a large abnormal bump caused by excessive upward displacement of the clavicle. The athlete is usually unable to move the arm and will hold it tightly against the body. To treat a first-degree sprain, the AT must use the PRICES method. A second- or third-degree sprain can be treated with PRICES initially, but the athlete must be referred to an orthopedist to rule out a fracture.

A physician can take two courses of action to treat a third-degree tear: surgery or harness. During surgery, the acromioclavicular joint is wired or screwed together. A harness straps the clavicle down to hold the joint together long enough to allow the ligament to heal.

Glenohumeral Ligament Sprain

The glenohumeral joint is especially vulnerable to sprains when it is placed in abduction and external rotation. With a third-degree sprain, a more serious problem such as subluxation or dislocation is likely. The athlete with a glenohumeral ligament sprain will have pain with motion. The athlete is treated using PRICES and is referred to a physician.

A shoulder dislocation or repetitive subluxations are the most likely causes of a **glenoid labrum** tear. The labrum is the disc of cartilage in the glenohumeral joint. When the labrum tears, it can obstruct the range of motion or allow excessive movement in the joint.

Initial care for a tear is to immobilize the shoulder. The physician will have to evaluate the shoulder to determine the extent of the injury. Conservative treatment would be to immobilize the shoulder with the hope that the labrum would reattach without surgical intervention. In many cases, the labrum must be surgically reattached or removed.

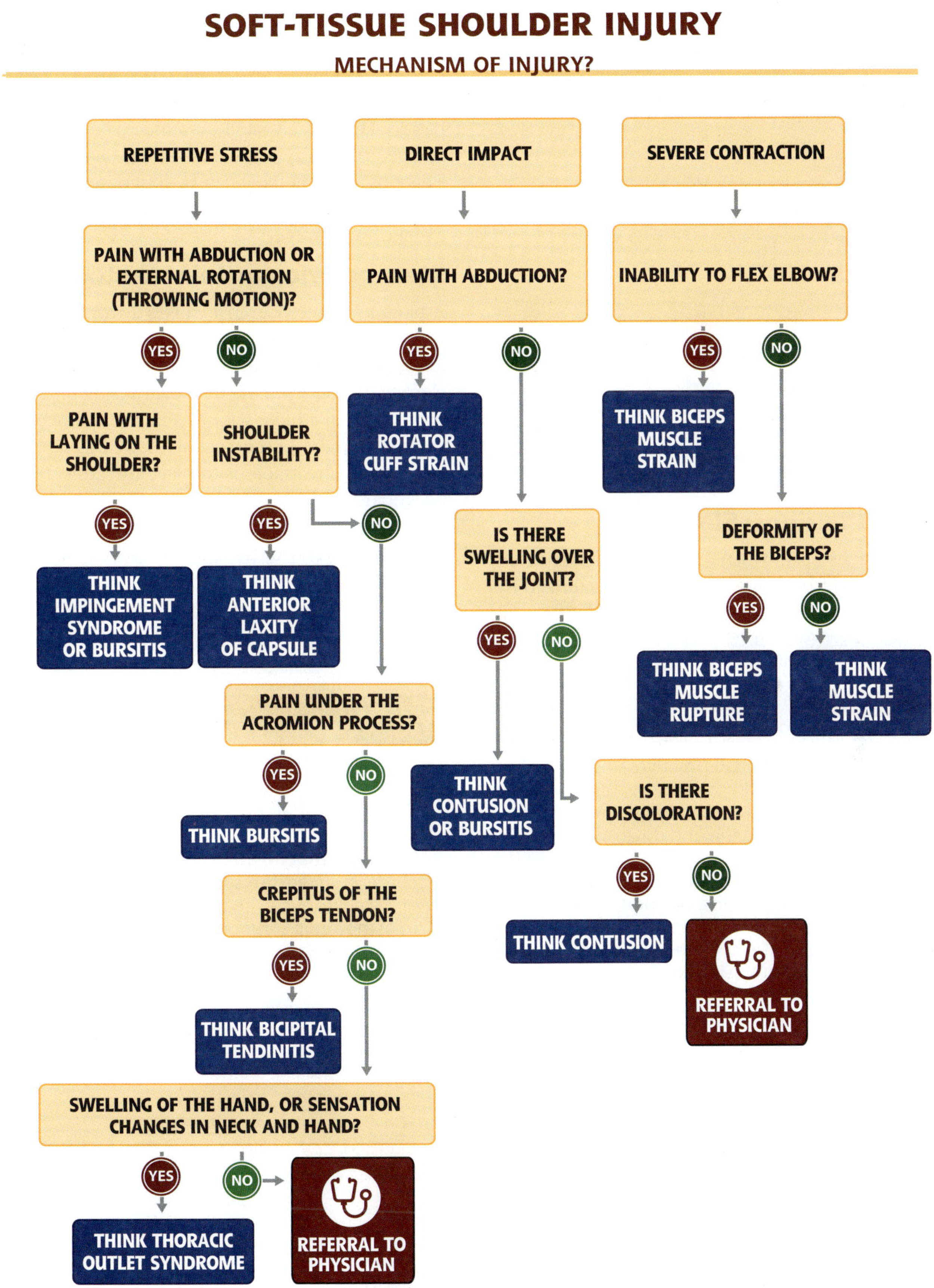

Figure 15.8 Distinguishing between soft-tissue shoulder injuries.

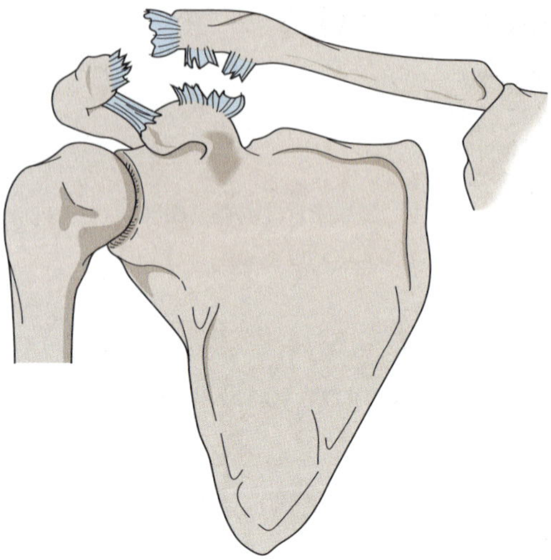

Figure 15.9 A shoulder separation occurs at the acromioclavicular joint. It is a sprain of the acromioclavicular ligament.

Labral Lesions: SLAP

SLAP lesions occur when the labrum has been torn or damaged (see figure 15.4). It is characterized by pain and clicking in the shoulder. SLAP lesions can be diagnosed with a clinical examination but are also diagnosed using advanced diagnostic testing. A high percentage (77%) of athletes who suffer with SLAP lesions also have other injuries, so it is important to have thorough diagnosis. NATA has looked closely at the evaluation, treatment, and return-to-play standards for the SLAP lesions. This position statement can be found in the online resources. SLAP lesions can be treated conservatively or with surgery.

Sternoclavicular Joint Dislocation

A blow to the clavicle that causes a rupture of the sternoclavicular joint ligaments can cause a posterior dislocation. A posterior dislocation of the clavicle can press on the trachea, causing difficulty breathing. An athlete with this injury will become anxious, and the AT must act to resolve this situation quickly. The treatment is to place the athlete on a backboard with the side of the affected shoulder off the board. With the shoulder below the board, the proximal end of the clavicle moves anteriorly away from the trachea. The athlete will have to see a physician for additional treatment.

The Real World

After a Tuesday football practice, a player reported mild shoulder pain. When the athlete removed his shirt, we could see that the end of his clavicle was pressing against his skin. The acromioclavicular ligament had been torn and no longer held the clavicle and the scapula together at the acromioclavicular joint. We could press the end down, but it would just shift upward again. We asked when he had injured it, and he said that the previous Saturday he had fallen off a snowmobile and hurt it. He had normal strength and range of motion, and though an orthopedic surgeon suggested surgery, he elected not to have surgery to screw the two bones together. We made him a custom pad to protect the acromioclavicular joint, and he was able to continue participating. The orthopedic surgeon convinced the athlete to have surgery after the season ended to avoid arthritis and any future cosmetic problems (i.e., a bony prominence over the shoulder).

Anonymous

Summary

The shoulder girdle has many ligaments; consequently, it is vulnerable to sprains. The glenohumeral joint relies on rotator cuff strength for stability, but a dislocation can occur, usually by forceful abduction and external rotation. The acromioclavicular joint can be sprained as well, resulting in a shoulder separation. A rotator cuff strain can be debilitating, and proper recovery is imperative before the athlete returns to competition. A strong rotator cuff and a well-conditioned shoulder will prevent many shoulder injuries. Other injuries such as dislocation and labral tears can plague an athlete. Prompt diagnosis, treatment, and rehabilitation are essential in managing this complex joint.

Key Terms

Define the following terms found in this chapter:

- glenoid labrum
- impingement syndrome
- rotator cuff
- shoulder separation
- SITS
- SLAP lesion
- Thrower's Ten

As an AT, you are responsible for preventing injuries as well as treatment and rehabilitation. What advice would you give the softball and baseball teams regarding stretching and strengthening to prevent rotator cuff injuries during the season? Provide an explanation of the major muscles of the rotator cuff and their primary functions.

To access supplementary material for this chapter, including the Understanding Check worksheet, vocabulary quizzes, extension activities, and chapter-specific resources and forms, visit the web resource: http://ancillaries.humankinetics.com/FundamentalsOfAthleticTrainingAndSportsMedicine5E

chapter 16

Elbow Injuries

Objectives

After completing this chapter, the student will be able to do the following:

- Describe the basic anatomy of the arm and elbow.
- Explain common arm and elbow injuries that occur with athletic participation.
- Identify signs and symptoms of arm and elbow injuries.
- Explain treatment parameters performed by ATs for elbow injuries.

The elbow functions with any upper-extremity movement. It is prone to muscle and tendon injuries because it is the site of many muscle attachments.

ANATOMY OF THE ELBOW

The elbow is a hinge joint involving three major bones: the humerus, radius, and ulna (see figure 16.1). The radius and ulna are the bones between the elbow and wrist. The distal end of the humerus becomes wider, similar to the distal end of the femur in the leg, and forms the medial and lateral epicondyles. The ulna is hooked to the end of the humerus and forms a tight joint. The radius is the bone on the thumb side of the forearm. It rests against the humerus and is able to rotate, allowing the forearm to pronate and supinate.

The elbow has anatomical triangles that provide bony points for assessment (figure 16.2). The first triangle is formed by the olecranon process, the medial epicondyle, and the lateral epicondyle.

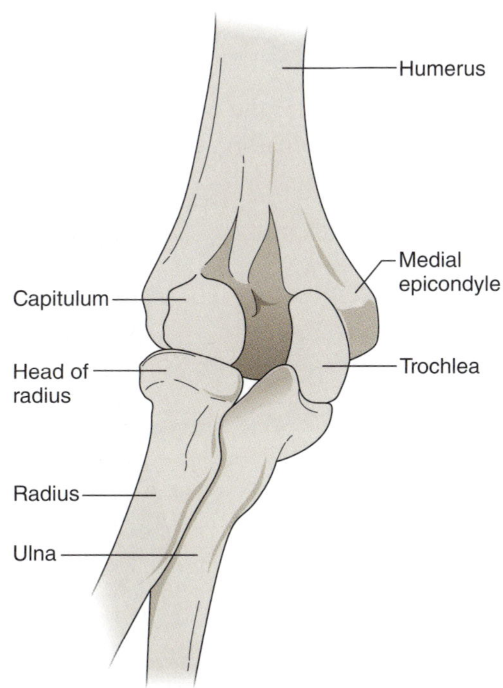

Figure 16.1 Anterior view of the elbow. The elbow is a tight joint held together by many ligaments.

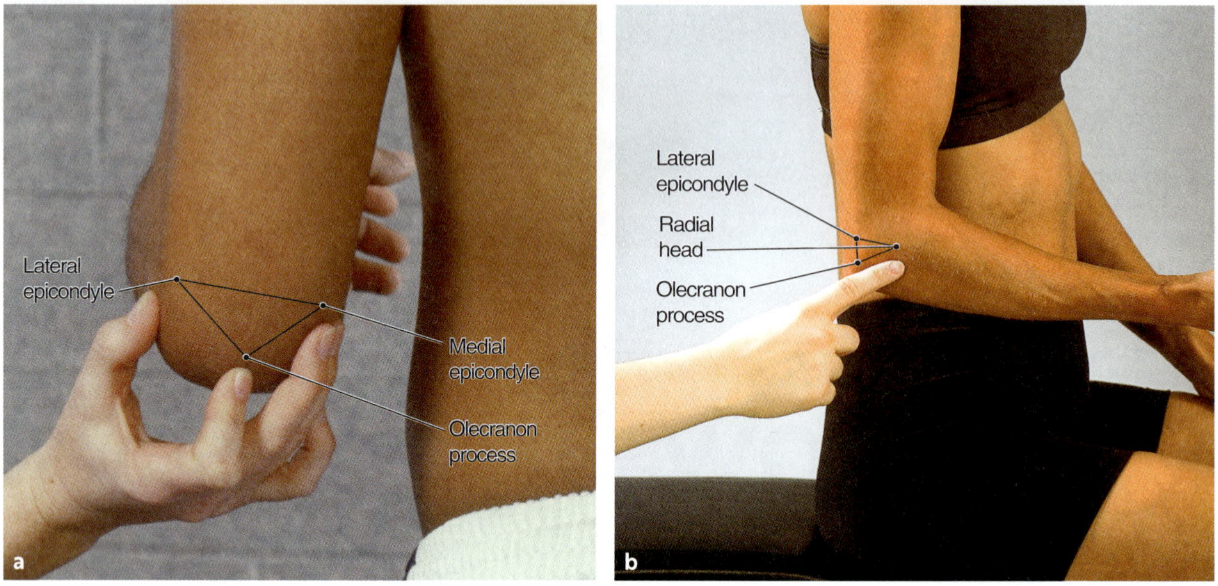

Figure 16.2 Triangles of the olecranon process.

(a) Reprinted by permission from S.J. Shultz, P.A. Houglum, and D.H. Perrin, *Examination of Musculoskeletal Injuries*, 4th ed. (Champaign, IL: Human Kinetics 2016), 311. (b) Reprinted by permission from R. Behnke, *Kinetic Anatomy*, 3rd ed. (Champaign, IL: Human Kinetics 2022), 69.

When viewed posteriorly, this triangle reveals that the epicondyles are level. The second triangle has the radial head, lateral epicondyle, and olecranon process. These triangles are important when assessing injuries of the elbow because when these bony prominences do not align, further assessment is necessary.

Muscles

As noted in chapter 15, the triceps muscle mostly performs elbow extension, whereas the biceps accomplishes elbow flexion. The wrist flexors attach at the medial epicondyle of the humerus and then run toward the hand. The wrist extensors attach to the lateral epicondyle of the humerus (figure 16.3*a-b*). These muscles help stabilize the elbow.

Several nerves and blood vessels pass through the small spaces and grooves around the elbow en route to the lower arm. Therefore, an injury occurring at the elbow must be assessed to determine if these blood vessels or nerves have been damaged. Checking for a pulse and ascertaining if an athlete

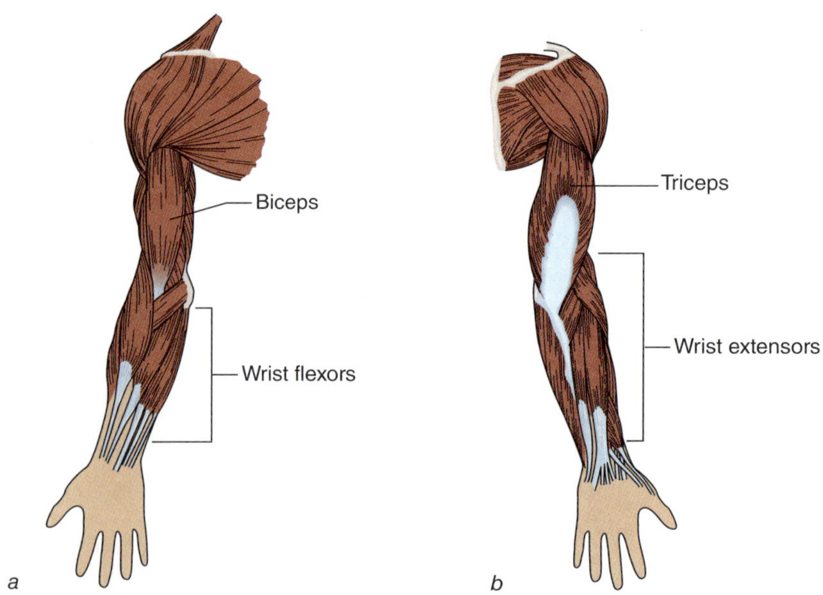

Figure 16.3 *(a)* Anterior and *(b)* posterior view of elbow and wrist musculature. Many muscles make up the wrist flexors and extensors that attach to the medial and lateral epicondyles of the humerus.

can feel their hand is a helpful procedure. Common pulse areas near the elbow are the brachial artery located on the medial surface of the mid humerus. The brachial nerve also courses through this region as well into the cubital fossa. The major nerves of the elbow are the ulnar nerve, median nerve, and radial nerve as they course through the elbow to the wrist and hand.

Muscles of the elbow often assist with shoulder and wrist and hand function in addition to their role at the elbow. Many of the muscles are classically grouped together and named for the function they have. For example, wrist flexors and wrist extensors are groups of muscles that perform these functions. As you get more advanced in anatomical knowledge, knowing the names will be important.

Ligaments

The joint capsule is a ligament that surrounds the elbow. It provides stability to the elbow joint, but the elbow also relies on several major ligaments for stability, particularly the ulnar collateral, radial collateral, and annular ligaments.

The ulnar collateral ligament helps to stabilize the inside, or medial, aspect of the elbow, whereas the radial collateral ligament helps to stabilize the outside, or lateral, aspect. These ligaments are also known as the medial and lateral collateral ligaments (figure 16.4*a-b*).

The annular ligament helps hold the radius and ulna together near the elbow joint. The radius and ulna are also supported by the interosseus membrane. This tissue joins the radius and the ulna from the elbow to the wrist and keeps the two bones from separating.

Bursa

The olecranon **bursa** is a thin, fluid-filled sac located at the posterior of the elbow, between the skin and the olecranon process. The purpose of this bursa is to allow smooth movement between the skin and the bone.

PREVENTING ELBOW INJURIES

The elbow is not injured frequently. Many injuries that ATs see at the elbow joint are caused by overuse—the repetitive movements and stresses delivered to the wrist and elbow over time eventually break down the tissue, causing chronic inflammation and pain. This is especially true in racket sports such as tennis and racquetball, where injuries to the lateral aspect of the elbow are most common. Many athletes pay a great deal of attention to strengthening the biceps and triceps muscles, but they fail to properly condition the smaller muscles such as the wrist flexors and extensors. Stretching and strengthening these structures is recommended to prevent overuse injuries. We describe stretches in chapter 22.

It is imperative for the AT to work with the coach to detect any improper techniques athletes are using, because these can eventually lead to

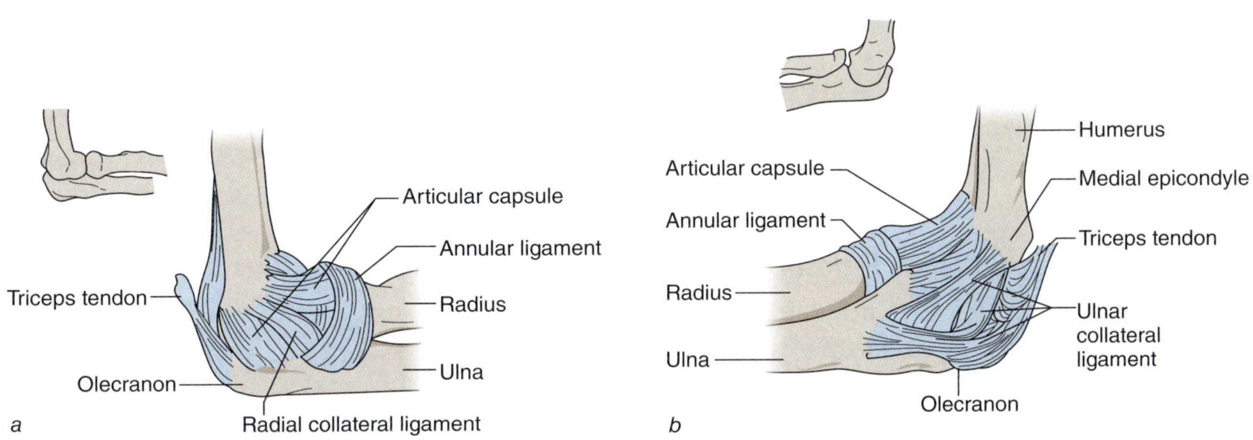

Figure 16.4 *(a)* Lateral and *(b)* medial views of the elbow. The ulna hooks on to the end of the humerus, whereas the radius rests against it.

overuse injuries. Equipment is also a factor preventing elbow injuries, especially in racket sports. For example, excessive stress on the elbow musculature can result from using a racket with a grip that is too small. The AT and the coach can work together to identify these problems and prevent such injuries.

Athletes who throw (such as baseball and softball players) should alter their activity and rest after long days of throwing. The rules limiting young pitchers' activity also help keep overuse problems of the elbow (and shoulder) to a minimum. ATs at industrial sites have reduced overuse injuries by instituting job-rotation programs whereby workers do a variety of jobs rather than the same job day after day. These modifications protect the elbow from repeated movements that cause overuse injuries.

TREATING ELBOW INJURIES AND CONDITIONS

The medial and lateral aspects of the elbow joint can suffer ligament sprains. Also, muscle and tendon injuries occur because the elbow and wrist are involved in repetitive stress during athletics. Fractures of the elbow can be extremely serious.

Bone Injuries

Bone fractures to the distal end of the humerus are not common in athletics. If they do occur, it is often due to powerful mechanisms of injury, such as the hand being planted on the ground and someone forcing the arm into excessive side bending. Fractures between the condyles of the humerus are also rare in sport, but if direct impact is the mechanism of injury and pain is located at the medial aspect of the elbow about 2 inches (5 cm) above the joint, a fracture should be suspected. If either type of fracture occurs, it is an absolute emergency because it can result in compression of an artery or nerve.

Epiphyseal and Avulsion Fractures

Epiphyseal and avulsion fractures are more common on the medial epicondyle or olecranon of the elbow (the olecranon is the process of the ulna projecting behind the elbow joint). An epiphyseal injury should be suspected whenever an athlete presents with swelling, pain, and loss of movement. Remember that a growing athlete is more likely to injure the growth plate than suffer a bone fracture or ligament injury. Severe pain and deformity indicate an avulsion fracture. If you suspect either of these injuries, refer the athlete to a physician.

> ***Understanding Diversity***
>
> For Native Americans, one's hair is often a sign of strength, power, and beauty, so cutting it could signify shame (Treuer 2012). If hair needs to be cut or shaved, this needs to be explained and permission should be given prior. Return the hair to the person after.

Ulnar Dislocations

The elbow is one of the most commonly dislocated joints in the body (see figure 16.5). As mentioned previously, the ulna hooks on to the end of the humerus, making the elbow a fairly tight joint. Therefore, it takes a traumatic injury to dislocate the ulna from the humerus. Usually, a violent hyperextension injury or a severe blow to the lateral aspect of the elbow will dislodge the ulna from the humerus; most often, it moves posteriorly. When a dislocation occurs, an obvious deformity will be noticed and the lateral olecranon triangle will become horizontal (see figure 16.6). The arm must

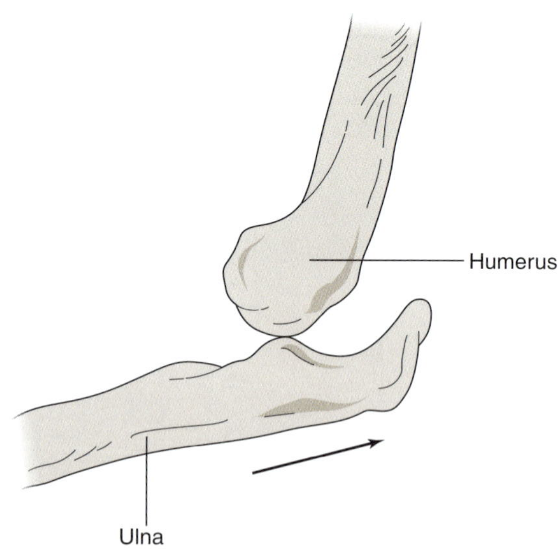

Figure 16.5 Elbow dislocations typically occur in a posterior direction.

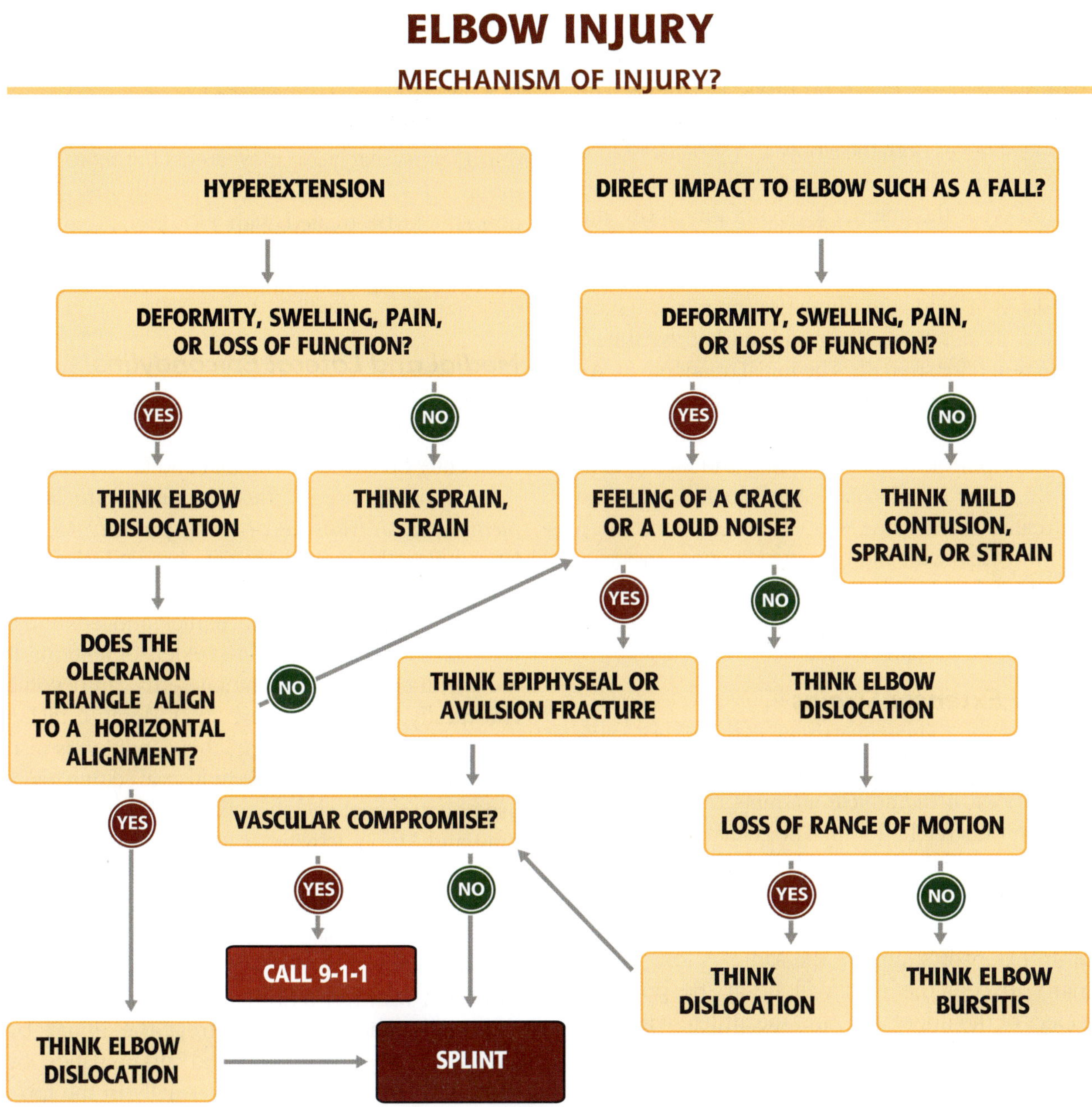

Figure 16.6 Dislocation or fracture of the elbow: signs and symptoms.

be immediately splinted in the position it is found in, and the athlete must be seen in the emergency room by a physician so that the dislocation can be treated.

Muscle and Tendon Injuries

Strains of elbow musculature are most often caused by either excessive resistive forces or overuse. Elbow strains can occur in the elbow flexor and extensor musculature as well as the wrist flexor and extensor musculature. As with strains discussed in previous chapters, they can be mild, moderate, or severe. A complete strain or rupture of a muscular structure, such as the biceps, is usually evident by the deformity caused when the muscle balls up due to the elasticity of the muscle.

Elbow Flexor Strains

Strains to the flexor muscles often are caused by a loaded movement that includes both the elbow and shoulder. The body's two-joint muscles—the muscles involved with creating movement at more than one joint—seem to be prone to strains. The biceps muscle is a perfect example of a two-joint muscle; it flexes both the elbow and shoulder joints. Minor elbow flexor strains are characterized by discomfort at the anterior aspect of the elbow and minimal swelling. The athlete will also demonstrate weakness and extra discomfort when elbow flexion is resisted. A moderate elbow flexor strain will have mild to moderate swelling and marked weakness when tested for strength. The initial treatment an AT may give for an elbow flexor strain is PRICES. When the initial inflammation has subsided, the athlete can then perform mild stretching and strengthening exercises as indicated. A moderate strain can be treated in the same way, but the AT must keep in mind that with more tissue damage, progress will often be slower. Complete muscle or tendon ruptures or suspected avulsion injuries should be referred to the team physician.

Elbow Extensor Strains

Excessive resistance to the triceps muscle often causes tissue damage to the elbow extensors. This can happen if the athlete attempts to break a fall with an outstretched arm. The injury needs to be assessed carefully because the triceps tendon can often pull a bit of bone away from the ulna at the point where the tendon attaches. The characteristics of an extensor strain are the same as for a flexor injury, except the pain will be at the posterior aspect of the upper arm, and the athlete will often experience more pain when the AT resists elbow extension. Treatment with PRICES is recommended, and after inflammation has subsided, the elbow extensor should be stretched mildly and strengthened as tolerated.

Wrist Flexor Strains

Wrist flexor strains at the elbow often result in pain over the medial epicondyle of the humerus or the front of the forearm. These strains can result from excessive resistance during wrist flexion movements or, more commonly, from overuse. Initially this condition should be treated with PRICES, and activity should be modified. Mild stretching can be performed by the athlete, and wrist curls and grip strengthening are helpful.

Wrist Extensor Strains

Wrist extensor strains at the elbow frequently result in pain over the lateral epicondyle of the humerus. These strains can result from excessive resistance during wrist extension movements but more commonly are caused by overuse. Initially this condition should be treated with PRICES, and activity should be modified. The athlete can also perform mild stretching, and doing reverse wrist curls can be helpful as well.

Medial and Lateral Epicondylitis

As noted previously, the elbow is prone to overuse conditions that create chronic inflammation, which frequently occurs at the medial and lateral epicondyles of the humerus. These conditions are called *medial epicondylitis* and *lateral epicondylitis*, the latter being the more frequent chronic inflammatory injury.

As a result of poor mechanics and continual use over a long time, the wrist extensor tendons at the lateral epicondyle of the humerus can become chronically inflamed (figure 16.7). Because racket sports are a common cause, this condition is also called **tennis elbow**. In the industrial setting, daily use of equipment such as a hammer and any gripping and lifting activities can cause lateral elbow inflammation.

Lateral epicondylitis is characterized by pain over the lateral epicondyle of the humerus. Minimal swelling is sometimes present. Pain with wrist extension with resistance is common.

Initially, the AT should treat the injury by attempting to reduce pain and inflammation by using PRICES. The support is usually in the form of a tennis elbow strap that is wrapped around the

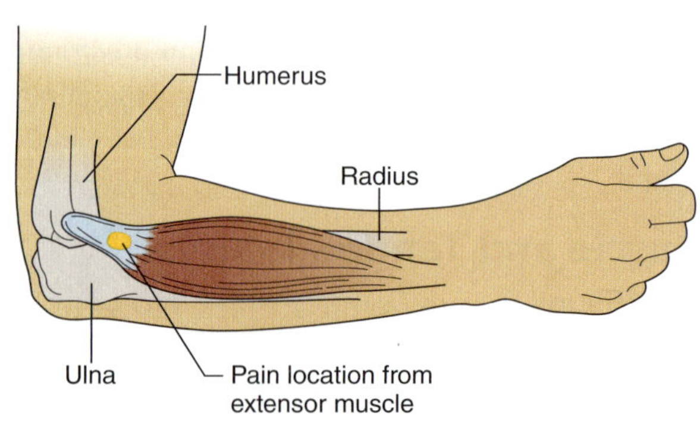

Figure 16.7 Pain from lateral epicondylitis.

elbow. Limiting activity that aggravates the condition is also wise. Mildly stretching the extensor tendons is helpful, and muscle strength and endurance should be improved as tolerated. The athlete should gradually be allowed to participate in further activity. The AT may reduce the number of repetitions the athlete performs and may also suggest using a two-handed backhand in racket sports. The team physician may choose to use medication to help resolve the condition.

Although not as common as lateral epicondylitis, many athletes get medial epicondylitis, often from repetitive throwing. This condition involves inflammation of the wrist flexor tendons where they attach to the humerus. Some people refer to medial epicondylitis as **Little League elbow**. Little League elbow is also suggested to be a separation of the epiphysis at the medial aspect of the humerus in younger athletes (usually between the ages of 9 and 12) from throwing (see figure 16.8).

Treatment for medial epicondylitis is similar to that of lateral epicondylitis—protection, rest, ice application, compression, and elevation. The athlete needs to decrease the amount of throwing and strengthen the wrist flexor muscles. The AT will monitor either condition. She will also perform a thorough evaluation because compression of the ulnar nerve is possible at the elbow joint, especially when a medial elbow injury has occurred. The AT will refer the athlete to a physician if a fracture is suspected or if the athlete is complaining of numbness, tingling, or excessive pain.

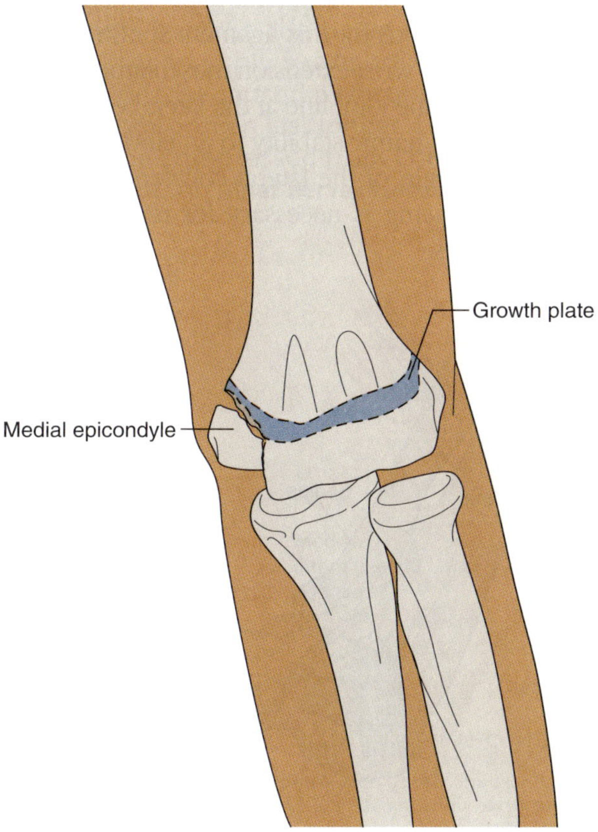

Figure 16.8 Little League elbow.

> **The Real World**
>
> While pitching during a college baseball game, our school's pitcher heard a pop. In obvious pain, he grabbed his elbow, fell off the pitcher's mound into the grass, and rolled around screaming that he had broken his elbow. With all that screaming, it was obvious the athlete was breathing and had a pulse. After calming him down, I determined that there were no obvious fractures around the elbow and that it would be okay for him to walk into the dugout for further examination. The athlete was apprehensive about moving the elbow during examination because it was painful, and he continued to insist that his elbow was broken. He had extreme tenderness throughout the medial side of the elbow, especially just distal to the medial epicondyle. I took his distal pulse, checked capillary refill, and performed sensory tests. Grip strength was good, and the arm was neurovascularly normal. On valgus stress to the elbow, the athlete had a great deal of instability, which indicated an injury to the ulnar collateral ligament. We decided to ice the athlete's elbow, place it in a sling, and refer him to his family orthopedist. It turned out that he had an ulnar collateral ligament rupture that required reconstructive surgery and extensive rehabilitation. Although he never pitched again, he was able to play competitive baseball as a first baseman.
>
> **Greg Ehlers, EdD, ATC**

Ligament Injuries

Elbow sprains, as with all sprains, are classified as first, second, and third degree. Any of the elbow ligaments can be sprained, including the ulnar collateral ligament and the radial collateral ligament. The annular ligament is seldom sprained due to its location and function.

seldom a disabling condition, the fluid buildup can become the size of a golf ball (see figure 16.11). The AT must apply compression wraps, and if the condition persists, the team physician may want to drain the fluid from the area. In any event, the elbow needs to be adequately protected with padding to avoid further contusions.

The radial nerve can also be injured, usually by becoming entrapped by a bone if a fracture occurs or by a muscle after an injury such as a strain. An injury to the radial nerve can palsy, meaning the nerve does not transmit electrical signals to muscles needed for contraction. See figure 16.12 for the neural anatomy of the elbow.

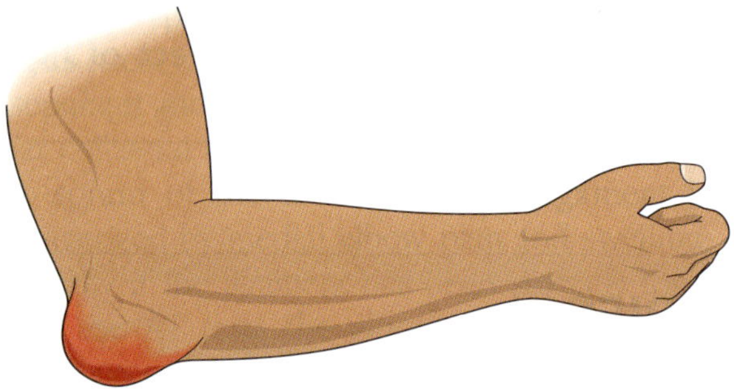

Figure 16.11 Olecranon bursitis.

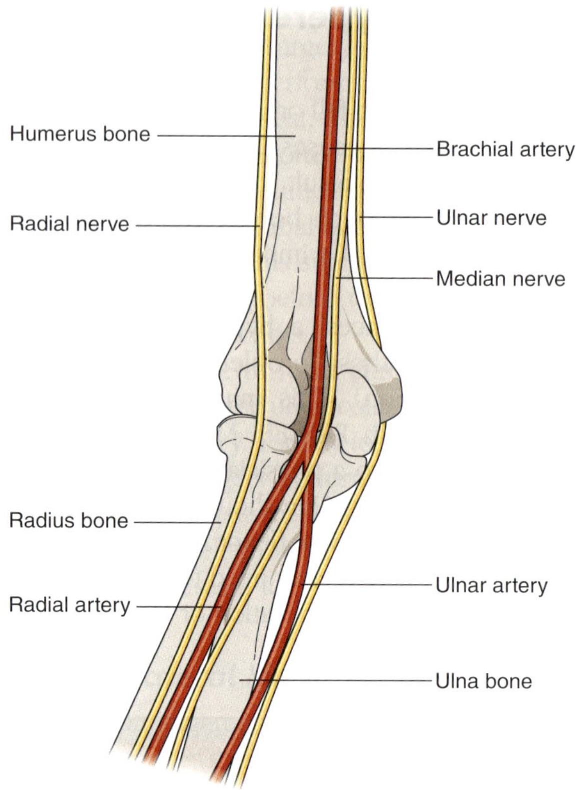

Figure 16.12 Nerves and arteries around the elbow joint.

RED FLAGS

Splint the injury and get the athlete to the emergency room for any of the following:

- Loss of function in the elbow
- Loss of sensation in the elbow
- Deformity of the elbow
- Lack of circulation in the hand after an elbow injury

Summary

The elbow is a hinge joint composed of the humerus of the upper arm and the radius and ulna of the lower arm. The biceps and triceps muscles flex and extend the elbow, respectively. The wrist flexor and extensor muscles extend across the elbow and attach to the humerus. The elbow is also stabilized by the radial collateral ligament at the lateral aspect of the joint and the ulnar collateral ligament at the medial aspect of the joint. These ligaments are sometimes sprained in much the same way that the medial and lateral collateral ligaments of the knee are sprained. The elbow is also subject to overuse injuries, such as tennis elbow. New procedures are emerging to treat, manage, and surgically repair injuries to the elbow.

Key Terms

Define the following terms found in this chapter:

- bursa
- Little League elbow
- tennis elbow
- Tommy John surgery
- ulnar nerve relocation
- valgus

A volleyball player landed on their elbow and says that it seems like there is a tennis ball under their skin. They say that it hurts to put any pressure on it and that when they put their elbows on the desk in school, it becomes super sore. What condition do you believe this athlete is experiencing? What would you advise the athlete to do to manage the pain and prevent further exacerbation of the problem?

To access supplementary material for this chapter, including the Understanding Check worksheet, vocabulary quizzes, extension activities, and chapter-specific resources and forms, visit the web resource: http://ancillaries.humankinetics.com/FundamentalsOfAthleticTrainingAndSportsMedicine5E

chapter 17

Wrist and Hand Injuries

Objectives

After completing this chapter, the student will be able to do the following:

- Understand the basic anatomy of the wrist and hand.
- Explain the various types of wrist and hand injuries.
- Understand common mechanisms that cause the injuries.
- Understand the signs and symptoms of wrist and hand fractures.
- Understand and appreciate the role of triangular fibrocartilage in the wrist.

Injuries to the wrist account for up to 9% of all sport-related injuries. Catching a ball, holding a club, falling on an outstretched arm, and grasping an opponent are essential tasks in sport. An injury to a wrist or hand can be exceedingly limiting and demoralizing for an athlete. Recognizing the type and extent of injury will help determine appropriate care and speed return to competition.

ANATOMY OF THE WRIST AND HAND

The wrist and hand contain a triangular fibrocartilage and many bones, muscles, ligaments, nerves, and blood vessels. All are necessary for the total function of the hand—one of the most active body parts—and if any anatomical part is injured, it will decrease an athlete's functional ability.

Bones and Joints

The wrist is the joint between the arm and the hand. It is made up of eight irregularly shaped carpal bones that articulate between the radius and ulna of the arm and the metacarpals of the hand to allow wrist movement (see figure 17.1). They are located in two rows: the proximal row has the scaphoid bone, lunate bone, triquetrum bone, and pisiform bone. The distal row has the trapezium bone, trapezoid bone, capitate bone, and hamate bone. The scaphoid, sometimes called the scaphoid navicular, is of particular importance. It has a blood supply

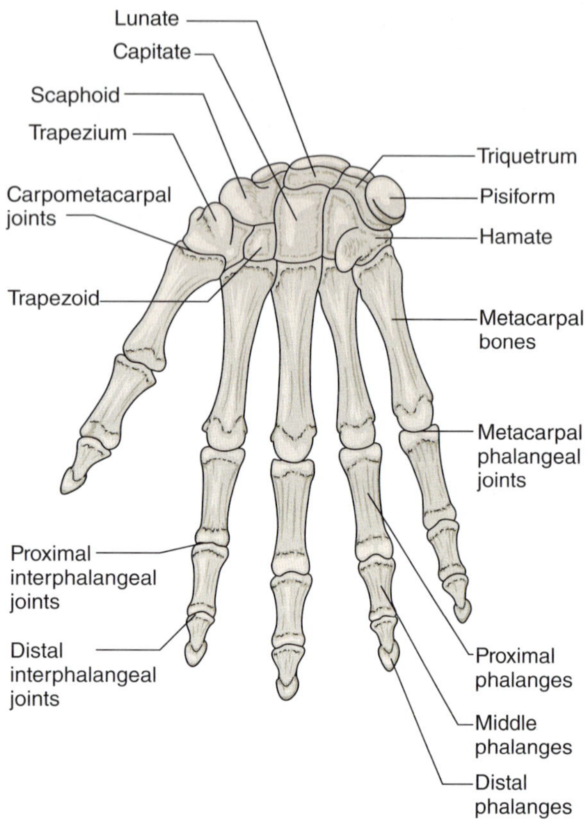

Figure 17.1 Bones and joints of the hand.

on only one end and therefore has difficulty healing when fractured. When the fingers are spread, the scaphoid sits in a depression at the wrist that is referred to as the *anatomical snuffbox*.

At the distal end, each of the five metacarpals joins with the proximal phalanx of one of the fingers. The metacarpals are numbered 1 through 5, beginning at the thumb side of the hand. The fingers have 14 phalanges.

Joints in the hand are named for the bones that compose them and whether they are distal or proximal. For example, the thumb has two joints: the metacarpophalangeal joint and the interphalangeal joint. Each of the second through fifth fingers has a metacarpophalangeal (MCP) joint, a proximal interphalangeal (PIP) joint, and a distal interphalangeal (DIP) joint.

Muscles

Wrist and hand movements are controlled by many muscles, which are categorized into extensor and flexor groups. The flexor muscle groups are found on the anterior surface of the forearm, and the extensor muscles are located on the posterior aspect of the forearm. Together they work to perform complex movements required by the wrist and hand.

Ligaments

The wrist and hand ligaments are intricate because of the many bones that must be connected. The wrist is stabilized by collateral ligaments medially and laterally. The ulnar collateral ligament attaches the distal end of the ulna to the triquetral and pisiform bones. The radial collateral ligament attaches the distal end of the radius to the trapezium and scaphoid bones.

Understanding Diversity

The palmaris longus muscle is absent in 12% to 20% of Caucasians (Ioannis et al. 2015). It is absent in approximately 14% of all persons. The lack of palmaris longus means that an athlete may be unable to forcefully flex the wrist. This can cause an athlete to be unable to adequately grip a racket, forcibly squeeze an object, and appropriately generate force to throw a ball.

Of particular importance to ATs is the flexor retinaculum, also known as the transverse carpal ligament. This structure is located on the anterior aspect of the carpal bones and lies over the wrist flexor tendons and median nerve. The retinaculum not only stabilizes the carpal bones but also provides a protective covering over the flexor tendons and median nerve that pass beneath it.

The thumb has several important ligaments. In particular, the ulnar collateral ligament of the thumb (also known as the medial collateral ligament) is located on the medial aspect, and the radial collateral ligament (also known as the lateral collateral ligament) is located on the lateral aspect (figure 17.2). These ligaments provide medial and lateral stability to the joint.

Triangular Fibrocartilage Complex (TFCC)

The TFCC is a group of cartilage and ligaments that connect the lunate, triquetrum, and ulnar head (see figure 17.3). It allows you to perform gripping actions with ease and stabilizes the ulnar side of

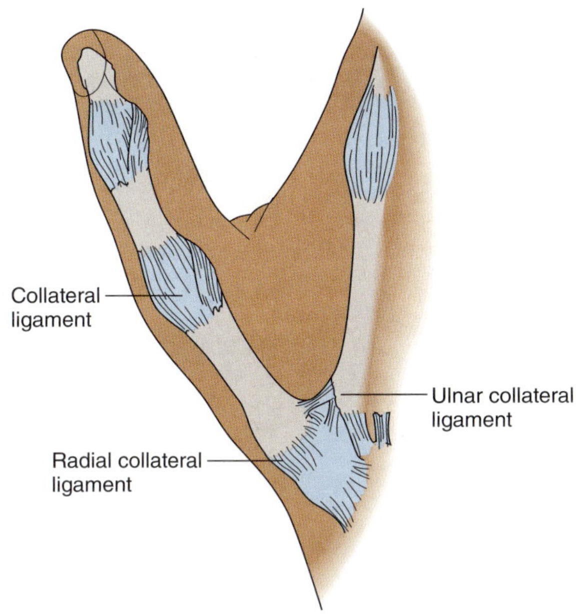

Figure 17.2 Thumb ligaments.

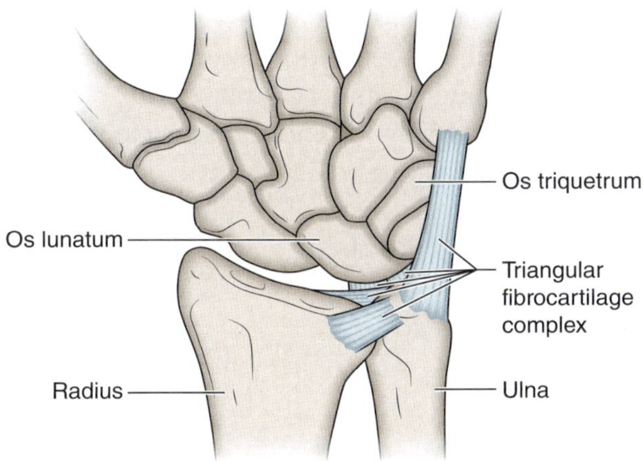

Figure 17.3 TFCC.

Adapted from Physiopedia. Available: https://www.physio-pedia.com/Triangular_Fibrocartilage_Complex_Injuries.

the wrist. When this structure is injured through overuse, a sudden twist to the wrist, or from a fall on an outstretched arm, the wrist becomes less stable.

PREVENTING WRIST AND HAND INJURIES

Commonly used protective equipment for the wrist and hand includes braces, tape, gloves, and padding. Wearing gloves or tape can protect the area from wounds, and padding can prevent contusions of the dorsal hand. Many football players wear thumb braces to protect against sprains. ATs can use plastic splints and braces to prevent injury for athletes who may be susceptible. In some sports, however, rules prohibit using protective equipment made of hard materials or allow the equipment only with a physician's note. Taping is typically permitted in most sports.

TREATING WRIST AND HAND INJURIES AND CONDITIONS

With a hand, one can manipulate objects and perform feats of astounding complexity. The slightest injury can change a movement or make it difficult for the athlete to participate in sport or perform activities of daily living. Prompt evaluation and treatment can preserve normal function in this region.

Bone Injuries

Any bone in the wrist and hand can fracture. Hands are used in all sports and are often put in harm's way. Direct impacts are the most frequent cause of the fractures. Swelling, pain, deformity, and disability are common with fractures. Two complications are associated with fractures: nonunion and death of the bone, which is also called **avascular necrosis** (death due to lack of blood flow). In the wrist, the scaphoid bone is most often associated with nonunion and avascular necrosis. All fractures should be cared for with splinting and should be evaluated by a physician.

Another common fracture occurs to the metacarpal region, specifically to the fourth or fifth metacarpal. A fracture to this area is called a **boxer's fracture** because it often occurs due to punching or hitting a hard object. An X-ray will confirm this diagnosis, and the athlete will be immobilized to allow the bone to heal.

A **Colles' fracture** occurs to the distal forearm. When both the radius and ulna are fractured, if an athlete reaches a hand out to catch a fall, the arm often bends into extension at the fracture site. This requires immediate immobilization and referral to a physician for casting or sometimes surgery.

Muscle and Tendon Injuries

Any of the numerous muscles of the wrist and hand can be strained by repetitive stress and stretching with activities of daily living or sports. Pain, swelling, weakness, and inability to move are common signs and symptoms. The AT will use range-of-motion testing to determine which muscle has been affected. Analysis of the athlete's movements can help determine the cause when repetitive stress is suspected. The AT should use the PRICES method and assign exercises to strengthen a weak muscle to prepare the athlete to return to competition. Taping the muscle for additional support can also be helpful. Sometimes, short periods of splinting are required to get the area to heal. Care should be avoided with prolonged immobilization without movement unless requested by the physician because the joint can lose mobility.

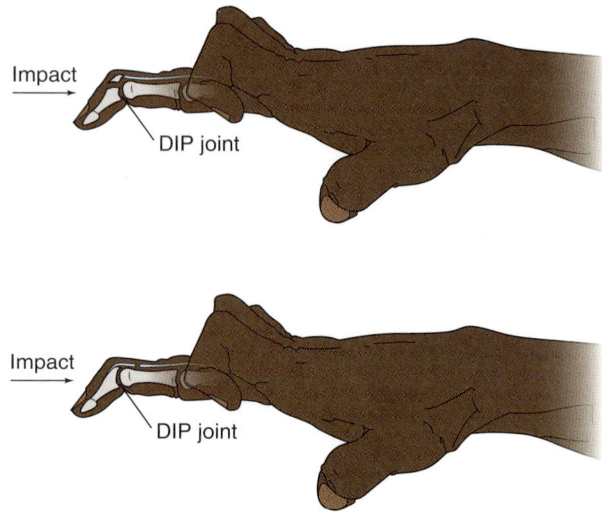

Figure 17.4 An avulsion fracture of the distal phalanx of the fingers results in a mallet finger. A mallet finger cannot be extended at the DIP joint.

Tendinitis

Tendinitis is defined as inflammation of the tendon. The cause of the inflammation can be overuse, stretching, or an impact. Because it is difficult to overcome, the AT's goal is to prevent tendinitis by increasing strength and flexibility, using padding, and avoiding repetitive injuries.

The thumb is vulnerable to **de Quervain's tendinitis**, which affects the abductor pollicis longus and extensor pollicis brevis. Shot-putters who hold the shot while the wrist is in radial deviation are prone to de Quervain's tendinitis. The athlete will have difficulty with abduction of the thumb and may experience swelling and crepitus. The athlete needs to discontinue the repetitive movements. The PRICES method of care is appropriate in this case.

Mallet Finger

Mallet finger (see figure 17.4) is the result of the fingertip receiving an impact. The impact causes the extensor tendon to tear from the bone. The distinguishing feature of this injury is that the fingertip is in flexion. The athlete cannot lift the tip of the finger to straighten the bone because the tendon is no longer attached; they will experience pain and swelling. The AT will splint the finger into extension and refer the athlete to a physician for care. The physician has two courses of action: Treat the injury surgically or keep the finger splinted. The tendon can heal back to the bone if it is kept still and extended. If the tendon is retracted too far from its attachment, surgery is required to reattach the tendon. In many instances, an athlete will not consider this injury to be important and may fail to report it. This negligence will result in a permanent flexion of the DIP joint.

Jersey Finger

Jersey finger is similar to mallet finger except that the flexor tendon tears from the fingertip. The athlete will not be able to flex the DIP joint of the finger. Injury occurs when the DIP joint is forcibly flexed, such as when the athlete is holding

> **? What Would You Do If . . .**
>
> A male gymnast was putting on his gymnastics pants. His hand slipped, and he noticed he could no longer lift the end of his finger. You explain this could be a mallet finger and should be seen by the AT and team physician. The athlete refuses. You tell him that it could result in a permanent injury. The athlete responds by saying, "That's why we have insurance."

an opponent's jersey in their fist and their finger is forced to extend, tearing the tendon. They will experience pain and swelling. Splinting and ice are good initial treatments. The finger will require an X-ray to determine the extent of the injury, and a physician will decide if the athlete needs surgery.

Boutonniere Deformity

A **boutonniere deformity** occurs at the PIP joint (see figure 17.5). A hard impact over the PIP joint can cause a tear in the joint capsule, which allows the extensor tendons to fall laterally. When the tendons are in the lateral position, they contract and force flexion of the DIP joint. The athlete will not be able to extend the PIP joint and will experience pain and swelling. The AT should splint the finger and refer the athlete to a physician for treatment. In many instances, the finger can be splinted, allowing the connective tissue that keeps the extensor tendons in place to heal. Otherwise, surgical intervention is necessary. For more on distinguishing between finger injuries, see figure 17.6.

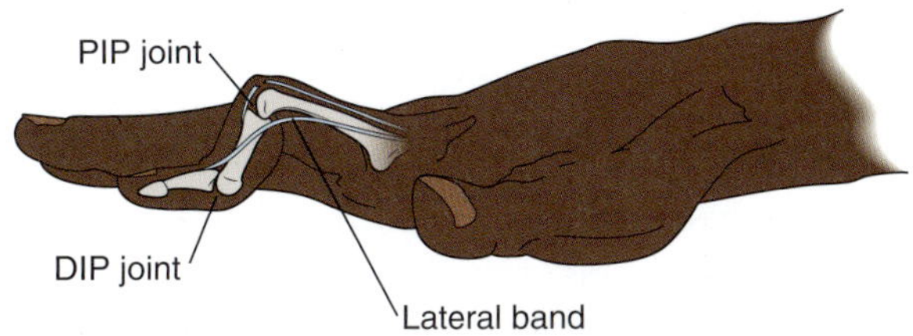

Figure 17.5 Boutonniere deformity. If the sheath that holds the extensor tendon on top of the finger is torn, causing the tendons to slide to the sides of the finger, the PIP joint flexes and the DIP joint hyperextends.

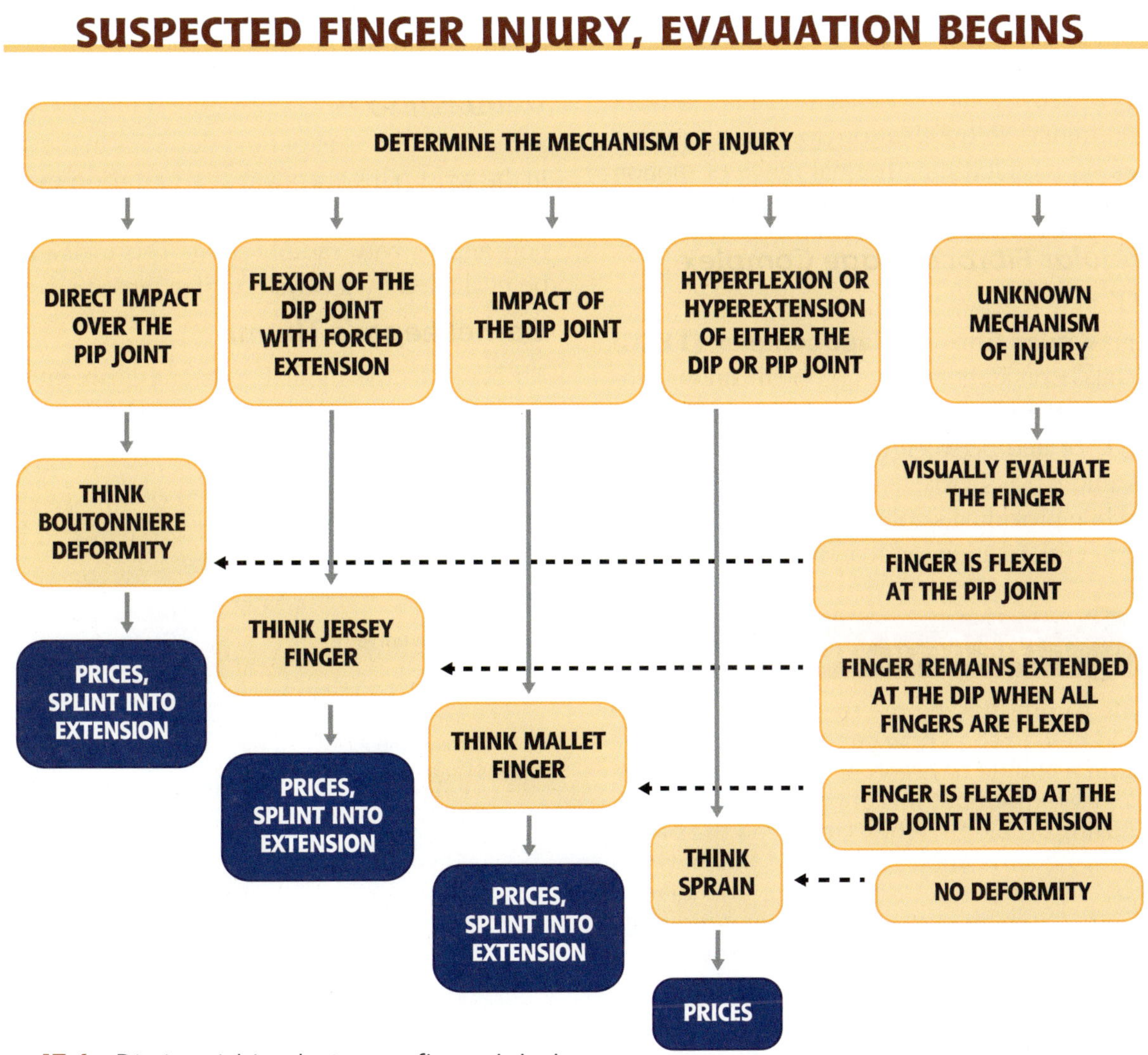

Figure 17.6 Distinguishing between finger injuries.

Ligament Injuries

Many sprains are not serious and can be treated with PRICES. One common misconception about sprains is that they must be pulled back into place. This is not true. Sprains are injured ligaments and pulling on an injured ligament can only cause more injury.

Wrist Sprain

Wrist sprains commonly occur from overuse, falls on an outstretched arm, and a forceful twisting motion. Which ligament is injured depends on the stress. An excessive amount of ulnar deviation at the wrist, for example, will injure the ligament on the radial side due to too much tension or overstretching, and excessive radial deviation at the wrist will injure the ligament on the medial side. The athlete will experience pain, possibly decreased range of motion, decreased grip strength, and swelling. The AT should recommend PRICES. When the athlete returns to activity, taping for support may prevent further injury. Rehabilitation for wrist sprains focuses on reestablishing normal range of motion and strength, including grip strength and function.

Triangular Fibrocartilage Complex Injury

The **triangular fibrocartilage complex (TFCC)** injury has been identified as a problem among athletes who sprain their wrists. The TFCC is a piece of cartilage located between the ulna and the carpal bones, and it plays a role in cushioning these structures while providing stability. The TFCC is injured with forceful rotation or hyperextension of the wrist. The athlete will experience pain, weakness, clicking, and loss of function in gripping actions. Treatment of this injury often involves immobilization followed by a rehabilitation plan to restore wrist range of motion and strength. In some instances, the TFCC must be surgically repaired. This injury is difficult to diagnose and requires careful evaluation.

> **The Real World**
>
> A male gymnast asked me to look at his hand. He said he had somehow cut his palm during a workout a couple days earlier. He had cared for the injury himself but was unhappy that he was still having problems. When I removed the bandages, it became apparent why he was having a problem—he had used a needle and black thread to stitch his own hand. Luckily, it did not appear to be infected. I sent the student to his family physician, who removed the stitches and placed him on antibiotics.
>
> **Lorin Cartwright, MS, ATC**

Dislocation of the Lunate

When an athlete falls on their hand, it can be in flexion or extension at the time of impact. Either motion can result in a dislocation of a carpal bone, most commonly the lunate. **Lunate dislocation** will cause deformity, and the third knuckle will look lower than the others. There will also be pain, swelling, and decreased range of motion (see figure 17.7). The dislocation of any carpal bone should be splinted and referred to a physician, who must relocate the bone. These are often casted to establish continuity during healing.

Ganglion Cyst

Sometimes a pocket of fluid develops in the sheath in the wrist. This is known as a **ganglion cyst** (see figure 17.8). Treatment often includes ice application and activity modification. The injury should be evaluated by a physician if symptoms persist.

Gamekeeper's Thumb

An injury to the medial collateral ligament of the thumb is known as **gamekeeper's thumb** (see

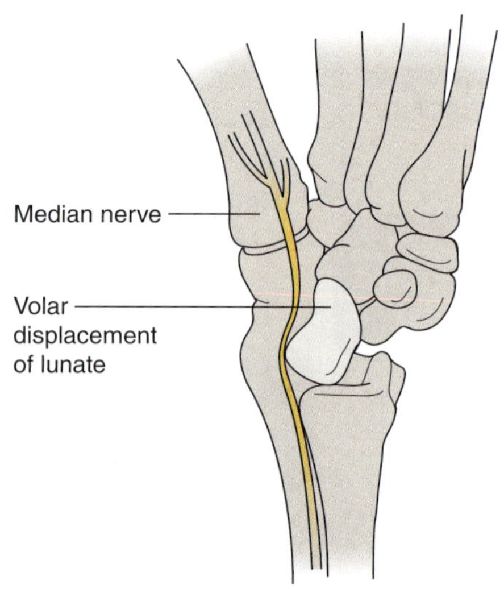

Figure 17.7 Lunate dislocation.

Reprinted by permission from S. Shultz, P. Houglum, and D. Perrin, *Examination of Musculoskeletal Injuries*, 4th ed. (Champaign, IL: Human Kinetics, 2016), 347.

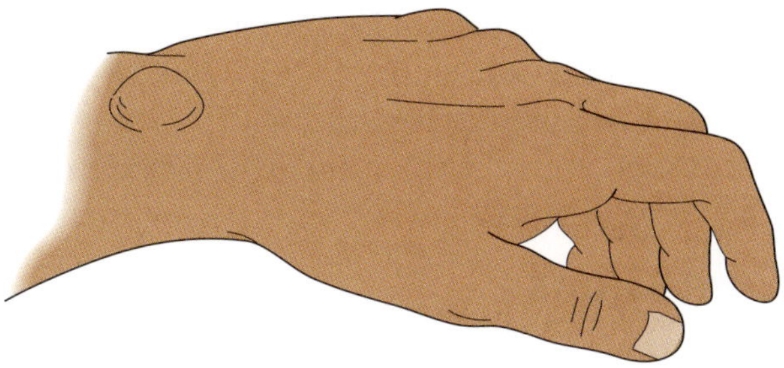

Figure 17.8 Ganglion cyst.

figure 17.9) and sometimes as skier's thumb. The term *gamekeeper's thumb* is an old one that was first used to describe farmers who injured the ligament when breaking the necks of birds intended for the cooking pot. This injury is also known as skier's thumb because the ski pole sometimes gets stuck and forces the thumb into abduction. In general, the ligament on the medial aspect of the thumb is injured when the thumb is forcefully abducted, such as when catching a basketball. The athlete will complain of pain over the joint, and the area may be swollen.

Treatment of the injury involves splinting the medial aspect of the thumb and icing. An X-ray will be necessary to determine if an avulsion fracture is associated with the ligament tear. Taping is often required when the athlete returns to play in order to protect the region from reinjury.

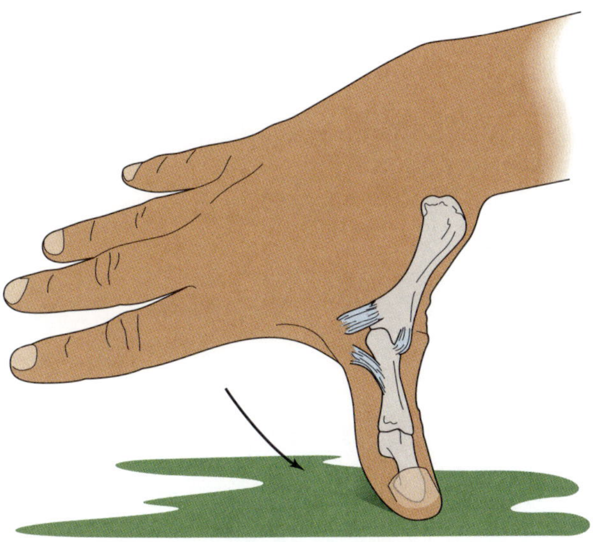

Figure 17.9 Gamekeeper's thumb and mechanism. When the thumb is pulled away from the finger, the ulnar collateral ligament can rupture.

Interphalangeal Collateral Ligament Sprain

A collateral ligament is located on the side of each interphalangeal joint. The ligaments provide stability when the phalanges are stressed, but they can be sprained when a joint is stressed beyond normal—for example, if the finger is hit by a ball, if the athlete lands with fingers curled or extended, or if the athlete accidentally catches a finger on an opponent's jersey. Injury to the collateral ligament is painful and disabling. The joint can swell and become discolored. The AT will confer with the team physician to determine if an X-ray is necessary to rule out a fracture. Ice application will keep the swelling to a minimum; if the finger swells too much, the athlete will be unable to bend it. When the athlete returns to competition, it is common to tape the injured finger to an uninjured neighbor (i.e., buddy taping). Padding may prevent additional injuries.

> **What Would You Do If . . .**
>
> A softball player slid headfirst into second base, and afterward her index finger did not look right. She tells you that she had another player pull her finger, and she felt it pop.

Dislocation of the Interphalangeal or Metacarpophalangeal Joint

When a dislocation of the interphalangeal or MCP joint occurs, one bone usually moves dorsal and one moves volar. The team physician should relocate all dislocated fingers and thumbs because tiny tendons, nerves, and blood vessels make their way through joint spaces. If the relocation is done incorrectly, there can be permanent damage to that finger. Some states permit ATs to reduce dislocations. Even though it is "just a finger," be sure to know the limits of practice in your state before reducing any dislocation.

With a dislocation, the ligament may tear, with possible fractures also occurring. We know of a softball player who dived for a ball and dislocated her finger. Her teammate pulled on the finger in an

RED FLAGS

Refer the athlete to a physician if they experience any of the following:

- Decreased sensation in the hand, fingers, or wrist
- Deformity compared to the noninjured side
- Increased joint laxity
- Loss of motion

attempt to help, driving the splintered bone pieces into the tendon and severing it. Four pins and one surgery later, the softball player has a straight finger that she will not let anyone touch.

Nerve Injury

As with the elbow, nerve injuries can occur in the wrist and hand. **Carpal tunnel syndrome** is a common injury to the median nerve that runs anterior to the carpal bones. In this area, the carpal bones form a tunnel along with the overlying ligamentous tissue. The median nerve travels through the tunnel into the hand. If this tunnel narrows due to overuse from gripping, typing, or any other repetitive movements, the nerve will be compressed. Compression of the median nerve causes pain, tingling, numbness, and weakness in the thumb, index finger, and third digit of the hand.

Treatment involves using a wrist splint, stretching the flexor muscles of the wrist, and medication. If this fails to work, a physician may inject the area with a steroid, or surgical procedures called carpal tunnel releases may be performed to open the space. During this procedure, the retinaculum holding the tendons and nerve in place will be surgically cut to release the pressure on those structures. After a short immobilization and rehabilitation, most athletes recover fully.

Contusions

A direct impact to the dorsal aspect of the hand can cause a great deal of swelling. The hand can swell and appear deformed. The AT will have to rule out a metacarpal fracture. The care for this type of injury is PRICES. When the athlete is able to return to competition, padding the hand is an important consideration.

A direct impact to the tip of the finger can cause bleeding under the fingernail. This is referred to as a **subungual hematoma**. When this occurs, the tip of the finger will swell, causing discoloration of the nail and significant pain. Because the pressure from the swelling causes so much pain, the AT may consider referring this athlete to the physician. The typical treatment of a subungual hematoma is to drain the area by drilling a hole in the fingernail. Typically, the hematoma will clear up on its own, and eventually the nail will fall off.

FYI

Volar

The palm side of the hand.

Dorsal

The back or posterior portion of the body in the anatomical position.

Summary

The wrist and hand are involved in every activity of daily living and athletic activity, so they are susceptible to numerous injuries that can range from minor to permanently disabling. An athlete who is trying to be helpful can increase the severity of an injury, such as by pulling on an injured finger. Because of the intricate structure of the wrist and hand, the signs and symptoms of many injuries are identical. To ensure the best possible outcome, the AT, coach, or team physician should be the first one to provide care. The physician should evaluate most sprains to rule out fractures. Any unresolved injury should be referred for comprehensive evaluation to ensure proper function in the region.

Key Terms

Define the following terms found in this chapter:

- avascular necrosis
- boutonniere deformity
- boxer's fracture
- carpal tunnel syndrome
- Colles' fracture
- de Quervain's tendinitis
- gamekeeper's thumb
- ganglion cyst
- jersey finger
- lunate dislocation
- mallet finger
- subungual hematoma
- triangular fibrocartilage complex (TFCC)

A track athlete barrels across the finish line and falls forward, landing on an outstretched arm. The athlete reports generalized wrist pain after the fall. What are the differential wrist diagnoses associated with this common mechanism of injury? Identify which injury could result in a vascular condition to the bone that could create poor healing and long-term complications.

To access supplementary material for this chapter, including the Understanding Check worksheet, vocabulary quizzes, extension activities, and chapter-specific resources and forms, visit the web resource: http://ancillaries.humankinetics.com/FundamentalsOfAthleticTrainingAndSportsMedicine5E

Unit V

Athletic-Related Injuries to the Lower Extremity

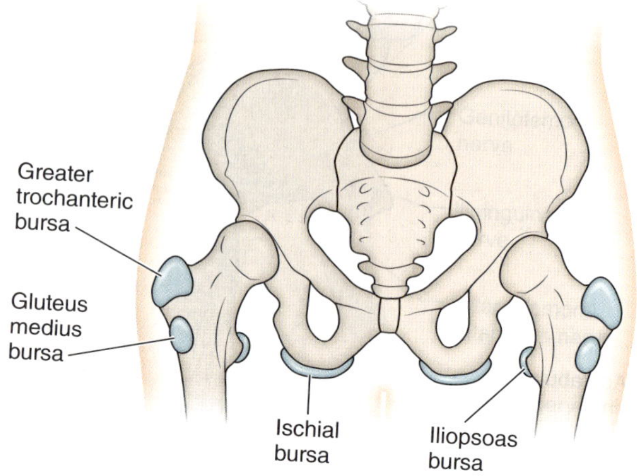

Figure 18.11 Bursa sacs.

wear a hip pad to cover this area. Proper strength training for any portion of the body can never be too strongly emphasized, and because the muscles around the hip and lower torso are considered the core region, strength in these muscles is necessary for balance and stability.

TREATING HIP, PELVIS, AND THIGH INJURIES AND CONDITIONS

Most injuries to the hip, pelvis, and thigh are strains and contusions. However, the area is not exempt from other injuries, such as fractures and dislocations.

Bone Injuries

Although pelvic fractures are not common, they can occur when excessive stress is placed on the bone tissue. Athletic-related fractures of the hip, pelvis, and femur often occur from an avulsion (the tendon pulling away the bone), disruption of the epiphysis (damage to the growth plate), stress, or trauma to the femur.

Hip Pointers

A **hip pointer** is a contusion of the iliac crest. The iliac crest is superficial and has little soft tissue covering it; however, many muscles attach near the crest, so when a serious force hits the bone, it can be debilitating. The area must be protected from further contact by a protective pad.

Labral Tears

It is not a common injury, but the labrum can tear if an acute injury occurs, though in most patients, the occurrence is insidious, meaning it occurs slowly with no specific mechanism of injury. A torn labrum can flip into the joint and result in catching, groin pain, and restricted range of motion at the hip. A labral tear will often need to be surgically repaired, but in some instances, the athlete can learn to manage the condition so the tear does not aggravate the joint.

Avulsions

Avulsion fractures occur from forceful muscle contractions that pull the bone away at the site where the tendon attaches. This may happen, for example, when a football player continues to run aggressively forward while a defender is holding his leg. The hip flexor may forcefully contract, causing a fracture.

Growth Plate Fractures

Epiphyseal fractures occur at the growth plates of bones, especially at the **capital femoral epiphysis**, where the neck of the femur joins the head. The head of the femur slips off the neck, causing pain in the groin, hip, and knee. According to experts, this injury is the most common hip disorder in active children between the ages of 10 and 15. When an AT suspects this condition, the athlete should be referred to a physician because treatment includes stopping the slippage and closing the growth plate with a surgical procedure.

Stress Fractures

Although uncommon, femoral stress fractures do occur in athletes who do a great deal of running. Stress fractures are caused by repetitive stress, typically from the pounding the lower extremity takes while running. This pounding can cause the femur to bend slightly. Just as if a pencil were bending, one side of the bone is compressed while the other side is stretched. When bone tissue is repeatedly stretched, small hairline fractures can develop, causing a great deal of pain and discomfort. Rest and an alternative activity such as aquatic therapy

What Would You Do If . . .

While at football practice, the AT and a student assistant are helping an injured player off the field. You see that another athlete seems to have injured his leg during a play—it appears to be externally rotated, and he is in a lot of pain. As you approach the athlete, another player starts to grab his teammate's injured leg, saying that it needs to be straightened out.

are indicated to reduce the stress on the fracture site so it can heal.

Femur Fractures

Because the femur is the largest bone in the body, the stress required to fracture it is often extreme. A femur fracture is characterized by severe pain and loss of function as well as internal bleeding, swelling, or tearing of muscles, tendons, nerves, and arteries. Typically, the athlete is unable to move the leg. A femur fracture often causes the leg to externally rotate. Initial treatment for a femur fracture includes immobilization and transportation to the hospital by EMS personnel. They will often use a traction splint that gently pulls the femur, reducing leg pain and spasm.

Coccyx Fractures

The coccyx is better known as the tailbone. Fracture of the coccyx is caused by a fall directly on the bone. This type of fracture is painful, and the athlete will find it difficult to sit. The initial care requires physician intervention and an X-ray. A donut-shaped pillow can aid the athlete with sitting.

Hip Dislocations

Extreme stress can cause a dislocation. Most hip dislocations occur posteriorly and accompany other trauma such as fractures. Severe damage can occur in this area because of the nerve and vascular structures. An athlete with a dislocated hip is likely to be in extreme pain, and the leg is often internally rotated (see figure 18.12). With such an injury, EMS should be called to transport the athlete to the hospital as soon as possible. Only a physician should reduce a hip dislocation. Significant follow-up treatment is required before the athlete can

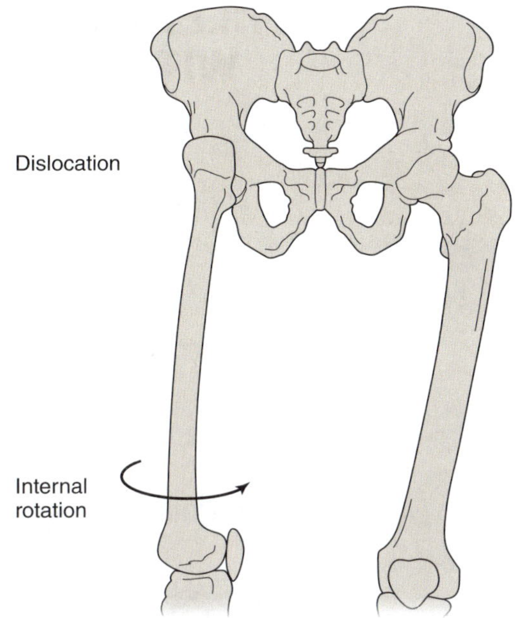

Figure 18.12 A hip dislocation. Note that the leg is internally rotated.

return to activity. Rehabilitation for a hip dislocation often begins with establishing normal range of motion and strength. Gait training, or relearning how to walk normally, will be necessary. As you can imagine, this is a long process. See figure 18.13 to learn to differentiate between a femur fracture and a dislocation.

Legg-Calvé-Perthes Disease

In some children and teens who are still growing, a disruption of blood flow to the head of the femur causes the tissue at the head of the femur to die, a condition known as **Legg-Calvé-Perthes disease**. Typical symptoms include groin or knee pain and walking with a limp. If this condition is suspected, the athlete should be referred to a physician immediately.

RED FLAGS

The following conditions and injuries require immediate physician referral:

- Hip dislocation
- Femur fracture
- Legg-Calvé-Perthes disease

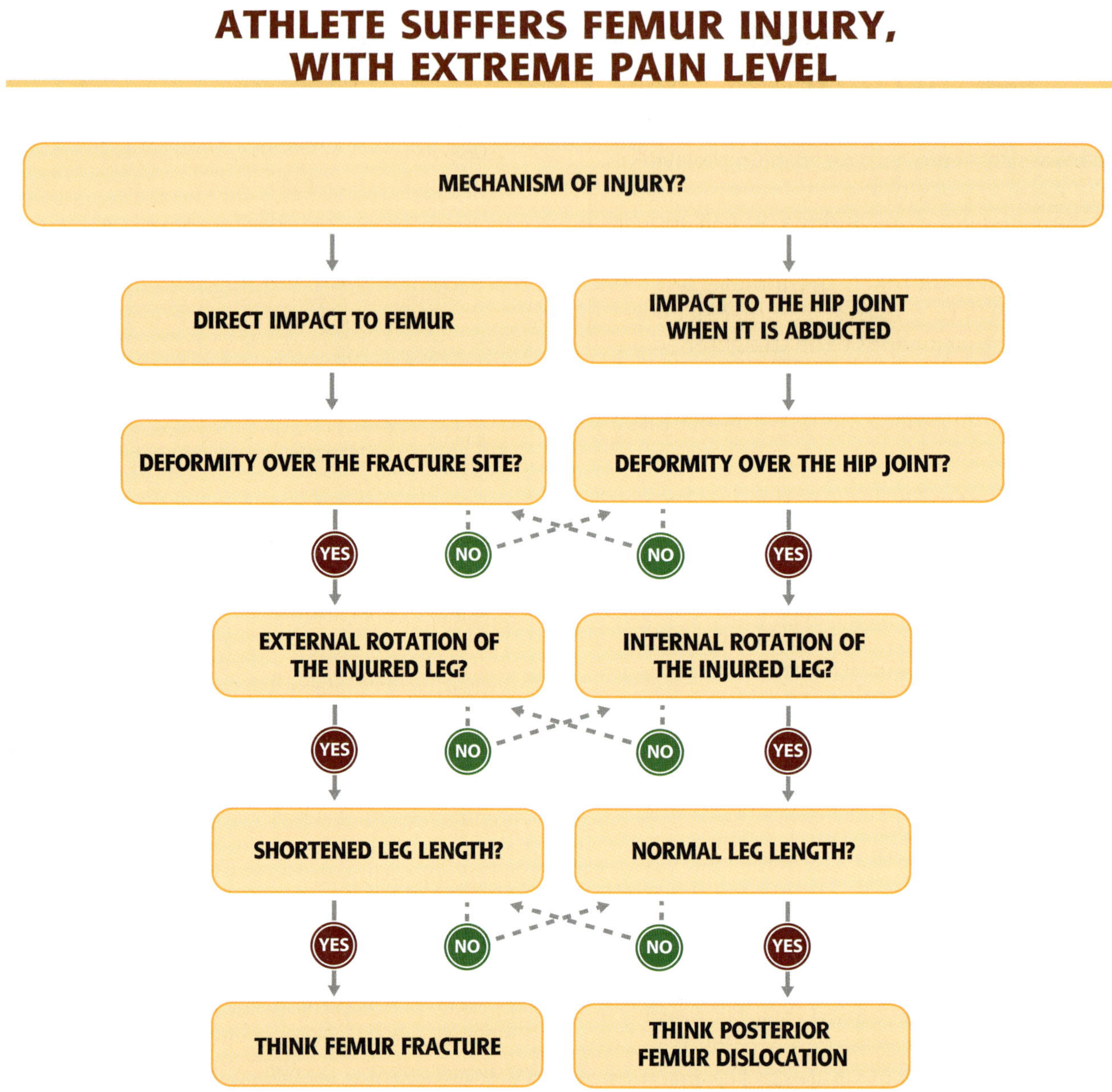

Figure 18.13 Differentiating between a femur fracture and a dislocation.

Understanding Diversity

The bones in Navajo Indians are less dense, making them more prone to fractures (Miller et al. 2016).

Muscle and Tendon Injuries

Thigh strains are common athletic injuries, especially to the hip flexor, extensor, and groin musculature. Many muscles in the leg cross two joints—for example, the hamstrings cross the back of the hip joint to help with extension and the knee joint to help with knee flexion—and some people see this as the cause of strains in the region. Another theory is that when a strength imbalance occurs, the stronger muscle group puts excessive tension on the opposing muscle group. For example, if an athlete has a great deal of strength in their quadriceps but has weak hamstrings, the hamstrings are prone to strains.

Strains should initially be treated with PRICES and wrapped with a supportive elastic bandage. Moderate and severe strains may need to be referred to a physician. Rehabilitation will focus on regaining strength and range of motion and enhancing flexibility before returning to play.

Hip and Thigh Muscle Contusions

Deep thigh contusions are common, especially in collision sports. In many contact sports, such as rugby or football, opponents collide with the athlete's thigh and compress the tissue. Thigh contusions can result in a lack of knee flexion due to tightness. Although many bruises suffered in athletics are minor, thigh contusions can cause disability. The more severe contusions can cause tissue tearing and extensive bleeding. If not managed appropriately, serious thigh contusions can cause a condition known as **myositis ossificans**, which is the formation of bone tissue in the muscle (see figure 18.14). Because bone tissue is not as extensible as muscle tissue, disability and loss of function are typical consequences.

When treating a thigh contusion, proceed with PRICES, but the knee should be flexed during the ice application. An AT may put the athlete in a hinged knee immobilizer with the knee locked into flexion, limiting the total loss of flexibility due to the injury. With a moderate to severe contusion, the athlete should be placed on crutches to minimize stress to the area and then referred to the team physician. Active rest, ice, and gentle stretching routines are effective in restoring mobility. Ultrasound (discussed in chapter 21) is often used to help reabsorb the blood that collects internally and to break up the bony tissue deposits. The AT must make certain that a protective pad is placed over the contusion to prevent repeated contusions to the area, because this also can create myositis ossificans.

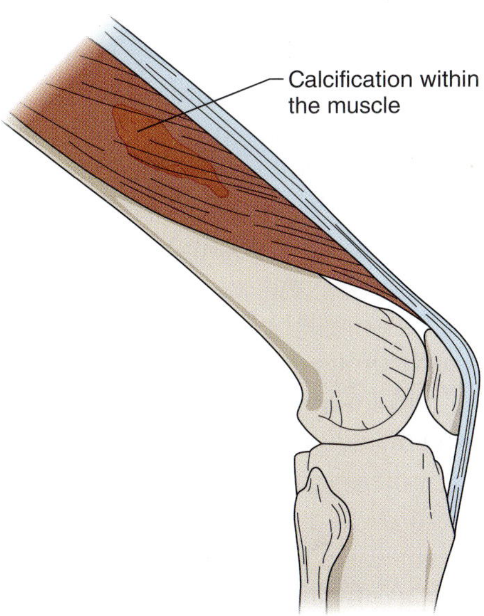

Figure 18.14 Myositis ossificans.

Iliopsoas Syndrome

The iliopsoas muscle originates at L5-S2 of the spine and inserts on the lessor trochanter of the femur. Two muscles combine to create the iliopsoas, the psoas and iliacus. The primary function is flexion of the spine and flexion of the hip.

Iliopsoas syndrome is attributed to the movement of the iliopsoas tendon over the bony prominence of the hip. The usual bony prominences include the head of the femur and the lessor trochanter. This hip movement is normal until pain is caused by overuse, a sudden contraction of the muscle, or direct contact. The athlete will experience pain deep in the low back, groin, or pelvic region. There can be pain with active range of motion, especially flexion of the hip or back. The iliopsoas syndrome may be accompanied by tendinitis and or bursitis. Iliopsoas syndrome treatment includes PRICES.

Ligament Injuries

The hip is a ball-and-socket joint that is extremely stable, mostly because the head of the femur sits so deeply in the pelvis. Thick ligamentous structures and strong muscles also surround the hip. The labrum is the cartilage that deepens the socket and allows the hip to move smoothly throughout the range of motion.

Neurologic Conditions

Neurological conditions of the hip can pose significant issues for patients. The hip is a weight-bearing bone, and pressure on the nerves can debilitate the patient. The AT will need to determine if the condition originates in the spine, hip, pelvis, or thigh.

Femoral Nerve Entrapment

The femoral nerve can become entrapped as it traverses from the spine along its course to muscles. The most common entrapment occurs as the nerve exits the spine at L2-3 or L3-4. The tingling, weakness, or pain is noted at the anterior medial aspect of the thigh and the medial aspect of the lower leg.

The most common form of entrapment occurs at the spine with spinal discs that prolapse and place pressure on the nerve. Treatment will be based on the point of the entrapment. Traction of the spine, stretching, anti-inflammatories, and rest may be the best first approach. Exercise will be needed to strengthen the muscles as the entrapment is released.

Piriformis Syndrome

Piriformis syndrome occurs when the sciatic nerve is entrapped between the piriformis muscle and the tissue around the ischial tuberosity. Piriformis syndrome mimics sciatic nerve pain, with pain shooting down the posterior of the leg. There will be gluteal pain, tingling, and numbness along the path of the sciatic nerve.

Diagnosis is to apply pressure to the nerves as well as stretching the piriformis muscle. A positive test is an indication of piriformis syndrome. Once the diagnosis is made, treatment includes rest, anti-inflammatories, range of motion activities, massage, trigger-point therapy, and stretching.

Inflammatory Conditions

Inflammatory conditions can be created by many conditions, including infections, swelling, and degenerative processes. Infections of the hip are caused by pathogens that are typically bacterial, viral, fungal, or parasitic. An infection in another part of the body may spread to the hip. Degenerative conditions usually occur when the articular and labrum cartilage deteriorates and the head of the femur rubs against the bony surface of the pelvis. The result is pain, decreased range of motion, and inflammation, leading to disability.

Trochanteric Bursitis

The lateral hip, specifically over the greater trochanter of the femur, can create pressure over the bursa. The bursa is a fluid-filled sac that reduces friction of tendons that cross this bony prominence. When the bursa is irritated by too much pressure from the tendons, it becomes inflamed. Athletes with **trochanteric bursitis** will report snapping of the hip when they climb stairs.

Osteitis Pubis

If the pubic symphysis is subjected to repeated stress, it can become inflamed and painful. This is known as **osteitis pubis**. The pain will radiate into the adductor muscles when an athlete is running or during any movement with adduction of the leg. Ultimately, the athlete will require PRICES with rehabilitation that takes pressure off the muscles. Full recovery may take a long time.

Osteomyelitis

An infection in the bone is characterized by pain at the site, fever, and malaise. Decreased range of motion, erythema, and purulence are also signs. The hip is a common site of this type of infection. **Osteomyelitis** can occur because of a traumatic injury, an open wound, or generalized infection. The *Staphylococcus* infection may spread through the blood, or it may occur after a direct injury in the area. The primary treatment involves referral to a physician, antibiotics, and debridement of the area.

Septic Arthritis

Septic arthritis is an infection in the synovial fluid. Common ways for the infection to invade the body are through an open fracture, an infected wound, a puncture wound, or an infection in the body. Staphylococcus is the common bacteria. Signs and symptoms include decreased range of motion, fever, and redness about the area.

The diagnosis is done through removal of fluid from the joint. Treatment may consist of draining the joint and antibiotics.

Osteoarthritis

Osteoarthritis of the hip is caused by the wearing away of the articular surface of the head of the femur and degradation of the labrum of the acetabulum. The result is the acetabulum and the femoral head grinding on one another, creating a roughened surface. Eventually, the roughening can lead to bone spurs, and the hip joint will become inflamed. There will be less range of motion and pain. Osteoarthritis can be treated conservatively with ice, anti-inflammatories, and pain medications; by losing weight; rest; range-of-motion exercises; strengthening; and using an assistive device (cane or crutches).

Significant cases of osteoarthritis may require referral to a physician. Hip replacement may be necessary if conservative treatment does not achieve the desired effect.

The Real World

I always look forward to the first football scrimmage of the year. I was watching as a defensive back came near the sideline to make a play on the wide receiver. A blocker for the wide receiver hit the defensive back in the hip with his shoulder pad in an attempt to block. The defensive back did the splits while being blocked and tackling the receiver. He was in severe pain, was supine with hip and knee flexion, and was unable to get up. After I assessed him, I determined he had dislocated his hip, and I called for emergency medical assistance. We placed him on a backboard with padding beneath his knee to maintain flexion. At the hospital, his hip was relocated. Unfortunately, a dislocated hip needs several months of rest and rehabilitation for proper healing—he never played in a game that year.

Lorin Cartwright, MS, ATC

Summary

The hip is a stable joint, not only because of its bony structure but also because it has strong muscles and ligaments surrounding it. The thigh has strong musculature but can receive deep contusions, especially to the quadriceps, if not properly protected. These injuries can be debilitating for the athlete and require immediate care. The AT must be aware that an adolescent athlete may develop Legg-Calvé-Perthes disease or growth plate fractures at the capital femoral epiphysis. The AT should take care to get a thorough history and observe the athlete's hip for joint position because this can help detect a fracture of the growth areas around the hip. Rehabilitation of the hip often involves reestablishing flexibility and muscle strength around the joint.

Key Terms

Define the following terms found in this chapter:

- acetabulum
- capital femoral epiphysis
- hip pointer
- iliopsoas syndrome
- labrum
- Legg-Calvé-Perthes disease
- myositis ossificans
- osteitis pubis
- osteoarthritis
- osteomyelitis
- piriformis syndrome
- septic arthritis
- trochanteric bursitis

As an AT, you are working with the school's track team. After assessing the previous year's injuries, you decide that there needs to be a stretching program. Working with the coach, you need to develop a preventive stretching program to prevent hamstring and hip injuries. Which type of stretching and what specific stretches would you recommend and why?

To access supplementary material for this chapter, including the Understanding Check worksheet, vocabulary quizzes, extension activities, and chapter-specific resources and forms, visit the web resource: http://ancillaries.humankinetics.com/FundamentalsOfAthleticTrainingAndSportsMedicine5E

chapter 19

Knee Injuries

Objectives

After completing this chapter, the student will be able to do the following:

- Describe the basic anatomy of the knee.
- Explain common knee injuries that occur with athletic participation.
- Identify signs and symptoms of knee injuries.
- Explain treatment parameters performed by an AT for specific knee injuries.

The knee is vulnerable to ligament sprains, tendon strains, and cartilage damage. In this chapter, we describe the basic anatomy of the knee and injuries common to athletes.

ANATOMY OF THE KNEE

The knee is a hinge joint at the articulation, or point of contact, of three bones. The joint is stabilized by four major ligaments, cartilage, and strong musculature. The knee is also able to rotate. The knee is made up of three compartments: medial, lateral, and patellofemoral.

Bones

The bones that form the knee joint are the femur, tibia, and patella (see figure 19.1). The primary movement of the knee occurs at the articulation of the tibia and femur, which is called the *tibiofemoral joint*. The patella is a sesamoid, or floating bone, and is embedded in the patellar tendon that attaches the quadriceps to the front of the tibia and protects the front of the joint. As the knee flexes and extends, the patella glides up and down on the front of the femur. This is called the *patellofemoral joint*.

Muscles

Knee muscles provide both movement and stability. The primary muscles spanning the knee are the quadriceps and hamstrings. Knee extension is performed by the four quadriceps muscles: the vastus medialis, vastus lateralis, vastus intermedius, and rectus femoris (see figure 19.2). The vastus muscles of the quadriceps originate on the femur, whereas the rectus femoris originates at the anterior aspect of the pelvis. The quadriceps run toward the patella and attach to the patellar tendon at the anterior knee. The patellar tendon crosses the anterior aspect of the knee joint and inserts on the superior aspect of the tibia. The lateral aspect of the knee is supported by the iliotibial band.

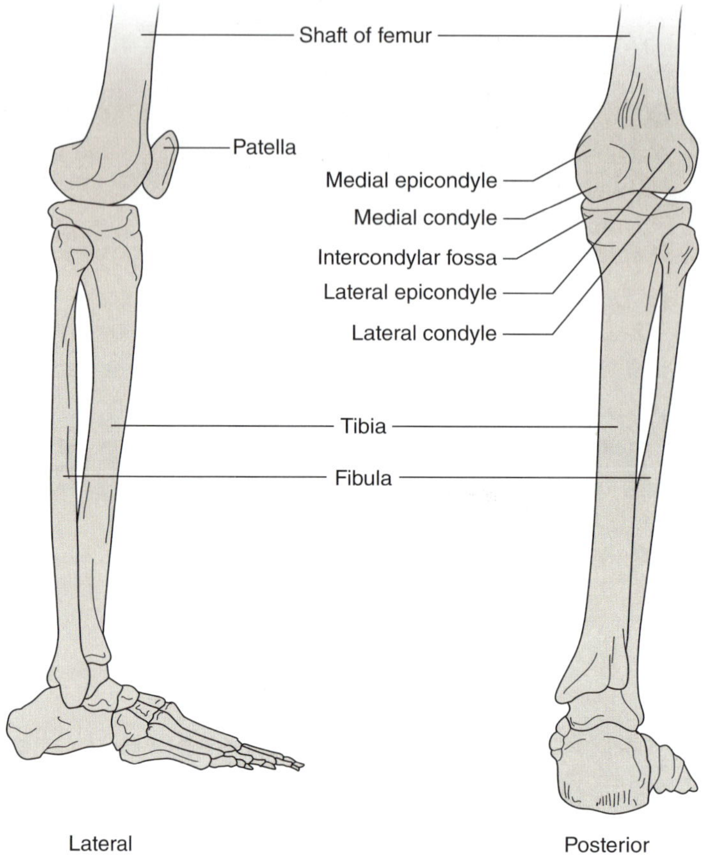

Figure 19.1 Lateral and posterior views of the knee.

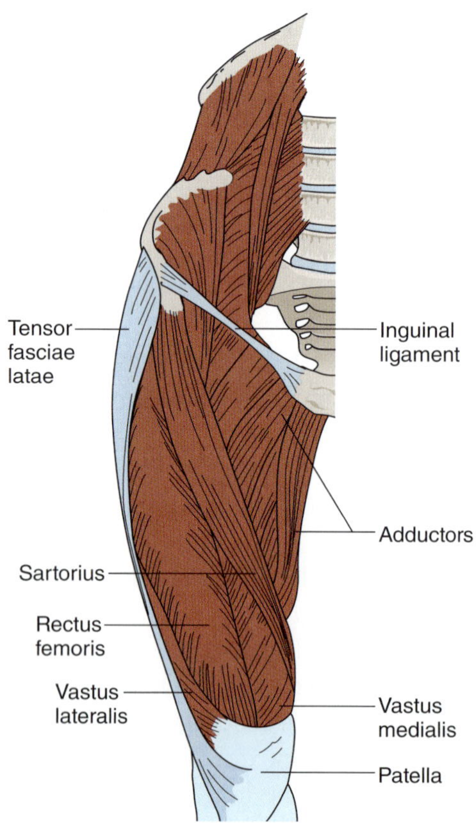

Figure 19.2 The quadriceps muscles.

Knee flexion is predominantly the result of contracting the hamstring muscles. The term **hamstrings** refers collectively to the biceps femoris, semimembranosus, and semitendinosus muscles (see figure 19.3). The three hamstring muscles attach on the posterior aspect of the lower pelvis and run down the back of the thigh and across the knee to their attachment on the tibia. The attachment location helps prevent forward movement of the tibia on the femur.

Besides the quadriceps and hamstrings, other important muscles around the knee joint allow movement and provide stability. Posteriorly, the gastrocnemius muscle crosses the knee joint, originating at the posterior aspect of the femur. The gastrocnemius is known mainly as a muscle that allows us to point our toes (plantar flexion), but it also functions with the popliteus muscle to flex the knee.

At the medial aspect of the knee, the gracilis muscle crosses the knee joint. This muscle originates near the groin and inserts on the medial tibia; its function is to adduct the femur. On the lateral

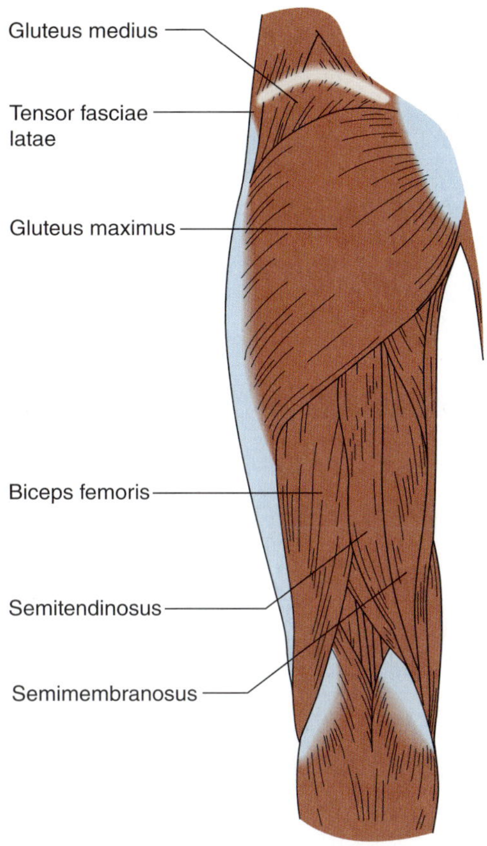

Figure 19.3 The hamstring muscles.

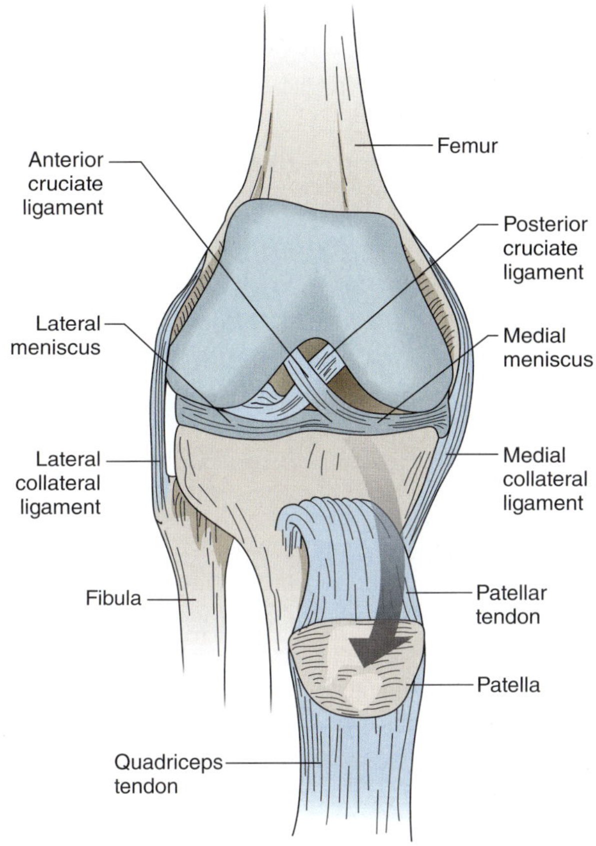

Figure 19.4 Major ligaments of the knee. Note how the cruciate ligaments cross in the center of the knee.

> **What Would You Do If . . .**
>
> An athlete has been treated in the athletic training room for jumper's knee. While you are getting the watercoolers set up for practice, you notice that the athlete is starting to play one-on-one with a teammate before warming up and stretching.

aspect of the knee, the iliotibial band crosses the knee joint. The iliotibial band is a tough connective tissue that the tensor fasciae latae and gluteus maximus of the hip merge into. These muscles help to abduct the hip.

Ligaments

There are four primary knee ligaments (see figure 19.4). The **medial collateral ligament (MCL)** helps stabilize the inside or medial aspect of the knee, and the **lateral collateral ligament (LCL)** helps stabilize the outside or lateral aspect of the knee. The **anterior cruciate ligament (ACL)** keeps the tibia from moving forward on the femur, and the **posterior cruciate ligament (PCL)** prevents the tibia from moving backward on the femur. The ACL and PCL pass through the middle of the knee joint and cross each other; hence the name *cruciate*, which means "cross shaped."

Cartilage

The ends of the tibia and the femur are covered and cushioned by pieces of tough cartilage tissue called the menisci (see figure 19.5). Without the menisci, the tibia and femur would rub against each other, which would cause the bone to wear down quickly. The menisci also help stabilize the knee joint. The top of the tibia is flat, like a tabletop. The end of the femur, specifically the condyles, is rounded, like an orange. Without something to stabilize the joint, the femur would move a great deal on the tibia—

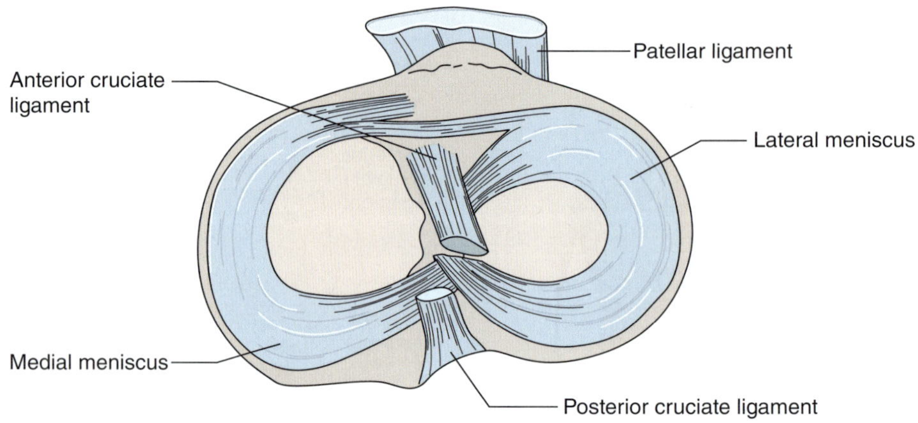

Figure 19.5 A top view of the medial and lateral menisci.

in other words, the orange would roll around on the tabletop. The menisci are thicker on the sides and thinner in the middle, forming a dish-shaped hollow. They are also attached to the top of the tibia, which provides a seat for the femoral condyles to sit in on top of the tibia—like putting the orange in a bowl on the table. The femur can move, but it will not roll off the tibia.

Innervation

The anterior aspect of the knee is innervated by the branches of the femoral nerve. The muscles innervated by the branches of the femoral nerve include sartorius, quadriceps, and pectineus.

Posterior innervation of the knee is covered by the tibial and common peroneal nerves. The hamstrings are innervated by the common peroneal nerve and the tibial nerve. The tibial nerve continues inferiorly into the lower leg, innervating the gastrocnemius. Figure 19.6 shows the innervation of the knee.

Circulation

The deep femoral and popliteal arteries provide blood supply to the posterior aspect of the knee. The anterior blood supply is provided by branches of the femoral artery. The medial aspect is the descending genicular, with a branch to the superior medial genicular and the inferior medial genicular. The lateral aspect of the knee consists of the superior lateral genicular and the inferior lateral genicular, a branch to the anterior and posterior tibial arteries. In figure 19.7, the circulation of the knee is shown.

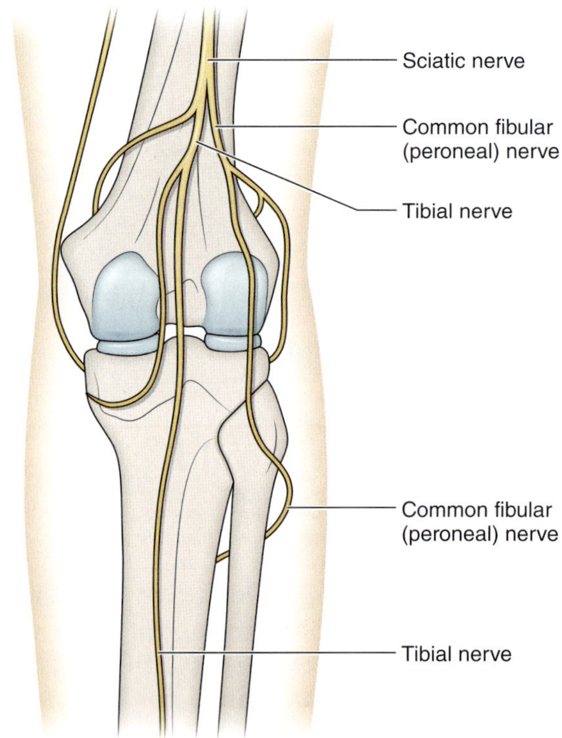

Figure 19.6 Innervation of the knee.

Bursa Sacs

The knee is also surrounded by approximately 14 bursa sacs—fluid-filled structures that provide cushioning or prevent friction. See figure 19.8 to see the bursa sacs. The most common bursa sacs are the prepatellar bursa (in front of the kneecap), infrapatellar bursa (underneath the kneecap), suprapatellar bursa (above the kneecap), pes anserine bursa (on the inner knee), and semimembranosus bursa (on the medial or inner knee posteriorly).

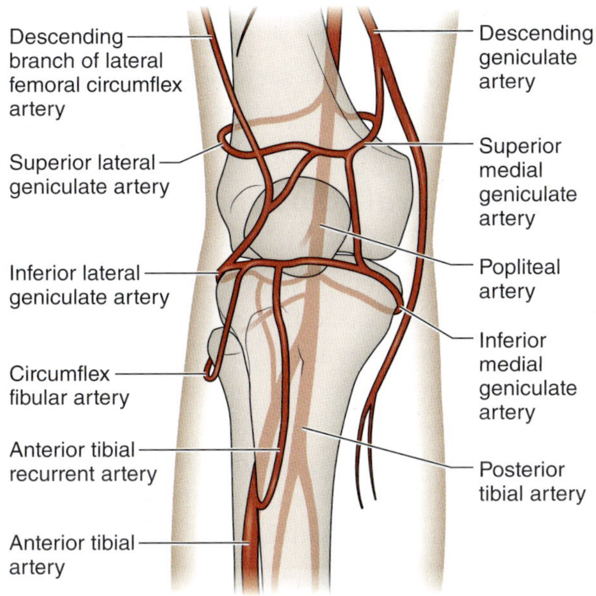

Figure 19.7 Arterial circulation of the knee.

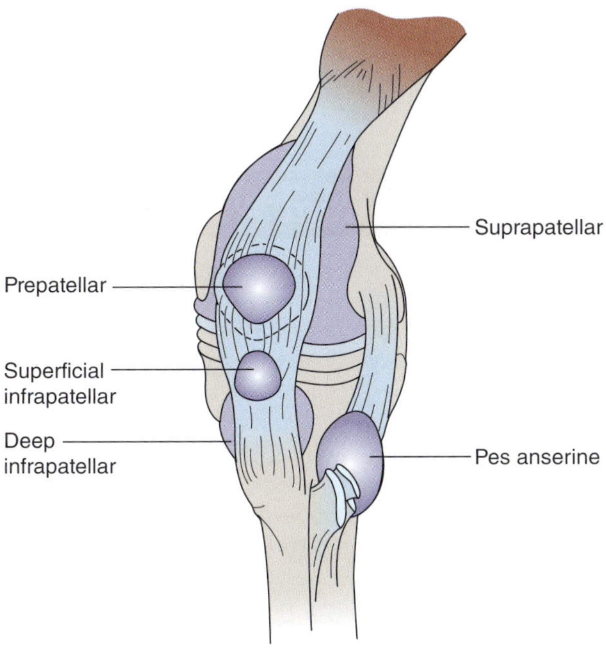

Figure 19.8 Bursa sacs of the knee.

Reprinted by permission from S. Shultz, P. Houglum, and D. Perrin, *Examination of Musculoskeletal Injuries*, 4th ed. (Champaign, IL: Human Kinetics, 2016), 472.

These important structures enhance the function of the knee.

PREVENTING KNEE INJURIES

Ligament sprains are among the most common injuries to the knee. Remembering that the muscles in this area provide stability to the knee and help resist abnormal bony movement, athletes should develop strength in these muscles (i.e., the quadriceps, hamstrings, gastrocnemius, and hip abductors and adductors). For instance, heel raises are a good way to strengthen the gastrocnemius, which is located at the back of the lower leg and helps to point the toes. Some ATs and athletes use preventive knee braces that are designed to protect the MCL (see figure 19.9); however, there is insufficient research to warrant using braces to prevent ligament injury.

If an athlete has problems with their knees, the AT should examine the leg structure to determine

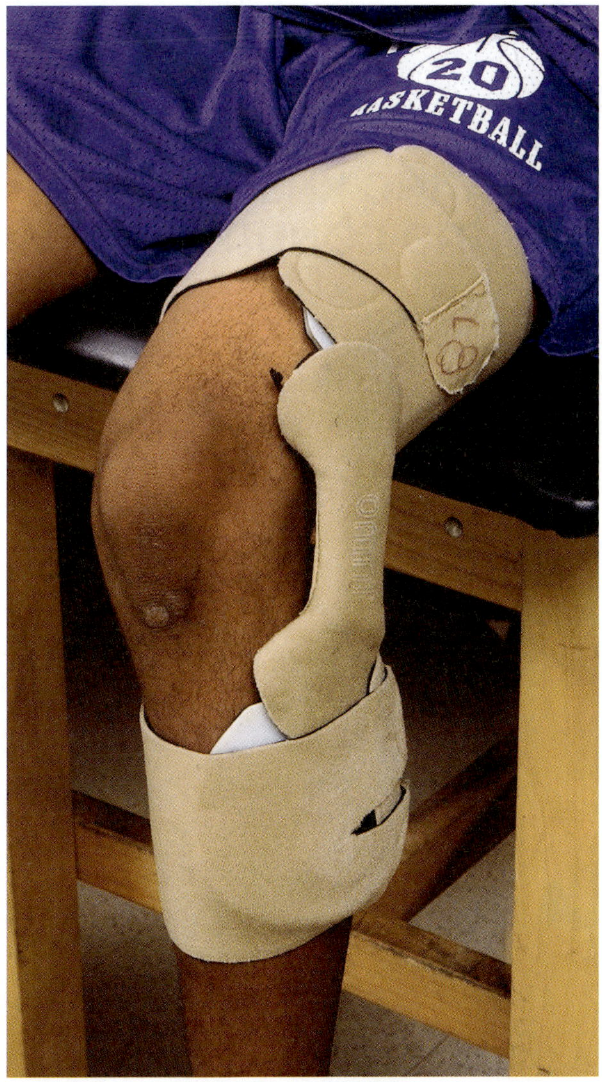

Figure 19.9 A protective knee brace is applied to an athlete's knee to prevent tearing of the MCL, which can result from a blow to the lateral side.

whether they have genu valgum, also known as knock-knees, or genu varum, also known as bowlegs (see figure 19.10). These conditions may provide insight into the type of knee problem the athlete is suffering. Also, knowing if one of these conditions is present will help in selecting appropriate equipment, such as knee braces or athletic shoes.

Current research has identified neuromuscular training as an effective way to prevent knee injuries, particularly injuries to the ACL. Neuromuscular training involves teaching athletes how to land from a jump, how to change directions while maintaining appropriate lower-extremity alignment (keep the knee over the foot), and how to flex the knee and hip during movements. It also involves balance training and proper deceleration in activities involving knee flexion.

TREATING KNEE INJURIES AND CONDITIONS

The knee is exposed to many forces. This makes it vulnerable to injuries, especially to the ligaments, but tendon and bone injuries also occur. The patella and menisci are subject to unique athletic-related injuries.

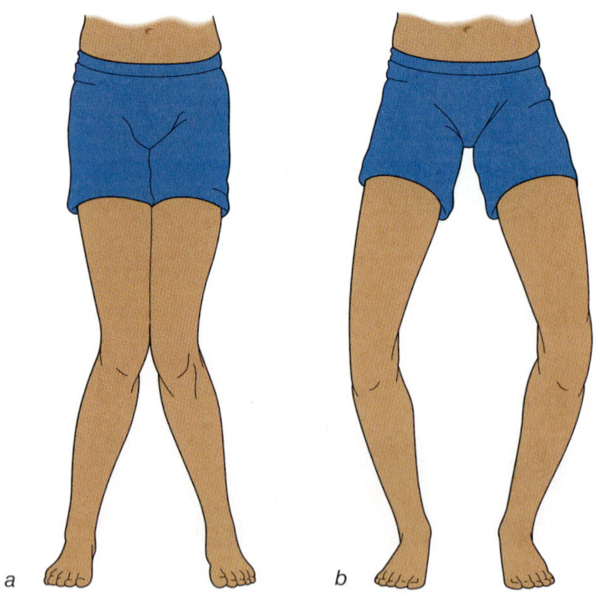

Figure 19.10 *(a)* Knock-knees and *(b)* bowlegs.

Bone Injuries

Although the patella is not immune to fracture, other bone injuries are more common. These include chondromalacia and patellar dislocations.

Patellofemoral Pain Syndrome

Patellofemoral pain syndrome involves a set of symptoms that include pain and discomfort around the patella, often caused by patellar tracking problems. As the knee bends, the patella is grated across the femur instead of riding smoothly, causing the cartilage on the back of the patella to soften or wear away. This is known as **chondromalacia** and is characterized by achiness around the patella, especially with prolonged sitting in the same position. The athlete will often report a grinding sensation with flexion and extension. If the AT places a hand over the patella as the athlete flexes and extends the knee, the grinding can even be felt. Treatment for chondromalacia involves correcting any problems with patellar tracking, strengthening the

> **The Real World**
>
> As an AT working at a large high school, I was summoned to the track and field area because an athlete had fallen over the hurdles. When I arrived at the track, I saw that the athlete was in pain and moaning that his knees were injured. I gently pulled up his pant legs to see what was wrong. There were obvious deformities at the anterior aspects of both knees. Where the patellae should have been were two large depressions, and the patellae themselves were sitting several inches above the knee joints, where the quadriceps had pulled them. We called EMS immediately. I acted calm and reassuring, knowing that if the young man panicked, things would only get worse. We immobilized his legs and treated him for shock. Once he was at the hospital, the surgeons determined that he had ruptured one patellar tendon and fractured his other patella in half. Although I had limited contact with this athlete afterward, his recovery looked positive because he received quick advanced care by physicians, and he was in good health.
>
> **Lisa V. Pitney, MSEd**

vastus medialis muscle, and improving flexibility of the quadriceps and hamstrings. Bent-leg activities should be avoided because they tend to aggravate the condition. Treatment for patellofemoral pain syndrome should also address any weakness around the hip joint since this has been identified as an effective intervention.

Patellar Dislocation

Occasionally an athlete's patella will be forced to the lateral aspect of the knee, usually while the knee is bent and forced to twist inward. This deformity is hard to overlook. The athlete is often in distress, and EMS must be called unless the team physician is present. Only a physician should reduce a dislocated patella; otherwise, complications may result, and the posterior aspect of the patella may be injured further. Treatment involves immobilizing the knee for a short time. Then the athlete should begin exercising to regain mobility and strength around the knee joint. Sometimes athletes are advised to wear a knee sleeve with a patellar hole to help keep the patella in place during activity.

Epiphyseal Plate Injury

The epiphyseal plate is located at the proximal end of the tibia. Remember that the epiphyseal plate is the area in the bone where cartilaginous cells transition into new bone cells. This area is the weakest place in the bone, which makes it vulnerable to fracture. If the epiphyseal plate is injured, it can result in interrupted bone growth, potentially altering full growth in that bone. Direct trauma or a sprain of the ligaments that attach near the plate can result in its damage.

The AT will splint or immobilize the area until a physician can determine the course of action and long-term care.

Patellar Fracture

Fractures of the patella can occur either by direct impact or noncontact. A helmet hitting the patella is an example of a direct-impact injury. A noncontact mechanism of injury can occur when there is a forcible contraction of the quadriceps, causing maximum stress on the patella and the tendon. A fractured patella will present with swelling and pain. Figure 19.11 is an X-ray of a patellar fracture. Immediate treatment includes PRICES, and a knee immobilizer and crutches provide additional knee protection. A follow-up with an orthopedist will be necessary.

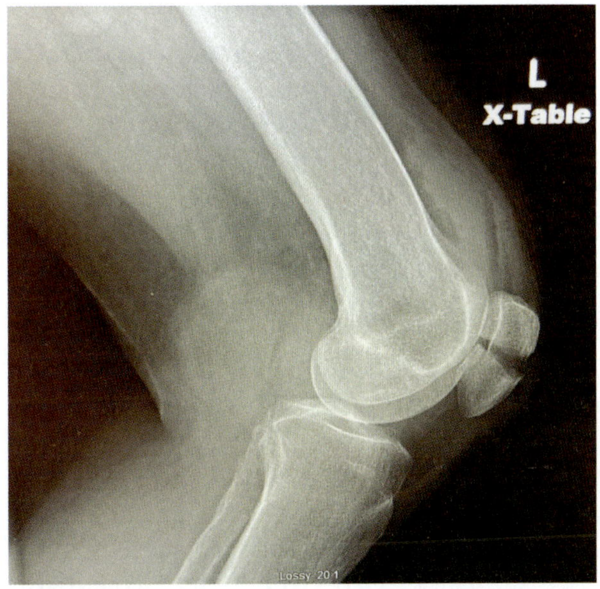

Figure 19.11 Fracture of the patella.
Reprinted by permission.

Muscle and Tendon Injuries

Many muscle and tendon injuries at the knee are chronic and are caused by overuse. The patellar tendon in particular is commonly involved.

Patellar Tendinitis

Patellar tendinitis is an overuse disorder characterized by quadriceps weakness, tenderness over the patellar tendon, and minimal swelling. The condition is also called *jumper's knee* because athletes who perform a lot of jumping (e.g., basketball and volleyball players) often get this condition. In the early stages, the athlete typically has pain after activity, but in the later stages, the condition can result in pain during activity as well as loss of strength. The AT will attempt to control inflammation by applying ice and modifying the athlete's activity level, usually restricting running and jumping. The rehabilitation program should address any quadriceps flexibility problems and leg weakness.

Although the term *tendinitis* is often used, the term *tendinosis* is often more appropriate. Tendinosis denotes a condition of the tendon, meaning it is degenerated, painful, and weak, but there is no inflammation.

If a tendon is already weak but the athlete continues to participate, a rupture can occur. A patellar tendon rupture means that the amount of stress applied to the tendon exceeded the ability of the tendon to withstand the force, ripping apart the fibers. With this injury, the elasticity of the quadriceps will retract the patella upward; thus, a deformity at the anterior knee will be present.

Osgood-Schlatter Disorder

Younger athletes who run and jump a lot sometimes develop an irritation at the site of the patellar tendon attachment to the front of the tibia, or the tibial tuberosity. Adolescent bones are still somewhat soft, and repeated stressful activity can sometimes cause the patellar tendon to partially pull away from the bone, an injury called **Osgood-Schlatter disorder**. It typically causes knee discomfort, swelling, tenderness, and pain during activity. Athletes with this condition should restrict their activity until it is resolved. However, this does not mean they should stop all activity. For example, although a basketball player should stop aggressive running and jumping, an alternative activity that may not irritate the injury is stationary bicycling. The athlete can maintain their fitness level without causing additional problems. Generally, pain should be used as a guide; that is, activity should be modified based on the athlete's pain level. If the athlete does not modify activity appropriately, they may experience prolonged periods of pain. Ice application before and after activity is also helpful. A special pad may need to be made to fit over the front of the tibia because this area becomes extremely tender. Osgood-Schlatter disorder often improves by age 16 or 17, but a bony growth may develop at the top of the tibia. Unfortunately, the bump remains even after the symptoms of the condition have disappeared.

Patellar Tendon Rupture

A direct blow to the patellar tendon can cause a partial or complete rupture. An example of such a direct blow is a defensive football player's face mask ramming into the knee of a hurdling running back. The sign is that the patella will be drawn in the superior direction when compared to the uninjured knee. Surgical repair is necessary for a significantly ruptured tendon.

Ligament Injuries

Like other joints, knee ligament sprains can be mild (first degree), moderate (second degree), or severe (third degree). The four primary ligaments are the most commonly sprained.

Anterior Cruciate Ligament Injuries

The ACL keeps the tibia from moving forward on the femur. If this ligament is injured (see figure 19.12), the athlete is often disabled, complaining of the knee giving way, collapsing, and popping. Injuries to the ACL are often the most serious of all knee ligament injuries, and the ACL ligament is most frequently surgically reconstructed.

The ACL is often injured as the athlete attempts to change directions quickly, decelerates, and twists the lower leg; they may hear a popping sound during the twisting mechanism. However, it can also be injured because of excessive hyperextension. Direct contact to the anterior of the knee forcing hyperextension is another mechanism of injury. Regardless of the mechanism, a torn ACL causes rapid swelling and loss of knee function. Immediate treatment includes PRICES, and a knee immobilizer and crutches provide additional knee protection. A follow-up with an orthopedist is necessary if a torn ACL is suspected.

An athlete rarely functions well with a torn ACL, and the injury often needs to be surgically reconstructed. However, the athlete, the surgeon, and

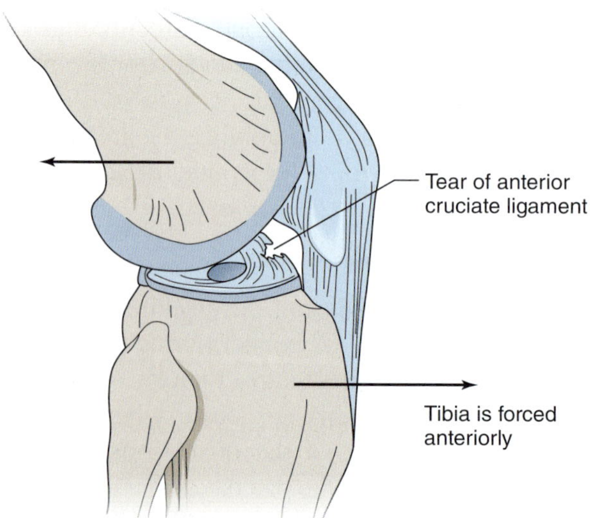

Figure 19.12 An ACL tear results from the tibia moving forward forcefully on the femur.

the athlete's family need to make this decision. The decision may depend on the amount of instability that exists, the level of function the athlete desires, and the age of the athlete.

Surgical reconstruction of the ACL can involve two types of tissues, autografts or allografts. An autograft involves a piece of tissue from the athlete's body. The tissues used in these instances will include either a portion (about one third) of the patellar tendon or a hamstring tendon (usually the semitendinosus). The tissue used for an allograft involves a portion of the athlete's patellar tendon, the athlete's Achilles tendon, a hamstring tendon, or a cadaver's patellar tendon. Cadaver allografts require irradiation to ensure sterilization before surgery. The surgical reconstruction and the determination of which type of graft to be used will be decided with the orthopedic surgeon.

ACL injury rehabilitation focuses on restoring range of motion and strengthening the hamstrings to help stabilize the tibia and regain full function. Even with an aggressive ACL rehabilitation program, it may be six months before the athlete can return to participation.

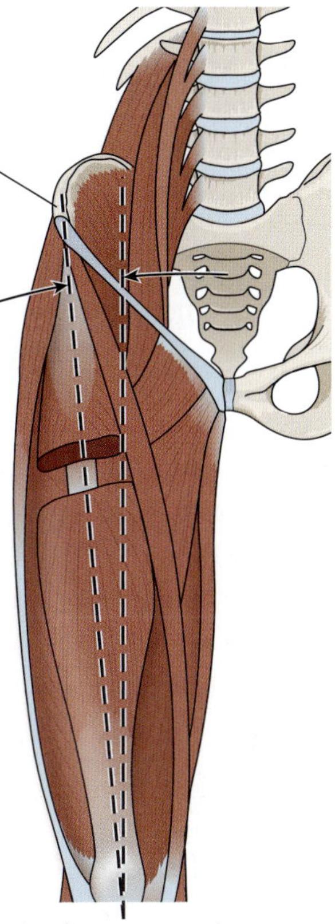

Figure 19.13 Landmarks for measuring Q-angle.

Reprinted by permission from R.S. Behnke and J. Plant, *Kinetic Anatomy*, 4th ed. (Champaign, IL: Human Kinetics, 2022), 227.

Posterior Cruciate Ligament Injuries

The PCL prevents posterior tibial movement on the femur. It is frequently injured when an athlete falls and a bent knee bears their full weight, when the knee is forcefully hyperflexed, or when a blow is delivered to the front of the tibia.

After determining the mechanism of the injury, the AT may suspect a PCL injury if the athlete reports having heard a pop. Surprisingly, there tends to be little swelling with PCL injuries. Initial treatment should include PRICES and a physician referral. A rehabilitation program for mild or moderate PCL sprains will focus on strengthening the quadriceps and regaining full function. Although physicians disagree about whether surgery should be performed on a severe PCL injury, even complete PCL tears can be rehabilitated without surgical intervention—many athletes can become functional again after the initial pain and swelling are controlled and the knee is strengthened.

> **Understanding Diversity**
>
> Female athletes are more prone to ACL injuries compared with male athletes. The reasons for this are varied. One theory is that female athletes have a higher Q-angle, which is the angle created by the femur and the tibia. Because females tend to have wider hips than males, the Q-angle is greater, resulting in the knee collapsing inward and forward during function (see figure 19.13). Another theory is that during the female menstrual cycle, hormones are released that create joint laxity, or looseness in the joints. If the joint is lax, it is more unstable, and the tibia may shift more on the femur. Lastly, it is thought that the landing mechanics of women are the cause—more stress is applied to the ACL instead of the surrounding muscles to absorb the impact forces.

Medial Collateral Ligament Sprains

The MCL is frequently injured when an athlete receives a blow to the outside of the knee. This causes the knee to bend inward (valgus stress) and stresses the MCL. A mild MCL sprain usually results in medial joint line pain, little if any swelling, no joint laxity when stressed by the AT, and full knee flexion and extension. A moderate MCL sprain often results in mild swelling, discomfort, and joint laxity when stressed by the AT during the injury assessment. A moderate or severe amount of swelling, loss of function, and a great deal of joint laxity often characterize a severe MCL injury.

Regardless of the severity of the injury, the athlete's knee should be treated with PRICES (see figure 19.14). A mild injury may require only an elastic wrap for compression and support. However, with a moderate or severe MCL injury, the knee should be put in an immobilizer. Rehabilitation considerations include strengthening the muscles that cross the medial aspect of the knee. If the knee has moderate or severe MCL damage, the AT should consider the possibility of damage to the menisci or an ACL injury.

Lateral Collateral Ligament Injuries

LCL injuries occur less frequently than MCL injuries do. The signs and symptoms are similar, except the discomfort is at the lateral aspect of the knee. Treatment for an LCL injury is the same as for an MCL injury. In terms of regaining joint stability, strengthening exercises should focus on the lateral thigh muscles and hamstrings.

Unhappy Triad

When evaluating ligament injuries, one must also consider if the meniscus has been injured. The unhappy triad comes about from a direct contact to the lateral aspect of the knee with the foot planted. The blow to the lateral knee translates energy across, causing inward (valgus) stress. This force tears the MCL, the medial meniscus, and the ACL. Treatment includes PRICES and referral to an orthopedic surgeon.

Cartilage Injuries

Each large piece of fibrous cartilage in the knee joint is a **meniscus**. The function of the menisci is shock absorption and stability. Unfortunately, the menisci are vulnerable to significant injury, specifically tears.

The most common injury to the meniscus is a tear, which can be on the outer edge, middle, inside edge, or ends (horns) of the meniscus. Meniscus tears typically happen with a twisting movement of the knee or with hyperflexion and hyperextension injuries. An athlete with a torn meniscus will often complain of pain at the joint line; have problems putting weight on the limb; complain of clicking,

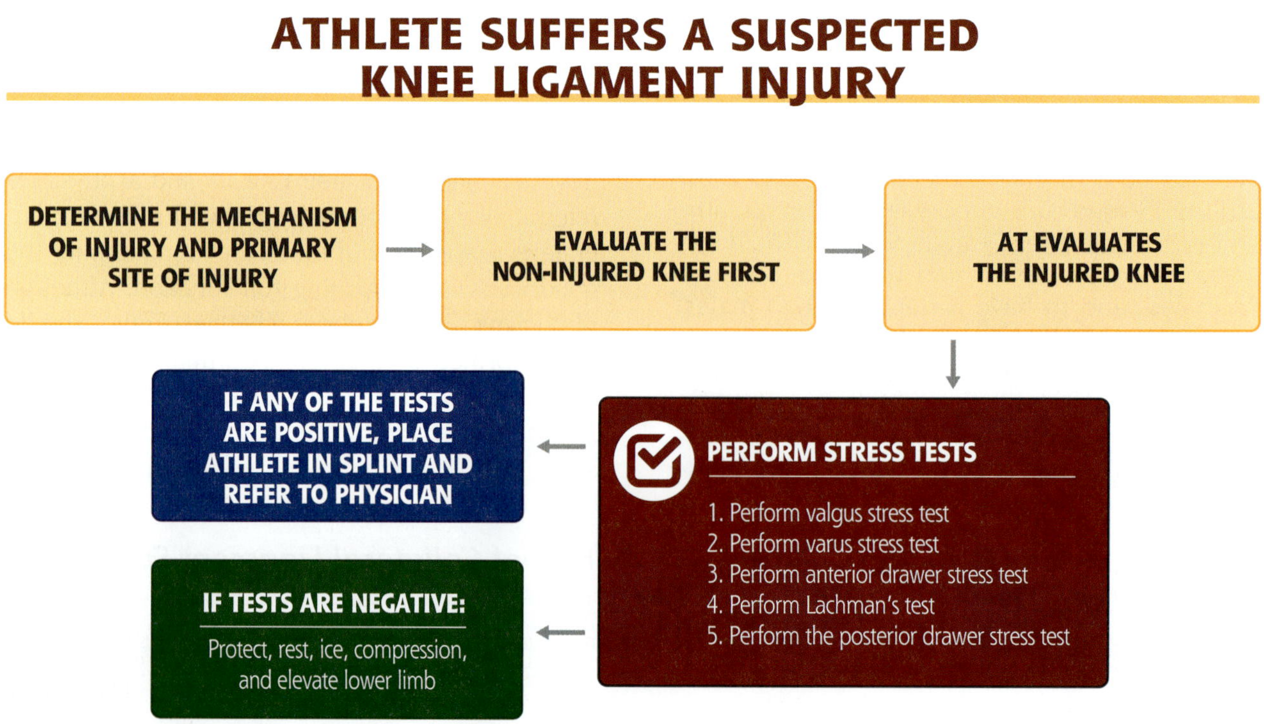

Figure 19.14 Acute knee ligament evaluation algorithm.

catching, or locking; and walk with a limp. He will be unable to fully extend and flex the knee and may have swelling.

Tears of the meniscus used to be treated by surgically removing the entire meniscus (called a **meniscectomy**). (See figure 19.15, which shows a bucket-handle tear, a type of meniscus injury.) However, due in part to the prevalence of **arthroscopic surgery**, where small surgical instruments are inserted into the knee through tiny holes, treatment of a torn meniscus often involves taking out only the small piece of tissue that has been torn. The consequence of a meniscectomy, whether full or partial, is early onset osteoarthritis. Ultimately the effect of osteoarthritis is knee replacement surgery.

Depending on where the meniscus is torn, sometimes surgeons are able to suture (sew) it back together. The benefit of repairing the meniscus is a shorter recovery time and a better long-term prognosis (Lee et al. 2019).

During rehabilitation after an injury to or surgery on the meniscus, an athlete initially will use exercises that do not involve placing weight on the injured leg. Aquatic therapy programs are ideal for helping to reestablish range of motion and strength. Then the athlete will progress slowly to more weight-bearing exercises as tolerated.

Fat Pad Syndrome

The infrapatellar fat pad lies behind and just beneath the patella and acts as a barrier and cushion between the patella and femur. When an athlete extends the knee, the fat pad can become trapped between these bones. **Fat pad syndrome** is sometimes referred to as **Hoffa's syndrome**. The signs and symptoms of this condition include tenderness beneath the knee, swelling, and pain with extension. The area should be rested and treated with ice and possibly needs an ultrasound.

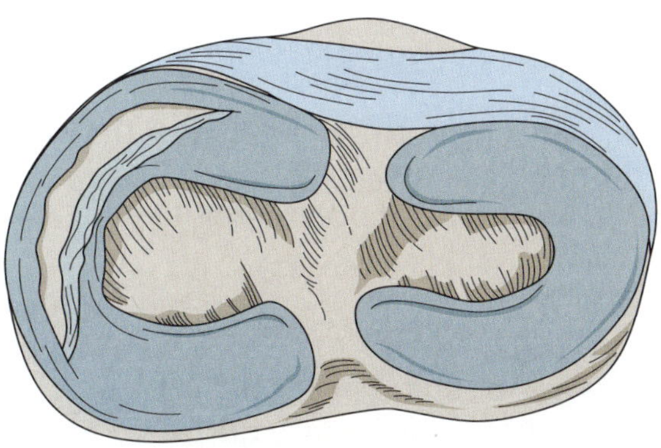

Figure 19.15 Bucket-handle tear of the meniscus.

> **RED FLAGS**
>
> Take the following actions if a knee is stuck or gives out:
>
> - Splint in place if the knee is stuck in an immovable position.
> - Send the athlete to a physician if the knee gives out.

Iliotibial Band Syndrome

An athlete who has tightness of the iliotibial band may experience pain over the lateral aspect of the knee. The knee pain may be accompanied by a snapping sensation as the band crosses over the lateral epicondyle of the femur. On examination, the AT will define the tightness of the band and pinpoint the pain to the lateral epicondyle. The treatment is stretching of the band, using a foam roller to massage the area, and rest as needed. Prevention is to effectively stretch the tendon and to use moderation when running. Overuse is a precipitating factor in iliotibial band syndrome.

Bursitis

When a bursa sac becomes inflamed, either from friction or a direct blow, it will swell and create pain in the knee. Bursitis can be managed with PRICES as well as compression wrapping. If the bursa sac swells to a great degree, a doctor may choose to drain the synovial fluid out of the bursa. Most often, though, bursitis responds well to conservative treatment and activity modification.

Popliteal Cyst

A popliteal cyst is better known by the name Baker's cyst. Sometimes when an injury or deterioration occurs in the knee joint, excess synovial fluid can accumulate in the posterior aspect of the knee. The popliteal bursa, which reduces friction during movement, may fill with the excessive fluid. A popliteal bursa filled with excessive fluid is called a cyst.

Injuries that may lead to a cyst include ACL or PCL tears, arthritis, or a meniscus tear. The athlete will describe knee pain, have swelling in the popliteal area and lower leg, and lack knee flexion and extension. Treatment is treating the initial cause of the swelling. Immediate treatment includes PRICES. Referral to a physician is appropriate. The physician may prescribe steroid medication and aspirate the fluid to bring about relief.

Degenerative Conditions

A degenerative condition occurs over a long time. These conditions can occur because of an injury and progress to a degeneration of the bony surfaces. Some degeneration occurs over time and from everyday movement. Degenerative conditions can become debilitating.

Osteoarthritis

The knee has three compartments: medial, lateral, and anterior. Each of these compartments are subject to osteoarthritis. Osteoarthritis is a degenerative arthritis of the knee. This form of arthritis takes place over years of wear and tear of the articular surface and meniscus. As surfaces degrade, they become roughened, which adds to the deterioration. Eventually the surface in the joint is bone on bone, causing swelling, pain, decreased range of motion, and bone spurs. The significance of the bone-to-bone surface can occur in one, two, or all three compartments. If all three compartments are involved, it is known as **tricompartment failure**. Conservative treatment includes PRICES, and a follow-up with an orthopedist will be necessary.

Post-Traumatic Arthritis

Post-traumatic arthritis develops after a knee injury that impairs movement or damages the bone or cartilaginous surfaces. Similar to osteoarthritis, the degradation of the joint surfaces occurs over time. Signs and symptoms include pain, swelling, decreased range of motion, and bone spurs. Treatment includes PRICES and referral to an orthopedic surgeon.

Summary

The knee is the joint between the femur, tibia, and patella. The quadriceps extend the knee, and the hamstrings flex it. The cartilage, or menisci, of the knee provides a cushion between the tibia and femur. Four primary ligaments aid in the stability of the knee: the MCL, LCL, ACL, and PCL. A complete tear to the ACL needs to be surgically repaired by an orthopedic surgeon.

Key Terms

Define the following terms found in this chapter:

- anterior cruciate ligament (ACL)
- arthroscopic surgery
- chondromalacia
- fat pad syndrome
- hamstrings
- Hoffa's syndrome
- lateral collateral ligament (LCL)
- medial collateral ligament (MCL)
- meniscectomy
- meniscus
- Osgood-Schlatter disorder
- patellar tendinitis
- posterior cruciate ligament (PCL)
- tricompartment failure

An athlete comes to you, the AT, and indicates they have a clicking in the knee, pain with steps, and buckling of the knee. What is your initial thought on what this injury might be? What evaluative techniques would you use to determine the injury? To what type of doctor would you refer this athlete to ensure specialized care?

To access supplementary material for this chapter, including the Understanding Check worksheet, vocabulary quizzes, extension activities, and chapter-specific resources and forms, visit the web resource: http://ancillaries.humankinetics.com/FundamentalsOfAthleticTrainingAndSportsMedicine5E

chapter 20

Foot, Ankle, and Lower-Leg Injuries

Objectives

After completing this chapter, the student will be able to do the following:

- Describe the basic anatomy of the foot, ankle, and lower leg.
- Explain common injuries that occur to the foot.
- Identify common injuries that occur to the ankle.
- Describe signs and symptoms of lower-leg injuries.
- Identify strategies for preventing injuries to the ankle and lower leg.

The foot, ankle, and lower leg support the body weight and transfer force as a person walks and runs. They work to maintain balance and adapt to various surfaces. Ankle injuries are among the most common injuries seen by team physicians and ATs; in fact, the ankle may be the most frequently injured joint.

ANATOMY OF THE FOOT, ANKLE, AND LOWER LEG

The lower leg, foot, and ankle play a critical role in balance, shock absorption, and movement. The bones provide structure and protection, while the muscles and tendons produce movement.

Bones and Joints

There are 28 bones in the foot (see figure 20.1). The bones in the toes are called **phalanges**. The toes are numbered 1 to 5, the great toe being number 1. Except for the great toe, each toe has three bones: the distal, middle, and proximal phalanges. (The great toe has only distal and proximal phalanges.) The toe joints are referred to as *interphalangeal joints*. Under the great toe are two small bones, the sesamoids, which assist with flexion of the toe. The **metatarsals** are the long bones of the foot; like the toes, they are numbered 1 to 5. The joints between the phalanges and the metatarsals are the metatarsophalangeal joints. The phalanges, metatarsals, and sesamoids are known as the forefoot.

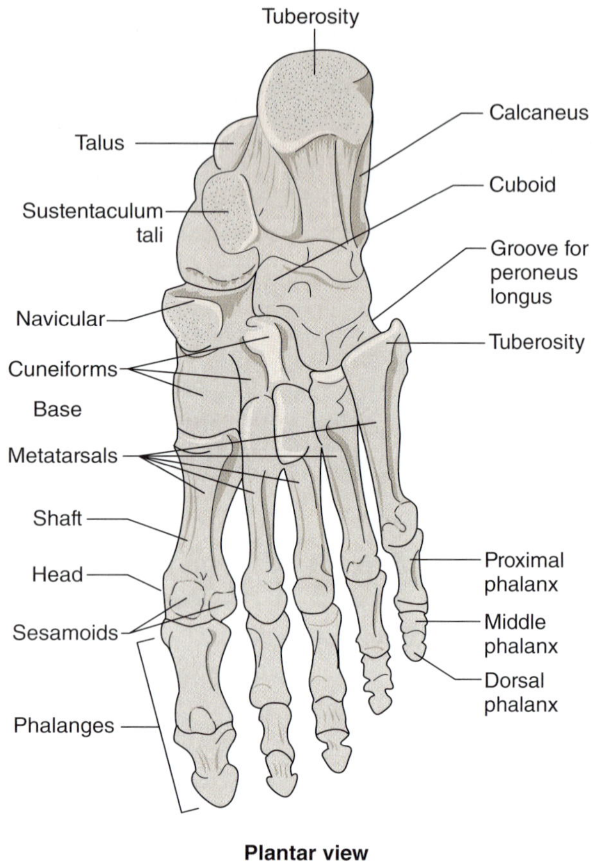

Figure 20.1 Bones of the foot.

The midfoot, which lies between the metatarsals and the **talus** and **calcaneus**, contains several small bones that articulate (join together at a joint) with one another, producing subtle movements. Bones in the midfoot include the navicular, cuboid, and cuneiforms. The hindfoot, the most posterior portion of the foot, has two bones: the talus and calcaneus.

The ankle is the joint between the talus and calcaneus of the foot and the fibula and tibia of the lower leg. The calcaneus, also known as the heel bone, is below the talus. The posterior portion of the calcaneus is the attachment point of the Achilles tendon. The tibia and fibula articulate at both distal and proximal ends, and muscles and ligaments between the two bones hold them together from one end to the other. The **medial malleolus** is the end of the tibia on the medial side, and the end of the fibula at the lateral aspect is known as the **lateral malleolus**. The ankle is held together by ligaments. The fibula extends past the ankle joint and stops severe eversion.

Understanding Diversity

The peroneus tertius muscle is missing in approximately 5% to 17% of white people (Patel and Patel 2021). The absence of the peroneus tertius means that the athlete may have difficulty dorsiflexing and everting the ankles.

Arches of the Foot

There are three arches on the **plantar surface** (bottom) of the foot that function as shock absorbers: the transverse, longitudinal, and metatarsal arches (see figure 20.2). The transverse arch is in front of the heel and goes from the fifth metatarsal to the navicular bone of the foot. The longitudinal arch runs from the calcaneus to the metatarsal heads. The metatarsal arch runs along the metatarsal heads.

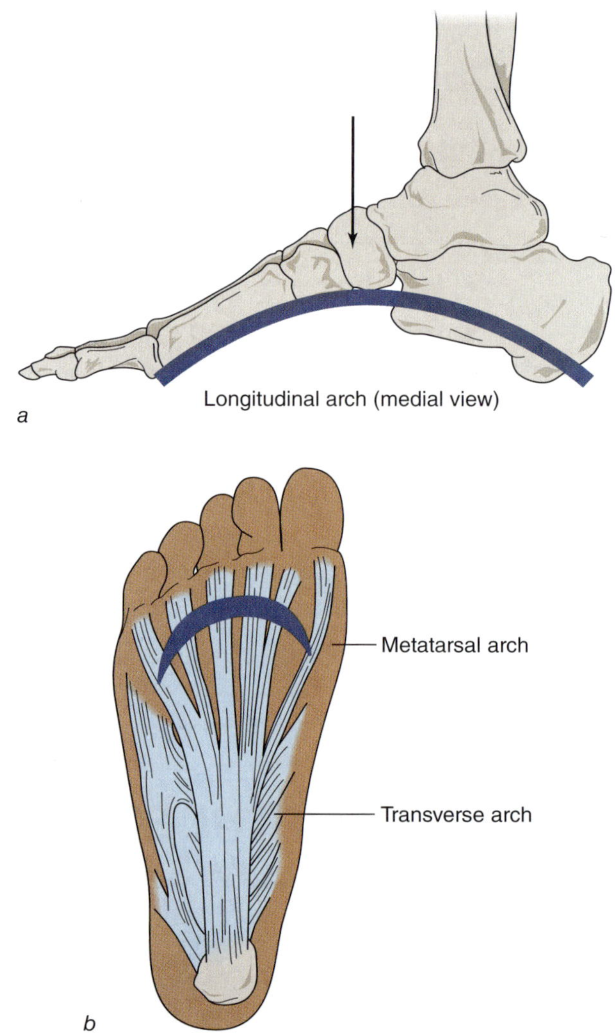

Figure 20.2 *(a)* Longitudinal and *(b)* metatarsal and transverse arches of the foot.

Muscles and Tendons

The muscles of the lower leg and ankle control movement of the foot and leg (see figure 20.3). The peroneal muscles, including the peroneus brevis and peroneus longus, attach to the lateral aspect of the lower leg and run a course to the lateral aspect and underside of the foot. This muscle group helps stabilize the lateral aspect of the ankle. The **gastrocnemius** is a powerful muscle in the calf that attaches by the **Achilles tendon** at the posterior aspect of the calcaneus bone. The gastrocnemius is not the only muscle that merges into the Achilles tendon; the **soleus** muscle also meshes into the Achilles. Together, the gastrocnemius and soleus act to flex the foot downward (plantar flexion) and allow athletes to propel themselves when running.

The Achilles tendon is extremely strong. It can withstand a tension force of several times the athlete's body weight while running.

The lower leg has four compartments that contain muscles, nerves, and vessels. The compartments are separated by fascia. The four compartments are the anterior, lateral, superficial posterior, and deep posterior.

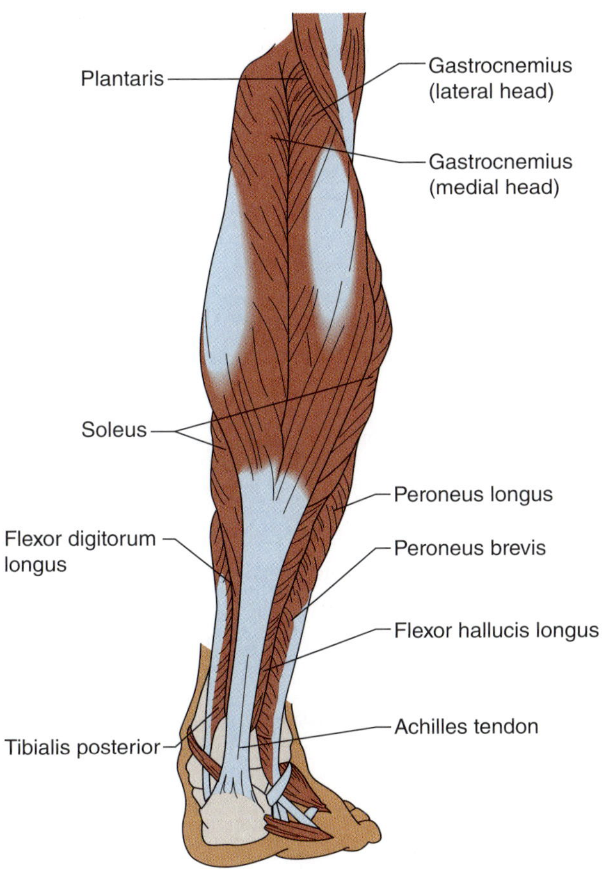

Figure 20.3 Major muscles of the lower leg.

Ligaments

Strong ligaments of the foot are located laterally, medially, and on the plantar surface. Many of the ligament names give the attachment points, making it easier to identify their locations. The lateral aspect of the ankle has numerous ligaments, including the anterior talofibular, posterior talofibular, and calcaneofibular ligaments (see figure 20.4*a*). The lateral ligaments hold the bony structures together on the lateral side but are not as strong as the medial ligament. The medial ligament is called the *deltoid* (see figure 20.4*b*). The deltoid covers the entire surface of the medial side of the ankle and maintains stability, especially during eversion. The deltoid ligament is stronger than all the lateral ligaments combined.

FYI

Sesamoids

Sesamoids are bones or cartilage located in a tendon, especially at a joint, that ease muscular movement over a bony surface.

Cartilage

Each bone in the foot and ankle has articular cartilage to create smooth movement between them. The articular surfaces in the ankle are subject to tremendous pressure because the joint is weight bearing.

Innervation

The anterior lower leg is innervated by the common peroneal. The posterior aspect of the lower leg and ankle is innervated by the tibial nerve. See figure 20.5 for the nerves of the lower leg.

Circulation

The ankle and lower leg are supplied by the anterior tibial artery. The posterior portion of the ankle and lower leg are supplied by the posterior tibial artery. In figure 20.6, a view of the circulation of the ankle and lower leg is available.

Bursa Sacs

There are three fluid-filled bursa sacs in the lower leg and ankle. The retrocalcaneal bursa is located

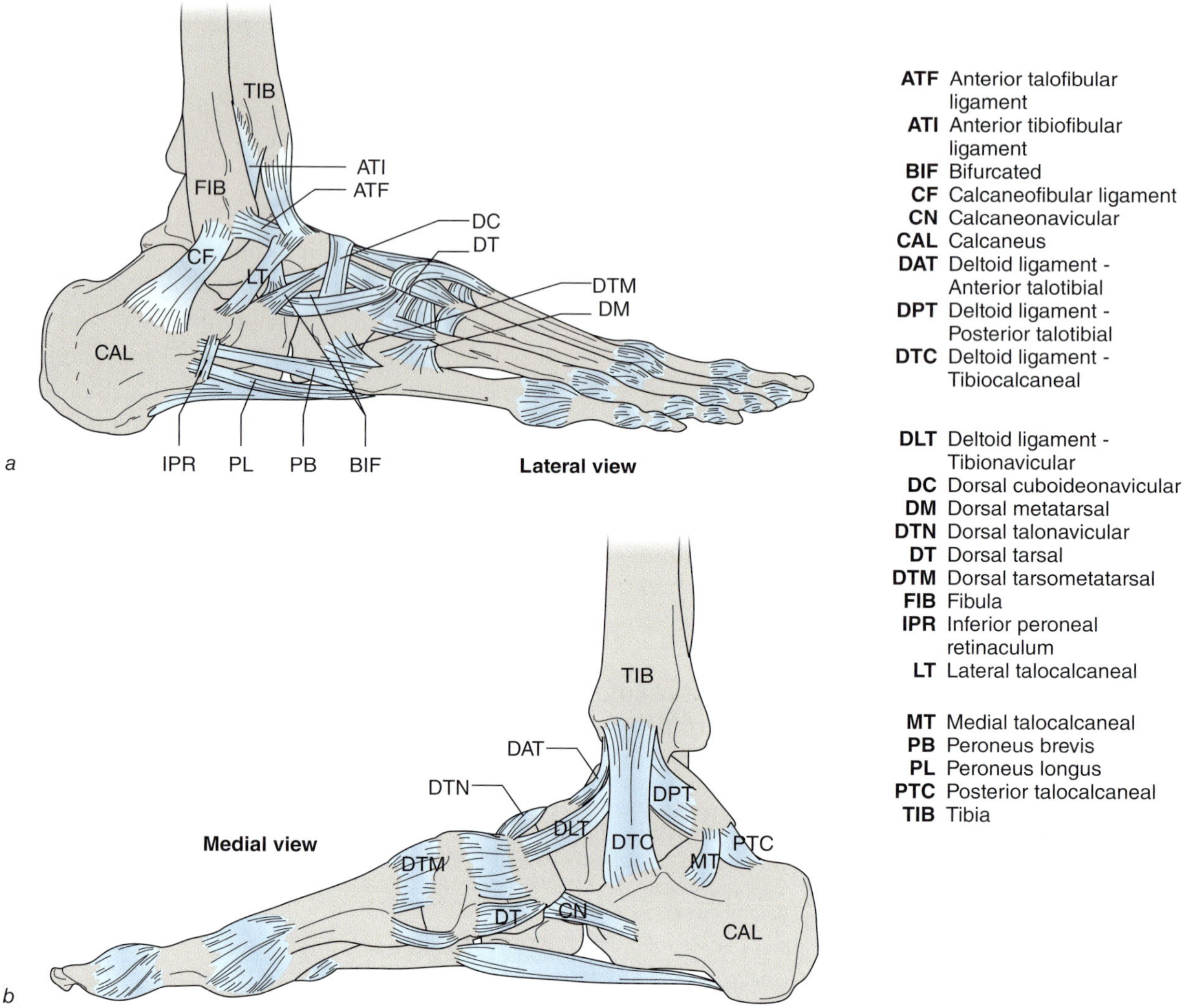

Figure 20.4 Ligaments of the foot: *(a)* lateral view and *(b)* medial view.

between the Achilles tendon and calcaneus. The bursa that lies between the skin and the Achilles tendon is the subcutaneous calcaneal (figure 20.7). The medial malleolar bursa lies between the skin and the medial malleolus.

Gait Cycle

When a person walks or runs, the lower leg and ankle go through a system of movements. The gait cycle has eight parts: heel strike, load phase, midstance, heel off, toe off, early swing, mid swing, and late swing. The heel strike occurs when the body weight is transferring to that leg. The load phase is a transfer of weight to that extremity. A complete transfer of weight will be on that leg at midstance. The heel off phase is when the heel begins to lift off the ground while the contralateral heel strikes the ground. When the toe pushes off the ground, this is the toe off phase. The early swing phase is when the hip and knee flex to allow clearance for the foot. When the flexed leg is vertically aligned with the contralateral leg, this is known as mid swing. The swing as the leg is coming through and just before heel strike is known as late swing. Figure 20.8 shows the eight phases of the gait cycle.

The gait cycle can be disrupted through orthopedic problems, neurological conditions, and medical disorders.

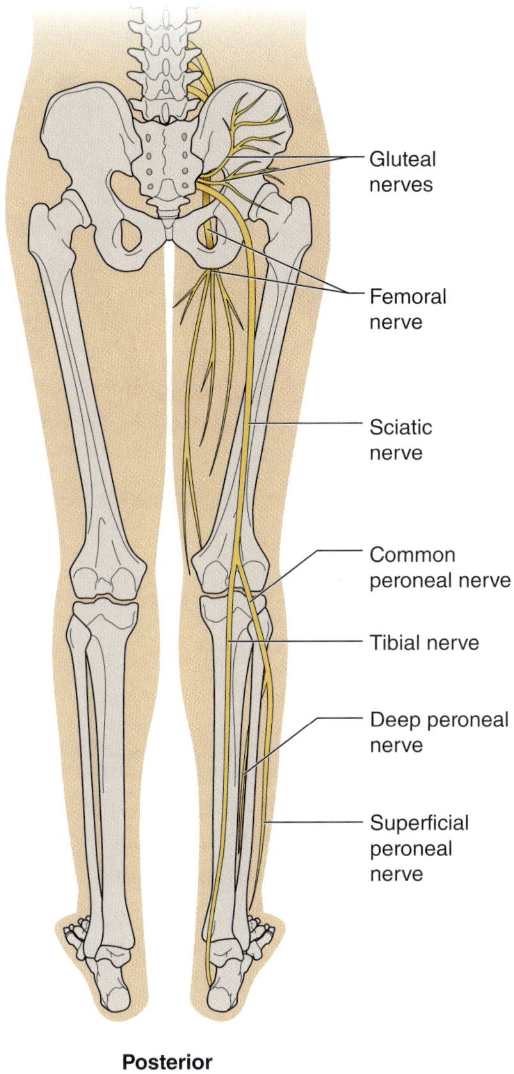

Figure 20.5 Nerves of the lower leg and foot.

Reprinted by permission from R.S. Behnke and J. Plant, *Kinetic Anatomy*, 4th ed. (Champaign, IL: Human Kinetics, 2022), 255.

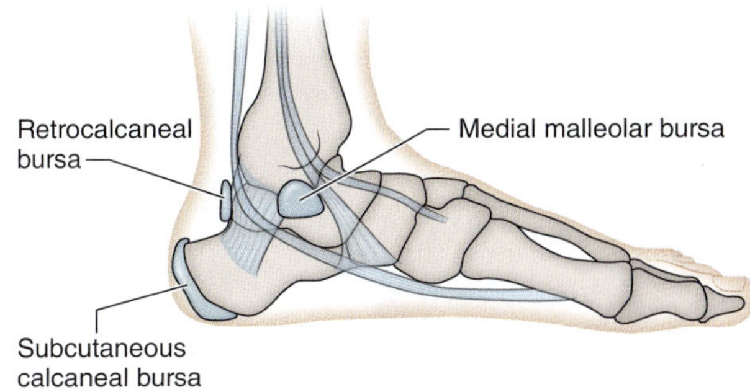

Figure 20.7 Bursa sacs of the foot.

Adapted from Aid My Bursa.com. Available: https://aidmybursa.com/bursitis-foot/foot-ankle-bursitis-overview.php.

PREVENTING FOOT, ANKLE, AND LOWER-LEG INJURIES

Taking care of the foot, ankle, and lower leg is essential to injury prevention and continuous athletic participation. Many athletes take protective measures such as wearing shoes that provide ankle and arch support, using supportive ankle taping (to prevent ankle inversion), and wearing shin guards (to prevent contusions of the lower leg). Strengthening and conditioning programs can also help to prevent injuries. If the team physician finds a weakness in the athlete's foot, ankle, or lower leg, the athlete should be placed on a rehabilitation program that emphasizes strengthening. In some instances, muscles that are very tight will need to be stretched.

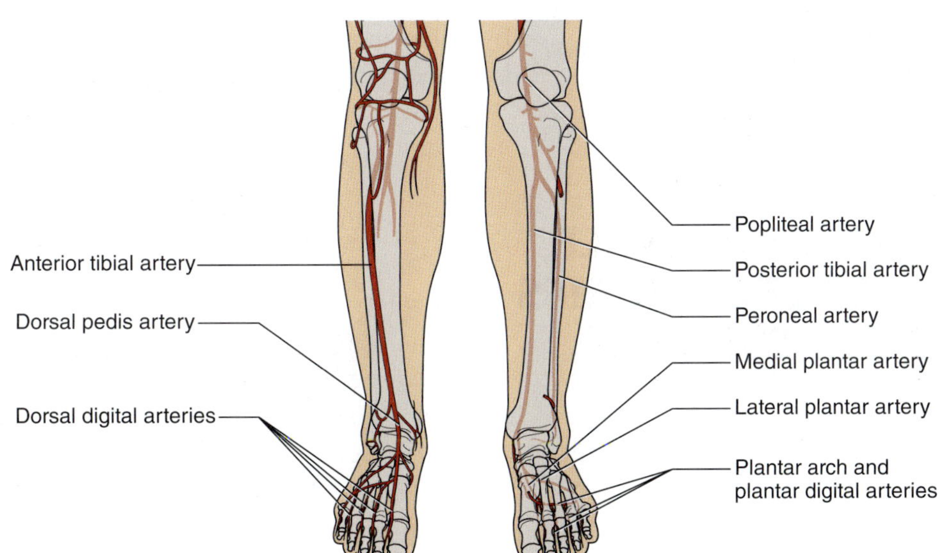

Figure 20.6 Arterial circulation of the lower leg and foot.

Reprinted by permission from S. Shultz, P. Houglum, and D. Perrin, *Examination of Musculoskeletal Injuries*, 4th ed. (Champaign, IL: Human Kinetics, 2016), 144.

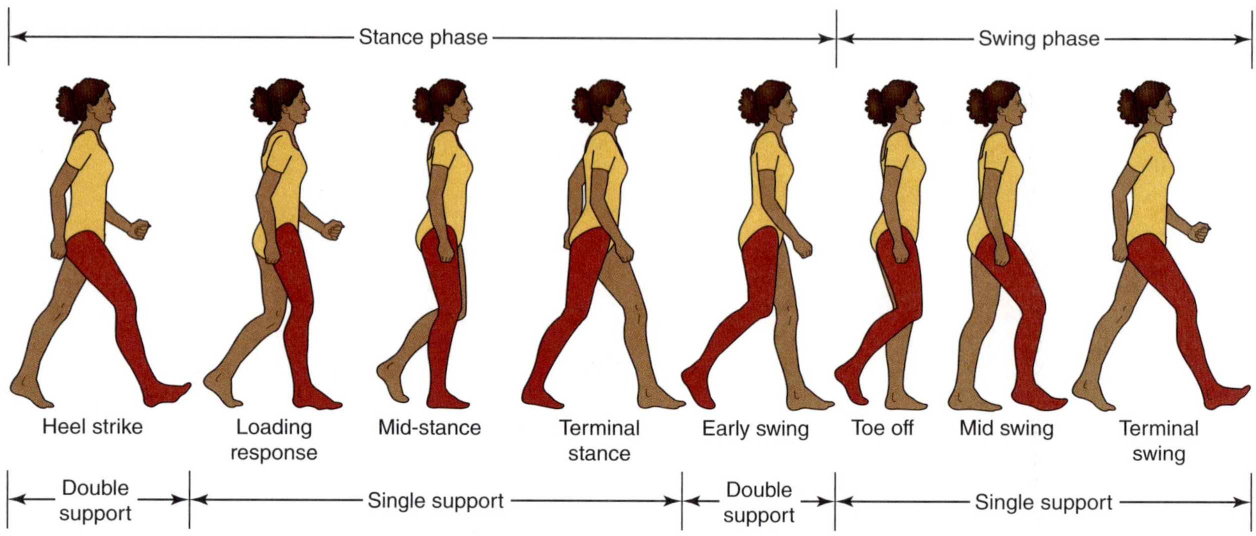

Figure 20.8 Eight phases of the gait cycle.

Reprinted by permission from W. Pirker and R. Katzenschlager, "Gait Disorders in Adults and the Elderly: A Clinical Guide," *Wiener Klinische Wochenschrift* 129 (2016). Distributed under the terms of the Creative Commons Attribution 4.0 International License (http://creativecommons.org/licenses/by/4.0/).

Conditioning under the guidance of a coach may prevent stress fractures. Proper footwear that can absorb shock has also been shown to reduce metatarsal stress fractures.

Balance training can reduce the onset of ankle sprains. As such, balance exercises should be incorporated into strength and conditioning programs for athletes.

> **What Would You Do If . . .**
>
> The AT has been caring for an athlete who has lower-leg pain. In gym class, you note that this athlete plays without shoes. He constantly limps during class and at practices.

TREATING FOOT, ANKLE, AND LOWER-LEG INJURIES AND CONDITIONS

The feet and legs form the foundation on which an athlete walks and runs. Injuries to ligaments, muscles, tendons, and bones in this area can be disabling.

Bone Injuries

Direct impacts to an area and repetitive use can cause fractures. Common symptoms include pain, pressure, and an inability to move the body part. The AT will discover crepitus, swelling, and possible bone displacement. After splinting, the athlete must be referred to a physician for X-rays and a cast. The base of the fifth metatarsal and the epiphyses of the distal tibia and fibula are common fracture sites. Stress fractures, which are caused by repetitive use, are often seen in several areas around the foot, ankle, and lower leg.

Jones Fracture

The most common avulsion fracture is of the fifth metatarsal—a **Jones fracture** (see figure 20.9). When an ankle is forced into inversion, the muscles contract so forcefully to stabilize the lateral aspect of the ankle that the peroneus brevis tendon pulls a part of the bone away at its attachment. The AT will

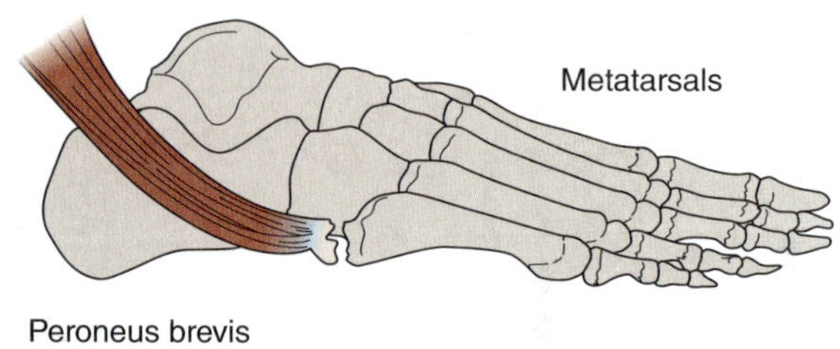

Figure 20.9 Jones fracture.

treat the injury using PRICES and refer the athlete to a physician. Many physicians will cast the ankle to allow the bone to heal.

Epiphyseal Injury of Distal Tibia and Fibula

The distal tibia and fibula epiphyses, or growth plates, can become injured when the ankle is forced into plantar flexion and inversion. The athlete will experience pain and swelling over the epiphysis and have difficulty walking or running because of the pain. The AT will splint the injury and refer the athlete to a physician for X-rays. This is a potentially serious injury because it is possible for the epiphysis to close prematurely, stunting bone growth at the site.

> **FYI**
>
> **Bone Scan**
>
> A bone scan is a diagnostic test performed with a radioactive substance that allows physicians to see small disruptions in the bone.

Stress Fracture

Stress fractures of the lower leg and foot most commonly occur to the tibia, fibula, and metatarsals, and repetitive stress due to running is usually the cause. The athlete will present with pain that becomes more intense at night and after activity. Pain and swelling will be located over the bone. Some physicians believe that a stress fracture can be distinguished by using a tuning fork—the vibrations from the tuning fork vibrate the bone but do not irritate muscles. The edge of one tine of the fork is struck against the assessor's knee, and the base of the tuning fork is placed on the injured site. If the athlete indicates pain, he most likely has a fracture. A bone scan can verify the diagnosis of a stress fracture. An X-ray will not show a stress fracture until two weeks after the initial injury, when a callus begins to form at the site. Stress fractures require four to six weeks of rest, and the athlete must see a physician. Although stress fractures are rarely casted, the athlete will be given crutches to eliminate pressure on the limb. If the injury is not detected early or the athlete fails to report it, a complete fracture may result, which could create serious complications.

Muscle and Tendon Injuries

Strains occur from overstretching or putting a muscle or tendon under excessive tension. **Tendinitis**, which is the inflammation of a tendon, typically results from a repetitive stress such as running or jumping. Common tendon injuries and strains in this region involve the tendons of the medial aspect of the tibia as well as the Achilles tendon.

Medial Tibial Stress Syndrome

Shin splints is a common term for pain in the lower leg. Some people use it to refer to muscle strains, stress fractures, and even tendinitis. However, to doctors, shin splints are known as *medial tibial stress syndrome*. The muscle fibers on the medial side of the tibia become torn and irritated. The athlete will complain of pain and the inability to run or walk properly. The pain will be located over the distal medial side of the tibia, although there may be swelling on the lateral side as well. The athlete will generally have tight calf muscles, wear older shoes, and be out of shape for the running they are currently doing. There are several successful methods of relieving shin splints, but PRICES is foremost. If the athlete limps, they must take a break from running and rest or at least change their training to something else, such as biking. When the athlete has permission to return to participation, the AT may wrap the medial side of the leg, pulling the soft tissue toward the bone, and recommend new shoes, stretching, and arch supports.

Achilles Tendinitis

The Achilles tendon is the strong tendon joining the gastrocnemius muscle to the heel. Any sport involving repeated running, jumping, and landing may cause cells in the tendon to break down prematurely, and this irritation or inflammation is referred to as *tendinitis*. During an evaluation, the AT will note swelling, tenderness, crepitus, and an expression of pain on the athlete's face when they palpate the Achilles tendon, especially with dorsiflexion. The athlete will also be weak when plantar flexion is resisted. The athlete must rest the tendon and apply ice and may need a referral to a physician for

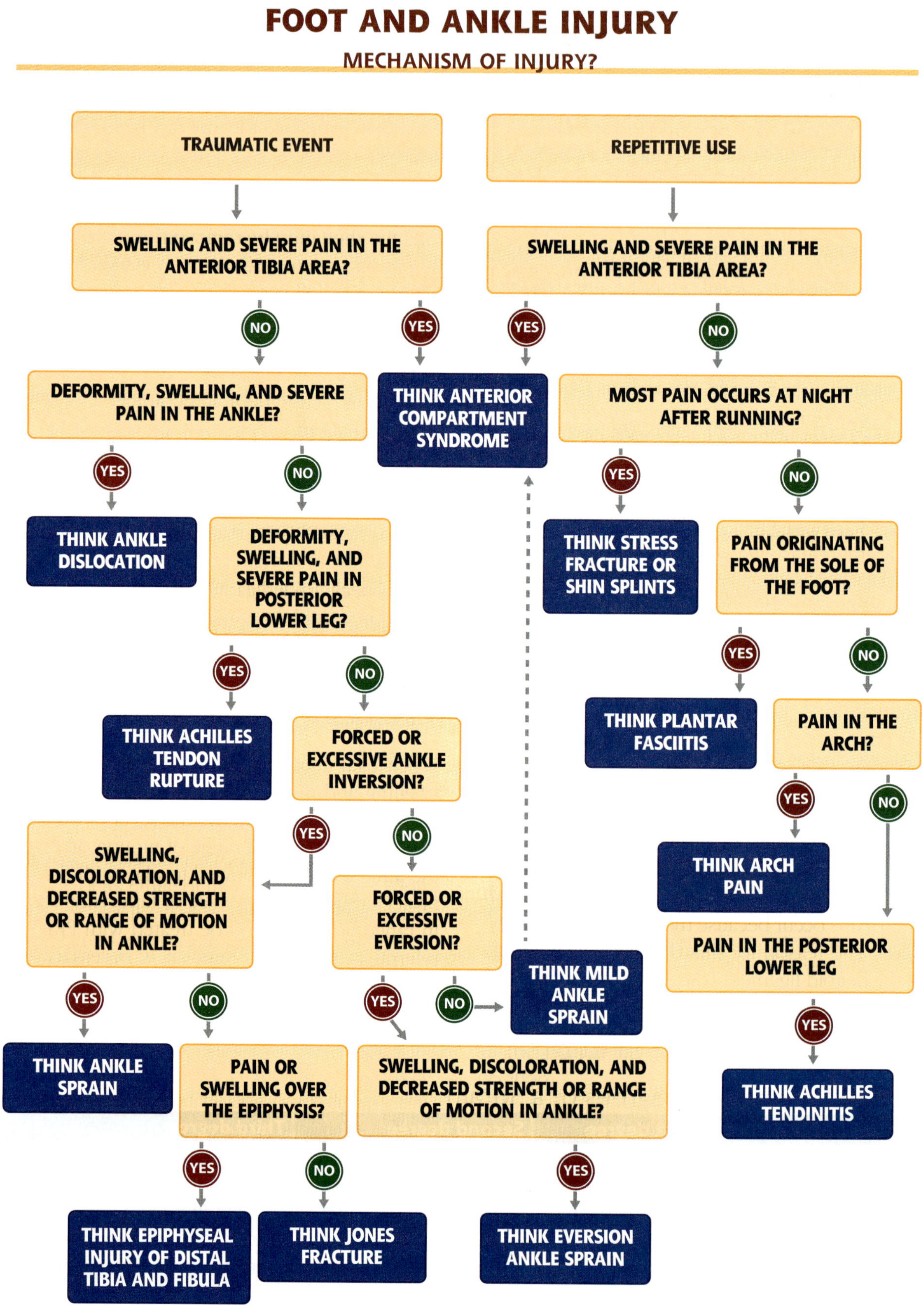

Figure 20.10 Assessment of a foot and ankle injury.

RED FLAGS

The following signs and symptoms of foot, ankle, and lower-leg injuries require immediate referral to a physician:

- Loss of pulse in the foot
- Loss of sensation in the foot
- Third-degree ankle sprain
- Complete Achilles tendon rupture
- Ankle dislocation
- All fractures
- Anterior compartment syndrome

Another type of ankle sprain is a syndesmosis sprain. This injury is also called a *high ankle sprain*. The **syndesmosis** binds the distal ends of the tibia and fibula together, and when the ankle is either severely everted, or rotated, the talus can force the tibia and fibula to spread apart and sprain the ankle. Syndesmotic ankle sprains often take longer to heal.

Ankle Dislocation

An ankle dislocation can occur either anteriorly or posteriorly. An anterior dislocation occurs when the heel of the foot strikes the ground forcefully. A posterior dislocation occurs with a blow to the anterior aspect of the leg while the ankle is in plantar flexion. The athlete will be in obvious pain and will refuse to move or allow the foot to be touched. There will be deformity and an inability to use the foot. Swelling will rapidly appear. It is important to act quickly in the case of an ankle dislocation. The AT should call 911, splint the lower leg and ankle, apply ice, and remove the athlete from the field. In addition to damaging the ligaments, nerves and blood vessels can be injured; this means a physician must put the bones back in place.

What Would You Do If . . .

A hockey player with an ankle sprain tells you that she does not need the help of an AT. She intends to use kerosene applications twice a day.

Tissue Injuries

The weight-bearing lower extremities are prone to various tissue injuries. These include contusions, toe injuries, and anterior compartment syndrome.

Contusions

Soccer and field hockey players are prone to contusions of the lower leg—thus the invention of the shin guard. The impact of a ball, stick, or foot on the shin will cause swelling, pain, and discoloration. The athlete may limp and have limited range of motion. The AT will recommend ice and rest until full range of motion is restored. The athlete will need additional padding, such as a donut, to protect the area from further impacts.

Toe Abnormalities

Toe deformities, such as **hammertoes** (see figure 20.11), can create difficulties for athletes. A hammertoe means that the middle joint of the toe is flexed and the metatarsal phalangeal and distal phalangeal joints are hyperextended. This deformity can become a problem, especially if a callus forms at the top of the flexed joint. **Hallux valgus**, also known as a **bunion**, is caused by excessive valgus stress (pressure toward the midline of the body) at the great toe (see figure 20.12). This deformity is often caused by poorly fitting footwear, usually shoes that are too tight. A common toe injury is an **ingrown toenail** (see figure 20.13), whereby the nail grows into the surrounding soft tissue. Ingrown toenails are often the result of poor trimming of

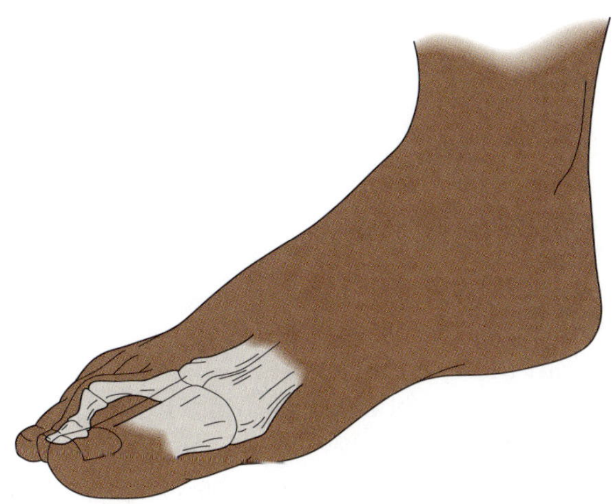

Figure 20.11 Hammertoe.

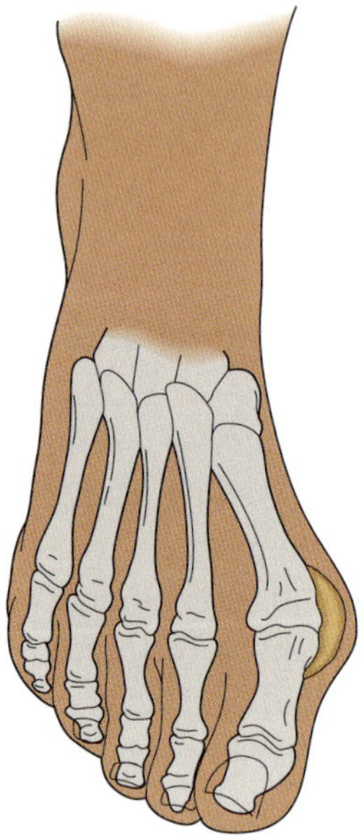

Figure 20.12 Bunion.

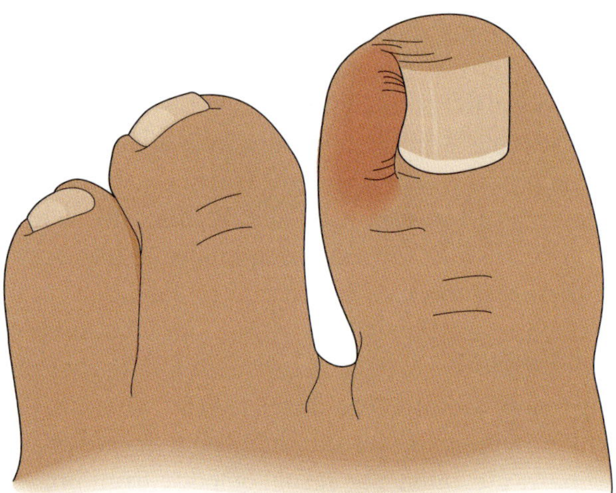

Figure 20.13 Ingrown toenail.

the nail, such as trimming in a rounded fashion rather than straight across or trimming the nail too short. In severe instances, a physician may need to extract a portion of the nail to reduce pain and inflammation.

Heel Bruises

Beneath the calcaneus exists a thick fat pad that helps to absorb shock as we walk. If there is too much impact on the heel, a contusion can result. This heel bruise is debilitating because we strike with our heels first as we walk, and the fat pad is tender when it is bruised. The area must be treated with ice and padded to help absorb shock to give it time to heal.

Anterior Compartment Syndrome

Anterior compartment syndrome is sometimes mistaken for shin splints, but as the name implies, it is an anterior compartment injury. The muscles to the anterior aspect of the tibia are enclosed in connective tissue. When the tissue in the compartment swells due to overuse or a severe impact, the swelling increases the pressure on the connective tissue, which causes severe pain that increases with activity and does not subside without activity. The AT will note heat, red skin, loss of foot motion, and hardness of the area. An inability to move the foot and severe pain are indicators of this problem. The athlete must be seen by a physician immediately to prevent nerve damage from the pressure. The physician will make an incision in the leg to relieve the pressure, and the athlete can return to activity while wearing a supportive brace or bandage.

Chronic Exertional Compartment Syndrome

Athletes who compete in repetitive exercise such as running are more likely to experience chronic exertional compartment syndrome. Those that experience chronic exertional compartment syndrome exhibit swelling and pain in a compartment of the lower leg. Athletes report their pain and swelling comes at about the same time during exercise. The syndrome is relieved with rest. PRICES is the best course of treatment. Decompression of the compartment may be necessary if PRICES is ineffective.

Neurological Conditions

Compression and repetitive use can cause neurological conditions. The AT is likely to find common symptoms that include pain, tingling, and numbness distal to the neurological injury. In the foot, two of the more common conditions neurologically are tarsal tunnel syndrome and Morton's neuroma.

Tarsal Tunnel Syndrome

The tarsal tunnel is the area posterior medial to the medial malleolus. This tunnel provides a path for the tendons; nerve and blood supply traverse distally to the foot. The flexor retinaculum, a tissue, acts as a protective covering holding the tendons, nerves, and arterial blood supply in the tunnel. An injury to the retinaculum, such as an eversion ankle sprain, can cause swelling or scar tissue. Any compromise of the tunnel can compress the tendons, nerve, or blood supply. The result the compression is referred to as **tarsal tunnel syndrome**.

Signs and symptoms include numbness in the longitudinal arch, shooting pain, and tingling. PRICES is the best initial treatment.

Morton's Neuroma

When the nerves that run under the transverse arch of the foot become impinged, it can lead to an irritation. The typical mechanism of injury is repetitive irritation of the nerve. The athlete will experience numbness in the toes and pain usually between the third and fourth metatarsal heads. PRICES is the best initial treatment.

Reflex Sympathetic Dystrophy Syndrome

The onset of reflex sympathetic dystrophy syndrome (RSDS) usually occurs after an injury, but the pain is regional and severe and does not match the level of the injury. University of Rochester Medical Center (2024) indicates that 1 to 2 percent of bone fractures and 2 to 5 percent of nerve injuries result in RSDS. This syndrome is also known as *complex regional pain syndrome (CRPS)*. Signs include skin color changes, swelling on the unaffected side, edema, changes in the bone, decreased strength, hair and nail changes at the site, motor dysfunction, skin temperature being hot or cold, decreased range of motion, and muscle tremors (University of Rochester Medical Center 2024; Stanford Medicine 2024). Symptoms may include hyperalgesia, a burning sensation, and severe pain (University of Rochester Medical Center 2024; Stanford Medicine 2024). Treatment for RSDS is a referral to a physician for possible intervention with medication. The belief is that the autonomic nervous system has a dysfunction.

Shoe Fitting

Shoes are critical pieces of equipment for any athlete. Selecting the right shoe will depend on the sport, the surface, and the athlete's individual need. To determine shoe size, use a Brannock device (see figure 20.14). This is the typical device found in a shoe store, which will measure the length and width of the foot. The athlete should get both feet measured at the end of the day, when the feet are at their fullest. Both feet should be measured with the type of sock they will wear during competition. Measure both feet, as some athletes have one foot larger than the other.

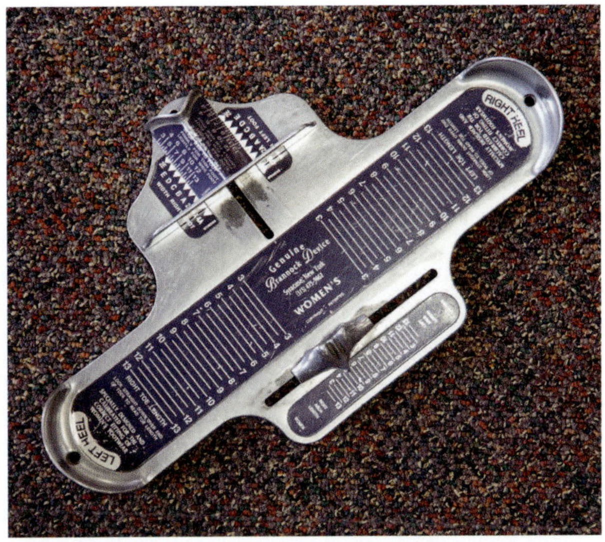

Figure 20.14 Brannock device for measuring foot size.

Once the foot size is determined, the athlete should try on a pair of shoes. The athlete should make sure that their toes have space in the toe box. Find the longest toe and make sure there is a space the width of 1 inch (25 mm) to the end of the shoe. The width of the shoe should not squeeze the toes and metatarsals. Figure 20.15 shows the anatomy of a shoe. The athlete should walk around in the shoes and test them for comfort and support. If the foot moves in the shoe, it is too large, and if the shoe is too tight, it is too small. The shoe may have to be modified if the athlete has foot issues, such as a bunion.

Orthotics

Orthotics are a custom-made medical device that fits inside shoes that corrects foot mechanics. Poor foot mechanics result in several injuries. Plantar fasciitis, ankle sprains, and heel spurs are a few foot injuries that can be treated by orthotics. Plastics, cork, or carbon fiber are the materials used to fashion orthotics. See figure 20.16 for a view of various orthotics types.

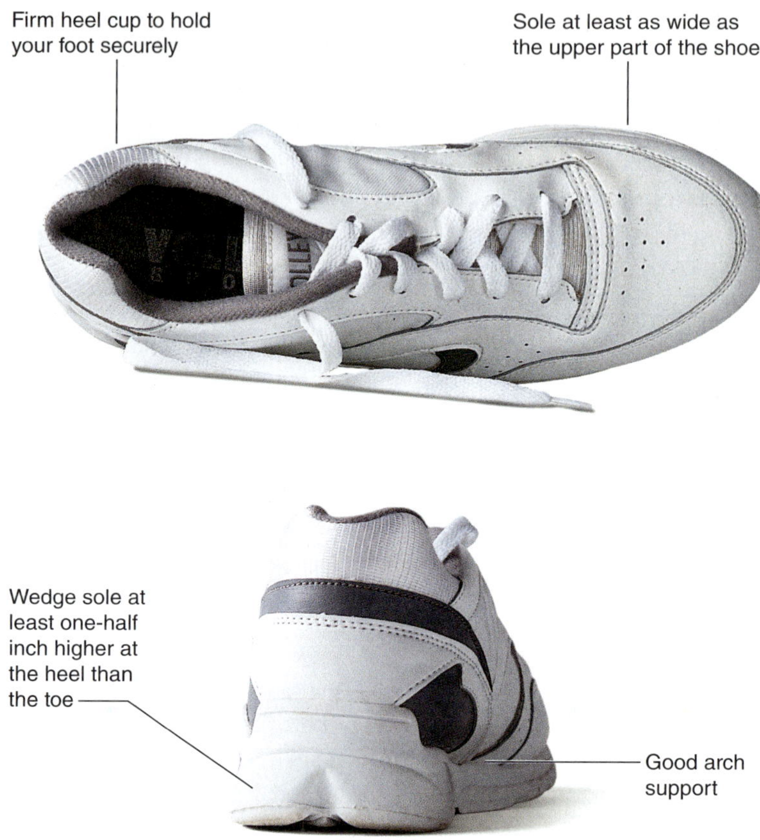

Figure 20.15 Anatomy of a shoe.

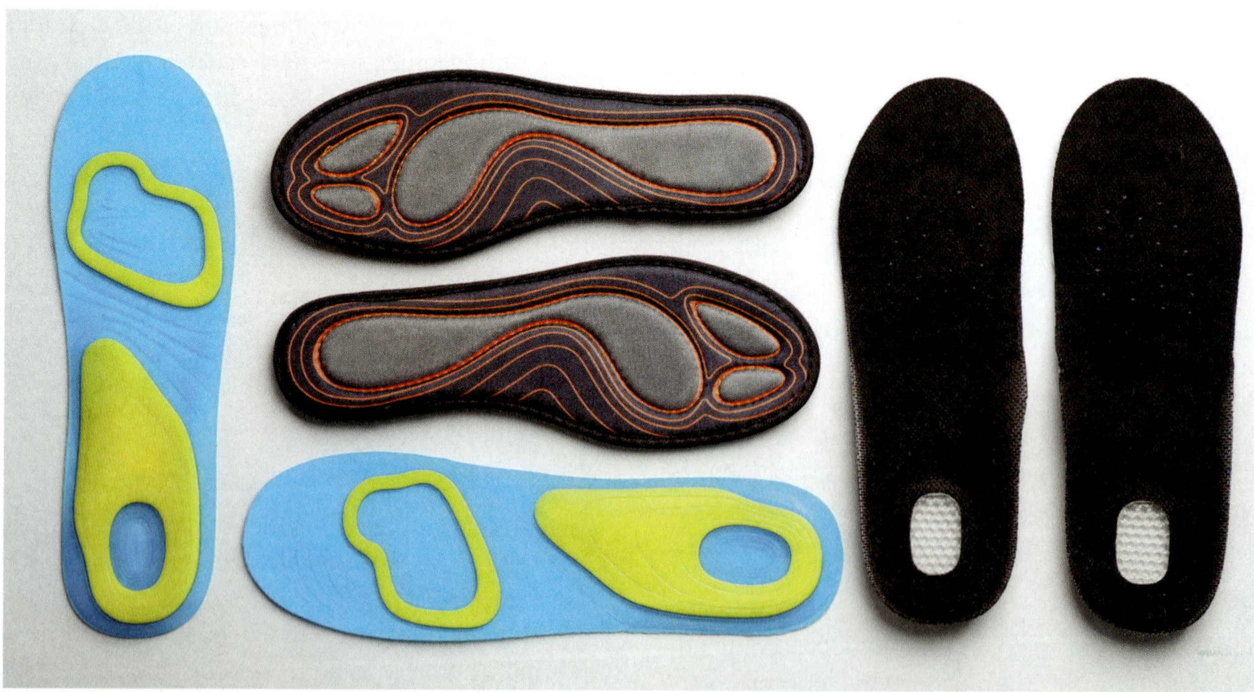

Figure 20.16 Various orthotics.
Liudmila Chernetska/iStock/Getty Images

Summary

In addition to fractures, sprains, and strains, injuries caused by stress and overuse are common in the lower leg, foot, and ankle. The bones, ligaments, and tendons must be aligned to prevent injury and to allow the joints to function. PRICES is used to care for injuries of the lower extremity. Proper footwear and good hygiene are necessary for preventing toe abnormalities.

Key Terms

Define the following terms found in this chapter:

- Achilles tendon
- bunion
- calcaneus
- gastrocnemius
- hallux valgus
- hammertoe
- heel spur
- ingrown toenail
- Jones fracture
- lateral malleolus
- medial malleolus
- metatarsals
- phalanges
- plantar fasciitis
- plantar surface
- shin splints
- soleus
- syndesmosis
- talus
- tarsal tunnel syndrome
- tendinitis

An athlete reports that they sprained their ankle about three days ago. Upon initial assessment the athlete reports that the original injury on the lateral side of the ankle is feeling better, but there is pain on the upper part of the lower leg about halfway up. What injury do you suspect? How does this injury differ from a lateral ankle sprain? What are your options for care?

To access supplementary material for this chapter, including the Understanding Check worksheet, vocabulary quizzes, extension activities, and chapter-specific resources and forms, visit the web resource: http://ancillaries.humankinetics.com/FundamentalsOfAthleticTrainingAndSportsMedicine5E

Plan of Action

Initial treatment: ICE, COMPRESSION, ELEVATION 20 MINUTES. ATHLETE INSTRUCTED TO REST THE AREA AND MAINTAIN COMPRESSION; ALSO FITTED FOR CRUTCHES AND INSTRUCTED IN THE USE OF CRUTCH WALKING.

The athlete will be: ☐ Referred to a physician ________

☐ Referred to school nurse ________ ☑ Treated by certified AT

Treatment will be: 4 days per week for 3 weeks

Treatment to consist of: ICE APPLICATION, STRENGTHENING EXERCISES, AND FUNCTIONAL ACTIVITY AS TOLERATED. THE AREA IS TO BE ICED POSTEXERCISE.

Short-term goals to be completed in 1 week(s): (1) ELIMINATE SWELLING, (2) ATTAIN NORMAL DORSIFLEXION AND INVERSION ROM, (3) BE ABLE TO WALK IN LAZY S AND Z PATTERN, (4) IMPROVE BALANCE TO 30 SECONDS, (5) REDUCE PAIN TO 2 RATING.

Intermediate goals to be completed in 1 week(s): WALK WITHOUT AID OF CRUTCHES.

Long-term goals to be completed in 2 week(s): (1) OBTAIN NORMAL STRENGTH FOR ALL MOVEMENTS; (2) JOG STRAIGHT, LAZY S, AND Z PATTERNS; (3) ELIMINATE PAIN; (4) IMPROVE BALANCE TO NORMAL.

Long-term goals to be completed in 3 week(s): (1) RUN LAZY S AND Z PATTERN, (2) SPRINT LAZY S AND Z PATTERN, (3) RETURN TO PRACTICE.

Parents contacted: ☒ YES

☐ NO Date: 6-1-25

Explain: ________

Signature: ________

Figure 21.1 Sample SOAP note. *(continued)*

1. Mobility
2. Flexibility
3. Proprioception
4. Muscular strength
5. Muscular endurance
6. Muscular power
7. Cardiorespiratory endurance
8. Sport-specific function

These elements allow athletes to be functional in their chosen sport.

Think of phases of treatment as the IMPRESS program (see figure 21.2): **i**nitial inflammatory phase, **m**obility restoration phase, **p**roprioception phase, **r**esistance training phase, **e**ndurance training

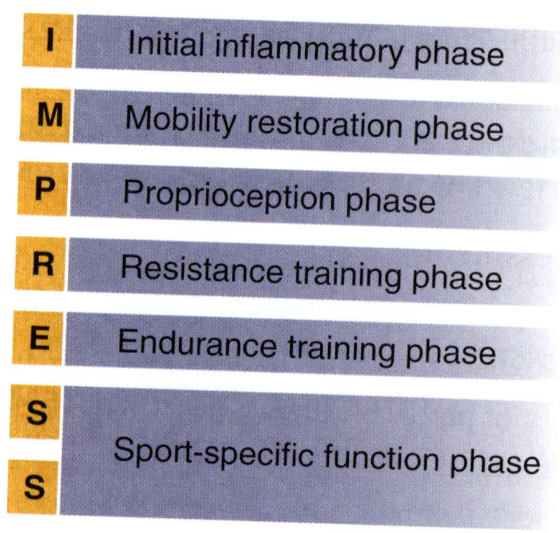

Figure 21.2 IMPRESS phases of treatment for organizing a rehabilitation program.

phase, and **s**port-**s**pecific function phase. Athletes should always try to maintain their cardiorespiratory endurance as much as possible during the program.

Although we have presented these phases of therapeutic exercises as a step-by-step process, in practice, the progression is not quite so clear. Each athlete is different and progresses at a different pace. For example, some people may be able to begin light strengthening exercises before establishing full flexibility. The sports medicine team will work with injured athletes to integrate them into practices before the establishment of full strength. Perhaps the most important thing to remember as a future AT is to be as progressive as you can when rehabilitating an athlete but never do anything that would cause harm.

Initial Inflammatory Phase

In the initial treatment phase, the AT's primary goal is to control the amount of inflammation. Inflammation results from the body's response to an injury and is characterized by warmth, redness, swelling, and pain. It is the mechanism by which damaged tissue begins to return to normal. Although inflammation is necessary for tissue healing to occur, if it gets out of hand, chronic inflammation can result.

Pain can significantly interfere with a person's ability to function. It results from an initial injury or trauma, particularly when nerve tissue is damaged. Even if nerve tissue is not directly damaged, pain can indicate that tissue damage has occurred. During the inflammatory process, the body releases chemicals that irritate nerve tissue; the swelling that results from the inflammatory process can put pressure on nerves, resulting in pain. Also, because the perception of pain warns the body of tissue damage, the body guards against further injury by causing muscle spasm. Muscle spasm itself can cause pain, and thus a pain-spasm-pain cycle occurs.

To control inflammation in the initial phase, prevent further damage and reduce swelling, pain, and edema. As we discuss in chapter 25, the critical treatment in this phase is PRICES, which stands for **p**rotected, **r**ested, **i**ced, **c**ompressed, **e**levated, and **s**upported.

Mobility Restoration Phase

Once inflammation is controlled—as characterized by improved comfort and decreased swelling, **edema** (a thick swelling caused by excessive serous protein), and pain—joint mobility can be restored. This is done with therapeutic exercises that progress from passive range of motion to active–assistive range of motion to active range of motion. Once range of motion is back to normal, flexibility training can begin.

Restoring Range of Motion

There are three phases in restoring normal range of motion:

1. ***Passive.*** When the AT moves an athlete's body segment through the range of motion and the athlete simply relaxes and produces no muscle contractions, **passive range of motion (PROM)** is being performed. Early pain-free PROM performed for an injury has been shown to be beneficial for tissue healing. However, PROM should not be done if it causes pain. In fact, most exercises should be done using pain as a guide—if the athlete complains of pain, the exercise should be stopped. PROM is most often used to keep the soft-tissue structures from becoming too tight following an injury.

2. ***Active–assistive.*** When the AT and the athlete move a body segment through the range of motion together, it is termed **active–assistive range of motion (AAROM)**. This is done when an injured athlete is strong enough (and pain is no longer a problem) to produce a muscle contraction but not strong enough to move the joint through a full range of motion. AAROM should also use pain as a guide.

3. ***Active.*** When an athlete can move a body segment through a full range of motion without assistance, they are performing **active range of motion (AROM)**. AROM is necessary before strengthening of the joint can begin. Once AROM is established, flexibility training can begin.

Establishing Flexibility

For an injured athlete, restoring mobility means getting flexibility back to normal. Note that range of motion and flexibility are not the same. **Flexibility** refers to the ability to move a joint through a full range of motion without restriction. Normal flexibility is needed for the body to function properly. To have normal range of motion, an athlete must have flexibility of the soft-tissue structures around a

The Real World

When I worked at a physical therapy clinic, I helped rehabilitate a patient who had just had minor knee surgery. His physician gave us orders to accelerate him through the program because the patient was getting married in three weeks and planned to snow ski in Lake Tahoe, Nevada. The athlete worked hard and was compliant. By the second week, he had gained full range of motion and normal strength in his knee. His balance and proprioception continued to improve, and by the time he was ready to leave for his wedding, his knee was fully functional. It just goes to show you that when an athlete is motivated, they can accomplish anything.

Anonymous

What Would You Do If . . .

You are assisting the AT in the athletic training room, and an athlete who has been doing extensive rehabilitation of her knee approaches you. She is disappointed that she is not allowed to return to practice even though she has normal range of motion and normal strength.

joint, including muscles, tendons, and skin. Stretching exercises often develop flexibility. These are covered in detail in chapter 22.

Proprioception Phase

Proprioception is the body's ability to get information to the brain in response to a stimulus arising in the body; it also refers to the body's ability to sense the position of its limbs at any moment. For example, an athlete who has gone airborne and then lands on an opponent's foot may injure their ankle if their brain does not sense that they are landing on someone's shoe and not the floor. Without proper proprioception, the body may not get the right muscles to fire at the right time to protect a joint. Because an athlete may have deficient proprioception due to an injury, many ATs believe that proprioception should be addressed in the early stages of a therapeutic exercise program, so many rehabilitation programs emphasize early proprioceptive training.

Proprioceptive training can be started early in a therapeutic exercise program by doing activities such as balance or coordination exercises.

Resistance Training Phase

Many programs can be used to improve an athlete's strength, or ability to exert force against a resistance, following an injury. **Resistance training** will strengthen not only the muscles but also surrounding tissues such as the ligaments and bone. Resistance training is a significant phase in the rehabilitation process. It can be done using free weights, resistive tubing, machines, and manual resistance. Resistance training is covered in chapter 22.

Endurance Phase

In addition to establishing or maintaining cardiorespiratory endurance, muscular endurance must be addressed. Muscles need not only to be strong for athletic participation but also to have **endurance**, or the ability to perform movements over time. Cardiorespiratory exercises should be performed as early as possible as long as the injury is not aggravated. Developing muscle endurance with weight training often involves performing a high number of repetitions with a low amount of weight.

Sport-Specific Function Phase

A therapeutic exercise program is not complete unless the athlete is fully prepared to meet the demands of sport. In this phase of the therapeutic exercise program, the athlete performs functional activities and is slowly integrated back into practices. Thus, it is necessary for the AT to be fully aware of the requirements of the sport, the movement patterns involved, and the degree of strength, speed, power, and endurance needed for the athlete to be successful.

The **sport-specific function** phase is marked by activities that mimic those the athlete will perform on the playing field or court. Athletes are required to run, jump, cut, and throw. They should generally progress from light functional exercises to heavy functional exercises and then to limited practice. Practices are often restricted, and the athlete can participate only if they have full range of motion, normal strength, normal flexibility, normal coordination, normal cardiorespiratory endurance, and the consent of the team physician.

RED FLAGS

Do not use therapeutic modalities in the following cases:

- There is no ground fault interrupter.
- The operator is untrained in that modality.
- The athlete has a contraindication for that modality.

THERAPEUTIC MODALITIES

Although the essential element of any rehabilitation program is exercise, many athletes cannot perform even minimally because their injuries become too painful or swollen. If the injured part is not used, however, the muscles may weaken and further complications may arise. To decrease pain and help with normal recovery, the AT will use therapeutic modalities.

Therapeutic modalities include heat, cold, ultrasound, and electrical muscle stimulation. They can be categorized as thermal, mechanical, or electrical. All therapeutic modalities must be used with extreme caution and, in some cases, only when prescribed by a physician.

Therapeutic modalities that require an electrical charge must be inspected annually to make sure they are operating properly. This entails having a bioelectrical technician inspect the modalities to make sure they meet safety standards.

Thermal Elements

Thermal elements transfer heat either into or out of body tissue. They are used to make the tissue either colder or warmer. The indications and contraindications for thermal modalities can be found in table 21.1.

Table 21.1 Indications and Contraindications for Thermal Modalities

Type of modality	Indications	Contraindications	Precautions*
Heat	Chronic inflammatory conditions Joint contracture Tightened tissue Chronic pain Chronic muscle spasm	Acute injuries Areas with sensory deficits Areas with circulation deficits Areas over tumors Peripheral vascular disease Open wounds	Heart disease
Cold	Acute injuries Pain Swelling Preparation for exercise Muscle spasms Inflammation	Cold-related allergies Open wounds Cardiovascular problems (heart disease) Areas with sensory deficits Cold hypersensitivity High blood pressure Respiratory problems Advanced diabetes or peripheral vascular disease Infection	Areas with superficial nerves Areas with circulation deficits

*Precautions means you can use the modality with extreme caution if the listed conditions exist.

Note: Disagreement exists among experts as to whether modalities are contraindicated or can be used with caution.

Data obtained from Kahanov and Payne (2022); Denegar, Saliba, and Saliba (2016).

FYI

Indications

Indications are the reasons a modality can be used on the body.

Contraindications

Contraindications are the reasons a modality should not be used for treatment.

Heating Modalities

Heating modalities warm body tissue to create a specific physiological response that helps the healing process. Heating modalities should be used only after the initial inflammatory response to injury is finished. Chronic (long-lasting) sprains and strains are injuries commonly treated with heat. Increasing the tissue temperature causes an increase in blood flow and in tissue extensibility, which helps to increase range of motion, increase healing potential, and reduce swelling. Heating modalities should not be used on acute injuries, areas of poor or impaired circulation, or areas of impaired sensation.

One of the most common heating modalities is a moist-heat pack such as the hydrocollator pack (see figure 21.3). These canvas packs are filled with a gel that retains heat after being activated in hot water. The packs are to be placed on an athlete only after they are wrapped in several layers of towels or placed in a special premade cover; otherwise, they may cause burns.

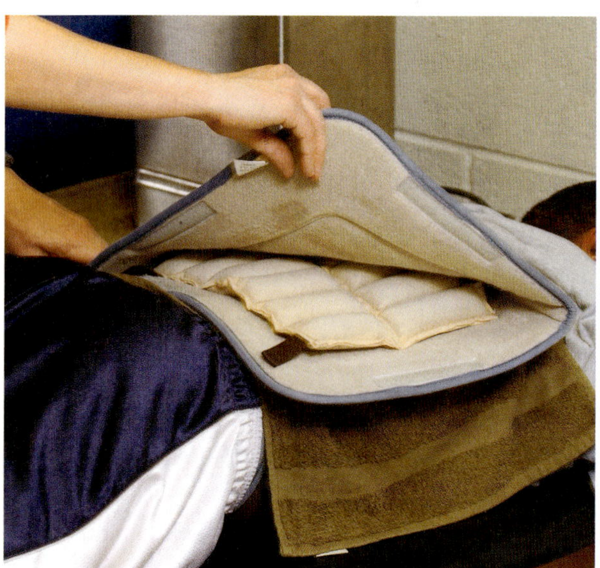

Figure 21.3 A hydrocollator pack being applied to an athlete. Note the extra layers of towels used to keep the back from getting too hot.

A warm **whirlpool** is another common method of heating tissue (see figure 21.4). Whirlpool application to an arm or leg can be performed for up to 20 minutes at a temperature ranging between 95 and 108 °F (35-42 °C). The same contraindications apply for whirlpools as for hot packs. Further, the whirlpool should not be turned on or off while the athlete is in the water, and the athlete receiving treatment should always be in view (electrocution or drowning are possible if precautions are not taken). The athlete should not be placed in a whirlpool if the water turbulence irritates the injury, if they have skin conditions or infected areas, or if they have a fever.

A **paraffin bath** is commonly used when treating the hands or the feet. Because these body regions are uneven, the area is dipped in the lique-

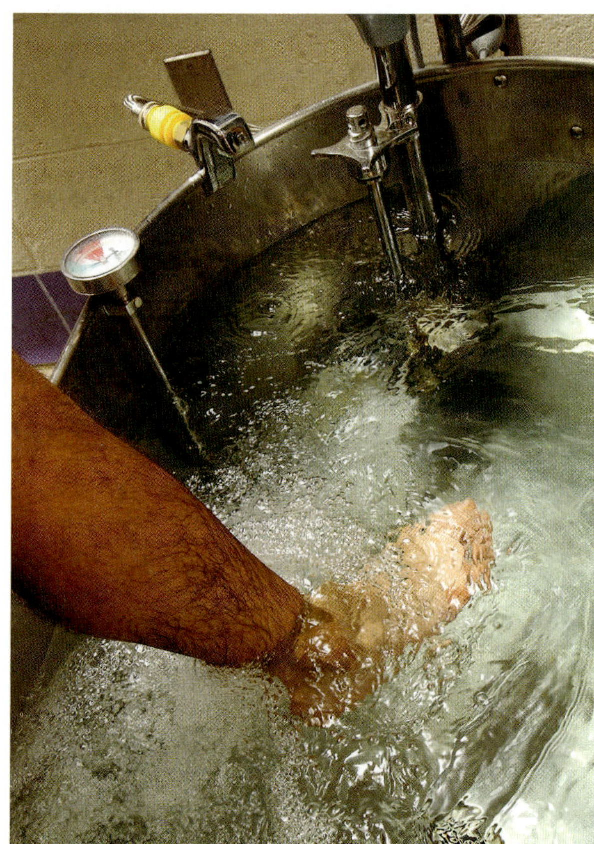

Figure 21.4 Whirlpool application to the foot.

fied paraffin and removed until the wax hardens on the skin (see figure 21.5). This is repeated 6 to 12 times, and then the body part is wrapped with a plastic bag and surrounded by layers of towels. The paraffin is kept on the body for 20 minutes and then peeled off.

Modalities that heat the tissue are often used to prepare the area for stretching or range-of-motion exercises.

Cooling Modalities

Cooling modalities cool the injured tissue, which constricts (narrows) blood vessels and decreases inflammation, cell metabolism, pain, and muscle spasm. Although cooling modalities are most commonly used to treat acute injures such as sprains and strains, they are also used during the rehabilitation process to decrease pain, thus allowing an injured athlete to perform exercises. **Cryotherapy** is using cold on the body to elicit specific physiological responses.

The most common cooling modality is the ice pack (see figure 21.6). Crushed or cubed ice in a plastic bag molds itself around injured body parts and can be easily secured in place. Ice packs should not be applied too tightly with an elastic wrap, and

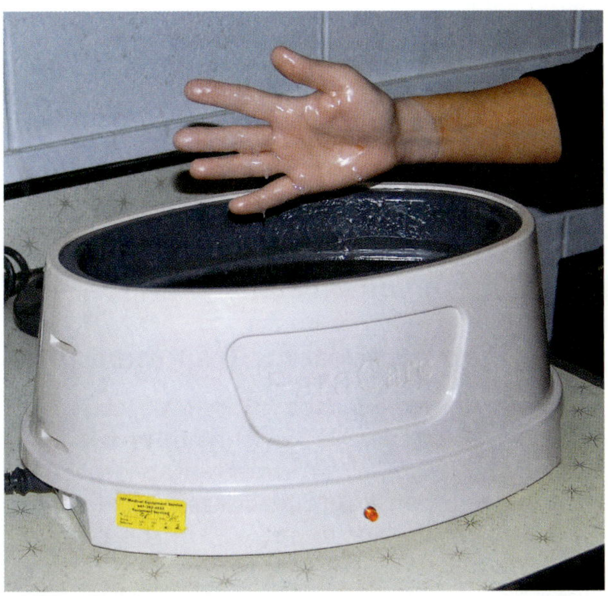

Figure 21.5 Paraffin bath showing a hand that was dipped into the wax and removed, allowing the wax to harden. This step is repeated 6 to 12 times.

Photo: Lorin A. Cartwright.

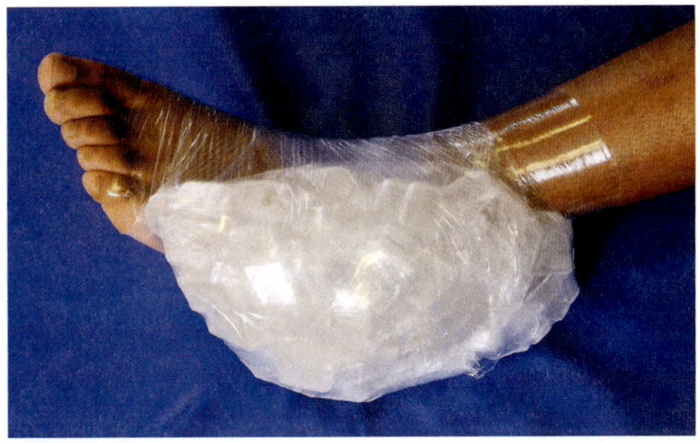

Figure 21.6 Ice packs are used for many injuries.

although the risk of frostbite is low, the athlete should be checked regularly. Cold should not be applied over open wounds, to areas of numbness, to someone who is overly sensitive to cold, or to an athlete who has cardiac or respiratory problems. The ice pack is applied for 20 to 30 minutes. When treating an acute injury, take the ice pack off after each 20- to 30-minute application and wait approximately 40 to 60 minutes before reapplying it. In other words, the ice is left off for twice the amount of time it was applied to the injured area. If the ice is left on too long, it can injure the skin or muscles.

Chemical cold packs are also popular because they can be stored in a freezer and reused. The AT must be careful, however, because chemical cold packs often get colder than 32 °F (0 °C) and could freeze tissue. When using such packs, be sure to place a barrier such as a towel between the pack and the skin surface. It is also helpful to check the skin several times during the application to make sure the athlete is not breaking out in a rash or developing a **blister**. Finally, the AT should make sure the pack is not leaking—if it is, it should not be used.

? What Would You Do If . . .

An athlete who injured his ankle yesterday has just entered the training room. He gets a hot pack and places it on his ankle.

Another common cooling method is an ice massage (see figure 21.7). Ice massage is performed by freezing water in a paper cup and then tearing the cup to expose the ice. The ice is then massaged over the injury site. Ice massage is not appropriate for acute injuries, but it is helpful when treating chronic injuries after exercise.

Whole-Body Cold-Water Immersion Whirlpool

For best postexercise results while using whole-body cold-water immersion, the water should be 50 to 59 °F (10-15 °C) (Machado et al. 2016). The athlete sits in a tub of water for 11 to 15 minutes without the agitation from the motor. It appears that muscle soreness and inflammation can be reduced using immersion modality. It is believed that immersion reduces blood flow to the area, thus reducing the inflammatory injury process caused by exercise, and athletes report less fatigue (Abaidia et al. 2017; Higgins et al. 2017).

Mechanical Elements

Mechanical elements produce a specific physiological effect with mechanical energy. They include ultrasound (acoustical energy), traction, massage, and intermittent compression devices. Indications and contraindications of mechanical elements can be found in table 21.2.

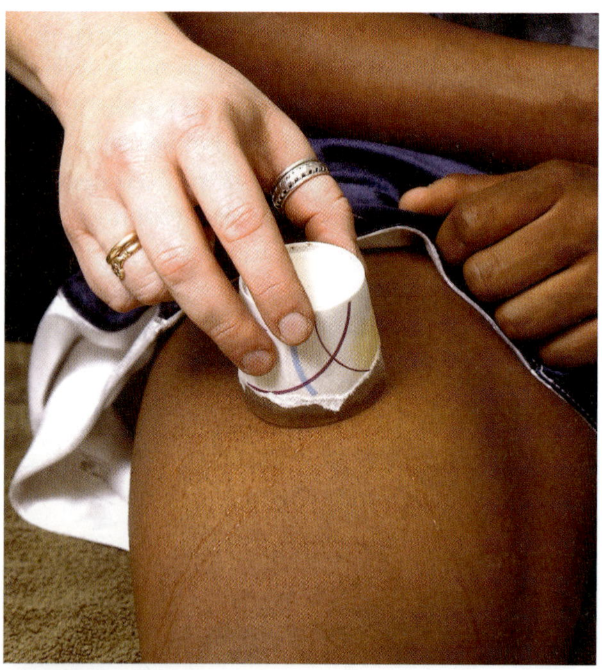

Figure 21.7 Ice massage.

Ultrasound

Ultrasound may be categorized as a thermal modality because it can produce a deep-heating effect, but it can also cause nonthermal reactions in the tissue. As sound waves pass through the tissue, heat is produced through a process known as conversion. If the sound waves are sporadic or intermittent, heat may not be produced. Ultrasound waves are extremely high frequency and cannot be heard by the human ear. Figure 21.8 shows ultrasound application.

Common ultrasound frequencies used in treating athletic injuries include 1 megahertz (MHz), 2 MHz, and 3 MHz. These are much higher frequencies than the human voice can produce. The frequency, not the amount of intensity, determines the depth of penetration of sound waves into the tissue. The 1 MHz frequency penetrates deeper than the 3 MHz. Therefore, the 3 MHz frequency may be better suited for injuries that are closer to the surface of the skin.

The effects of heating the tissue with ultrasound are the same as for a hot pack. Ultrasound, however, can affect deeper tissue than a hot pack can. In fact, 1 MHz ultrasound can penetrate up to 2 inches (5 cm) of tissue. For the ultrasound to create heat, the machine must be set for a continuous emission—that is, sound waves need to be flowing 100% of the time. A pulsed setting interrupts the flow of sound waves and reduces the thermal effects.

Understanding Diversity

Hijab Removal for Treatment

Women who wear hijabs do so as part of their Muslim religion. If the AT needs to provide an assessment or care, it is important to know the patient. Rehman and colleagues (2022) indicate that it is important to share with the patient why it is necessary to remove the hijab. Ask the woman to remove the hijab herself. Allow for privacy by limiting the number of people who can view her when the hijab is off.

Table 21.2 Indications and Contraindications for Mechanical Modalities

Type of modality	Indications	Contraindications
Ultrasound	Chronic inflammation Acute injuries (nonthermal application) Chronic injuries Muscle strains Ligament sprains Bruises, muscle spasm Tightened soft tissue Scar tissue	Areas with circulation deficits Areas with sensory deficits Over tumors Over growth plates in children Over heart, eyes, or nerve plexus Acute injuries, using the continuous heat setting Pregnancy Vascular problems Over spinal cord
Traction	Spinal disc protrusion Degenerative disc disease Degenerative joint disease Soft-tissue stiffness Nerve root compression Muscle spasm Joint tightness Intervertebral disc pain	Infection of the spine Osteoporosis Malignant tumors Acute injuries Pregnancy Rheumatoid arthritis Fractured vertebra Spinal hypermobility Cardiopulmonary problems Hiatal hernia (lumbar traction) Vascular problems
Massage	Promotion of relaxation Muscle spasm Pain Soft-tissue stiffness When increased circulation is needed Edema	Nonunion fracture sites Over open wounds Over dermatological conditions Acute injuries Over tumors
Intermittent compression	Postacute edema Lymphedema	Acute injuries Skin irritation When a fracture has not been ruled out Peripheral vascular disorders Compartment syndromes Infection Thrombophlebitis
Low-level light therapy	Open wounds Neck and back pain Arthritis Trigger points Carpal tunnel syndrome	Over cancerous tumors Pregnancy Over thyroid glands Children

Note: Because machines vary, manufacturers' guidelines should always be followed.

Disagreement exists among experts as to whether modalities are contraindicated or can be used with caution.

Data obtained from Kahanov and Payne (2022); Denegar, Saliba, and Saliba (2016).

When applying continuous ultrasound, the AT must move the sound head slowly and continuously. When pulsed ultrasound is applied, the sound head can be kept still. In either case, ultrasound must be applied using a coupling medium such as water, lotion, or gel. When the sound head is applied on the body part through the coupling medium, direct ultrasound is being applied. Direct application should be used only if the area is smooth. Irregularly shaped areas such as the hand, ankle, and elbow may need ultrasound applied indirectly (see figure 21.9). Indirect ultrasound is usually applied underwater in a plastic tub. When applying ultrasound underwater, the sound head must be fully immersed and placed about 0.5 to 1.0 inch (1.5-2.5 cm) away from the tissue, and the ultrasound

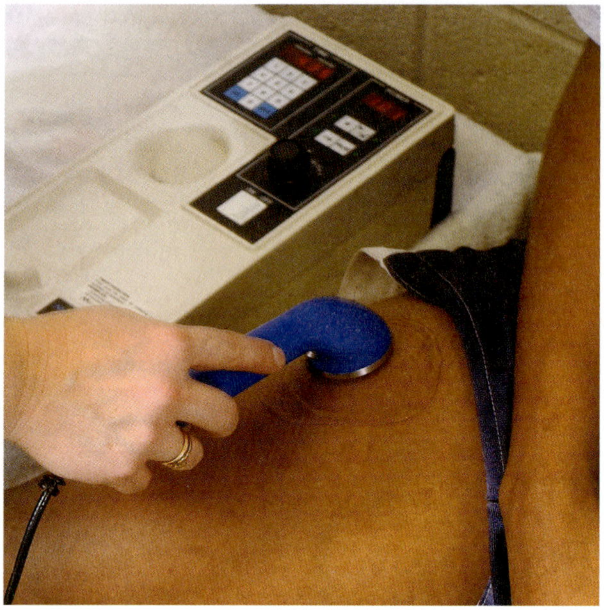

Figure 21.8 An ultrasound treatment provides benefits, but it must be used carefully or it can damage tissue.

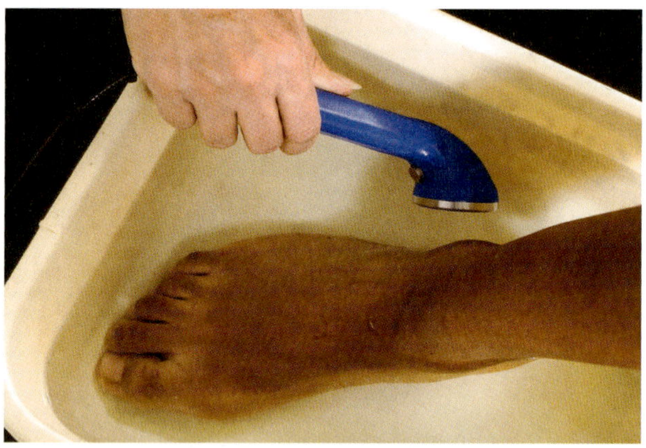

Figure 21.9 Indirect ultrasound application. Ultrasound can be applied underwater. This is especially helpful when the body area being treated is bumpy and the sound head will not stay flat against the tissue.

intensity must be increased. There are many contraindications for using ultrasound; therefore, it should be used with caution and only when prescribed by a physician. Refer to table 21.2.

Traction

Traction is a pulling force. In this context, it refers to deliberately attempting to separate the joints of the body if they have been compressed or if they have become stiff over time. It is most commonly done to vertebrae. Traction can be performed to both the cervical and lumbar spine and can be done either mechanically (with a machine) or manually (by the AT). For example, if an AT were given permission by a physician to perform cervical spine traction on an athlete, the athlete would lie on their back. The AT would place one hand under the back of their head and the other under their chin. The AT would then gently pull on the neck to gradually separate the vertebrae. This technique must be performed with extreme caution and only with a physician's permission.

Traction not only separates bones that have been pushed too close together but also minimally stretches the ligaments and muscles in the area. It may also help resolve a disc protrusion, which is discussed in chapter 14. It is thought that separating the vertebrae creates a suction force that can cause the protruded disc matter to move toward the center of the disc, where it belongs. Additionally, separating the vertebrae opens the space where the nerve roots exit the spinal cord (see figure 21.10). By increasing this space, pressure can be removed from the nerve root, helping to decrease pain and facilitate healing.

As a precaution, patients should be monitored during their first treatment to ensure that no complications arise, such as increased pain, discomfort, muscle spasm, numbness, or tingling (figure 21.11). Also, it is important to perform traction in a quiet

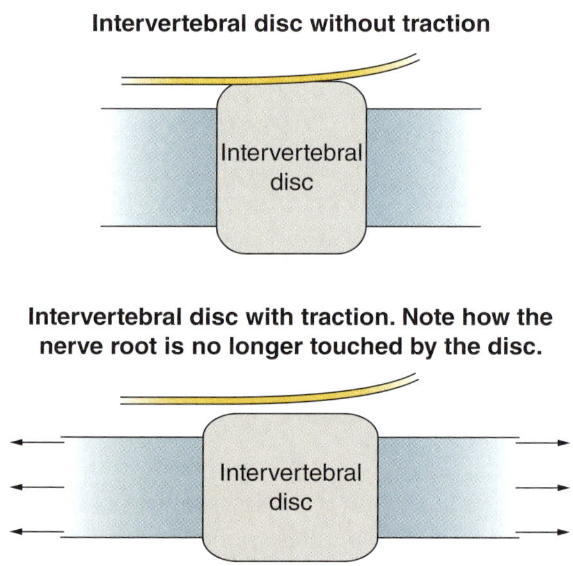

Figure 21.10 The effects of spinal traction. Traction pulls the joints apart and is helpful for relieving pressure on nerve roots at the spinal cord. Traction must be used cautiously and only if all contraindications have been ruled out.

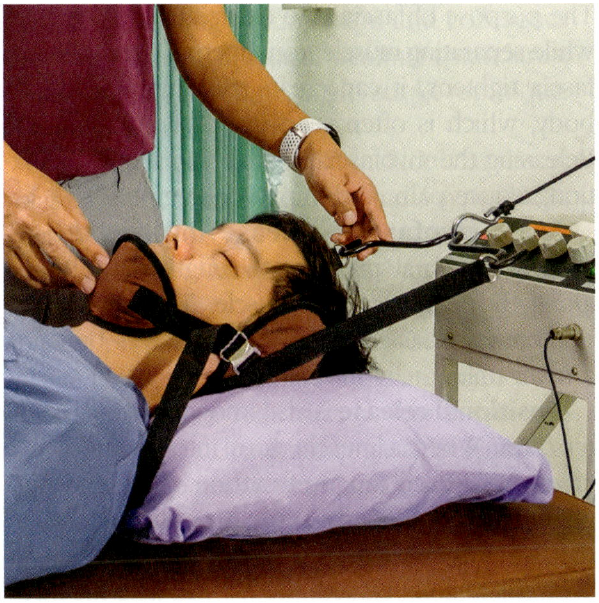

Figure 21.11 Mechanical spinal traction.
Six Characters/E+/Getty Images

area where the patient can relax. The indications and contraindications for cervical and lumbar traction are summarized in table 21.2. A physician should check the athlete before they receive traction and again before they return to participation.

Manual Therapy

ATs use manual therapy techniques to improve circulation, increase relaxation, improve range of motion, and reduce pain. Some of the skills in manual therapy include massage, trigger-point therapy, myofascial release, and positional release. These techniques do not use any machines, just the AT's hands. The AT will have to determine which manual therapy will work best to provide relief. Athletic trainers often need specialized training to perform these skills effectively.

Massage is the methodical kneading and stroking of the soft tissues. It is used to increase circulation, decrease muscle spasm, and relieve swelling. Massage is accomplished by long strokes that start distally and move toward the heart. The long strokes move from distal to proximal. Massage aids in removing metabolites from the muscles and reducing edema (Prentice 2021).

If the goal is to decrease swelling, the massage strokes must move from below the injury site toward the heart. Massage strokes include effleurage, petrissage, vibration, percussion, and friction.

Effleurage consists of stroking the tissue with the palm of the hand in a smooth, rhythmical manner (see figure 21.12*a*). Effleurage is often done at the beginning and end of a massage session. **Petrissage** is often described as kneading of the tissue as the skin, muscle, and fasciae are squeezed between the hands (see figure 21.12*b*).

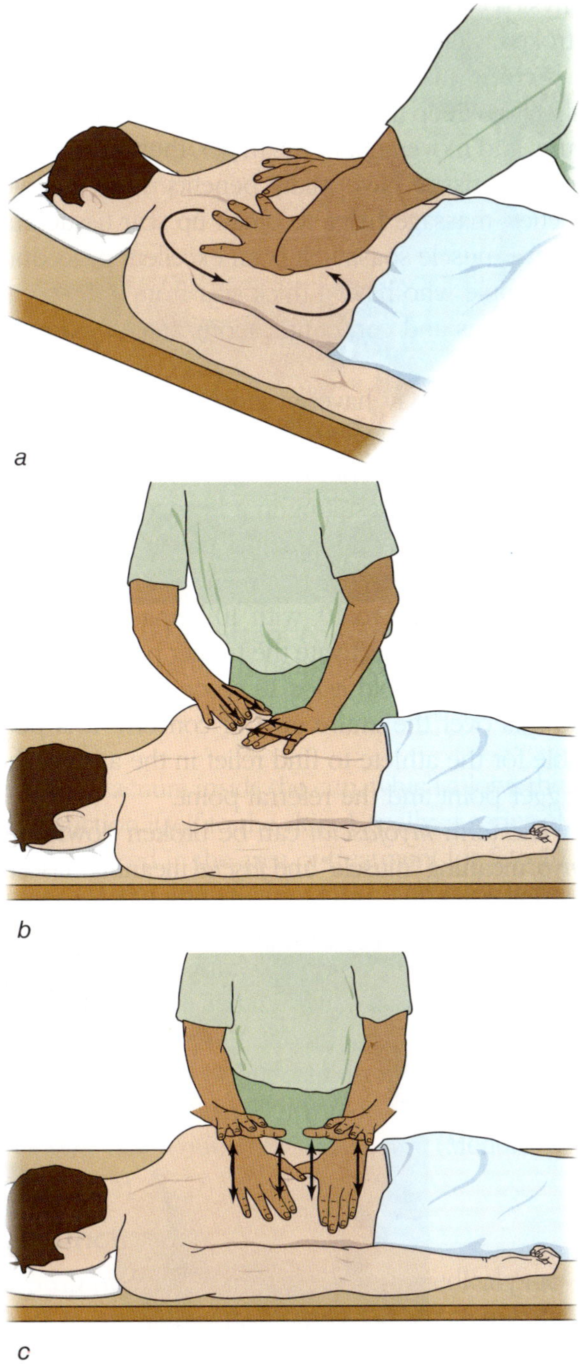

Figure 21.12 *(a)* Effleurage, *(b)* petrissage, and *(c)* percussion or tapotement massage strokes.

and yang forces are balanced (Dao), the person is healthy and when forces are unbalanced, the person is unhealthy (UC San Diego Center for Integrative Medicine 2017). Various conditions can be treated by acupuncture, including knee pain, sciatica, tennis elbow, nausea, upset stomach, depression, headaches, lower-back pain, and hypertension (UC San Diego Center for Integrative Medicine 2017).

Using acupuncture helps improve the flow of qi though the meridians. There are 365 points on the meridian where needles are placed to relieve the aforementioned conditions (see figure 21.15). Treatment time is usually one hour, and more than one treatment may be required to achieve the desired outcome.

Dry Needling

Dry needling is a Western medical practice that involves acupuncture needles placed into myofascial trigger points. The needles, although the same as acupuncture, are utilized differently. The needles are placed in the trigger point of a muscle or tissue in an area that is injured. The needles are inserted for a few seconds up to 15 minutes and then removed. Pain relief may occur within a day or may require several treatments. Contraindications include abnormal bleeding, vascular disease, diabetes, pregnancy, epilepsy, allergy to metals, children (under the age of 16), inability to tolerate the procedure, altered mental health status, or compromised immune system (Unverzagt, Berglund, and Thomas 2015).

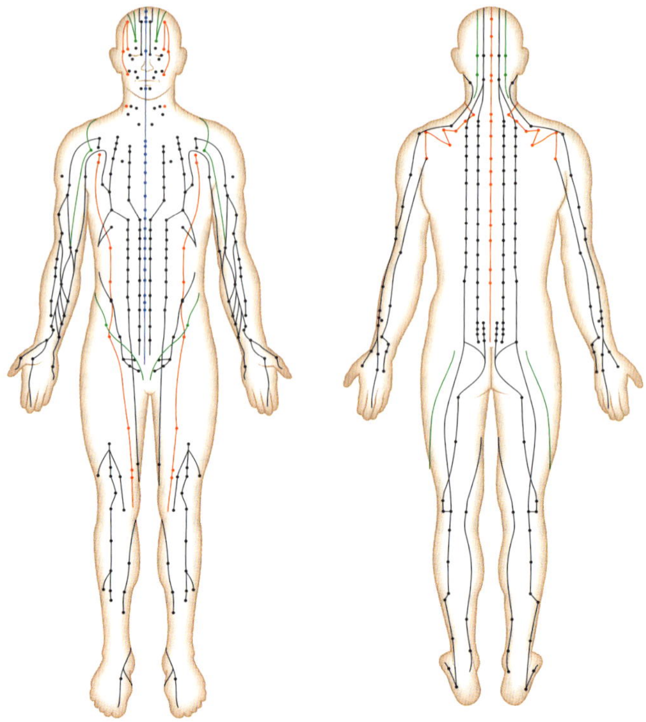

Figure 21.15 Meridians.

Dry needling is used to deactivate trigger points and increase blood flow, which in turn reduces pain and restores function. Stretching may be suggested as a post-treatment procedure.

Low-Level Light Therapy (LLLT) Laser

A laser used for low-level light therapy (LLLT) does not emit heat like lasers that are used for cutting materials. The LLLT laser is a cold laser and emits

SELECTING THE CORRECT MODALITY

- Have a confirmed diagnosis and know the underlying issues.
- Make sure the modality will help achieve goals and outcomes.
- Understand the physiological needs that will promote healing.
- Know psychological aspects of the patient.
- Know your patient's tolerance of the modality.
- Understand the timing for using the modality (using cryotherapy early and thermotherapy later).
- Know the effects a modality will create.
- Know the indications and contraindications of the modality.
- Determine the alternative modalities.

energy into the soft tissues in the area of use. The soft tissues may vibrate, increasing function in acute musculoskeletal injury, pain relief, and tissue repair (Anderson and Barnum 2022). LLLT has been found to be effective for low-back pain, carpal tunnel syndrome, myofascial pain, osteoarthritis, and neck pain (Anderson and Barnum 2022).

The common uses of LLLT include analgesia, wound healing, and as an anti-inflammatory (Kahanov and Payne 2022). The head of the laser is the probe. The athlete and AT should wear safety goggles to prevent eye damage. The probe is placed over the area with direct contact with the skin and then moved (Kahanov and Payne 2022; see figure 21.16). The AT will determine the dosage and length of time when using LLLT based on the type of injury and the athlete's goals. Denegar, Saliba, and Saliba (2016) indicate three techniques for application: point, scanning, and grid. Point application is used with the laser over a trigger point. Scanning follows imaginary lines over the area placed 1 centimeter (0.4 in.) apart. The grid technique traces lines in a grid pattern made of 1-centimeter (0.4 in.) squares.

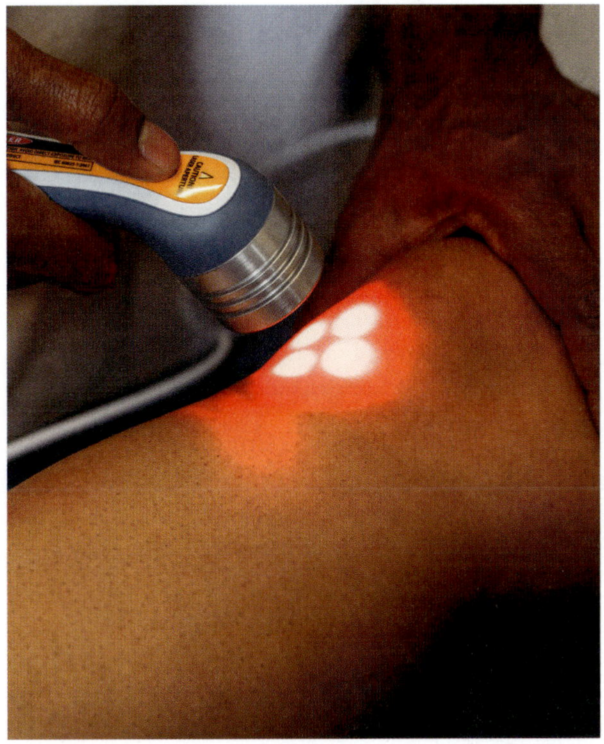

Figure 21.16 Low-level laser.

Electrical Elements

It may come as a shock to learn that electricity can be therapeutic. Many useful physiological changes occur when electricity is safely passed through tissue. Understanding these changes requires a familiarity with electricity. Again, we must warn of the dangers that can exist when using electrical modalities (see table 21.3). Such modalities should be used only by people who have been trained and only with a physician's prescription.

Electricity is the flow of electrons (negatively charged particles) through a circuit. A circuit is a path through which electricity flows, such as a wire in a house. Some circuits allow electrons to flow easily, whereas other circuits offer more resistance. Given a choice, electricity will always choose the path of least resistance. In the body, the tissues create a circuit. Tissues with high water content, such as muscles, conduct electricity well, whereas bones do not.

Table 21.3 Indications and Contraindications for Electrical Modalities

Indications	Contraindications
Pain	During pregnancy
Edema	When there is an unknown cause of pain
Preventing muscle weakness	Over infected sites
Reducing muscle spasm	Over heart, eyes, carotid sinus, upper airway, wound care, open wounds, or tumors
Reeducating muscle function	Pacemakers
Increasing local circulation	Over some fracture sites

Note: Because machines vary, manufacturer guidelines should always be followed.

Disagreement exists among some experts as to whether modalities are contraindicated or can be used with caution.

Data obtained from Kahanov and Payne (2022); Denegar, Saliba, and Saliba (2016).

FYI

Nerve Root Impingement

A spinal nerve root impingement means that something, such as part of a disc or swelling, puts pressure on the nerve where it exits the spinal cord.

Diastolic Blood Pressure

The diastolic blood pressure is the pressure in an artery while the heart is relaxed. It is the bottom number of a blood pressure reading.

The electron flow, or current, moves from a negative pole to a positive pole. Electrical currents can be either direct or alternating. With a **direct current (DC)**, electricity moves in one direction as it passes through the tissue circuit. Picture a simple DC electrical generator with two electrodes (positive and negative) placed on your forearm, one near your wrist and the other near your elbow. If the electrode pad nearest your wrist is the negative pole and the one nearest your elbow is the positive pole, a direct current of electricity will flow from your wrist to your elbow.

With an **alternating current (AC)**, electricity moves back and forth between electrodes, changing the direction in which it moves through a circuit. The AC generator is sophisticated and can switch an electrode from positive to negative. Using the previous example, if an AC current were applied to the body, electricity would constantly change directions between electrodes, moving toward your elbow one moment and toward your wrist the next.

Direct and alternating currents are applied to the body in either an interrupted (i.e., pulsed) or uninterrupted (i.e., continuous) pattern. A pulsed current simply means that the flow of electricity is consistently stopped and restarted. A continuous current is not stopped until the treatment is terminated.

Many types of electrical currents are used during the rehabilitation process, and they all require electrical pads placed on the surface of the skin (see figure 21.17). The type of current used and how it is applied to the body depends on the rehabilitation goals. For example, an AT may apply electricity to reduce pain, muscle spasm, or swelling, or they may apply it to increase strength and healing potential.

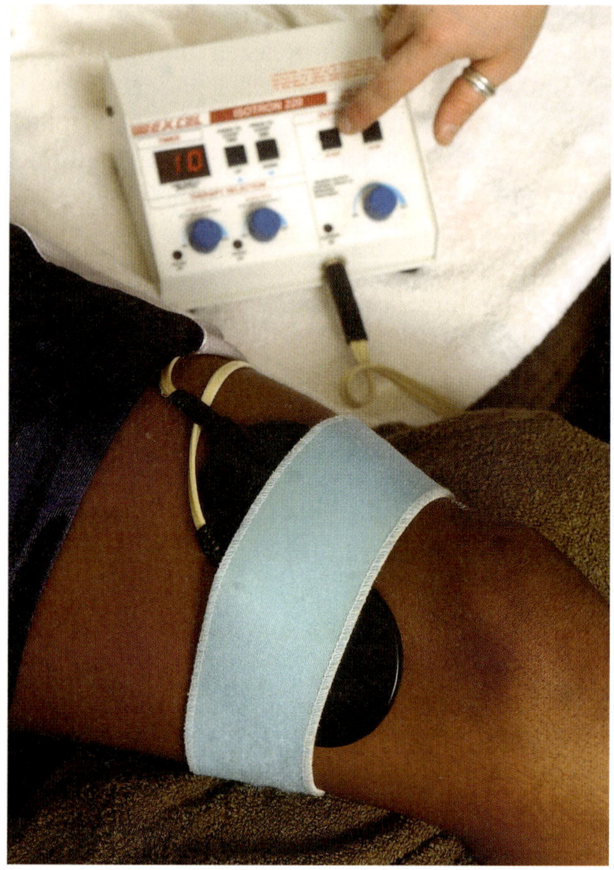

Figure 21.17 Electrical muscle stimulation helps reduce spasm and pain and can also help prevent weakness.

Types of electrical stimulation include high-voltage pulsed electrical muscle stimulation, low-intensity stimulation, interferential current, and transcutaneous electrical nerve stimulation.

Passing an electrical current over the body can create several physiological effects depending on the type, intensity, and duration of the current. For example, high-voltage pulsed direct stimulation can cause a muscle contraction, which helps prevent a muscle from weakening when recovering from an injury. The muscle contractions can also create a pumping action to reduce swelling and edema. Applying electrical current to the body at an intensity that can be felt but is insufficient for causing a muscle contraction is often helpful for reducing pain. When the muscle is stimulated to contract, it does so without help from the athlete. Although this sounds terrific, it will not make a person physically fit or help them lose weight.

Low-intensity stimulation, also known as microcurrent, introduces a low level of electricity into the tissue; the athlete does not even feel the current passing through the body. Low-intensity stimulation is thought to mimic the body's natural electrical flow and promote tissue healing.

Interferential current is created when two electrical currents cross one another, thus interfering with the flow of electricity. Although this sounds counterproductive, the interference creates an appropriate current that stimulates the tissue to create a muscle contraction, thus reducing pain and edema. Most treatments to help reduce pain, however, use **transcutaneous electrical nerve stimulation (TENS)**. TENS creates an electrical current that moves across the skin, resulting in a pins-and-needles sensation. This stimulus of the sensory nerves can cause pain to be gated or stopped in the spinal cord rather than transmitted to the brain, where pain perception occurs.

Summary

A SOAP note documents the findings of an injury assessment and structures an action plan for a rehabilitation program. In rehabilitation, ATs try to help an athlete attain normal function by regaining mobility, proprioception, strength, endurance, and sport-specific function. To aid the recovery process, ATs use therapeutic modalities such as heat, cold, ultrasound, electricity, and massage.

Key Terms

Define the following terms found in this chapter:

- active–assistive range of motion (AAROM)
- active range of motion (AROM)
- acupuncture
- alternating current (AC)
- blister
- cryotherapy
- cupping
- direct current (DC)
- edema
- effleurage
- endurance
- flexibility
- friction massage
- intermittent compression
- massage
- myofascial release
- paraffin bath
- passive range of motion (PROM)
- percussion massage
- petrissage
- positional release
- progression
- proprioception
- resistance training
- sport-specific function
- traction
- transcutaneous electrical nerve stimulation (TENS)
- trigger-point therapy
- ultrasound
- vibration massage
- whirlpool

You have just taken a new job as an AT. The first person comes to see you with an injury. As you begin the preliminary introduction you realize the person does not speak your language and vice versa. What options do you have to ensure that you are able to get the necessary information from the patient so that a proper assessment is done and treatment can be implemented? What are the available resources at a school, hospital, and occupational setting to assist in this situation?

To access supplementary material for this chapter, including the Understanding Check worksheet, vocabulary quizzes, extension activities, and chapter-specific resources and forms, visit the web resource: http://ancillaries.humankinetics.com/FundamentalsOfAthleticTrainingAndSportsMedicine5E

chapter 22

Strength Training and Reconditioning

Objectives

After completing this chapter, the student will be able to do the following:

- Explain the principles of strength training.
- Identify the various ways to develop strength.
- Compare muscular strength and endurance and explain how to develop each.
- Discuss the principles behind developing cardiorespiratory fitness.
- Identify appropriate exercises for rehabilitating specific conditions of the upper quarter, lower quarter, and trunk.
- Explain how technology can be incorporated into fitness programs.
- Identify common safety procedures for weight training.

Reconditioning an athlete during rehabilitation is the same as conditioning in the sense that both programs use the same principles. The primary goal of reconditioning is to help the athlete get back to their preinjury level of fitness. It is important to keep an athlete motivated during the rehabilitation program by using a variety of exercises to maintain fitness.

STRENGTH AND CONDITIONING PRINCIPLES

Injured athletes must get fit to successfully return to participation; therefore, their physical conditioning must be addressed. As discussed with the IMPRESS program in chapter 21, this includes strength, muscular endurance, **cardiorespiratory endurance**, and flexibility. Primary principles for strength and conditioning are progressive resistive exercise, overload, and specificity.

Progressive Resistive Exercise

When the goal is to develop an athlete's strength, **progressive resistive exercise (PRE)** is common. PRE involves progressively increasing the load (i.e., weight or number of repetitions), both during the training session and over time. By advancing the resistance training appropriately, further injury can be avoided and the body can adapt to the demands of the activity.

Overload Principle

The **overload principle** means that for muscle to gain strength or endurance, it must be stressed beyond the demands of previous activity. For example, if an athlete bench-presses 50 pounds (23 kg) for 10 repetitions every other day for 3 weeks, they may not significantly improve strength because they are not overloading the muscle. However, if the athlete lifts 50 pounds (23 kg) for 10 repetitions one day and then lifts 55 pounds (25 kg) two days later, they probably will stress their muscles beyond the demands of the previous bench press.

Weight is not the only factor we can increase, however. Many variables can be adjusted to overload the muscle, including workout frequency, the exercise intensity, the length of the workout, and the type of exercise performed. The variable the coach or AT changes will depend on the goal of the exercise. For example, if the athlete requires cardiorespiratory endurance for biking, the time spent biking during workouts should be increased. If the goal is to develop muscular endurance, the athlete will need to lift less weight for a higher number of repetitions; if the goal is to develop strength, the athlete should use more weight and fewer repetitions.

Specificity of Training

Specificity means that the body systems will adapt to the specific demands placed on them. For example, if an athlete wants to become a better runner, the training should consist mostly of running. But if the athlete wants to become a better hockey player, training should consist mostly of hockey and ice-skating activities. When an athlete does nothing more than lift weights, it is doubtful that their body will improve its cardiorespiratory function; likewise, if they only ride a bike, the upper body probably will not become stronger.

In the context of strength training, a muscle gets used to the specific activities required of it. Take the athlete who bench-presses 50 pounds (23 kg) for 10 repetitions every other day for 3 weeks. Although lifting this amount of weight for the first few days is difficult, it will become easy by the third week. Their muscles will adapt to the specific exercise (bench press) and the demands placed on them (50 pounds for 10 repetitions).

Data-Driven Strength Programs

Data-driven strength programs are based on objective data (current strength and goals), subjective data (how the athlete feels), training load for strength, and monitoring of recovery progress. An AT or fit-

> **What Would You Do If . . .**
>
> The AT asks you to give a message to an athlete who is working out in the weight room. When you enter the weight room, you notice that the athlete is alone, performing a bench press with a weight bar that has about 200 pounds (91 kg) on it.

ness expert will continuously adapt the training load based on the subjective data, recovery progress, and improvement in strength.

It is important to know baseline information in data-driven strength programs. Some basic questions are height, weight, and biological sex. A baseline for current strength is important in fitness. The one-repetition maximum (1 RM) is commonly used to determine an individual's strength and a starting point for a training program.

There are applications that will provide data-driven strength programs. An example of a data-driven app is the Juggernaut AI app. With these apps, a person can work on their progress and optimize their training by targeting weak areas, the frequency of their workouts, the amount of work necessary, and periodization. Apps work on algorithms and determine what is best for the athlete based on the input they receive daily. Apps provide a video of each exercise showing proper technique.

TYPES OF MUSCLE ACTIONS

Muscles function in various ways. At times, the muscles must contract simply to hold a joint still and not allow it to move. At other times, the muscle must contract to move a limb through a whole motion, such as when a softball player throws a ball. The three types of muscle actions are isotonic, isometric, and isokinetic. Regardless of which type an athlete performs, the goal is to overload the muscles to produce strength gains.

Isotonics

Isotonic contractions occur when moving a joint through a range of motion with a fixed amount of resistance. Performing an exercise with a free weight is a perfect example. Isotonic resistance training involves movement at the joint, and the muscles shorten and lengthen against resistance. When a muscle shortens against resistance, it is a concentric contraction; when a muscle lengthens against resistance, it is an eccentric contraction. Adolescent athletes should refrain from doing only eccentric weight training because it places a great deal of stress on the muscles and tendons.

Isometrics

When an **isometric contraction** is performed, there is no joint movement. Picture yourself pushing against a brick wall. Although the muscles in your arms and chest contract, no joint motion is produced. Because there is no motion at the joint, the joint is less likely to become irritated or painful. Therefore, isometric exercises are extremely useful for preventing weakness in the early stages following an injury.

Isokinetics

When an **isokinetic contraction** is performed, speed of movement is controlled. Isokinetics are typically performed using sophisticated equipment that controls the speed at which an athlete will work—no matter how much force they exert against the machine, they can make it move only at a predetermined speed. It is similar to trying to pull a canoe paddle through the water—you can pull easy or hard, but its speed does not change.

Kinetic Chain Movements

Besides isotonic and isometric contractions, there are other considerations when moving the body. Sometimes a limb moves openly in space and other times it is fixed firmly to the ground.

When you are moving your arm in the air, such as when throwing a baseball, your arm is functioning in an **open kinetic chain**. If you were to place yourself in a push-up position with your hands on the ground and bearing weight, you would be functioning in a **closed kinetic chain**.

As an AT chooses exercises for an injured athlete to perform, deciding whether to include open or closed kinetic chain exercises is important. Often open chain exercises are used early in a rehabilitation program because an athlete is not able to bear their body weight. Later in the program, the athlete can bear more weight, and closed kinetic chain exercises can be used.

MUSCULAR DEVELOPMENT PROGRAMS

Although many resistance training programs exist, the premise of each is the same. The purpose of

RESISTANCE TRAINING PROGRESSION FOR HEALTHY ADULTS

The American College of Sports Medicine (ACSM 2013) has the following recommendations:

1. Concentric, eccentric, and isometric muscle actions should be included in a resistance training program.
2. People at the beginner and intermediate levels should use a load of about 70% to 85% of what they could lift only one time for an exercise, or **one-repetition maximum (1RM)**. More advanced athletes should use about 70% to 100% of 1RM.
3. Use 1 to 3 sets of 8 to 12 repetitions during exercise to increase strength and power for a novice and intermediate level and 3 to 6 sets of 1 to 12 repetitions for advanced lifters (ACSM 2013).
4. Use 2 to 4 sets of 10 to 25 repetitions during exercise to improve muscular fitness (ACSM 2013).
5. Beginners should use 1 to 3 sets when starting a resistance training program.
6. Both one-sided (unilateral) and two-sided (bilateral) exercises should be performed during training. As an example, flexing one elbow while holding a dumbbell is a unilateral exercise, whereas flexing both elbows while holding a long bar with plates is a bilateral exercise. Also, exercises that use single-joint movements (e.g., only elbow flexion and extension) should be used as well as multijoint movements (e.g., a push-up that not only flexes and extends the elbow but also requires movement at the shoulder joint and scapula).
7. People at the beginner and intermediate levels should use both free-weight exercises and machines, whereas advanced athletes should focus on free weights.
8. Large muscle groups should be trained before small muscle groups. An example is working the deltoid and pectoralis major of the shoulder girdle before exercising the rotator cuff muscles.
9. Large muscle groups should be trained at least twice each week (Schoenfeld, Ogborn, and Krieger Medicine 2016).
10. Multijoint exercises should be performed before single-joint exercises.
11. A 2- to 3-minute rest between core exercises, such as the bench press or squats using high loads, is recommended. Only 1 to 2 minutes of rest are needed between sets of noncore exercises such as biceps curls.
12. Beginners should use slow to moderate speeds during resistance exercises. Intermediate lifters should use moderate speeds, and advanced athletes should use a variety of speeds, including fast speeds.
13. Novice lifters should exercise 2 or 3 days per week, and intermediate athletes should lift 3 days per week if it is a total-body workout (ACSM 2013). An intermediate athlete can train 4 days per week if splitting between upper- and lower-body workouts. In instances where an athlete may perform only lower-body exercises one day and upper-body exercises another day (split routine), each major muscle group should be trained once or twice per week.

The strength training guidelines should be modified for young athletes. Each young athlete needs a program tailored to their needs based on technical competency, training age, and maturity level (Haff and Triplett 2016). Technical competency refers to one's ability to do a resistance training technique properly. How long an athlete has been in a formal resistance program is called *training age*. *Maturity level* refers to the growth and physical stature of the individual. Also, Haff and Triplett (2016) recommend 1 to 3 sets of 6 to 15 repetitions.

such programs is to overload the muscles in a specific manner using isotonic, isokinetic, or isometric movements. However, most muscular development programs use isotonic movements and free weights.

Muscular Strength

Muscular strength is the ability to exert force against a resistance. Developing strength often also leads to developing muscular endurance and power. Generally, an athlete develops strength by using a heavy weight for a low number of repetitions. To accomplish this, the athlete may find it helpful to use a constant set method—that is, using the same amount of weight for the same number of sets and repetitions, such as 40 pounds (18 kg) performed in 4 sets of 4 repetitions. The ACSM released a 2009 position statement describing how to progress resistance training programs for healthy adults (see the sidebar, Resistance Training Progression for Healthy Adults).

The **DeLorme method** of PRE is an example of an ascending pyramid method. It requires the athlete to perform 3 sets in a progressive manner. Let's say that the maximum an athlete can military press for 10 repetitions is 200 pounds (91 kg). In the DeLorme method, the 200 pounds is called the *10-repetition maximum* weight, or 10RM, and the athlete does 3 sets of 10 repetitions at 50%, 75%, and 100% of 10RM. Thus, the athlete would perform the first set of 10 repetitions at 50% of 10RM, or 100 pounds (45 kg). This would be considered a warm-up. They would perform the second set at 150 pounds (68 kg), or 75% of 10RM, for 10 repetitions. The third set would be performed at the maximum weight of 200 pounds (91 kg), which is 100% of 10RM. DeLorme's program of 3 sets of 10 repetitions continues to be a popular method of strength training.

Another common method of training is the Nautilus method of weight training. In this method, a person performs a set of an exercise to fatigue, which is when they can no longer perform the exercise.

The **pyramid method** uses multiple sets (at least three and sometimes up to five or six) in which the weight is increased or decreased with each set (see figure 22.1). The athlete may use an ascending pyramid method when they want to build up to lifting the higher amount of weight with less chance of hurting themselves. It is thought that using a descending pyramid technique works the muscle against a higher amount of weight earlier, when it is not as fatigued. Performing multiple sets, for example by doing both sides of a pyramid, is thought to facilitate maximum strength gains. Provided that the muscle is overloaded, however, strength gains can be made regardless of the type of program the athlete follows.

Pyramid training involves about 5 sets of a given exercise. When an athlete ascends the pyramid (increases the weight per set), they are using the DeLorme method. When an athlete descends the pyramid (decreases the weight per set), they are using the Oxford technique. If they follow the bottom of the pyramid (maintains the same weight per set), they are using the constant set method.

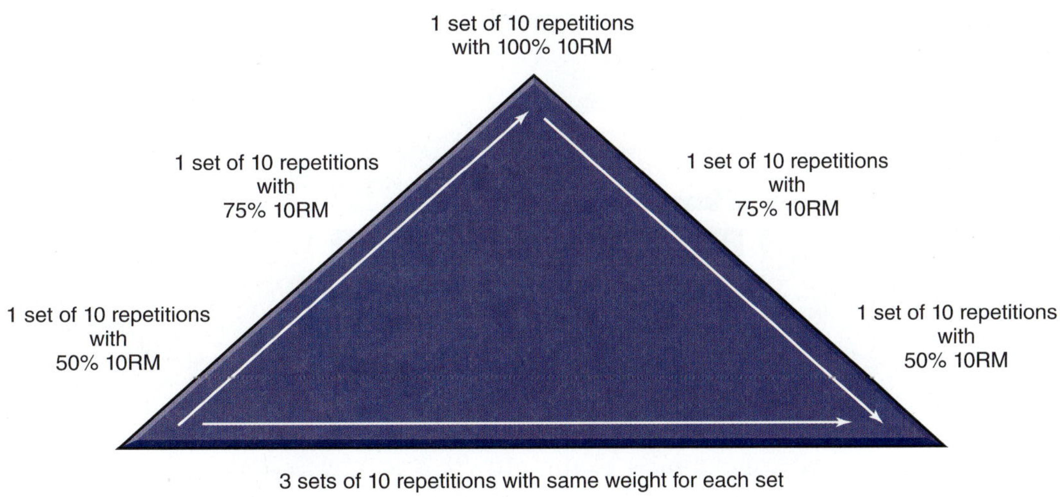

Figure 22.1 Pyramid training.

Muscular Endurance

The ability of a muscle to perform repetitive movements for an extended time is referred to as **muscular endurance**. Activities that require a significant amount of muscular endurance include cross country running, cross-country skiing, and many swimming events. An athlete can develop muscular endurance using the programs for building strength. However, using a lower amount of weight and performing a higher number of repetitions develops muscular endurance more efficiently.

Circuit training is a popular and effective method of developing muscular endurance as well as overall fitness. **Circuit training** involves exercising at multiple stations (usually 8-20) that often target a full-body workout (exercises to work all major muscle groups are selected). The athlete rotates from station to station, either performing a given number of repetitions or exercising for a given length of time (e.g., 30 seconds) at each station. It is wise to select stations that target alternate body parts so that the same muscles are not used at consecutive stations.

Power

Muscular power refers to the ability to exert force quickly. Many programs that focus on developing power do so by using heavy weights and a low number of repetitions; the movements, however, are performed quickly. For example, a football lineman must be able to react quickly once the ball is snapped by exploding off the line of scrimmage and pushing his opponent. The result is fast movement against resistance, but the play does not last long.

Plyometrics

Speed and force during muscle movement create muscular power. **Plyometric** movements stretch muscles, then go through eccentric contraction, amortization, and concentric contraction (Haff and Triplett 2016). This type of exercise improves strength, agility, stability, and balance (Healthline 2019). Plyometrics can improve power in the arms, legs, and hips. An example of leg, hip, and arm plyometrics can be found in figure 22.2.

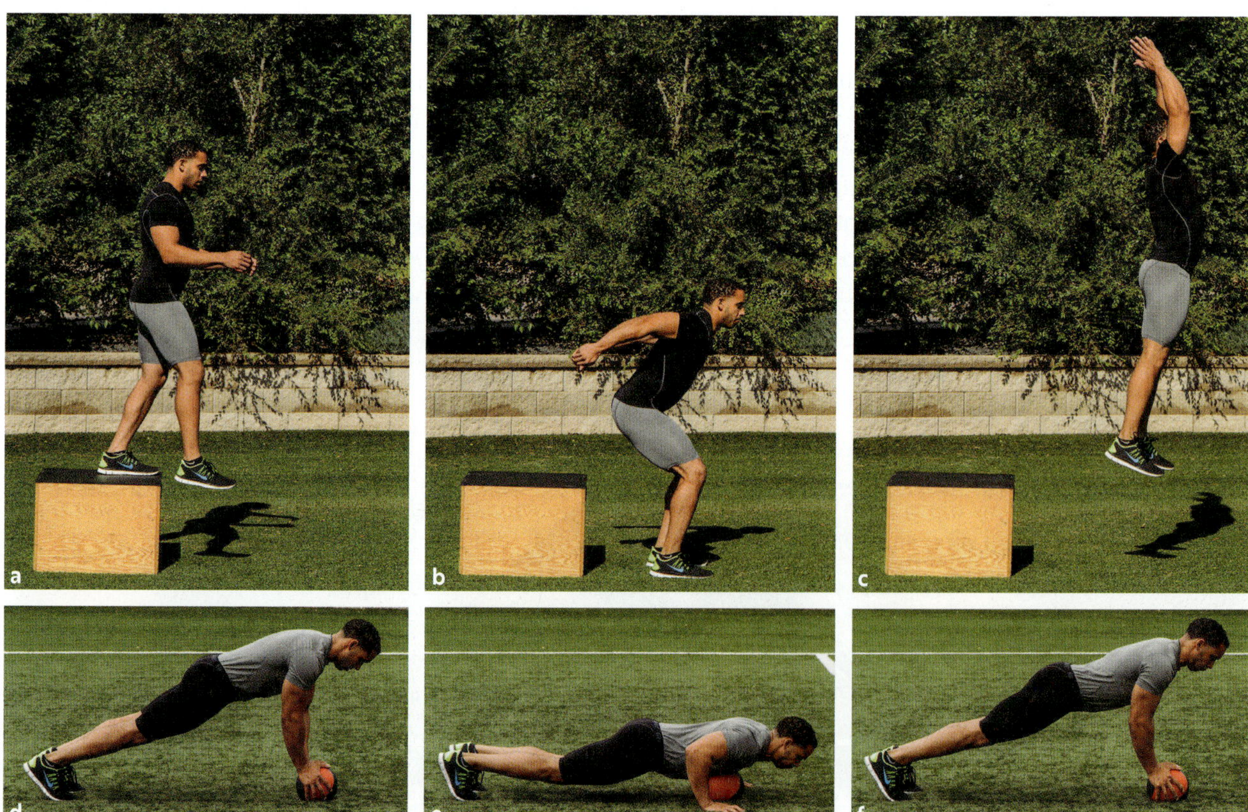

Figure 22.2 Plyometrics. Leg and hip: *(a)* The athlete stands on top of the box, *(b)* jumps off the box onto the floor, and then *(c)* jumps upward and performs arm plyometric. Depth push-up: *(d)* The athlete is in the push-up position with a medicine ball between his hands. *(e)* He lowers himself to the surface, hands on the surface, and then *(f)* pushes up off the surface and into the air, his hands back on the ball.

Kettlebells

Kettlebells are cast-iron balls with handles (see figure 22.3). There are various sizes and weights for kettlebells. Typical exercises can be done while using kettlebells as an additional element. Exercises in which a kettlebell can be incorporated include goblet squats, deadlifts, lunges, rows, cleans, overhead presses, swings, and snatches.

Kettlebell swings are popular. The swing is done with two hands and starts with the kettlebell between the legs on the ground. The athlete picks up the kettlebell by slightly squatting, moving to a more upright position, and swinging it posteriorly between their legs. The kettlebell then swings forward in an upward arc. The arms are kept in extension throughout. The kettlebell will reach eye level, and gravity will bring it back down and eventually between the legs again (see figure 22.4). This cycle is repeated. The swinging of the kettlebell, when done properly, can have a cardiorespiratory fitness component.

Otto and colleagues (2012) researched a weightlifting program versus kettlebell training for improvement in back squat strength and vertical jump. The results found that weight training was better at improving back squat strength and vertical jumping.

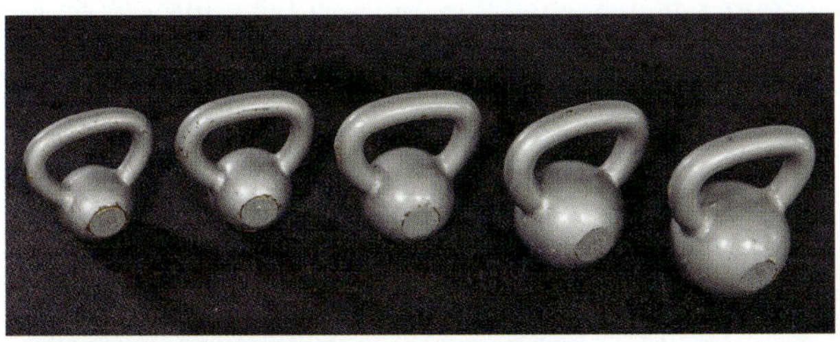

Figure 22.3 Cast-iron kettlebells.

CrossFit

CrossFit is a branded fitness program adopted by fitness gyms across the country. The program began in 2000 and is considered a high-intensity interval program. According to CrossFit (2002-2020), this program is designed to optimize physical competence in cardiorespiratory endurance, stamina, strength, flexibility, power, speed, coordination, agility, balance, and accuracy.

It utilizes functional daily movements performed at a high-intensity level. Typical daily movements might be pushing, squats, overhead reach, twisting, and walking and running. Workouts are designed to mimic everyday movement, especially two-joint movements. Things such as push-ups, squats, pull-ups, overhead press, and kipping are exercises that can be used as part of CrossFit. Each exercise has a high-intensity component and a time frame in which to complete the task. Experienced athletes may have to intensify their workout, and those who are less fit may have to reduce the intensity or repetitions. The CrossFit workout is varied daily, and days of rest are part of programming. Some equipment used in CrossFit are stationary bars, free-weight bars, kettlebells, medicine balls, ladders, rowing machines, biking, boxing, battle ropes, and gymnastics equipment.

CrossFit also has a nutrition program that is part of the training, which includes meat, vegetables,

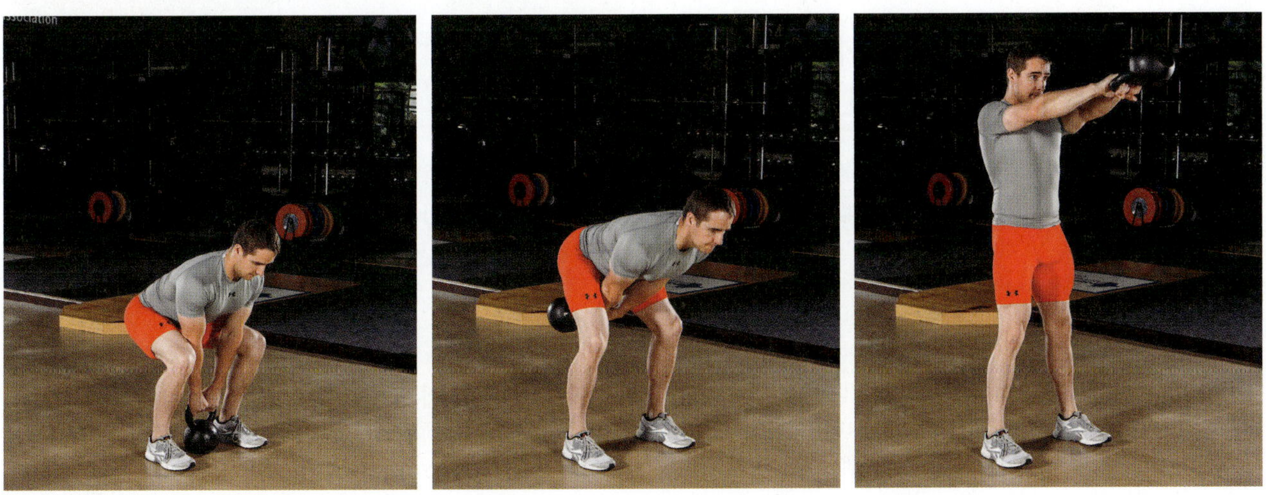

Figure 22.4 Two-arm kettlebell swing.

some fruits, nuts, and seeds, and being low in starches. Sugar is excluded from the CrossFit diet plan (CrossFit 2002-2020). The diet is 30% lean protein, 40% low-glycemic carbohydrates, and 30% fat from whole food (CrossFit 2002-2020).

Battle Ropes

Battle ropes improve aerobic capacity (Antony et al. 2015; Kuklick et al. 2013), upper-body and trunk muscular endurance (Bornath and Kenno 2022), and lower-body power (Antony et al. 2015). The length of a battle rope is up to the user, but they come in lengths from 10 to 50 feet (3-5 m). The thickness of the rope varies from 1.5 inches (4 cm) to 2.5 inches (6 cm). The weight of the rope will vary depending on the length and thickness of the rope.

The rope is doubled over and then tied to a stationary object with the athlete using both ends of the rope. Exercises that can be performed include a double-arm wave, side-to-side wave, alternating waves, in-out waves, and hip toss. The double-arm wave is accomplished with the athlete standing and waving the ropes in both hands synchronized, rapidly moving the hands from the thighs to the chest. The side-to-side wave occurs with the athlete standing and waving the ropes from side to side at waist level. Alternating waves are like double-arm waves, but instead of synchronized arms, the arms alternate, left, right, left, right. In-out waves occur when both elbows abduct then adduct in repetition. A hip toss is when the hands are together, the hips alternatively rotating left and right with the ropes slamming to the floor each time.

STRETCHING TO IMPROVE JOINT FLEXIBILITY

Stretching lengthens tissue that has been shortened from lack of use, such as when an athlete is immobilized in a cast. Stretching should be performed if range of motion is limited because of soft-tissue tightness around a joint. A stretch should not produce pain; instead, it should be comfortable. Stretching should be done before and after heavy athletic activity, but it is necessary to perform a light warm-up (aerobic activity) before stretching—stretching a cold muscle might lead to injury.

There are four types of stretches. The first is **static stretching**—the muscle is isolated, stretched, and held in the stretch for approximately 15 to 30 seconds. Static stretching develops flexibility; it should be done 3 times in each exercise session for 30 seconds at a time, addressing each muscle. Static stretching should be done after a light warm-up. The second type is **ballistic stretching**. Ballistic stretching is when a specific muscle is isolated and quickly stretched and relaxed repetitively, as though the athlete is bouncing. This form of stretching is not recommended because it can aggravate an existing injury or cause a new injury. **Dynamic stretching**, the third form, is done by simply moving a limb or part of the body through its range of motion. An example of dynamic stretching is swinging the leg forward and backward to stretch the hip. Proprioceptive neuromuscular facilitation stretching (PNF) involves taking the muscle actively to its end point, holding it there for 10 seconds, and then contracting it against resistance; this series is repeated (Haff and Triplett 2016). This is typically a partner stretch. See figure 22.5 for an example of a PNF stretch for the hamstring.

If the AT is going to individualize a warm-up program to increase flexibility, a baseline has to be established. The range of motion can be measured by using a goniometer. Record an individual's range of motion at various major joints; monitor the range of motion as the stretching and flexibility program is utilized. Some people will need extra stretching in particular areas based on their specific needs. These factors affect how much flexibility a particular joint will be able to obtain (Haff and Triplett 2016):

- Joint structure and type
- Age
- Sex
- Muscle tissue
- Stretch tolerance
- Resistance training
- Muscle size
- Activity level

A ball-and-socket joint such as the shoulder will have greater motion than a hinge joint such as a knee. As a person ages, they lose range of motion. For example, a person may develop arthritis in

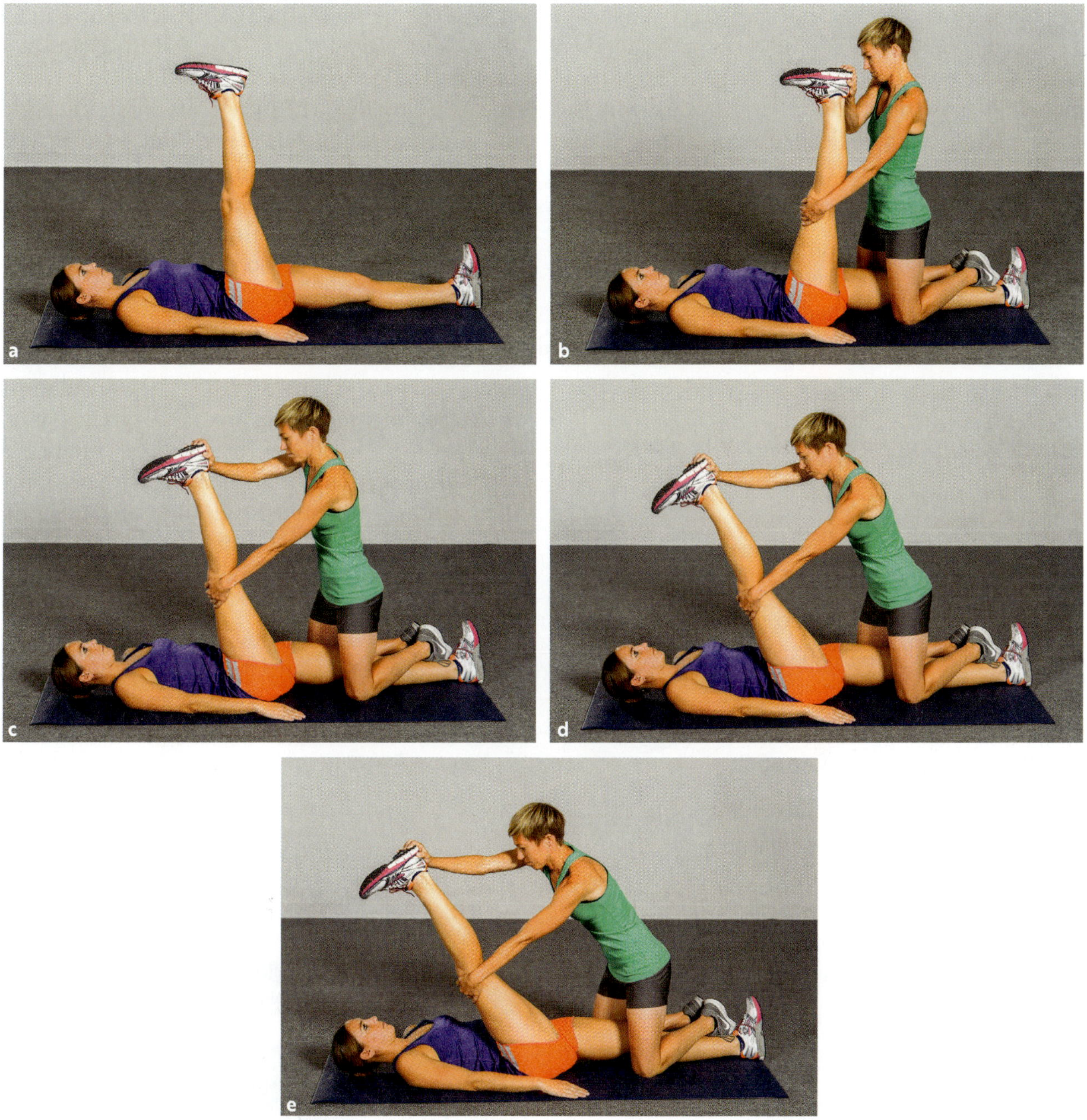

Figure 22.5 Hamstring PNF stretch: *(a)* Starting position; *(b)* partner and subject hand and leg positions; *(c)* passive prestretch of the hamstrings during hold-relax PNF hamstring stretch; *(d)* isometric action during hold-relax PNF hamstring stretch; *(e)* increased ROM during passive stretch of hold-relax PNF hamstring stretch.

a joint, which decreases the range that can be obtained at that joint. Females tend to be more flexible based on differences in the joint (Haff and Triplett 2016). Tissues in the body can contribute to a person's range of motion. If a tissue has been injured, for example, it may no longer have the same elasticity. Stretch tolerance is one's ability to tolerate the discomfort associated with stretching a muscle group (Haff and Triplett 2016). Those that have good stretch tolerance tend to have greater range of motion (Haff and Triplett 2016). When a person does resistance training, it is important to develop both the anterior and posterior muscle groups equally; failure to do so will decrease one's range of motion. Bulky muscles can impede an athlete's range of motion. Muscle size versus range of motion needs to be considered based on the need of the sport (Haff and Triplett 2016). An individual who is active tends to be more flexible than a person who is sedentary. Follow these guidelines to prepare a stretching program (Johnson 2012):

1. Determine the current range of motion at each joint for the area.
2. What is their baseline?
3. What is the objective?
4. What method of stretching is best for the objective?
5. Does the patient have any contraindications?
6. Set goals for each area.
7. Create a plan.
8. Reassess and document daily stretching.

There may be people who should not stretch. These are the contraindications to stretching (Johnson 2012):

- An acute injury or blood clot
- Those at risk of fracture
- Cancer
- When stretching causes pain
- Inflammatory conditions
- If stretching impairs the progress of another treatment
- An unstable joint that increasing flexibility would contribute to more instability
- If stretching would delay the healing process

Warm-Up

Warm-ups are important before physical activity. A warm-up prevents injuries, increases blood flow, reduces pain, and increases flexibility at a joint. The warm-up should be designed to gradually increase the body movement to the intensity the athlete will encounter during practice or an event. Even though the warm-up adds to the amount of time an individual is physically active, it is important for the athlete's body, so it should be taken seriously.

When designing a warm-up, the AT must determine the type of activity. The warm-up should be specifically designed to meet the needs of the athlete and be sport-specific. The warm-up should be 10 to 20 minutes long; less than that does not provide the necessary effects for the body (Haff and Triplett 2016). The two forms of warm-up are static and dynamic. Static stretching is when the individual takes a joint through a stretch with a hold for no longer than 30 seconds. Static stretching has not shown to enhance an athlete's performance before physical activity, so dynamic stretching has increased in popularity.

Dynamic stretching takes the athlete through an active range of motion similar to what the athlete will experience during exercise. The athlete starts with easy warm-up exercises and progresses in intensity. An example of dynamic stretching for a football player may be to do jumping jacks, jogging and then touching the ground, alternating leg swings across body, and large arm swings similar to those that they would be doing during a football game. These dynamic stretches can be made specific to the position and sport. A sport-specific dynamic stretch routine for a long jumper could include high knees, butt kicks, leg swings, squats, hip rotation, and alternating arm circles.

Figures 22.6 through 22.16 show dynamic warm-up stretches.

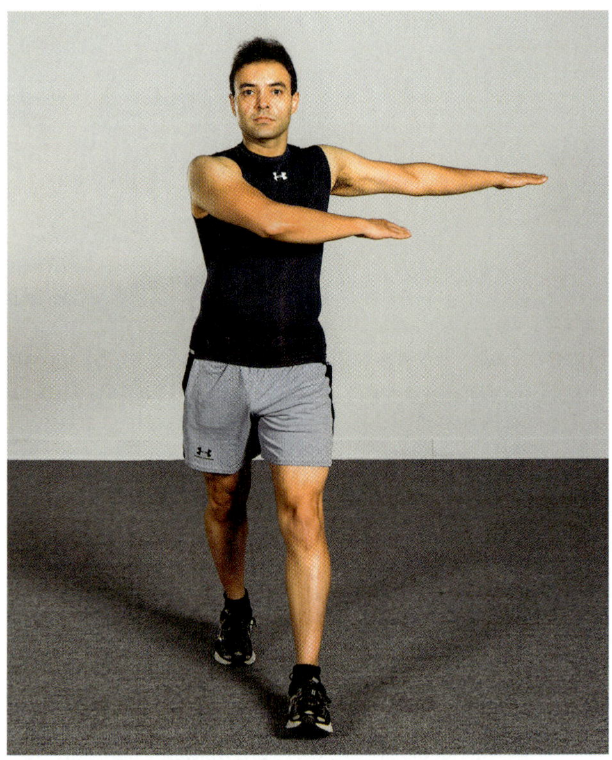

Figure 22.6 Arm swings.

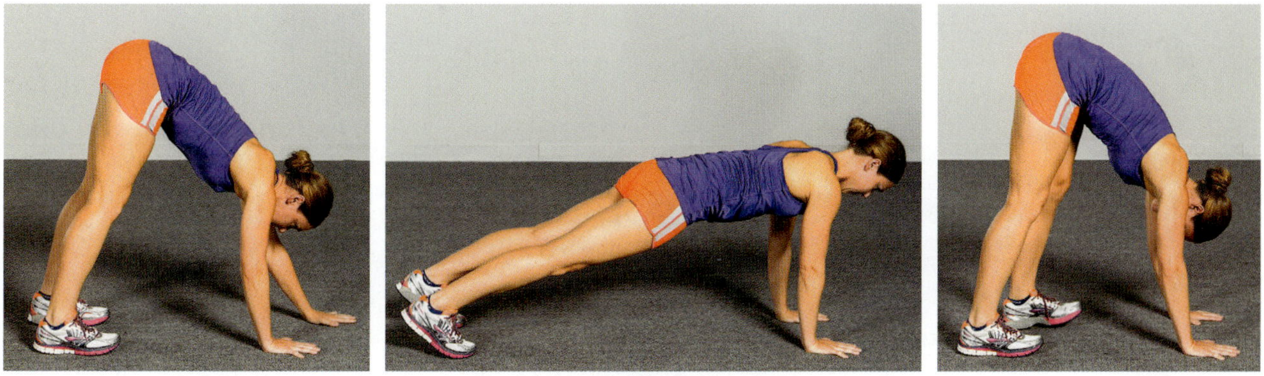

Figure 22.7 Inchworm.

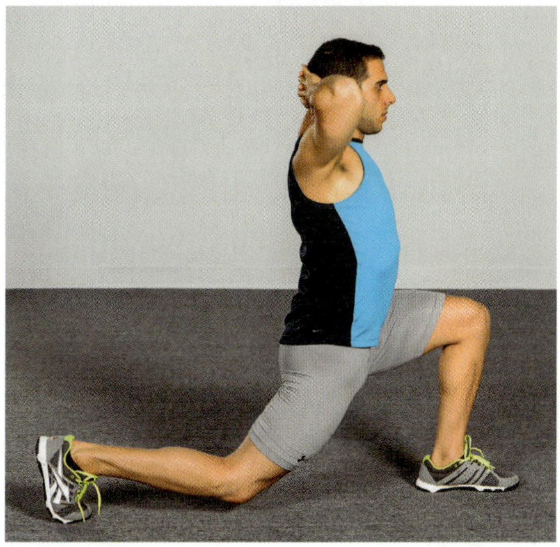

Figure 22.8 Lunge walk.

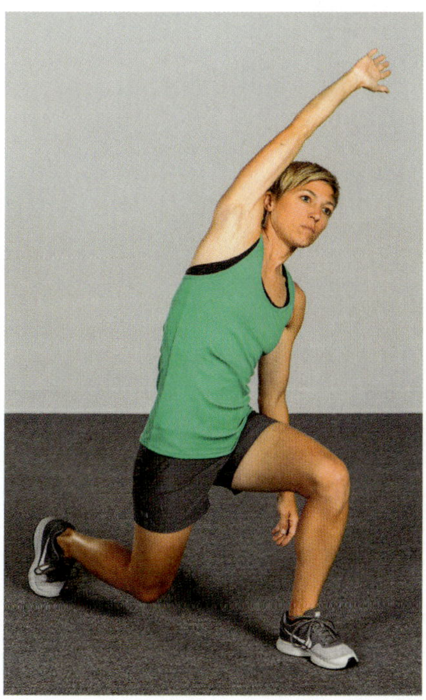

Figure 22.9 Lunge with overhead side reach.

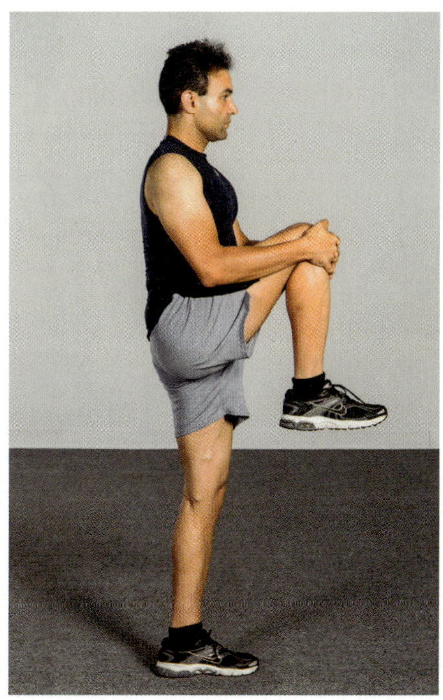

Figure 22.10 Walking knee lift.

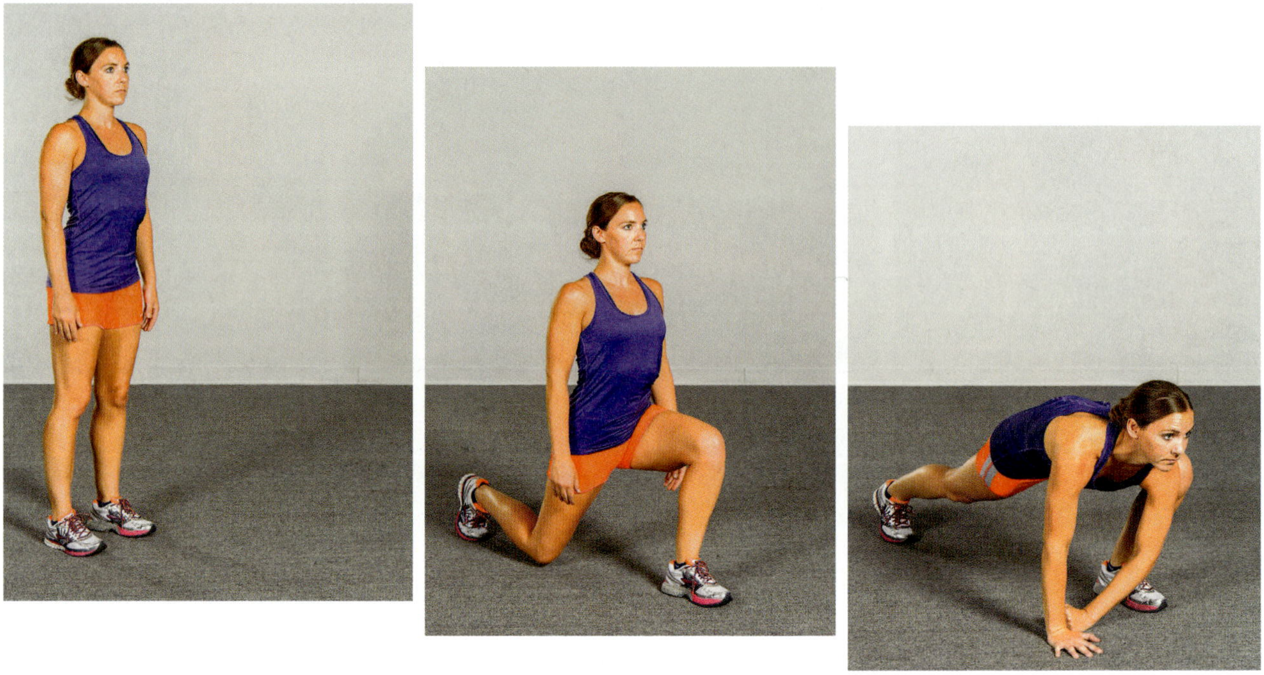

Figure 22.11 Forward lunge with elbow to instep.

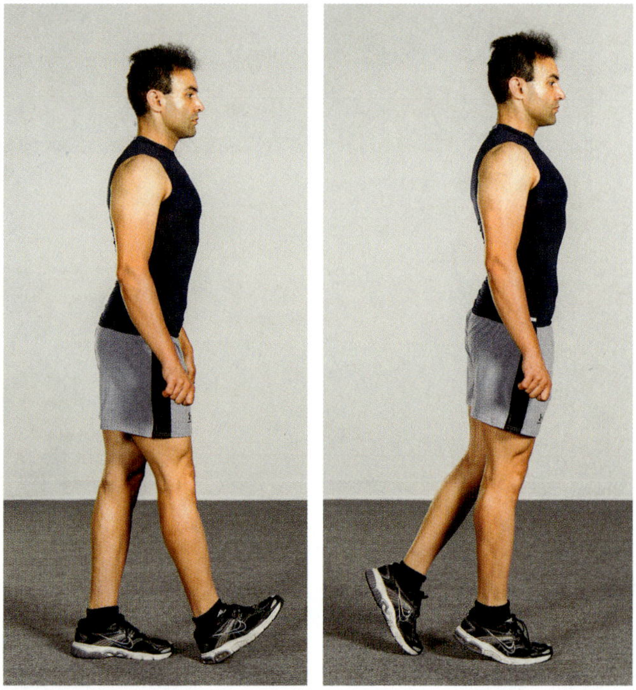

Figure 22.12 Heel-to-toe walk.

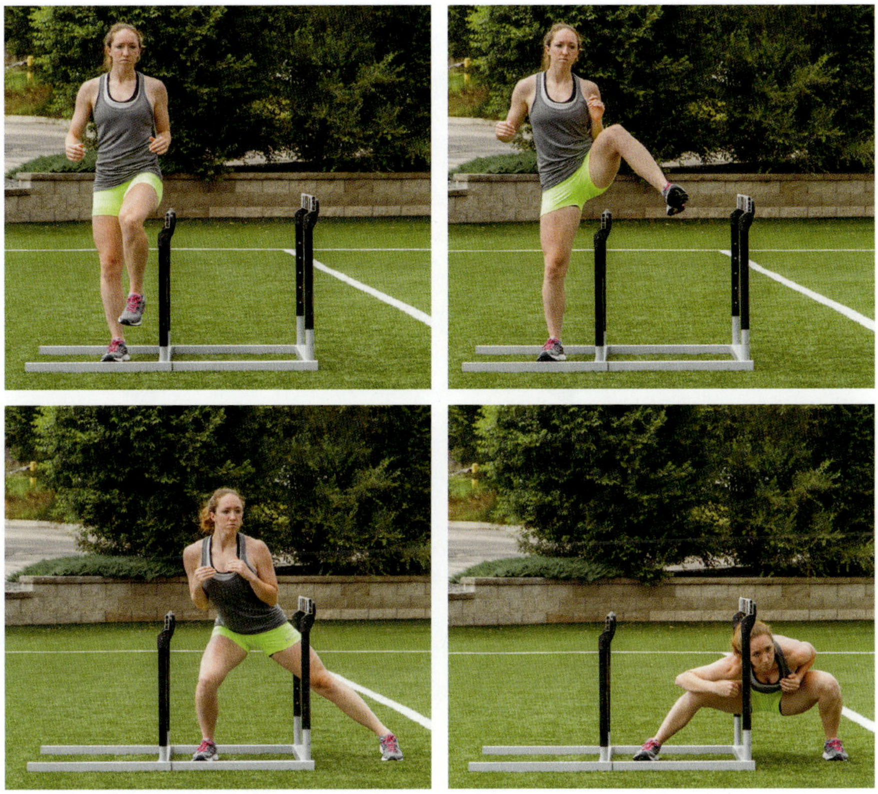

Figure 22.13 Walking over and under.

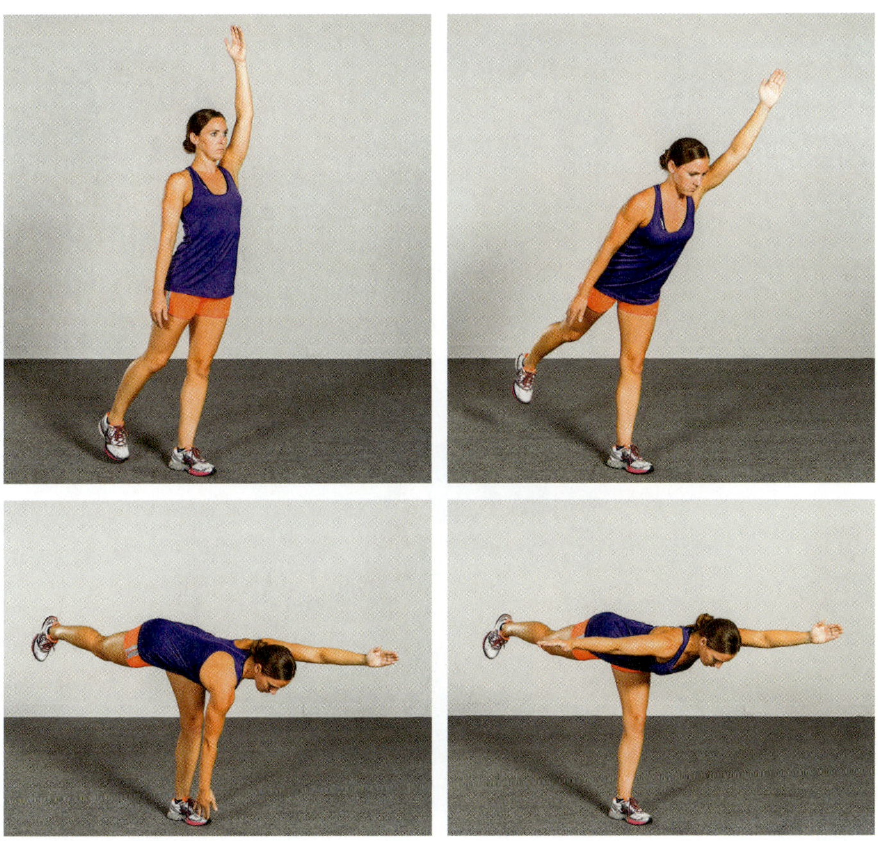

Figure 22.14 Inverted hamstring stretch.

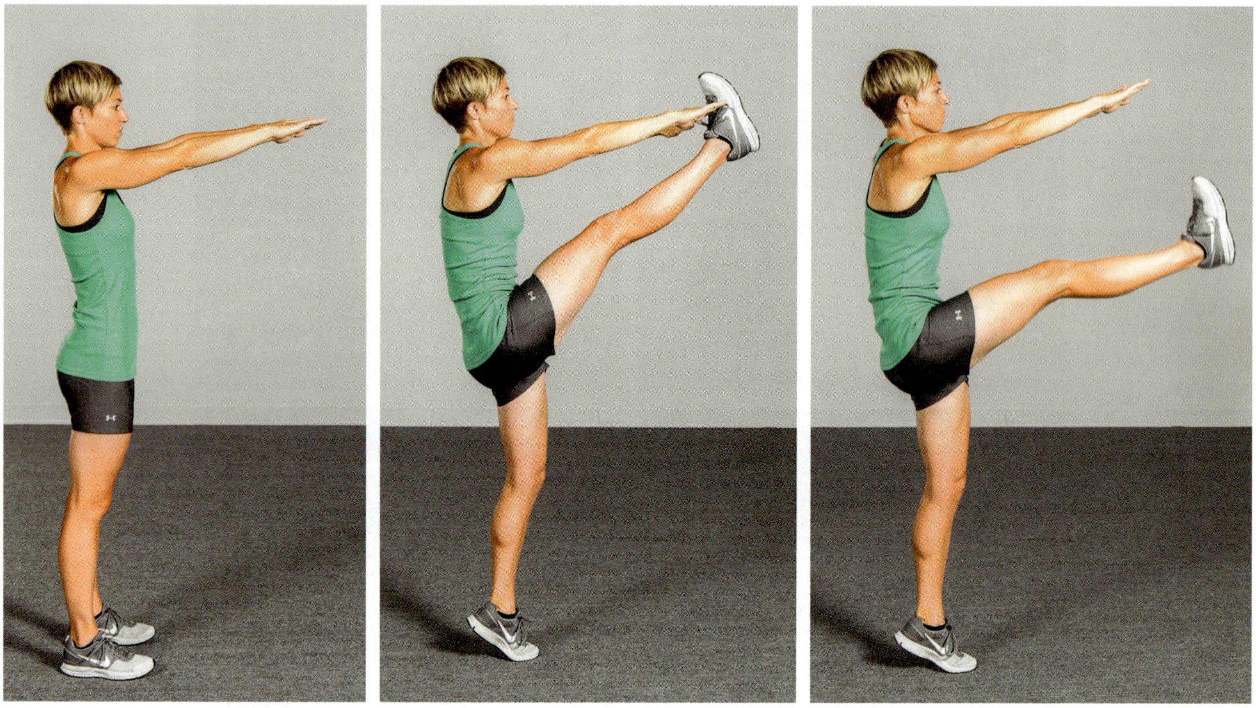

Figure 22.15 Straight-leg march.

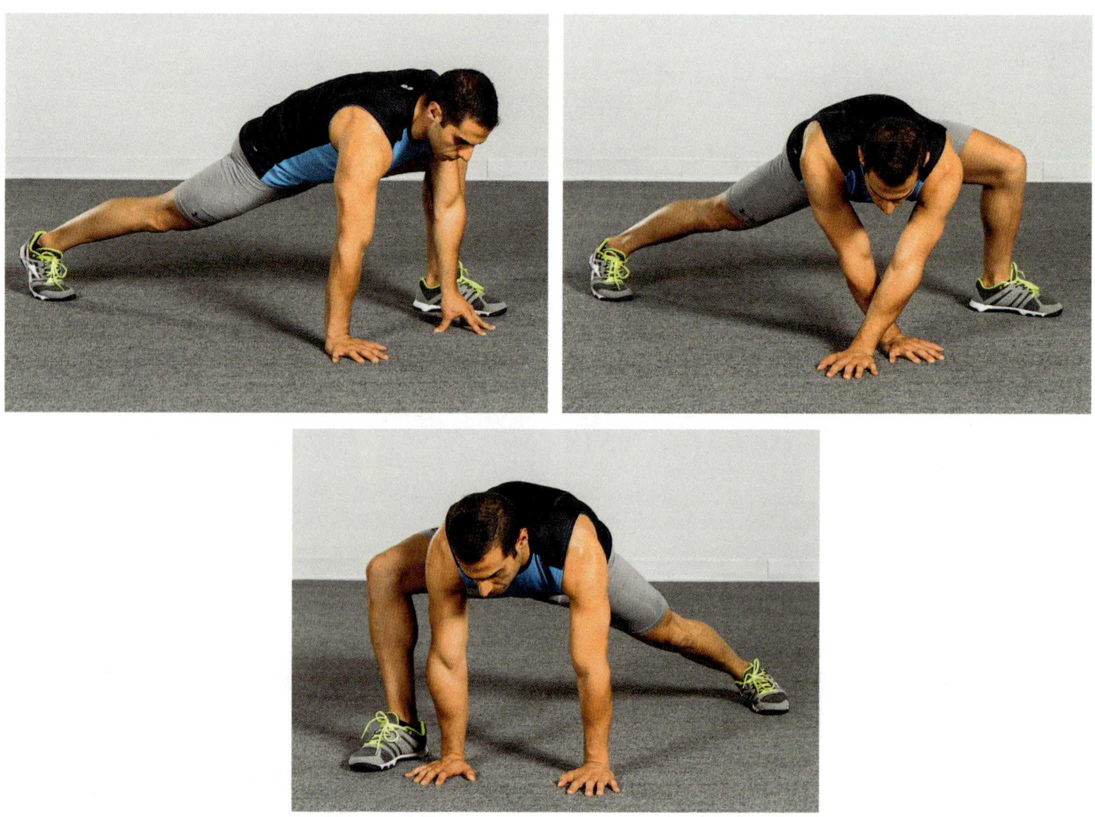

Figure 22.16 Spiderman crawl.

Stretching a body segment to gain range of motion can be done in one of two ways: active or passive. Active stretching is when the athlete applies the force to their body. Passive stretching is when someone else applies the force to the athlete's body.

Cool-Down

The cool-down should be utilized to reduce the heart rate, remove lactic acid buildup, and increase muscle elasticity while the muscles are warm. The dynamic cool-down is the reverse of the warm-up, with higher intensity leading to lower intensity. Static cool-down can be used as long as the stretch is no longer than a 30-second hold (Cleveland Clinic 2020). Figures 22.17 through 22.36 are static stretches that can be used in the cool-down phase.

NECK

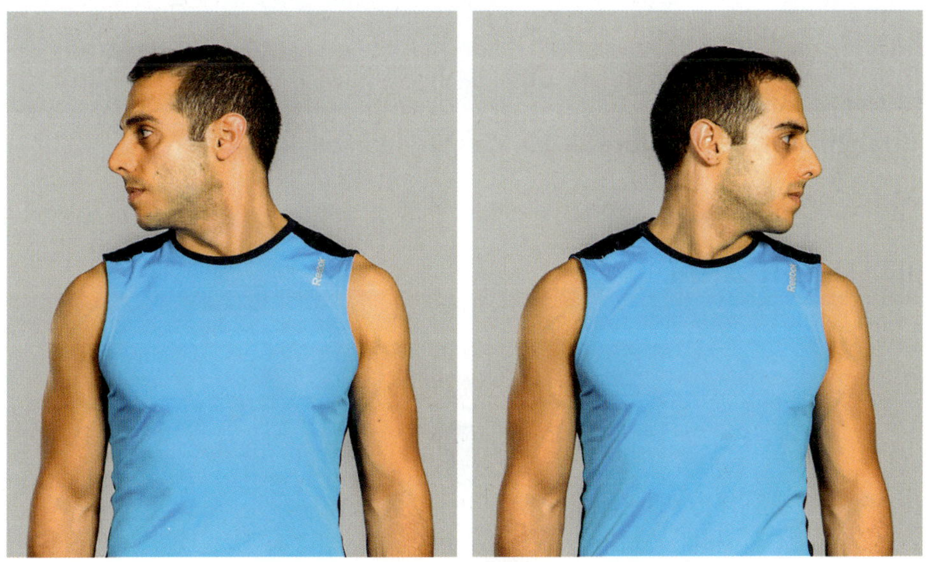

Figure 22.17 Look right and left.

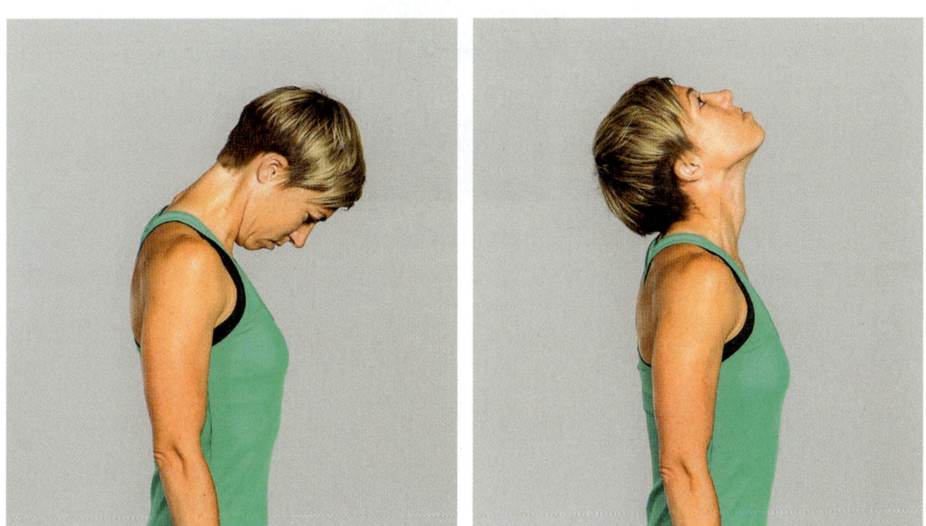

Figure 22.18 Flexion and extension.

SHOULDERS AND CHEST

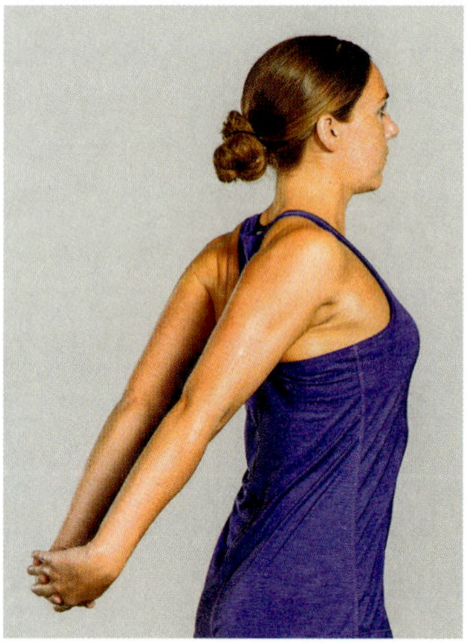

Figure 22.19 Straight arms behind back.

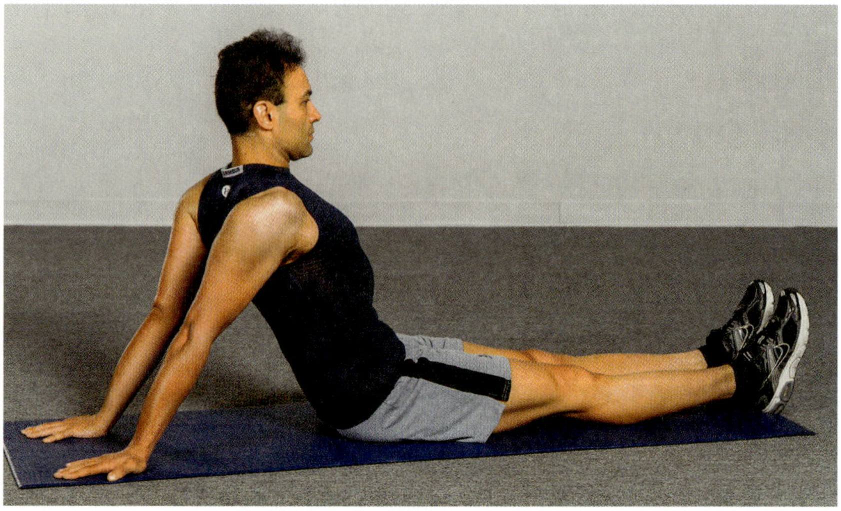

Figure 22.20 Seated lean back.

POSTERIOR UPPER ARM

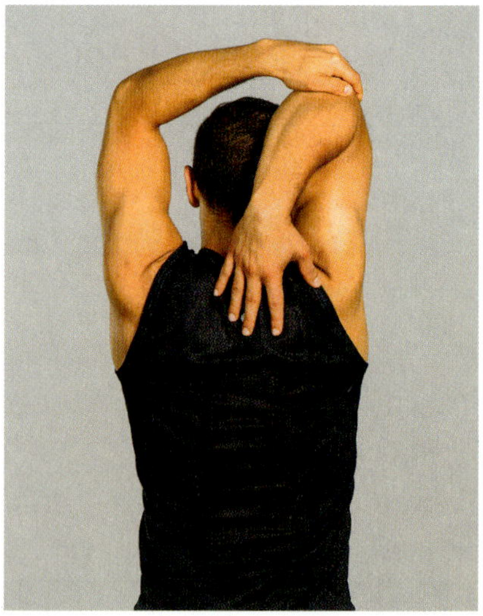

Figure 22.21 Behind-the-neck stretch.

UPPER BACK

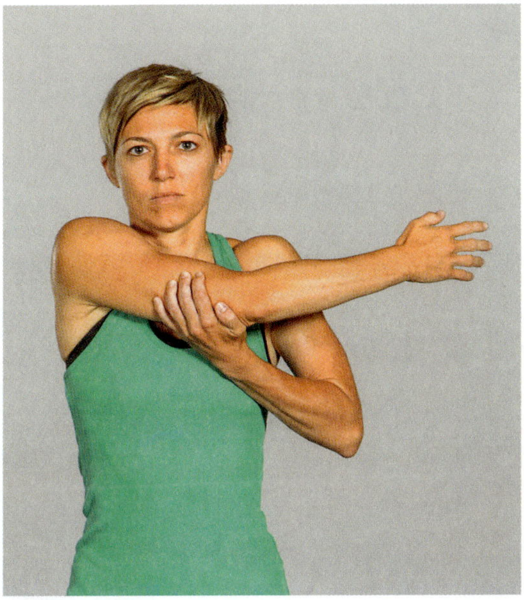

Figure 22.22 Cross arm in front of chest.

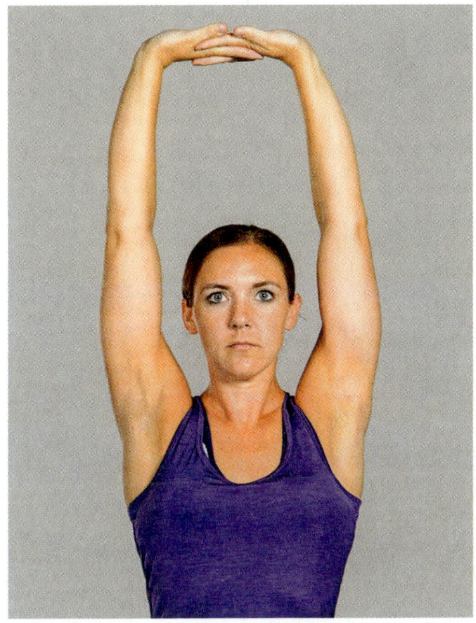

Figure 22.23 Arms straight up above head (pillar).

LOWER BACK

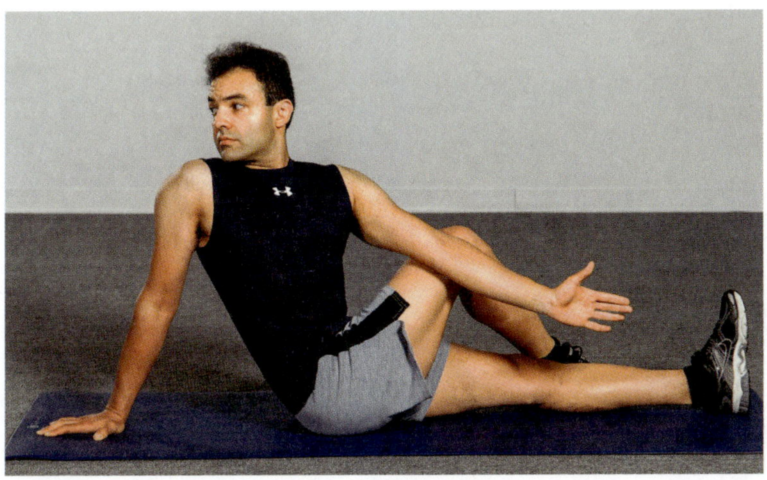

Figure 22.24 Spinal twist (pretzel).

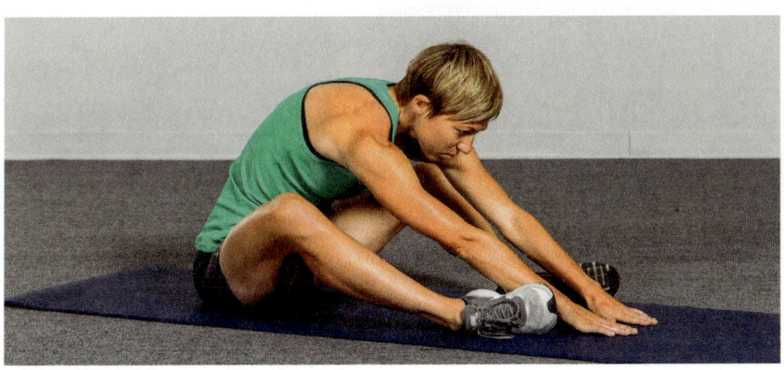

Figure 22.25 Semi-leg straddle.

HIPS

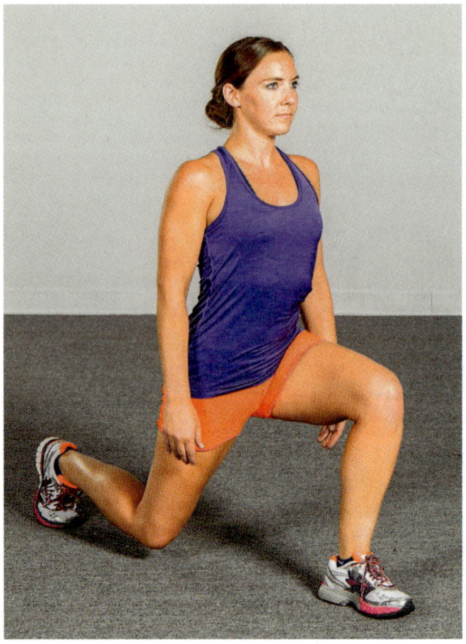

Figure 22.26 Forward lunge (fencer).

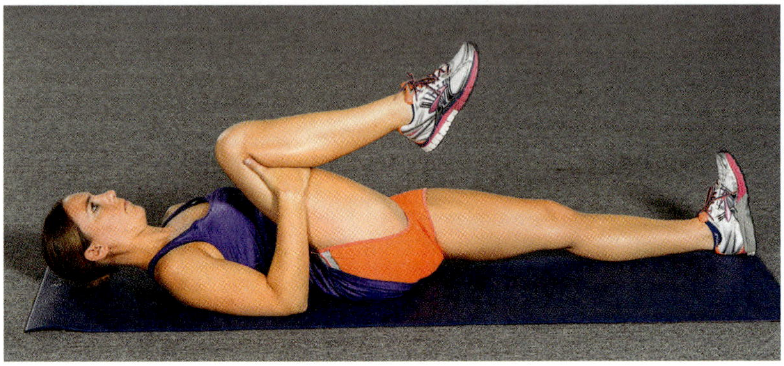

Figure 22.27 Supine knee flex.

TORSO

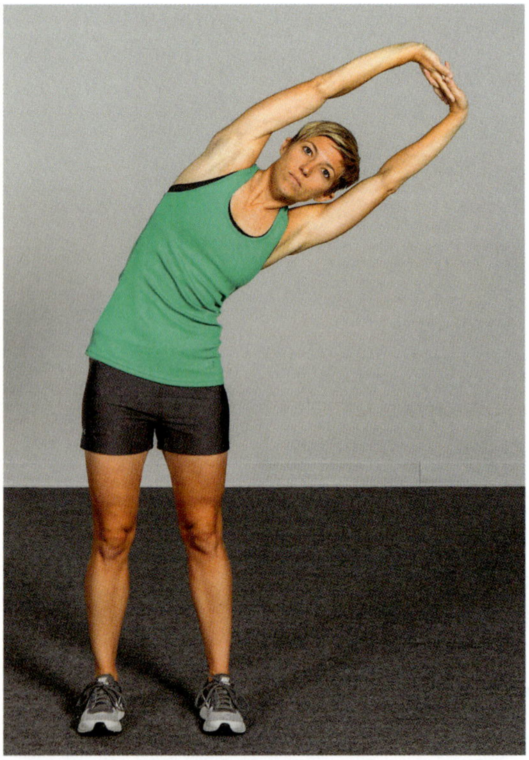

Figure 22.28 Side bend with straight arms.

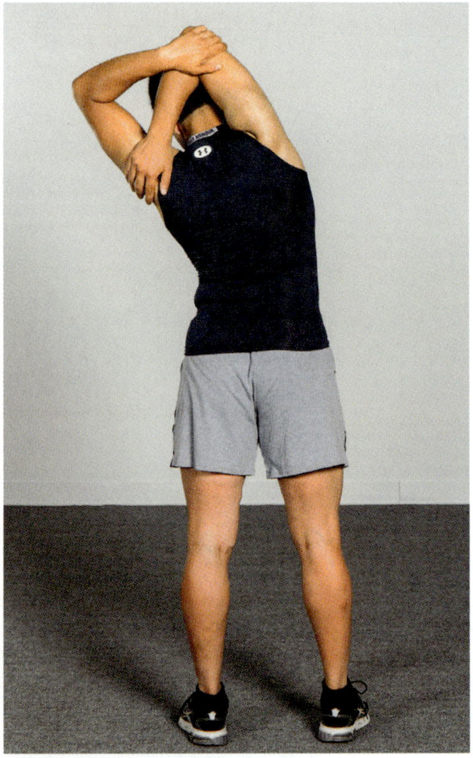

Figure 22.29 Side bend with bent arms.

THIGH

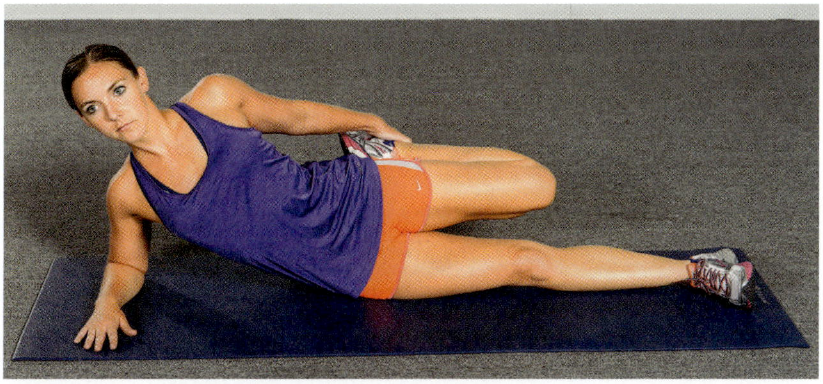

Figure 22.30 Side quadriceps stretch.

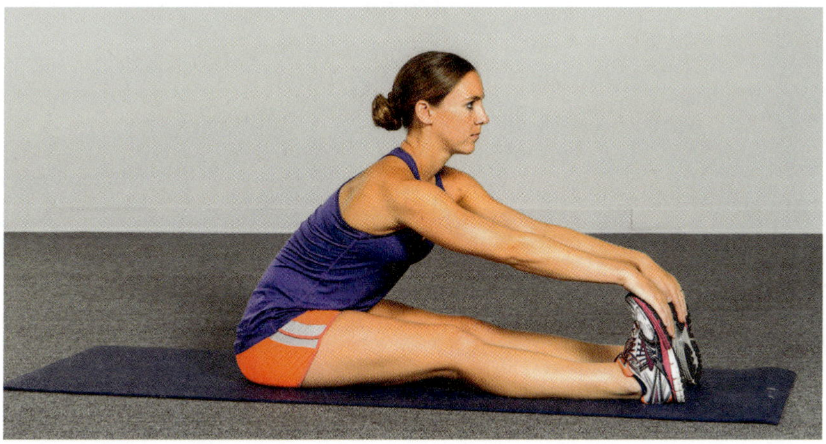

Figure 22.31 Sitting toe stretch.

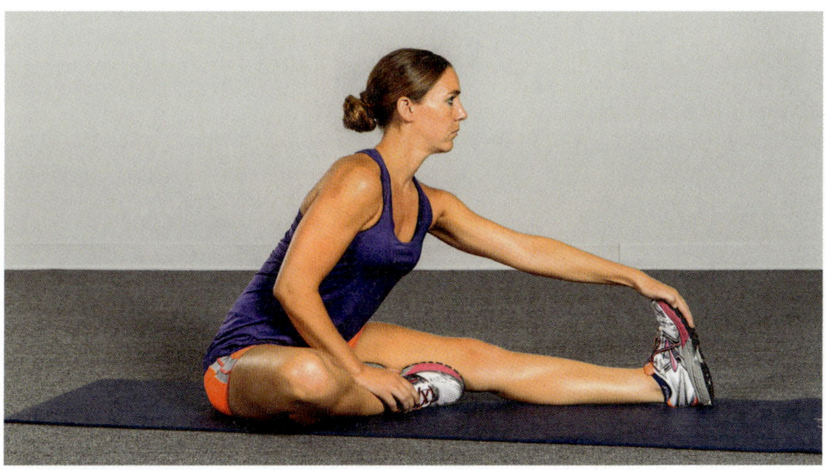

Figure 22.32 Figure four stretch (semi-straddle).

GROIN

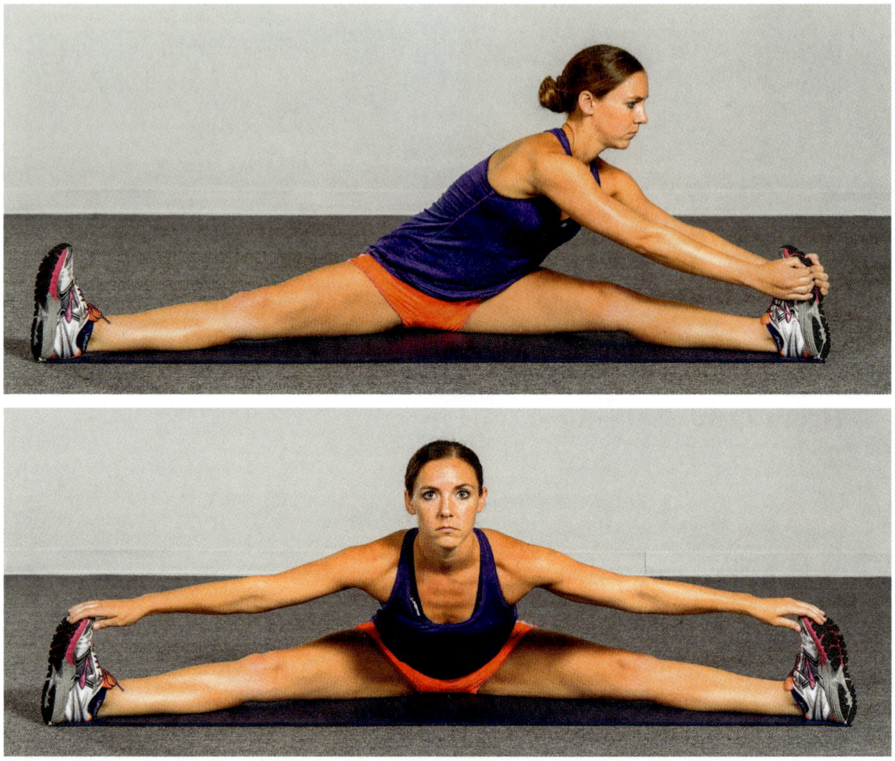

Figure 22.33 Straddle.

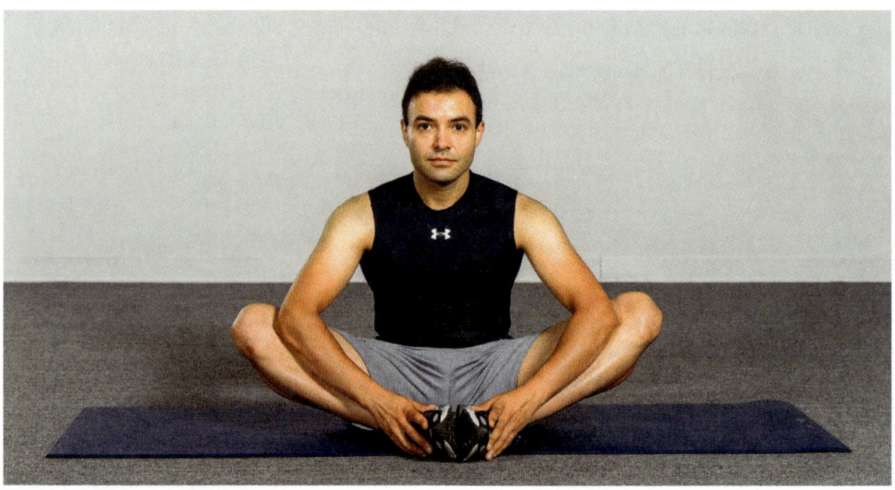

Figure 22.34 Butterfly.

CALF

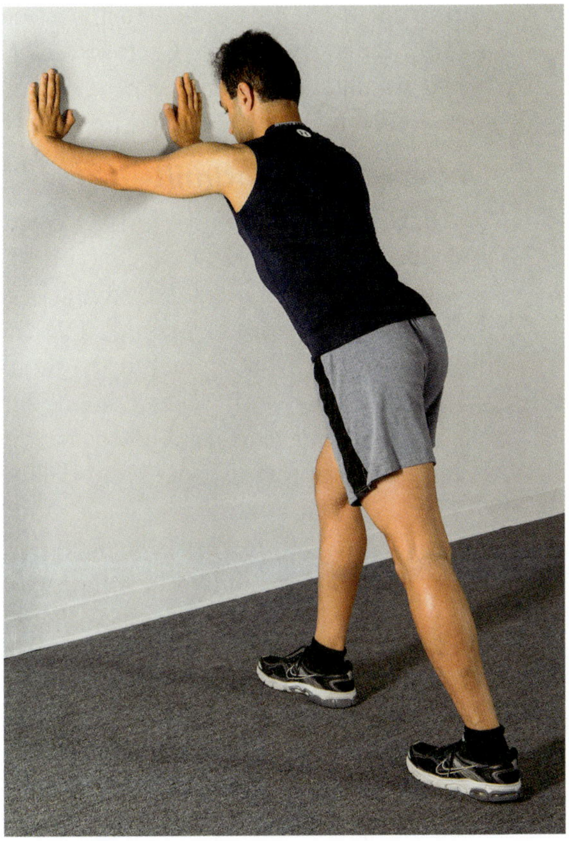

Figure 22.35 Wall stretch.

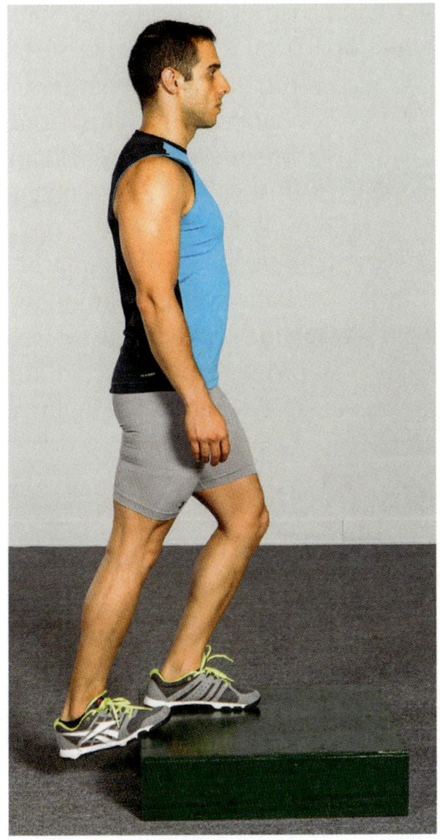

Figure 22.36 Step stretch.

EXERCISES FOR RECONDITIONING MUSCLES

Because there are many exercises for injuries, the AT and the athlete need to decide which exercises to perform. Although it is beyond the scope of this text to provide a comprehensive list of exercises, we provide information about basic exercises for reconditioning athletes following an injury and helping them develop general strength and mobility.

Reconditioning Techniques for the Lower Extremity

When rehabilitating the lower quarter, strengthening and establishing proprioception are major concerns. Balancing activities such as working on wobble boards and stork standing are excellent for regaining proprioception, even if the athlete can tolerate only partial weight bearing (see figure 22.37).

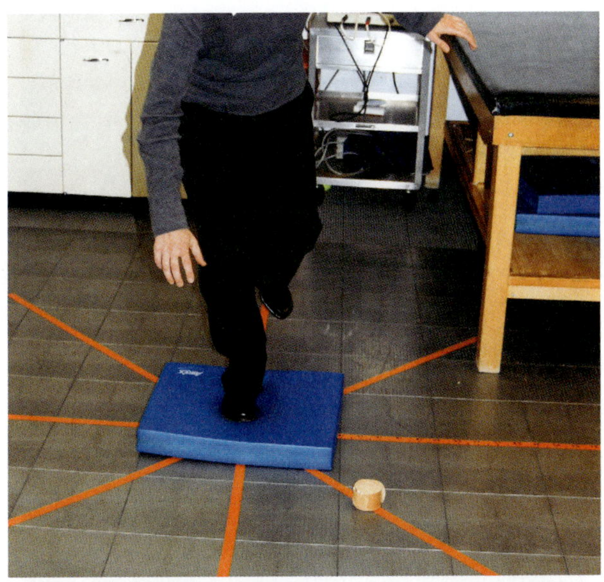

Figure 22.37 Balance exercise. The patient can initially stand still and then progress to reaching for objects placed on each line of the floor pattern.

Photo: Lorin A. Cartwright.

Balance exercises should be progressed carefully. Typically, an AT will have an injured athlete stand with a wide base of support (legs spread to shoulder-width apart) on a firm, stable surface. If the athlete is successful, the AT will progress them to a narrow base of support (feet close together) and then to an unstable surface such as a foam pad. Once successful in this position, the athlete can progress to standing on one leg using a stable and then an unstable surface. More dynamic balance exercises can be used afterward, meaning the athlete will begin moving their body while maintaining balance. Failure to properly progress an athlete's balance can result in a reinjury. See figure 22.37 for an example of a balance exercise progression.

Antigravity Treadmill

The antigravity treadmill requires the athlete to wear special shorts that connect to the air bladder of the machine. The air bladder seals and fills with air (see figure 22.38). The treadmill can be set to relieve up to 100% of the athlete's body weight. It can also be set for a particular speed (forward or backward) and an incline.

An antigravity treadmill allows an athlete who is rehabilitating their lower extremity to take a percentage of their body weight off that limb during a run or walk. With less pressure on the extremity, the athlete can focus on improving their gait, improving their fitness, increasing strength, and gaining range of motion. Clear panels all around the treadmill allow the AT to observe the gait and make recommendations based on observations.

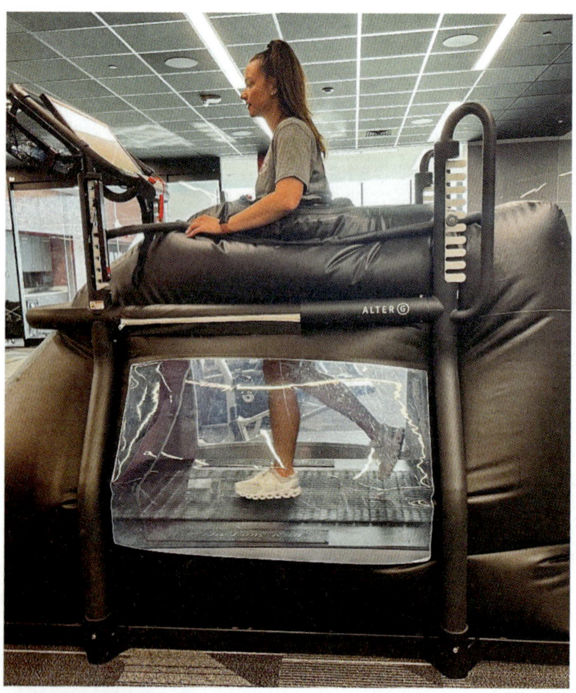

Figure 22.38 Antigravity treadmill.
Photo: Timothy Rood.

Underwater Treadmill

The underwater treadmill can be a built-in (like a pool) or portable model that sits on the floor. The treadmill allows the athlete to maintain their fitness level if they have been injured. The treadmill is filled with water from an inch up to shoulder level. Buoyancy of the body takes the pressure off the injured body part. This helps alleviate pain and joint stress while improving fitness and balance.

The user can control the speed and elevation of the treadmill to increase the workout intensity. Some underwater treadmills offer water jets to increase the resistance during a workout. Another feature is a massage therapy wand that can target certain muscles for therapy. The AT can view gait patterns, work on balance, and make corrections while the athlete is running or walking.

The Foot, Ankle, and Lower Leg

Rehabilitation procedures of the foot, ankle, and lower leg involve reestablishing flexibility and strength with active range-of-motion activities such as using a wobble board or calf stretches (see figure 22.39*a-b*) and writing the ABCs with the foot while it is hanging off the end of a table. Strength can be regained by using elastic bands while resistance is applied as the athlete inverts, everts, plantar flexes, and dorsiflexes his foot (see figure 22.39*c-f*). If another person is not available, the bands can be made into loops and securely fastened around hooks mounted on the floor, wall, table leg, or table edge. These exercises are excellent for many ankle sprains and strains.

Understanding Diversity

In Middle Eastern culture, showing the sole of the foot is considered rude and bad manners (Commisceo Global 2022). Crossing one's legs so others can see the sole is not appropriate.

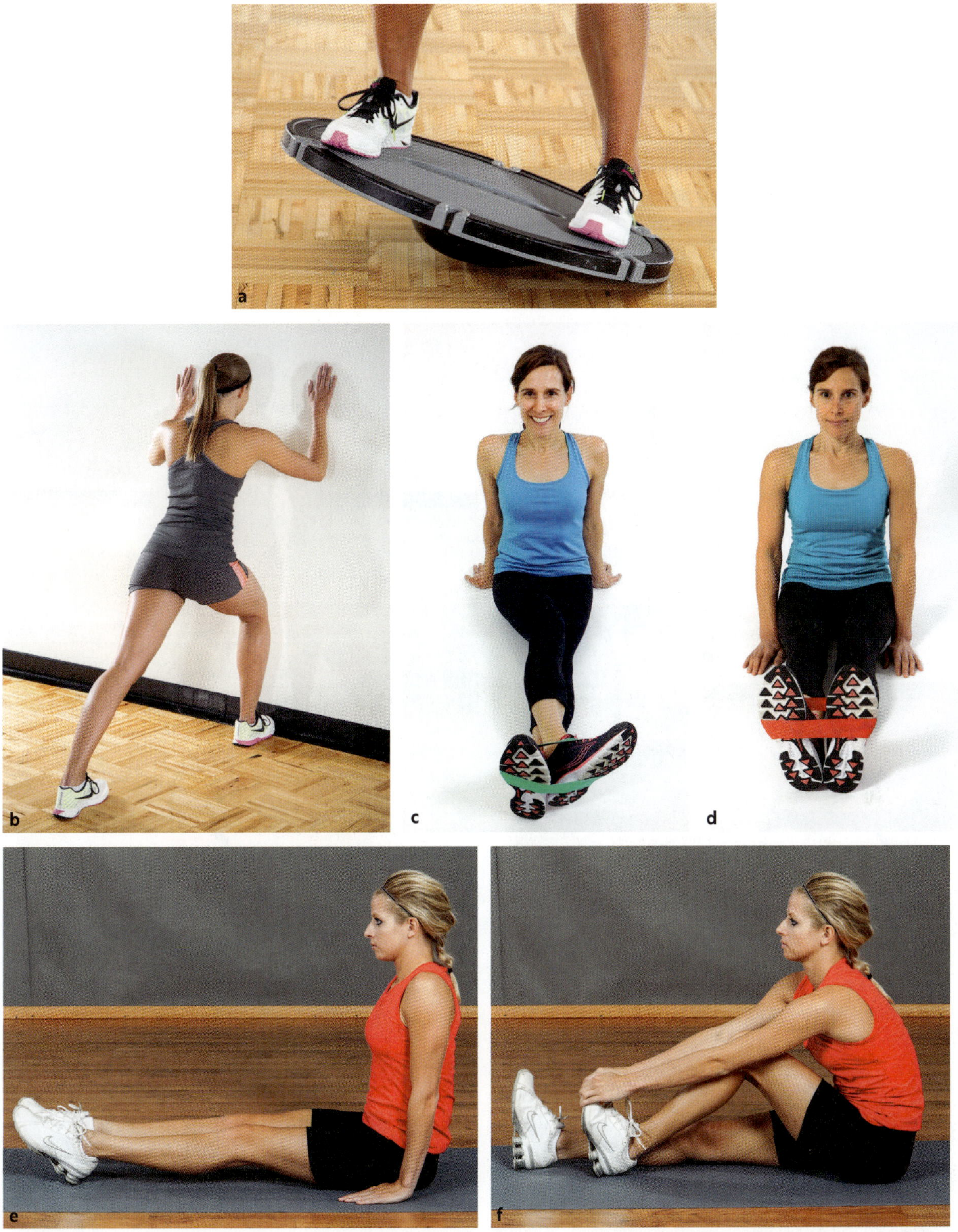

Figure 22.39 *(a)* Balance activities and wobble boards are helpful for regaining normal proprioception. *(b)* Calf stretches. Ankle strength can be improved using resistive tubing while the athlete moves the ankle into *(c)* inversion, *(d)* eversion, *(e)* plantar flexion, and *(f)* dorsiflexion.

The Knee, Hip, and Pelvis

To improve flexibility of the muscular structures around the knee, the athlete should perform static stretching of the involved muscle groups, specifically the quadriceps, groin, and hamstrings (see figure 22.40*a-c*). These stretching exercises are especially helpful for improving range of motion. The knee and hip musculature can be strengthened initially by using the weight of the limb itself with straight-leg raises (figure 22.40*d*) and later progressing to resistive exercise tubing (see figure 22.41*a-b*). Isotonic exercises with a knee and thigh machine can be done as well as forward lunges and wall squats (see figure 22.41*c-f*). Beginning with straight-leg raises helps to develop basic strength for athletes who are weak. As soon as possible, however, the athlete should perform strengthening exercises in a standing position (for example, with resistive tubing).

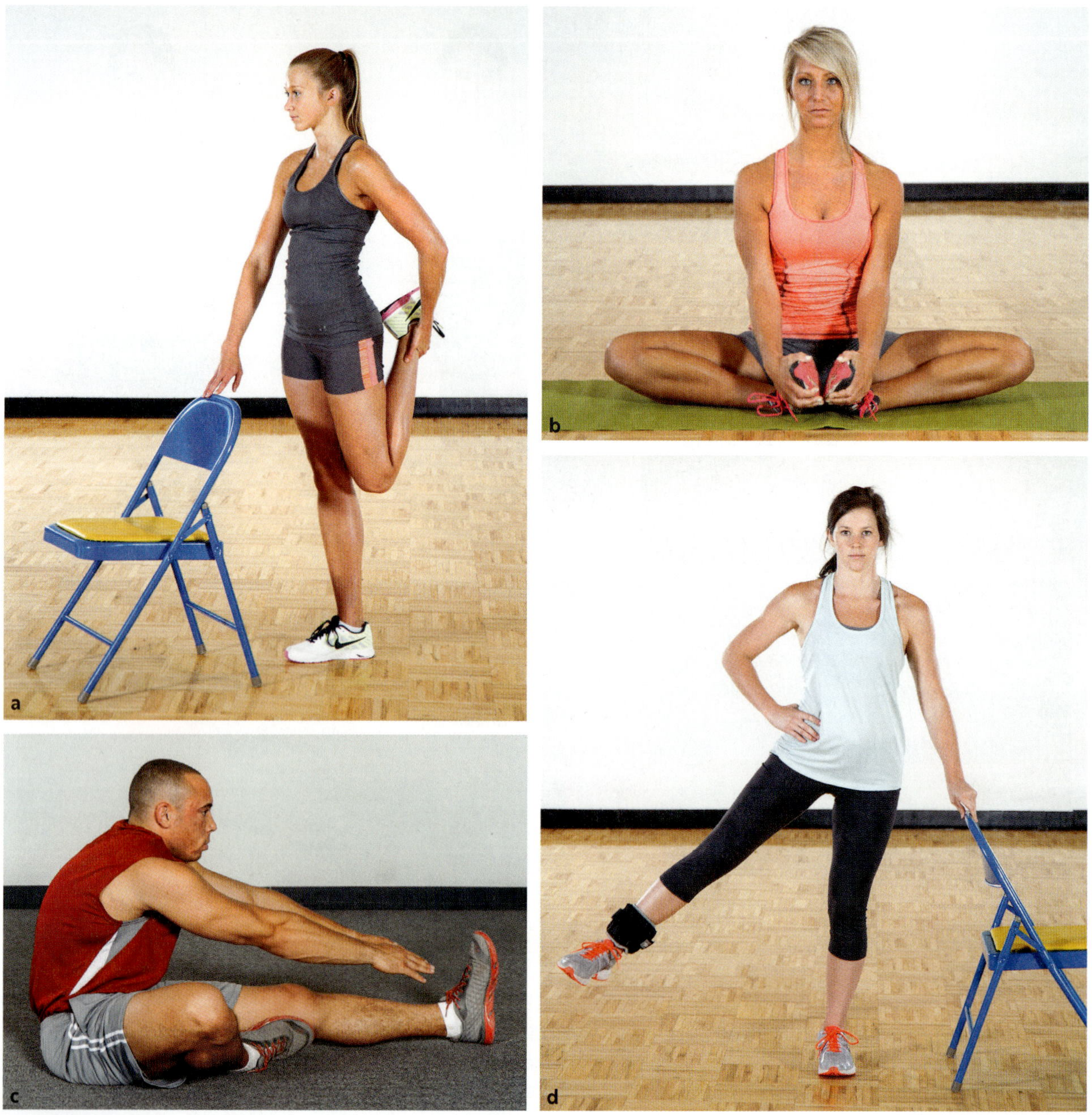

Figure 22.40 *(a)* Quadriceps, *(b)* groin, and *(c)* hamstring stretches. *(d)* Straight-leg raises performed against body weight or while lying down to strengthen the hip and knee.

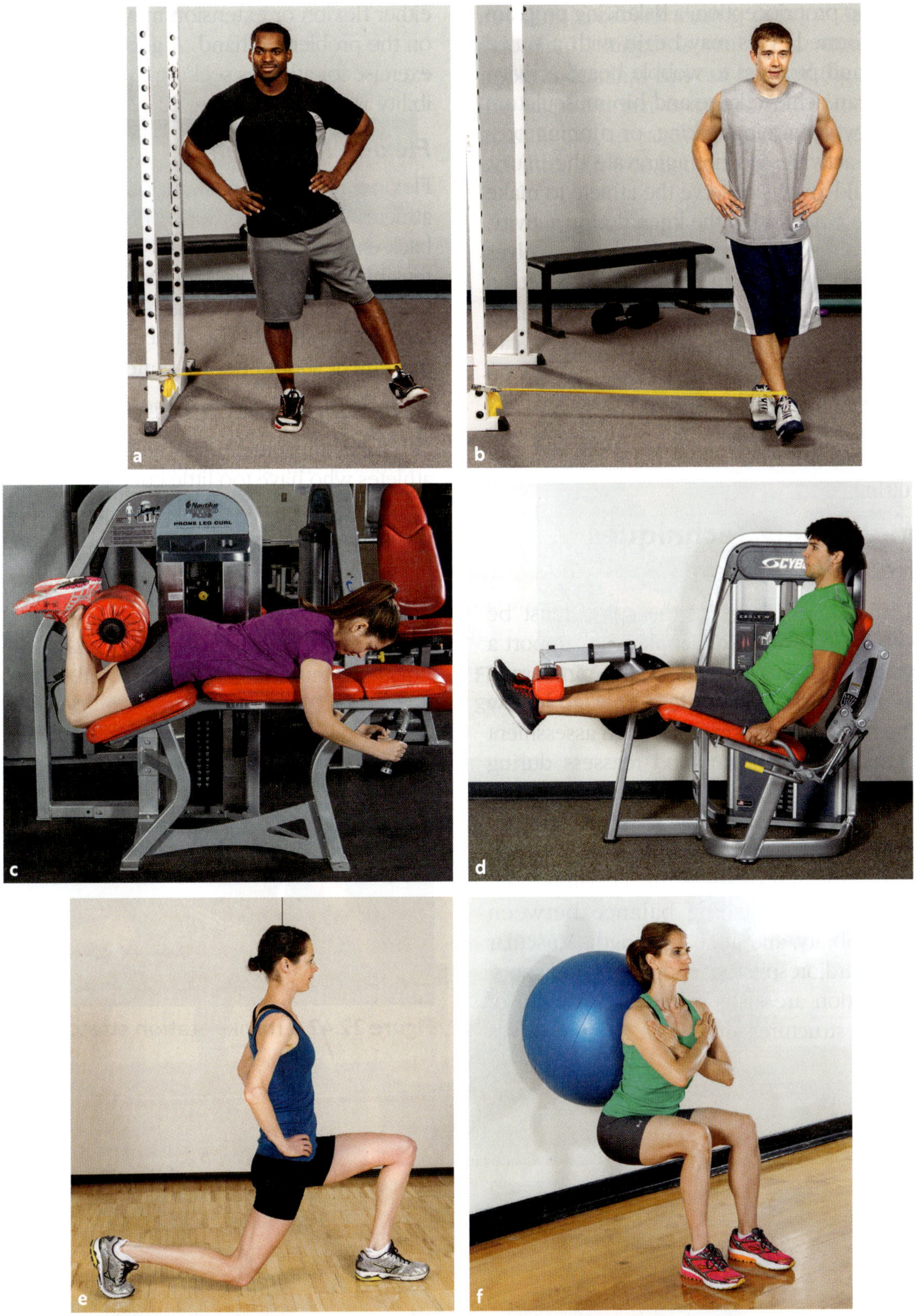

Figure 22.41 *(a-b)* Straight-leg raises performed against resistive tubing while standing are helpful for regaining hip and knee strength. *(c-d)* In the later stages of rehabilitation, isotonic movement can be done with weight machines to develop quadriceps and hamstring strength. *(e)* Forward lunges and *(f)* wall squats are a great functional way of strengthening the lower quarter.

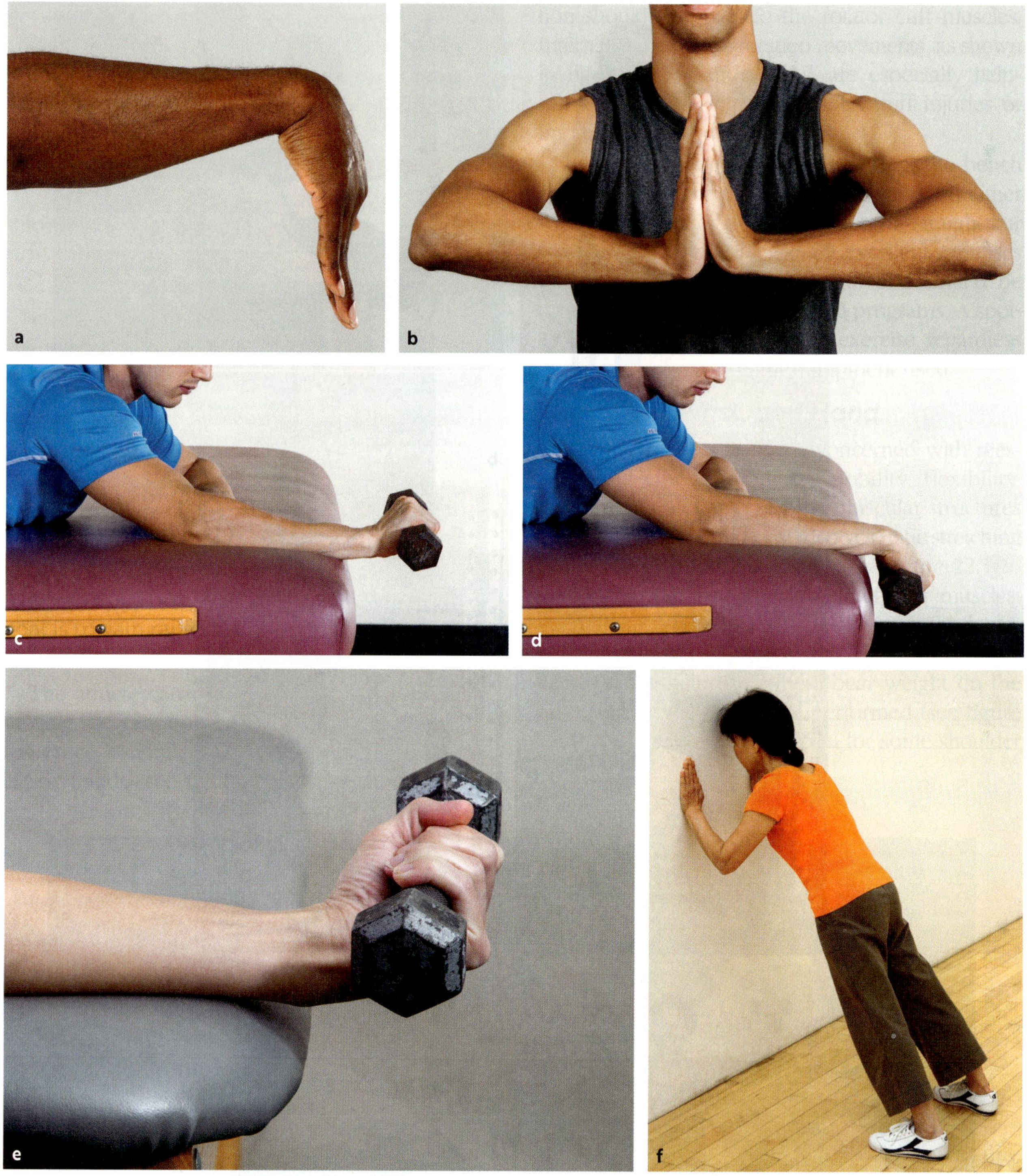

Figure 22.54 *(a-b)* Wrist extensor and flexor stretch. *(c-e)* Wrist and elbow strengthening exercises. *(f)* Wall push-ups help an athlete begin to bear weight on the upper extremity.

The biceps and triceps must not be neglected; they can be strengthened by performing triceps pull-downs and biceps curls (see figure 22.55*a-b*). Hand injuries may also require that an athlete attempt to improve grip strength by squeezing a racquetball or tennis ball, or they can squeeze putty between their fingers (see figure 22.55*c*). As long as the injury is not aggravated, elbow and wrist muscular endurance can be achieved by performing a high number of repetitions while lifting weights or

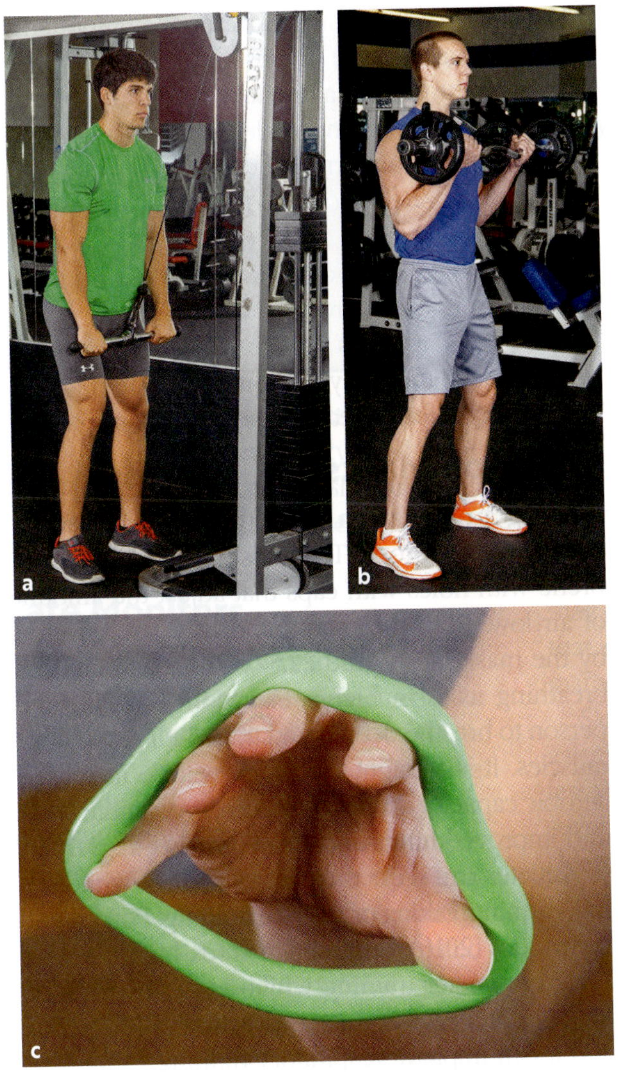

Figure 22.55 *(a)* Triceps pull-downs and *(b)* biceps curls are especially helpful for strengthening the upper arm. *(c)* Putty can be used to strengthen the fingers and hand.

by swimming, biking, or running. The AT should always observe the athlete to make sure that they are not aggravating the elbow or wrist injury during activity. The athlete can get back into sport activity by throwing, beginning with short distances at slow speeds and progressing to longer distances at higher speeds.

Although we have presented the contents of this section according to body region, the reality is that many joints work together to achieve a functional outcome. When we perform an athletic movement of the upper extremity, for example, the legs and trunk are often required to move simultaneously. With this concept in mind, many ATs focus on function so an athlete is ready for the demands of the sport.

Functional exercises take many forms, but the premise is to use sport-specific movements. As an example, if an athlete is performing a lunge to strengthen the legs, they can easily include an arm movement, such as a military press, and perform it at the same time. Another example is to have an athlete balance on a foam pad while performing biceps curls—that is working not only on upper-body strength but also balance.

CARDIORESPIRATORY CONDITIONING

Just as proper resistance training taxes and overloads the musculoskeletal system and makes it stronger, properly administered aerobic training can enhance an athlete's **cardiorespiratory endurance** in preparation for returning to play. The ACSM (n.d.) currently recommends training for 3 to 5 days a week to improve cardiorespiratory endurance. Training more than this can lead to overuse injuries because time must be taken to rest and recover throughout the week. The intensity of the exercise should elevate the heart rate to between 50% and 85% of the maximum heart rate (ACSM n.d.). To determine maximum heart rate, subtract the athlete's age from 220. For example, let's determine the target heart rate for a 16-year-old cross country runner. Using the formula to determine maximum heart rate gives us 220 – 16 = 204. If the athlete is new to running, we may choose to start easy and increase the intensity as they get in better shape. Therefore, if the runner begins training at 50% of maximal heart rate of 204 beats per minute, they must elevate their heart rate to about 104 beats per minute to get a training effect.

The duration, or amount of time, an athlete trains each session is another variable that can be controlled. To achieve maximum benefit, the exercise should be performed at the proper intensity for 20 to 60 minutes each session. As the intensity increases, the duration generally decreases.

The type of exercise selected to improve, maintain, or reestablish cardiorespiratory endurance for progress to standing and reaching across the body and then going up and down stairs.

Accelerometers and gyroscopes can now be found in smartwatches and smartphones. This technology can be used to analyze postural sway and gait. The accelerometer measures acceleration while the gyroscope measures orientation. The technology can measure balance when a person moves from sitting to standing and when working through balance exercises. Several vendors have applications that can be downloaded to the patient's smartphone that can help with monitoring balance. Some smartphones and smartwatches can detect falls and contact emergency services.

Vestibular Ocular Motor Screening (VOMS)

The **vestibular ocular motor screening** test is used to test the systems for concussions. Areas tested are vision, balance, and movement. The AT needs three items for the test: a target (a tongue depressor and their finger), a centimeter tape measure, and a metronome. There are five tests: smooth pursuit, saccades, convergence, vestibular ocular reflex, and visual motion sensitivity. The AT records symptoms on a scale of 0 to 10 before and during each test. The symptoms being assessed are headache, nausea, fogginess, and dizziness.

The smooth pursuit test allows the AT to test the athlete as their eyes follow a horizontal moving target. The athlete is seated, and the AT provides a fingertip as the target to follow three feet from the athlete's face. The AT moves their finger horizontally in an arc 1.5 feet (0.5 m) to the athlete's right, back to the middle, and 1.5 feet (0.5 m) to the athlete's left. This portion of the test should be repeated twice, and each repetition should take two seconds to complete. The second part of the test is similar, except the fingertip target moves vertically 1.5 feet (0.5 m) above the athlete's eye level and then 1.5 feet (0.5 m) below eye level.

The saccades test has a horizontal and a vertical component. The AT puts up 2 fingertips in the horizonal plane at 3 feet (1 m) from the athlete. The fingertips are at 30° on each side of the eye level. The athlete moves their eyes as rapidly as possible left and right for 10 repetitions. The vertical component entails placing the fingertips at 30° angles from the eye level and having the athlete move their eyes rapidly up and down for 10 repetitions.

An abnormal convergence test is where the near point to one's face is greater than or equal to 2 inches (6 cm) from the athlete's nose. The test is performed by placing a 14-point font on a tongue depressor. It is held at eye level, and the athlete brings the depressor toward their nose. The athlete stops the movement of the depressor when they see two images that must be distinct, not blurry. The measurement is taken where the distinct image occurs. This test is repeated three times.

During the vestibular ocular reflex test, a metronome is used and set at 180 beats per minute. The athlete focuses on an image that is 3 feet (1 m) away at eye level. The athlete moves their head 20° left, back to midline, and 20° right. The athlete's eyes remain focused on the image while the head turns to each beat of the metronome. Ten horizonal repetitions are performed. The vertical component of this test is performed with the same image at eye level at the midline. The head moves up and down to the beat of the metronome while the eyes remain focused on the image.

The final portion of the VOMS test is the visual motion sensitivity test. The athlete holds their arm out in front of them with their thumb up. The metronome is set at 50 beats per minute. The athlete rotates their body (including shoulders, head, and eyes), 80° left, then 80° to the right. The rotation is one beat of the metronome to the left and one beat to the right. Five repetitions complete this test.

According to Anzalone and colleagues (2016), the VOMS test is an effective tool when used with other tools. It has been found to be a predictor of recovery time for those who have suffered concussions.

Benign Paroxysmal Positional Vertigo (BPPV)

Benign paroxysmal positional vertigo symptoms are spinning or dizziness, nausea, and lightheadedness. Some signs can be difficulty walking in a straight line or eye twitching, known as nystagmus. Hyperextension of the neck and rolling over may set the signs and symptoms in motion. Another characteristic of BPPV is that as long as the head is in the horizontal plane, the vertigo symptoms are limited. The signs and symptoms can be mild or up to debilitating.

The cause of BPPV may be idiopathic or an impact to the head. There are three semicircular canals as part of the inner ear: the anterior, middle, and posterior. Calcium crystals are contained in fluid contained within the ultricle. When the crystals move out of the canals, the vestibular system does not function properly, and the athlete may experience headaches, spinning, balance issues, and the inability to walk in a straight line. It is imperative to have the crystals move back into their canal to help the athlete get back to normal.

When testing an athlete for BPPV, the AT may use Frenzel goggles. The Frenzel goggles are attached to a monitor. The goggles have mini cameras that are pointed at the eyes of the athlete. This is an easy way for the AT to see the eye movement (nystagmus) during the Epley maneuver.

The **Epley maneuver** is used to determine in which ear the crystals are not aligned as well as to move them back into their proper place. The athlete sits with their body at a 90-degree angle with pillows on the table that will allow for hyperextension of the neck. The pillows are arranged so that they contact the shoulders. For a right-side BPPV, the athlete will place their head at a 45-degree angle to the right, chin tucked, pause for a short period, and then lay back quickly onto the pillows (head still at 45°). There should be nystagmus at this point. The athlete must leave their eyes open so the AT can see when the nystagmus stops. When the nystagmus stops, the athlete remains in this position for one minute. After that minute ends, the athlete slowly rotates their head 90° to the left. If nystagmus occurs, the AT monitors it until it stops and then the athlete remains in that position for one minute. Next, the athlete rolls onto their left side, keeping their chin tucked with pillows under the shoulder. The athlete may experience nystagmus and stays in this position for one minute after the nystagmus ends. At that time, the athlete slowly sits upright, chin tucked and eyes straight ahead, and stays seated for 5 minutes. This Epley maneuver can be repeated twice, but then the athlete must keep their head at a 90-degree angle for the next two hours for it to be effective. For left-sided BPPV, the movements start seated with the head at a 45-degree angle to the left and chin tucked. Then follow the same routine opposite of the right-sided BPPV.

It may require a few days of doing the Epley maneuver to recover from BPPV. The BPPV may reoccur, but there is no way to predict when or if it will return. The Epley maneuver is seen in figure 22.58.

A WORD ON SAFETY

Safety during training should always be a chief concern. Do not let people using dumbbells act like dumbbells. Safety procedures must be established and faithfully followed.

Whether athletes are weight training or performing a cardiorespiratory workout, to prevent injury, they need a proper warm-up to prepare the body for the demands of the sport and a cool-down to help the body recover from the exercise. The warm-up and cool-down should include light cardiorespiratory work followed by stretching of the major muscle groups. Just how long the warm-up or cool-down should last is hotly debated among professionals, and the length is likely to vary from coach to coach and athlete to athlete. However, 10 to 15 minutes for each should be acceptable.

Athletes should follow several safety precautions when weight training. An athlete should always train with a partner who should know the exercise to be performed as well as the number of repetitions and be ready to assist when needed. The athlete should not hold their breath while performing

The Real World

A student of mine shared a video of a competitive powerlifter's weight training session. The athlete was performing a squat with about 550 pounds (250 kg) of weight on the bar. While he was squatting, his knee buckled and gave way. He collapsed to one side and lost control of the weight. Thankfully, his two spotters grabbed the bar, or he would have been badly hurt. Everyone watching the film got the message: Always train with a partner—or in some cases, two.

Bill Pitney, EdD, ATC

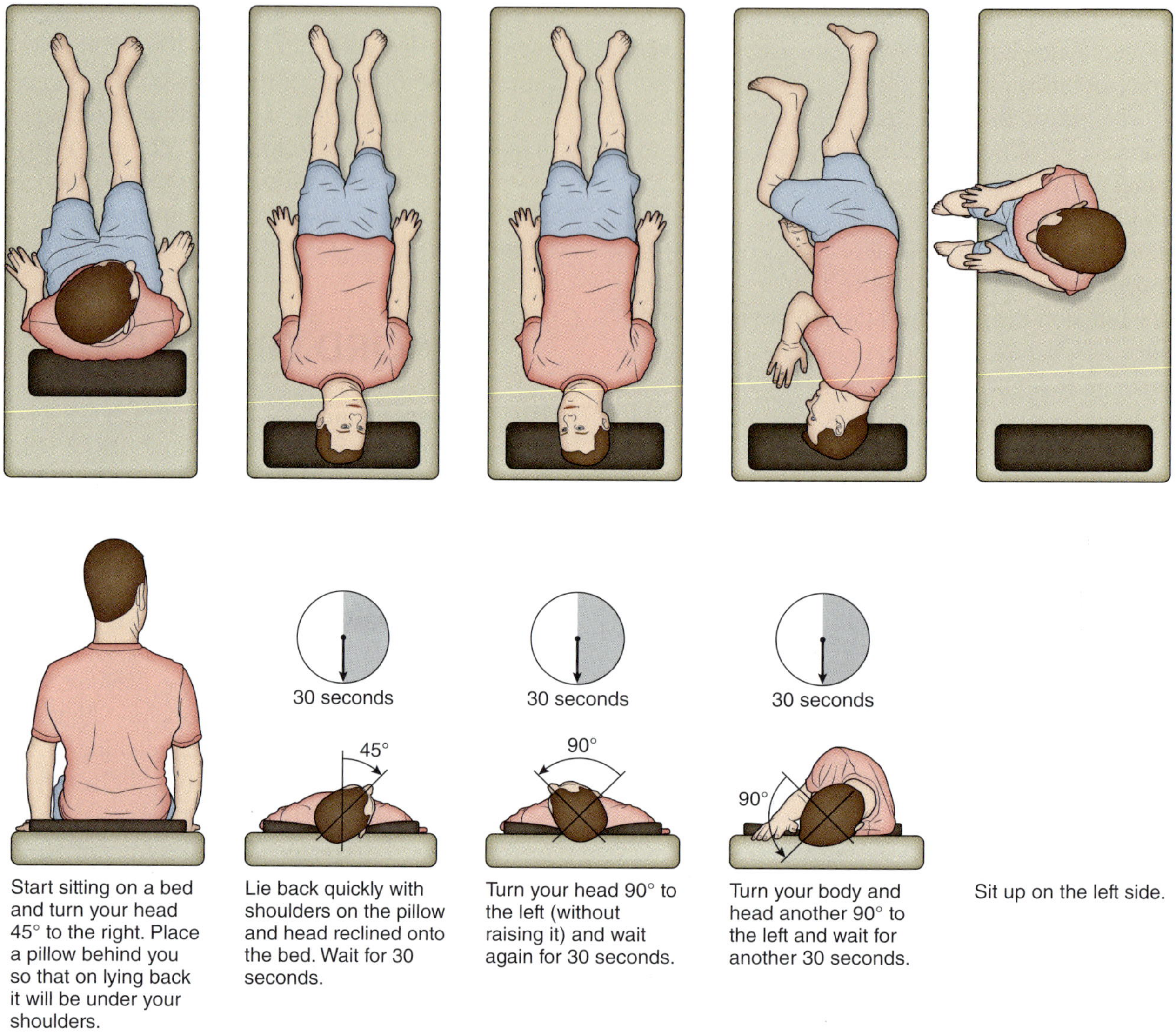

Figure 22.58 Epley maneuver for right-sided BPPV.
Adapted from A. Radtke, H. Neuhauser, M. von Brevern, and T. Lempert, Neurologische Klinik, Charité Berlin, Germany (1999).

an exercise; instead, they should exhale during concentric contractions (while exerting force) and inhale during eccentric contractions. Any time a bar is used, the weights should be secured with a collar. Exercise form should never be compromised, especially when the person is trying to lift a heavier weight. No horseplay in the training area should be tolerated—athletes must not be bumped while performing an exercise. Lastly, be careful when moving weights and weight stacks; it is easy to injure a finger or hand if you inadvertently catch it between the weights.

Proper weightlifting form has several components. The athlete should be stable—that is, when standing, lying, or sitting on a bench, they should always maintain balance and be able to control the weight. This means they should raise and lower the weight at a slow, easy pace, usually raising the weight for 2 seconds and lowering it for 4 seconds. An athlete should never cheat on their form just to be able to lift a weight.

When training for improved cardiorespiratory function, it is also a good idea to train with a partner. Training partners check on each other's water consumption and keep each other at an appropriate training level. Coaches and ATs should always monitor the heat index to be sure the environment is safe for training.

Summary

The AT should always follow PRE, overload, and specificity principles to ensure that a reconditioning program is both safe and effective. A complete conditioning program includes aerobic activity for cardiorespiratory endurance that allows the athlete to reach the target heart rate. Various programs can keep the athlete's interest while doing different things (battle ropes, CrossFit, or fitness drumming). New technology provides real-time analysis of current fitness levels and adjustments as needed. Stretching should be static to avoid injury in the warm-up, which should gradually raise the heart rate before the exercise program. Stretching should also be done in the cool-down, which should gradually lower the heart rate back to normal. For those with neurological issues, reconditioning is also necessary. Using special glasses or exercises can support the athlete's return. Safety rules and guidelines must be implemented and followed to avoid potential injury during weight training and conditioning.

Key Terms

Define the following terms found in this chapter:

- ballistic stretching
- benign paroxysmal positional vertigo
- cardiorespiratory endurance
- circuit training
- closed kinetic chain
- CrossFit
- DeLorme method
- dynamic stretching
- elevation mask
- Epley maneuver
- isokinetic contraction
- isometric contraction
- isotonic contraction
- muscular endurance
- muscular power
- muscular strength
- one-repetition maximum (1RM)
- open kinetic chain
- overload principle
- plyometric
- progressive resistive exercise (PRE)
- pyramid method
- specificity
- static stretching
- vestibular ocular motor screening

As an AT, you know that athletes are required to stay fit and conditioned throughout the entire year. Part of staying ready for a sport requires aerobic and anaerobic training. The soccer team needs their off-season training program. What aerobic and anaerobic exercises should you recommend? Provide a rationale for each exercise and include the benefit for the athlete.

To access supplementary material for this chapter, including the Understanding Check worksheet, vocabulary quizzes, extension activities, and chapter-specific resources and forms, visit the web resource: http://ancillaries.humankinetics.com/FundamentalsOfAthleticTrainingAndSportsMedicine5E

chapter 23

Psychosocial Aspects of Athletic Training

Objectives

After completing this chapter, the student will be able to do the following:

- Have a broad understanding of and appreciation for sport psychology.
- Understand relaxation and imagery techniques that are often used with athletes.
- Explain the athlete's perspective of an injury and typical emotional reactions.
- Identify the types and symptoms of eating disorders.
- Describe practical strategies to help an athlete better cope with an injury.

Athletes and ATs are beginning to understand that physical considerations are not the only factors in sport injury and rehabilitation; psychological factors such as stress play a major role as well. Therefore, ATs and athletes should learn the basics of sport psychology.

Sport psychology is the study of how variables such as life stress, mood, and motivation affect sport performance and sport-related injury. Sport psychologists and sport psychology consultants try to improve the mental well-being of athletes. They have many roles, such as the following:

- Researching to better understand how these variables affect athletes
- Teaching coaches, athletes, and ATs psychological techniques to improve performance
- Working directly with athletes in a clinical setting to help them deal with stress and improve sport performance

Many ATs are excellent at providing physical treatment and care to injured athletes. However, they also need to be aware that injuries can cause psychological problems that inhibit not only performance but also proper recovery. The most successful ATs have a clear understanding of an athlete's psychology, whether that athlete is injured or not.

MENTAL HEALTH RISK INDICATORS

Certain factors put an athlete more at risk for mental health issues. Knowing which athletes have a higher prevalence of risk factors will help the AT identify the athletes who need preventive care. Serious mental illness occurs in about 14.2 million people age 18 and older in the United States (National Institute of Mental Health 2022). Here are risk factors:

- Ages 18 to 25 have the highest mental illness prevalence (National Institute of Mental Health 2022)
- Being of two or more races increases risk of mental illness (National Institute of Mental Health 2022)
- Being LGBTQ
- History of mental illness
- History of abuse (Mayo Clinic 2022b)
- Genetically inherited mental health conditions
- Those with chronic health issues

Understanding Diversity

Mental illness can occur at any age. The American Psychiatric Association (2023) shows that 50% of all mental illness occurs before a person reaches age 14 and 75% by age 24.

Crisis Intervention

Purcell and colleagues (2019) suggest a model for crisis intervention: preventive or foundation components, indicated (at risk) prevention components, early intervention, and specialist mental health care.

- ***Preventive component.*** Educate athletes about mental health, remove the stigma around mental health, have the athlete focus on their goals, and provide athletes with feedback on things they should look for if there are mental health struggles.
- ***Indicated (at-risk) prevention components.*** Provide mental health programs for those who are at risk. Help coaches, teammates, and other ATs notice the subtle changes in an athlete's behavior by educating them on those things. Have a reporting mechanism to the AT that encourages early reporting.
- ***Early intervention.*** The AT needs to intervene with mental health support that's within their scope.
- ***Specialist mental health care.*** The AT will need mental health professionals who know how to deal with athletes and the specific condition.

ATs Care and CISM

While the AT can assist their athletes with mental health issues, an AT can also need support. In 2014, the National Athletic Trainer's Association formed a committee to support ATs in the event of a crisis. ATs Care provides peer-to-peer support to help ATs. The program involves training people in critical incident stress management (CISM). The International Critical Incident Stress Foundation teaches CISM all over the country. ATs interested in taking the training should contact the ICISF. Once trained in CISM, the AT can apply to become a part of their state ATs Care team. When an incident occurs, the ATs Care team in the state helps the AT through the stress management process.

The ATs Care team will help the AT assess how they are feeling now, will share information about how to cope, will provide typical signs and symptoms of stress, and will educate the AT about stress reactions. The ATs Care team can also recommend additional therapy with a therapist who specializes in trauma.

Scope of Practice for ATs

When dealing with mental health issues, the AT needs to understand that they have a finite set of skills. Recognition of mental health issues is the primary responsibility of the AT. The AT must be aware of their state practice acts, which may define what kinds of mental health issues they can directly work with. The AT must also be aware of the practice acts of mental health professionals to avoid legal issues.

Providing counseling for conditions such as anorexia, suicide, depression, and more should be left to licensed professionals who have had extensive training. The AT needs a list of professionals who care for various mental health conditions and have vetted them before an emergency. The AT should know what kinds of health insurance each professional accepts, their hours of availability, emergency phone numbers, and the need for referral and directions. Use the information in the Red Flag section to determine what constitutes an emergency.

REFERRING AN ATHLETE FOR PROFESSIONAL HELP

Although ATs have basic skills in counseling athletes, sometimes an athlete will need to be referred to another professional who specializes in a certain form of help. Issues that need referral are the following:

- Anxiety
- Generalized anxiety disorder
- Attention-deficit/hyperactivity disorder (ADHD)
- Burnout
- Depression
- Obsessive-compulsive disorder
- Panic disorder
- Post-traumatic response
- Suicidal thoughts
- Eating disorders
- Overwhelming life stressors
- Life-altering significant injury
- Mental health disorders
- Any situation the AT does not feel comfortable handling

The AT can refer athletes to various experts, such as the following:

- Psychiatrist—physician who specializes in mental health
- Psychologist—person who specializes in psychology and individual educational testing
- Social worker—person who specializes in group or individual therapy
- Sport psychologist—person who improves an athlete's performance using psychology

FYI

Mental Health Credentials

- Psychiatrist: MD or DO
- Psychologist: PsyD or PhD
- Master of social work: MSW
- Licensed social worker: LSW
- Licensed mental health counselor: LMHC
- National certified counselor: NCC

Anxiety

As you might imagine, high school athletes must deal with many pressures. Although few students could say they've never been stressed or anxious, athletes must cope with the expectations of their peers, coaches, and parents regarding their sport performance in addition to the everyday stress of school and social life. Because of these stresses, many athletes become anxious before sport participation. Although ATs are not sport psychologists, they spend a lot of time with the athletes and are in a good position to talk to them when necessary. The AT must be able to counsel an athlete who is too anxious.

Athletes need to be taught how deal with pregame anxiety, and in an interview with sports psychologist Chris Carr, Quinn (2020) suggested relaxation, self-control, and mindfulness.

Generalized Anxiety Disorder

Anxiety is fear of the unknown. Some people may have an anxiety that is temporary—for example, "Did I pass the test?" or "Will my parents ground me when they find out I was in a fight?" Those with generalized anxiety disorder have their worry repeatedly over six months for most days in the week (National Institute of Mental Health 2018). Signs and symptoms include irritability, sleep difficulty, restlessness, worrying, and muscle tension (National Institute of Mental Health 2018).

Treatment may consist of **cognitive behavioral therapy**, mindfulness training, meditation, coping skills, and medication. Cognitive behavioral therapy involves learning to recognize thought patterns that are specifically not based in fact and can intensify anxiety and stress and using skills to manage those thinking patterns (American Psychological Association 2022). With increased self-awareness of negative thoughts, the athlete can utilize problem-solving skills to help decrease anxiety, learning to be confident in their new skills and using strategies to cope with stressors (American Psychological Association 2022).

Attention-Deficit Hyperactivity Disorder

Attention-deficit hyperactivity disorder (ADHD) is a brain development disorder (Hyun Han et al. 2019). Like the name indicates, the athlete may have inattentive issues or hyperactivity, or both, which makes it difficult to function socially. Symptoms must be present in multiple life areas, such as academic, work, and sport. An athlete who fidgets, cannot sit still, and cannot listen to the coach's explanation is an example of one life area that may lead one to believe an athlete may have ADHD. Although the example seems minor, the pattern of behavior for those with ADHD persists for at least six months (Hyun Han et al. 2019). ADHD affects 6.4 million school-aged children; in adults, men are affected more than women (Kahanov and Payne 2022).

The physician will diagnose the athlete and refer for treatment. ADHD management may include therapy and medication. The medication used for treatment is a banned substance in the NCAA. An athlete taking the medication must have documentation in their medical record of their diagnosis. When the athlete is drug tested, they must inform the tester of the medication prescribed. When the drug test comes back positive, the documentation of ADHD will be in their record and an exception can be requested.

Burnout

Burnout has taken such a toll on athletes that they leave the sport they once loved. Neal (2015) defined burnout as "a syndrome of continual training and sport attention stress, resulting in staleness, overtraining, and eventually burnout." The signs and symptoms the AT should be aware of include a lack of desire to participate, a lack of interest, physical exhaustion, mental exhaustion, depression, and anxiety (Weinberg and Gould 2024). The AT can use the Maslach Burnout Inventory to measure the level, if any, of the burnout.

The treatment of burnout starts with prevention by resting and taking time away from sport (Neal 2016). An athlete who needs help should be referred to their physician and a licensed mental health care provider.

Depression

Depression is a feeling of despair or hopelessness that causes behavior such as not wanting to be around other people, not being excited about things that might normally be exciting, not taking the initiative to do things, and not talking much to anyone. Many theories exist about what causes a person to become depressed. Professionals think that depression is caused by biological (e.g., genetics), environmental (e.g., a traumatic childhood), or sociological (e.g., losing a spot on a team) factors. Along with feelings of hopelessness, a depressed athlete may exhibit many other signs and symptoms, including lack of appetite, nausea and indigestion, headaches, dizziness, and susceptibility to colds and other illnesses.

Panic Attack

A panic attack is a sudden uncontrolled fear when there is no real danger (Mayo Clinic 2022d). Panic attack signs and symptoms are shaking, fear, chest pain, sweating, difficulty breathing, rapid heart rate, and lightheadedness. Because the signs and symptoms mimic a heart attack, the AT should follow emergency procedures.

The cause of a panic attack is usually unknown. Athletes that have reoccurrences need to be referred to a physician and a therapist. If a diagnosis of recurring panic attacks is made, the usual treatment is therapy and medication (Mayo Clinic 2022d).

Obsessive-Compulsive Disorder

An obsession is having repetitive unwanted thoughts that cause the individual to feel distressed. A compulsion is the behavior in an attempt to stop the feeling of distress. The cycle repeats itself, with the obsession to compulsion recurring repeatedly. It is a mental health issue that can be disruptive to one's life if the cycle cannot be broken. An example of an obsession is a fear of germs; the compulsion may be constantly washing one's hands. The diagnosis of obsessive-compulsive disorder has three parts: psychological evaluation, meeting diagnostic criteria, and a physical examination (Mayo Clinic 2022c).

Treatment can consist of therapy and medication. Some individuals may require inpatient therapy (Mayo Clinic 2022c).

Post-Traumatic Response

A **post-traumatic response** is a sustained emotional disorder that results from a traumatic experience. For instance, a football player who was involved in a serious car accident in which a friend died might experience depression, problems with personal relationships, and impaired concentration, or he might even attempt suicide. Post-traumatic stress does not just happen to athletes; for example, an AT may experience post-traumatic stress disorder (PTSD) after working with an athlete who suffered a serious spinal cord injury. They may become fearful and unable to work well. They might also sleep a lot, refrain from eating, and avoid situations that are similar to the one that caused the initial stress.

COVID-19 is another example of a traumatic event that has caused PTSD for some. An athlete who was not able to participate in a sport they played every day, having family or teammates ill, or being isolated from friends and family was traumatic. Some athletes suffered the consequences, exhibiting PTSD. Treatment for PTSD is therapy and medication.

Suicidal Thoughts

Because of the many pressures that come with being a student, the AT working at a high school should be concerned about suicide. A person who attempts suicide has usually been through a stressful experience and is also suffering from depression. Warning signs of suicide include the following:

- Change in an athlete's eating and sleeping patterns
- Statements indicating the person wants to die
- Depression
- Anxiety
- Recent loss, such as a death in the family, a broken relationship, or the loss of a job
- Family history of suicide
- Lack of support from friends and family

If a student suspects that someone may be suicidal, they should tell the school counselor that they are concerned about that person. If an athlete has made a suicide attempt, the AT should call 911. If the athlete has serious suicidal thoughts and is not thinking clearly or exhibits suicidal warning signs but denies being suicidal, they should see a counselor as soon as possible.

People more likely to be at risk for suicide include the following:

- Those who have made previous suicide attempts
- Those who have a plan for their suicide
- Those who are lesbian, gay, bisexual, transgender, or queer (Hedegaard, Curtin, and Warner 2018)
- Those who have eating disorders
- Those who are isolated

An athletic injury need not be severe to create stress and discomfort for an athlete. A study by Yang and colleagues (2014) indicates that more than 80% of injured athletes relied on the social support of the

RED FLAGS

Call 911 if an athlete exhibits these signs of being suicidal:

- Makes clear statements about wanting to hurt themselves*
- Cannot state that they will not hurt themselves*
- Have a plan how they will commit suicide*
- Out of touch with reality
- Makes statements of hopelessness

*Must call if any one of these exists.

According to the Mayo Clinic (2022a), the body parts most obsessed with include face, hair, skin, veins, breast size, muscle size, and genitalia. It is necessary to get treatment for these athletes because BDD does not get better on its own.

Risk factors for BDD are having family members with it and their thoughts about what societal expectations are regarding body image, having other mental health conditions, or certain personality traits (Mayo Clinic 2022a). BDD usually starts in teenage years, and when an AT recognizes BDD early, a treatment plan can begin early (Mayo Clinic 2022a). Treatment includes cognitive behavioral therapy and medication.

Overwhelming Life Stressors

Every person experiences stress in life, but how one handles stress makes the difference. For an athlete, stressors can include illness or death of a friend or family member, parents getting divorced, transition to another academic or athletic level, internal pressure to perform, fear of failure, playing time, managing time, and identity issues.

Despite all the injury prevention strategies and other measures ATs take to ensure athlete safety, sometimes things go terribly wrong. Although it may not happen on the court or on the field, the death of an athlete is a tragic event that leaves coaches, teammates, and parents with a devastating loss. An athlete who needs to talk about the loss of a teammate may confide in the AT, who holds a position of help and trust.

The AT should understand that an athlete may express a great deal of anger during this time. The emotions that an athlete goes through when a peer dies are similar to those they will experience when they are injured.

The AT will understand that the athlete is experiencing stressors and support them either by providing a referral or stress management techniques. Techniques that can be used to help an athlete cope are guided meditation, breathing exercises, physical exercises, good nutrition, decreased social media use, and staying connected with supportive people (Hesler 2023). In some instances, medication may be needed to support the coping mechanism.

When an athlete's self-talk is negative, it is important to reframe that thinking to be more positive. The three-step process includes the following (St. Bonaventure University 2022):

1. Recognizing the negative thought
2. Determining the negative thoughts to reframe
3. Reframing the negative thought with a positive one

An example of this process is having the negative thought of "I'll never start a game." The athlete will recognize that this thought is unhelpful, say "Stop," and then reframe it by thinking, "One play at a time, and I'm getting better every day."

Some athletes may find it more comfortable to reduce stress through meditation, breathing exercises, or progressive relaxation. In the initial phases of learning meditation, breathing exercises, and progressive relaxation, it is best to find a place that is quiet, comfortable, and without interruption.

- ***Meditation.*** The athlete should find a comfortable position, either seated or lying on their back. A person must decide if closing their eyes or staring without focus feels like the best option. Next, the athlete should allow their body to relax and then push all outside thoughts from the mind. Some people like to chant a couple of words, such as "Just relax," either out loud or silently. Breathing should slow down as relaxation deepens.
- ***Breathing exercises.*** Like meditation, the goal of breathing exercises is to slow down the breathing pattern so thoughts are chased from the mind. Exhalation should be longer than the inhale. There is a longer pause between each inhalation. The eyes may be open or closed.
- ***Progressive relaxation.*** This technique addresses each body part, telling it to relax. To make it easy, start at the toes and work to the head. Tense the body part and then relax it. Do this at least twice per body part. Controlling one's breathing to a slower pace is also an essential part of the process.

An athlete who is subject to anxiety will benefit from learning self-control techniques.

Significant Injury

To understand the psychology of an injured athlete, we examine the classic five-stage theory Kubler-

Ross presented in the late 1960s. These stages represent the emotional response of an athlete and how they may act after an injury or loss. The stages are denial, anger, bargaining, depression, and acceptance. This theory has been widely referred to in much of the literature on psychological response to athletic injury. Although many athletes will progress through these stages in sequence, keep in mind that everyone is different, and some may exhibit these stages out of order.

- ***Denial.*** When an athlete is first injured, it is not uncommon for them to deny that there is a serious problem. Many athletes will tell themselves that things will soon be better. Unfortunately, when the athlete does not soon improve following a significant injury, they will feel anxious. They may also be emotionally disorganized, and the AT may hear them make unrealistic statements such as, "I will be fine. I'll be walking by tomorrow," when that may not be the case.
- ***Anger.*** Another response is anger, especially when the athlete realizes that the injury is real and potentially serious. They will often direct this anger at the nearest person, who may be a student assistant or AT. The athletic training staff and other members of the sports medicine team must not take the anger personally. They must remember that this is not a personal attack but rather an emotional release. Listen to the athlete and continue to respect them as an individual.
- ***Bargaining.*** Once an athlete's anger has diminished, they will begin to bargain with the AT, coach, team physician, God, and even themselves. They will attempt to make a deal with the AT, such as "If I can play at least one quarter of the basketball game, I will do all my exercises until my ankle is healed." When limits are set with the injured athlete, they may become depressed.
- ***Depression.*** The student assistant is in a good position to see if the athlete is depressed. The depression phase brings a lack of motivation and a feeling of hopelessness. This becomes a big challenge for the athletic training staff because athletes can become noncompliant with their treatment, which is a concern to both sport psychologists and ATs. The AT needs to be supportive, motivational, and understanding to get the athlete to comply with the treatment plan. In addition, if the AT takes the time to educate the athlete about the injury and why certain signs and symptoms exist, they can help them become more compliant with the rehabilitation program.
- ***Acceptance.*** When an injured athlete finally takes responsibility for their injury, they have come to the stage of acceptance. Accepting an injury means that the athlete has finally realized what it will take to get back to normal—or that they may never get back to what was normal, depending on the seriousness of the injury.

Many athletes become anxious when it comes time to return to participation. The AT must see to it that the athlete in a rehabilitation program progresses gradually from simple to more complex exercises to build confidence. Moreover, an AT is wise to allow the athlete opportunities to be with their teammates so that they can maintain contact and not feel isolated. In addition, a decisive therapeutic exercise program helps the athlete eliminate many fears of returning to play.

Mental Health Disorders

Some athletes will have mental health conditions. These conditions are divided into two categories: neurosis and psychosis. A **neurosis** is a mild form of mental health disorder, such as anxiety, fears, depression, anger issues, compulsive disorders, obsessions, and low self-worth. These people can be helped with medication and therapy.

The Real World

Many ATs deal with eating disorders as part of the job. One of my softball players was severely anorexic. I teamed with our psychologist and physician and encouraged the athlete to receive inpatient treatment. After three weeks and a gradual return to the sport, it appeared that the treatment was successful. The athlete graduated with honors, finished her softball career, and went on to get a master's degree. Sadly, this athlete stopped by my office six years later with a feeding tube in her nose. Eating disorders are crippling diseases.

Gretchen Schlabach, PhD, ATC

When someone loses touch with reality, it is known as a **psychosis**. The person with a psychosis may have an episode known as a psychotic break where they can see or hear things that do not exist (National Institute of Mental Health n.d.). Some psychotic forms of illness include bipolar disorder, schizophrenia, or severe depression. The treatment for a psychosis can include antipsychotic medication, psychotherapy, family support, and hospitalization.

The AT is one of the first people with an opportunity to respond to these kinds of mental health conditions. The AT is trained to recognize issues of mental health and refer the patient for the appropriate treatment.

RELATIONSHIP BUILDING

ATs are likely to deal with athletes from various racial and sociocultural backgrounds. Though the details of these backgrounds may not be fully understood, ATs should work to build positive relationships with all athletes, parents, and coaches. The most effective ATs are good listeners. Being a good listener means that the AT is fully invested in that athlete at that time. Thinking about other things or being distracted will take away from the positive relationship-building process.

An athlete needs to feel that the AT respects them and knows what to do and when to do it. Mutual respect will develop trust, which is important to the athlete. Doing what is in the best interest of the athlete does not mean the athlete will agree. The AT must also be consistent when working with athletes so that there is no perceived preferential treatment toward one athlete or another.

One thing an AT can do is try to see things from the athlete's perspective. For some athletes, an injury can be traumatizing. Before returning the athlete to competition, the AT will want to do some desensitizing work or refer the athlete to a social worker and make sure the athlete is mentally ready to return and has no fear of getting injured.

Some athletes will be relieved at getting hurt and not being able to play. These athletes may not have been totally invested, and the AT may have to work to get the athlete to determine if participation is what they want. If an athlete is not invested, they are more prone to injury and will find ways to malinger and use the AT's time unnecessarily.

Other athletes may view their injury as a reason to avoid working hard. These athletes will find ways to fake an injury or will be less than enthusiastic about doing rehabilitation. The AT needs to have a keen awareness of this type of athlete. Being able to push this athlete to fight through the supposed injury and get them back into competition is a delicate balance. Being an AT does not mean making athletes happy; it's about doing the right thing. The AT also must be careful to avoid assuming that the athlete is faking it each time they complain of being injured.

For other athletes, the injury may make them feel that they are no longer part of the team. These athletes need to be assured that they need to attend practices and encourage their teammates.

Sometimes athletes try to convince the AT to allow them to return to competition. If the AT has a good relationship with the athlete, it will be easier to explain why the athlete should not return. If there is no respect or trust, the athlete will look for another source that agrees with their desired outcome.

> **? What Would You Do If . . .**
>
> The AT has asked you to come up with ideas to make the athletic training room bright and cheerful.

PRACTICAL SUGGESTIONS

The AT can do many practical things in the athletic training room to help injured athletes cope with the injuries they have sustained. These include modeling, maintaining a good physical environment, and encouraging relaxation.

Modeling

Modeling means that an injured athlete can observe a successfully rehabilitated athlete who had a similar injury. The idea is that once the athlete sees someone with a similar injury who is doing well, they may become less discouraged and more motivated to work at their rehabilitation program. The AT and the student assistant should become positive, upbeat influences—another aspect of modeling. They should be cheerful and helpful to the athletes and treat the athletes as they would want to be treated.

Physical Environment

Imagine walking into a doctor's office that is dark, noisy, and smelly. Would you want to be there? Would you ever go back? Would you be comfortable performing exercises there? The same is true of the athletic training room. It is important to have a bright, clean, cheerful, and physically inviting atmosphere in which to treat athletes. In such an environment, the athletes may not feel that what they're doing is work; rather, it may be pleasant for them.

Relaxation

If you go to a high school track meet, look at the athletes preparing for an event. You will see some of them listening to music, others standing quietly with their eyes shut while gently moving their bodies through various patterns, and others lying down and taking deep breaths or stretching. Helping athletes relax helps them alleviate stress and cope with the demands of sport and sport injury. Several relaxation techniques can be found in the literature: breathing techniques, meditation, imagery, music therapy, massage, and muscle relaxation. Among these techniques, we discuss imagery and muscle relaxation.

Imagery

In the world of sport psychology, imagery is also known as visualization, mental training, and mental rehearsal. Imagery is used in athletics to help reduce stress. Several specific imagery techniques can be employed, but generally an athlete pictures themselves successfully completing a game, match, play, or event. Many sport psychologists describe the mental imagery process as creating a motion picture. The person doing the imaging is the writer, actor, producer, and director, all at once. They create the scene, the athletic movement, and the outcome that can help them visualize success. Imagery can also be done in the athletic training room to aid in rehabilitation.

Muscle Relaxation

Progressive muscle relaxation is a common relaxation method. It originated in the early 1900s with a physician named Edmund Jacobson. The routine has a series of muscle contractions and relaxations. The athlete assumes a comfortable position, probably lying down, and begins by contracting a muscle group (e.g., calves) at 100% effort for about 5 seconds and then relaxes them for a longer time, sometimes up to 45 seconds. Next, the athlete contracts the same muscles at 50% effort, followed by a rest period. Finally, the athlete gently contracts the muscle group for 5 seconds and then rests. The athlete should select each main muscle group and work their way through his body, concentrating on smooth, rhythmic breathing.

Summary

Athletes experience not only physical injuries but also psychological stresses that can be hard to manage. Sport psychologists can help athletes overcome many of the stresses they encounter with imagery and muscle relaxation techniques. Because ATs get to know athletes well and work with them every day, they can also help the athletes overcome anxiety. However, the AT must understand what an athlete will experience emotionally following an injury as well as the warning signs of mental health concerns.

Key Terms

Define the following terms found in this chapter:

- anorexia nervosa
- attention-deficit hyperactivity disorder
- bulimia nervosa
- burnout
- cognitive behavioral therapy
- depression (psychological)
- neurosis
- post-traumatic response
- psychosis
- sport psychology

An athlete has recently experienced a season-ending injury and will not be able to complete their senior year of sports. How can you, as the AT, help the athlete cope during the stages of grieving that the athlete might experience? Are there other professionals who may assist the athlete in dealing with loss?

To access supplementary material for this chapter, including the Understanding Check worksheet, vocabulary quizzes, extension activities, and chapter-specific resources and forms, visit the web resource: http://ancillaries.humankinetics.com/FundamentalsOfAthleticTrainingAndSportsMedicine5E

Unit VII

Providing Emergency Care

chapter 24

Planning for Emergencies

Objectives

After completing this chapter, the student will be able to do the following:

- Describe the principles of developing an emergency action plan.
- Explain why emergency action plans are necessary.
- Design a basic emergency action plan and pandemic plan.
- Understand the role of the student assistant during a crisis.

This chapter focuses on how to plan for emergencies and explains the role of the AT during a crisis. There may be times when student assistants will have to help a coach or AT care for a seriously injured athlete or deal with a potentially hazardous situation. To be sure that the sports medicine team and coaches perform to the best of their abilities, it is necessary to have an emergency action plan in place before an emergency happens.

Every athletic organization should develop and document a written emergency action plan that is practiced regularly. The plan should identify the roles and responsibilities of various personnel as well as the type and location of necessary emergency equipment. The emergency action plan should be specific for various locations (athletic fields or buildings) and mechanisms for clear communication should be established. Facilities that could be used to provide care to injured people should be included in the plan, and local EMS personnel should consult in the design of the plan. The emergency action plan should identify who will document the actions taken during the emergency as well as how the plan will be evaluated. Many people in the community and athletic organization have a responsibility to participate in creating and implementing an emergency action plan, and the finished plan should be reviewed by the school's administrators and legal counsel.

MEDICAL EMERGENCY CARDS

In most instances, an emergency will not be a mass casualty but will involve only one person at a time. To assist with the quality of care provided to the person, good planning involves using medical emergency cards. Many school districts require these cards. They contain important medical information as well as contact information in case of an emergency. See figure 24.1 for a sample card.

THE EMERGENCY ACTION PLAN

The **emergency action plan** will enable the central **sports medicine team** to cope with emergency situations. It should be shared with all school personnel (i.e., ATs, team physician, coaches, school nurse, campus police, team dentist, or social worker) and emergency medical responders. The emergency action plan for each venue should be posted in each facility (see figure 24.2). The emergency action plan should be practiced regularly in all facilities. Also, the sports medicine team should anticipate problems that could arise in various circumstances and with various personnel. If the AT is a per diem person or a visiting team AT, how will they be made aware of the emergency action plan? Will the emergency action plan change if it is a special holiday? If so, how will it change? Is there an emergency action plan for when you are traveling with the team?

Most often, the AT deals with a controlled situation, and the emergency action plan is simple. The plan becomes intricate when there are serious injuries. Before an emergency occurs, the sports medicine team should answer the following questions:

Doe, Jane

Emergency medical card

Date of issue: 03/04/25

Address: 456 7th St. Anywhere, IL 01234	**Date of birth:** 01/02/10 **Sex:** Female **Blood type:** B+	**Emergency contact:** John Doe **Relationship: Father** 555-123-4567 Cell: 555-345-5437
Preexisting conditions Asthma	**Medications** Advair twice a day Epinephrine as needed	**Emergency contact:** Janet Doe **Relationship: Mother** 555-789-1234 Cell: 555-345-5432
Allergies Peanuts Sulfa drugs Bee stings	**Physician** Dr. John Eod Phone: 555-543-2109	**Other** Insurance carrier: NatCoverage PPO

Figure 24.1 An emergency card should be available so an AT can quickly determine whether an athlete has any preexisting conditions or needs medications in a crisis.

Pioneer High School Sports Medicine

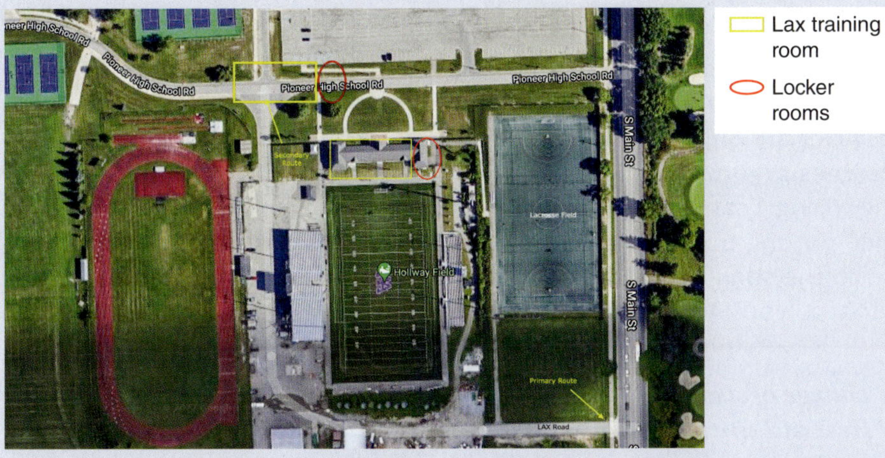

Emergency Action Plan

Lacrosse Stadium

Venue Address: 601 W. STADIUM BLVD., ANN ARBOR, MI 48103

Access Address: 1243 LAX ROAD, ANN ARBOR, MI 48103

Emergency Communications

Police/Fire/EMS 911

Poison Control 800-222-1222

Suicide Hotline 800-273-8255

Lax Athletic Training Room 734-124-4567

Landline Location 734-987-6543

Access Points

Primary Route: LAX ROAD SOUTH OF FIELD THROUGH DOUBLE GATE

Secondary Route: PIONEER HIGH SCHOOL ROAD WEST OF FIELD THROUGH SINGLE GATE

Emergency Equipment Locations

AED LACROSSE TRAINING ROOM LEFT SIDE OF ENTRY DOOR, MOUNTED ON WALL

Stretcher LACROSSE TRAINING ROOM LEFT SIDE 5′ FROM ENTRY DOOR, STANDING UP

Backboard LACROSSE TRAINING ROOM LEFT SIDE 6′ FROM ENTRY DOOR, STANDING UP

Splints LACROSSE TRAINING ROOM LEFT SIDE 5′ FROM ENTRY DOOR ON FLOOR

Cold Immersion Tank OUTSIDE THE LACROSSE TRAINING ROOM DOOR

Ice LACROSSE TRAINING ROOM, 20′ STRAIGHT AHEAD

Severe Weather Location

HOME AND AWAY TEAM LOCKER ROOMS

Figure 24.2 Emergency action plan for a lacrosse facility.

Adapted from Pioneer High School, Ann Arbor, Michigan. Imagery ©2024 Airbus, Maxar Technologies, Map data ©2024 Google.

What Would You Do If . . .

A football player has suffered a head injury. At the scene, you are asked to locate the player's parent. After arriving at the sideline, the parent becomes argumentative, saying, "There's nothing wrong. I came all this way to watch the game—put the boy back in!" Then the parent says to the son, "Why did you let that player do that to you? Are you dumb?"

1. ***Who is in charge of assessing an injury and beginning first aid until the proper help arrives?*** In order, the person in charge is (1) the team physician, (2) the AT, (3) the coach, and (4) the person with the most training in first aid and CPR. Do not delay rendering care while waiting for the AT to arrive. A student assistant who is certified in first aid and CPR can begin giving care until someone who is better trained takes over. Once the team physician or AT arrives, the first person at the scene should give a full account of what has been done and then be ready to perform other duties as assigned. The individual who ultimately runs the emergency action plan should be the person who understands and has the skills for it. For example, the team physician may not know how to put the air splint on because they are usually the ones who remove the splint to begin their orthopedic assessment at the hospital.

2. ***Is a phone available and is the emergency number known?*** Emergency phone numbers change when the team travels to away games. It is important to confirm the numbers before the start of a game—do not wait until something happens. If the AT uses a cellular phone, the battery must be charged and the bill must be paid on time. If the telephone service is cut off, how can you call for help? It is also important to have home and work phone contacts for all parents. For sporting events, it is helpful to have a landline available (in case cell phone service is disabled for some reason). Also, if a bomb threat is made at a facility, it is important to use a landline to contact EMS since a cell phone may trigger an explosion if the bomb is real.

Understanding Diversity

Emergency Phone Numbers

Too many phone numbers? Dial 211. You will be connected to a service center to get you routed to the right place.

- Life-threatening emergencies: 911
- Life-threatening emergencies in Europe: 112
- National Suicide Prevention Lifeline: 988
- Crisis Text Line: Text START to 741741
- Trevor Project LGBTQIA+ Hotline: 1-866-488-7386
- Trans Lifeline: 1-877-565-8860
- National Runaway Safeline: 1-800-RUNAWAY
- U.S. National Domestic Violence Hotline: 1-800-799-7233
- Rape Abuse and Incest Network: 1-800-656-HOPE
- National Human Trafficking Hotline: 1-888-373-7888
- National Child Abuse Hotline: 1-800-422-4453
- The National Council of Problem Gambling: 1-800-GAMBLER
- Substance Abuse Mental Health Service Administration: 1-800-662-HELP or text 435748
- Eating Disorders Awareness and Prevention: 1-800-931-2237
- Teen Hope Line: www.thehopeline.com/teenhopeline/ for a live chat
- National Maternal Mental Health Hotline: 1-833-TLC-MAMA
- Self-Abuse Finally Ends (S.A.F.E.): 1-800-DONT-CUT

3. ***Who will call for an ambulance?*** Ideally, the person who calls the ambulance is not directly responsible for giving care or getting supplies. To ensure that the caller does not panic and gives the right information, keep a list of emergency telephone procedures readily available for the caller to use. The ideal order of people who should call for an ambulance is coach, student assistant, and athletic director.

4. ***Who will control the crowd?*** Crowd control is best done by someone who is not directly responsible for giving care or getting supplies. It is difficult for those giving care when people are hovering over them, so anyone who is not a caregiver needs to be moved away. On the field, team captains must take charge and move the team away. If possible, the team should practice or play on another field while care is being given so they will not get in the way of the caregivers. A coach, student, game supervisor, or athletic director usually is available to control the crowd. Parents should be allowed to talk with their injured son or daughter, and someone should be prepared to give them support, drive them to the hospital, or remove them from the scene if necessary.

5. ***Is spectator safety accounted for?*** An emergency action plan must always consider spectator safety. Several facility-related items must be in place. First, the plan must move large masses of people from one location to the next. Consider, for example, a lightning storm occurring during a football game. An announcement must be prepared to communicate the situation to the spectators and tell them where to go and how to get there.

Second, signs must be in place to show people how to exit a facility. Any ushers or facility staff must provide directions that are consistent with the announcement and the signs.

Third, appropriate lighting will be necessary to ensure the movement of people from one area to the next. Emergency lighting systems are used in public facilities for this reason. If the power goes out, the emergency lighting is activated, allowing people to see the exits and signs.

6. ***Is a safe facility available for inclement weather?*** If spectators must be evacuated because of environmental conditions, a safe location must be identified in advance so their safety is secured. An ideal area to occupy in the event of lightning, for example, is a substantial enclosed building with indoor plumbing, electricity, and telephone communication. If there is a tornado, the ideal area is free of windows, as is an area belowground within the structure.

7. ***Who will bring supplies and equipment, and what supplies are needed?*** Be sure that the supplies in the training kits, golf carts, splint bags, and so forth are always stocked and the equipment is in working order. If the AT or coach receives a report of an injury, conducts an on-field evaluation, and determines that the athlete will need an injury splinted and crutches, having a student assistant who can read the universal signals that tell what equipment to bring out to the injured athlete can save valuable time (figure 24.3). If the AT discovers that they need more equipment than was brought to the accident scene, they can simply signal the

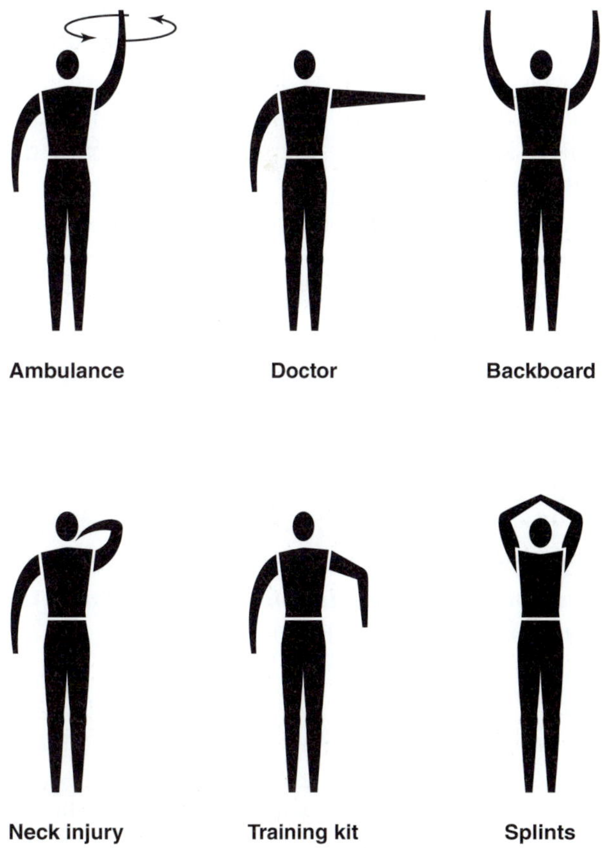

Figure 24.3 The AT can use sideline signals so that prompt care of the athlete can occur. The student assistant will read the signals of the AT and jump into action, getting equipment, getting the team physician, or calling for help.

assistant, who is stationed within sight but as close to the athletic training room as possible, to bring whatever is necessary.

8. ***Is an automated external defibrillator (AED) available?*** An AED is necessary to restart the heart in instances of sudden cardiac arrest. Physician Drezner and colleagues (2013) found that in schools without an AED, the survival rate for sudden cardiac arrest patients is 5% to 10%, while in those with an AED, the survival rate is 55% to 60%.

9. ***Who will transport or assist the athlete from the field of play?*** Sometimes an athlete is too severely injured to move. We discuss these situations in chapter 27. But most often, the injured athlete can be moved, and the AT can assist them from the field, perhaps with a golf cart, a stretcher, or crutches. If the athlete is too tall or too heavy for the AT to assist alone, the AT can recruit a couple of athletes and direct them in getting their injured teammate to the sideline. If the injured athlete is taken to the hospital, someone from the school must travel with them. This person can be the athletic director, a coach, or an AT. If the injured athlete who needs the ambulance is from an opposing team, the visiting coach is responsible for contacting the athlete's parents. Be sure that the athletic director, medical director, and school principal know which hospital the athlete has been sent to because they will get phone calls from people concerned about the athlete.

10. ***Which is the best hospital for the injury?*** Fortunately, most injuries do not require a level 1 trauma hospital. Which hospital in your area provides the highest level of trauma care and does your athlete need it?

11. ***Where is the safest and easiest access for emergency services to the area where the injured athlete is?*** The area around the injured athlete should be clear of materials, cars, and so forth, and any locks barring access to the area should be unlocked. If an athlete has to be transported by emergency helicopter, you will need to know where it will land. Know the GPS coordinates to the site in advance so they can be communicated immediately. Will spectators have to be removed because of the wind from the propellers, and will someone be able to travel with the injured athlete?

12. ***Who will direct the emergency services to the injured athlete?*** A coach, student, or athletic director usually is available to direct an ambulance to the area. A person should be stationed at every possible point where the ambulance might approach the scene, and each of these people should be instructed in the proper technique for signaling and guiding the emergency vehicle.

13. ***Who will notify the parents that their child has been injured?*** It is always best to let the athlete call and tell their parents that they have been injured. If they are in no condition to call, the AT, coach, or team physician should do so. Ask the athlete which family member is best to talk with (i.e., the person who will remain calm and be able to make medical decisions). The caller will tell that person what happened, what is being done, and who is caring for the athlete. They will find out which hospital is preferred by the family and will tell the parents where to meet emergency personnel. The AT should see to it that an emergency card, which gives emergency personnel permission to treat each athlete, is always with every athletic team. The emergency card should also give secondary contact information if the parents cannot be reached.

14. ***If more than one athlete is injured, what area will be used for triage, and how will athletes get to this facility?*** Most often the **triage** area, which is where decisions are made about which injuries must be treated first, is the training room or nurse's office. For a mass casualty situation, the best triage site may be a gym or an open field space. There may be times when the normal triage facilities are not available (e.g., fire, locked doors), so an alternative must be set up and its location communicated. In many instances where a large catastrophe has occurred at the school, the gymnasium may be used as a triage facility.

The AT plays a huge role in triage. The AT's medical background and preparation in injury assessment allow them to determine which people are suffering the severest injuries and need to be treated first. Communication is essential. Make sure everyone on the emergency team has a walkie-talkie/cell phone with charged batteries. Getting hurt people to the triage site may not be an easy task, especially if the injuries have occurred in an area that is difficult to reach because of locked doors and no keys, multiple stairways, or remoteness. Plan for the best way to move the injured, such as by wheelchair, crutches, backboard, stretcher, executive chair with wheels, or whatever is available. See figure 24.4 for more on the order of triage.

15. ***What personnel are available in the event of a mass casualty?*** How many faculty members, coaches, or students have been trained in first aid and CPR? Who can assist? If they are not on campus, can they be reached to help? At the beginning of the school year, a seminar should be held to train all faculty in first aid and CPR. Get a list of those faculty members who want to be a part of the emergency medical responder team. Decide who will be responsible for first aid kits, flashlights (if the electricity goes out), the emergency action plan, and first aid care for each area of the building (see the sidebar, Items Needed in an Emergency). It is important to have people in charge of the section of the building where they normally work. There may be no outside access to parts of the building, such as in the case of an explosion; therefore, there must be people inside who know what to do.

16. ***Where is the reunification site after a mass casualty?*** When there is a mass casualty, the tendency is for family and friends to rush to the site to find their loved ones. It is best to set aside a site where people can be reunited so it will not cause traffic congestion. The site should be a large area with a parking lot—for example, a church.

17. ***Who will fill out an accident report form and get statements from other witnesses?*** It is best to have someone document what is being done as it is going on.

18. ***How will the emergency medical response team work around known obstacles?*** Try to anticipate obstacles that will be common in an emergency situation, such as cars obstructing a driveway, stairways, pools, poisonous gas, locked doors, smoke, no lights, no phone, foul weather, equipment failure, communication problems, lots of

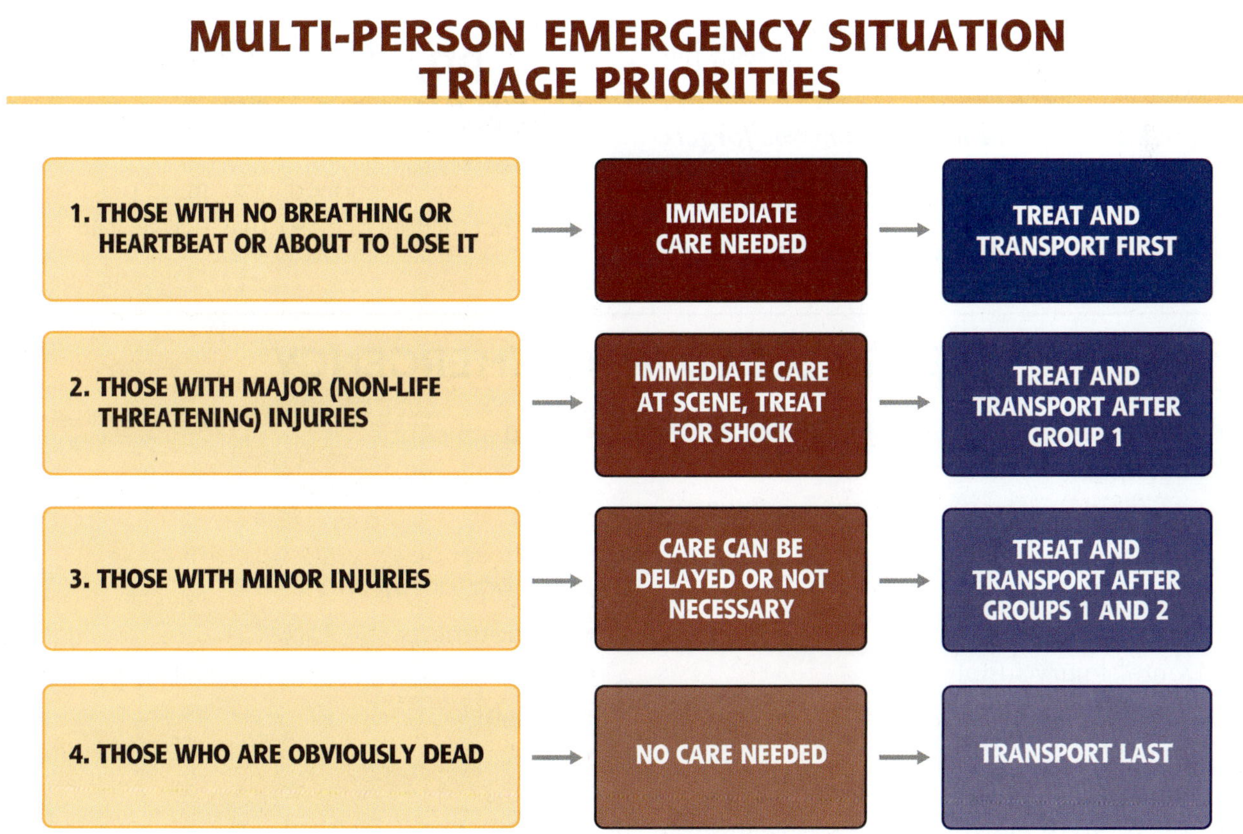
MULTI-PERSON EMERGENCY SITUATION TRIAGE PRIORITIES
1. THOSE WITH NO BREATHING OR HEARTBEAT OR ABOUT TO LOSE IT
IMMEDIATE CARE NEEDED
TREAT AND TRANSPORT FIRST
2. THOSE WITH MAJOR (NON-LIFE THREATENING) INJURIES
IMMEDIATE CARE AT SCENE, TREAT FOR SHOCK
TREAT AND TRANSPORT AFTER GROUP 1
3. THOSE WITH MINOR INJURIES
CARE CAN BE DELAYED OR NOT NECESSARY
TREAT AND TRANSPORT AFTER GROUPS 1 AND 2
4. THOSE WHO ARE OBVIOUSLY DEAD
NO CARE NEEDED
TRANSPORT LAST

Figure 24.4 The order of triage.

injuries and no help, and so on. The plan should include each of these obstacles and any others you can think of. If the plan is to remove an athlete from the field by a golf cart, but it is snowing and the golf cart will not go, be prepared with an alternative plan. Make sure that all the people in the response team have keys to the areas they will be responsible for. Everyone should have access to a walkie-talkie and a lantern.

19. ***How will the emergency action plan change for each facility (e.g., pool, gym, outdoors, game, practice, ski hill, ice arena)?*** Make sure people who can carry out the emergency action plan are located in each facility for which the response team is responsible.

20. ***How will the facilities be evacuated?*** Evacuation is difficult because some spectators know nothing about the facility. In the building, evacuation instructions should be posted in every room. The outdoors must be evacuated when lightning storms, tornadoes, or hurricanes are headed into the area. The evacuation plan should include the site where each team should go for protection and accounting purposes. Hold practice evacuations so that everyone becomes familiar with the procedures.

21. ***What should be done if someone forgets what to do?*** The emergency action plan should be available to all members of the emergency medical response team and coaching staff. Because all team members have walkie-talkies, if someone forgets what to do, another member can read the plan page by page to help get through it.

22. ***How will the emergency action plan interact with campus police and their plan?*** Each department will have their own emergency action plans and what are considered priorities for them. Securing an area and making sure it's safe may be their priority over the care of the injured. The AT must make sure the two emergency plans are not in conflict.

23. ***Who should talk to the press?*** The school system normally designates who will give information to the press and to the faculty and student body. Let the information person give the facts to the press. A fact sheet can be given to all staff members at school to keep rumors to a minimum.

24. ***Who will give counseling to those who need it?*** School counselors are usually designated to help with counseling. Most situations do not require counseling, but often it is helpful to talk over a situation and review what happened.

PRACTICING THE EMERGENCY ACTION PLAN

As previously mentioned, you must practice an emergency action plan so that people can learn

ITEMS NEEDED IN AN EMERGENCY

- Walkie-talkie or cellular phone
- First aid kit
- Wound care supplies
- Splints
- Scissors
- Eye-care supplies
- Dental-injury supplies
- Gloves
- Penlight
- Tweezers
- Pocket mask
- Hand antiseptic
- Elastic wraps
- Tape
- Stethoscope
- Blood pressure cuff
- Thermometer
- Ice
- Crutches
- Backboard
- Towels
- Notepad

their roles and so that potential problems can be recognized early and then corrected. Parts of the emergency action plan should be practiced daily. Involve different people in the plan and put them in different roles so they feel comfortable. Practice the plan at different sites, under various weather conditions and with variables (locked gates, no communication source, lack of personnel, multiple injuries, delayed transport, or lack of equipment). The following is an example of a practice session. The web resource has a reproducible sheet to assist you in practicing your emergency action plan.

First, athletic training staff should meet with EMS personnel to discuss everyone's role and make sure the equipment used is compatible. Second, once the roles have been clarified, set a date when a mock injury scenario can be practiced. In this situation, a student assistant can pretend they are an injured athlete who needs emergency medical care. The AT can initiate the emergency action plan, and a coach can contact EMS, alerting them that this is the practice drill for the emergency action plan. The AT can assess and monitor the athlete and direct another student assistant or coach to bring specific medical supplies (e.g., splints). At this time, another member of the crisis team should place people at appropriate locations to direct EMS personnel into the school. Once EMS arrives, the crisis team can determine the following:

- Did an appropriate person assess the victim and direct someone to call EMS?
- Was the assigned person able to find the nearest phone and give appropriate information to EMS?
- Were assigned people able to find and deliver appropriate medical supplies to the emergency site?
- Were people able to locate themselves appropriately so that EMS could enter the site and get to the victim?

These questions allow the crisis team to identify problems. However, the practice is not quite finished. The crisis team should perform the following mock actions:

1. Call the athlete's parents.
2. Complete an injury report.
3. Identify who will speak with the press.
4. Identify how counseling services will be activated.

At minimum, the practice session should facilitate communication between the people involved in managing a crisis and help uncover obstacles. Any problems should be discussed and decisions should be made about how best to solve them.

? What Would You Do If . . .

At a gymnastics meet, an athlete loses control, flies off the high bar, and lands on her back. The AT does an assessment and determines that she could have a spinal cord injury. You are instructed to call 911. A person comes out of the crowd and stops you, saying, "There is nothing wrong with the athlete."

! RED FLAGS

You may need to update your emergency action plan if you note any of the following:

- No secondary or tertiary backups are noted in the plan.
- The plan is written for only one type of emergency situation.
- The plan is more than three years old.
- The plan does not account for multiple victims at one time.
- The plan does not account for environmental factors (e.g., rain, tornado).
- The plan does not account for the type of surface (e.g., ice, grass, turf).

The Real World

One of the rules in cross country is to never touch a runner unless it is absolutely clear that they will not be able to finish the race; otherwise, you will disqualify them. We had spent a long day working a cross country meet, and the last race of the day was a combined boys' and girls' middle school race. I was responsible for an area on an uphill slope. As a young girl approached the hill, she began to cry. I encouraged her to keep going. Instead, she lay down on the grass and kept crying. I again encouraged her to get up and finish the race, but she just lay there.

Suddenly she stopped crying and appeared to have fallen asleep. I stood next to her and tried to elicit a response by talking to her, but she did not respond. At this point, I had to touch her. I checked her breathing and heartbeat, and everything was normal. I radioed to our central location to try to get more information. Her coach did not know if the girl had any illness that would put her in this condition. The coach was on her way to us when the girl's grandmother arrived. The grandmother stated that she was a nurse, and the girl would be fine with more air. Suddenly the anxious woman slapped her grandchild across the face so hard, her head rocked. Then she began giving the girl mouth-to-mouth breathing. I radioed for help, but before anyone else arrived, the girl became conscious and walked away with her grandmother. I never saw her again. To this day, I wish I had had the authority to intervene, and I still wonder if the girl was ill or if she just hated running.

Anonymous

PANDEMIC MANAGEMENT PLAN

A pandemic is usually caused by an infectious disease that spreads rapidly, and medication is not available to stop the spread. Characteristics of a **pandemic** include that they are rare; most people do not have immunity; healthy people are at risk for complications; health care providers and hospitals are overwhelmed; medication supply is inadequate; medical visits increase; increased complications and high death rates; and impact to the public, business, and world economies (Centers for Disease Control and Prevention 2019).

Having a pandemic management plan can help the AT act quickly and effectively. In preparation for a pandemic, FEMA (2020) suggests the following:

1. Determine how the illness is spread.
2. Take action to prevent the spread—determine who will lead each segment of the plan.
3. Prepare for virtual work, telemedicine, and school.
4. Gather supplies needed for the long-term: food, prescriptions, water, cleaning supplies, gloves, masks, and so on.
5. Understand the coverage provided by insurance carriers.
6. To prevent fraud, create password-protected documents.
7. Prepare a place for testing and vaccinating individuals.
8. Be prepared to isolate individuals who become ill and designate an area for this.
9. Know your responsibility regarding reporting.
10. Have a plan for contract tracing.

The Centers for Disease Control and Prevention (2020) suggests:

1. Stay healthy—protect yourself and your family
2. Stay connected
3. Remain calm
4. Find reliable health and news sources

Summary

To be the best AT, coach, or student assistant, it is important to have an emergency action plan and pandemic plan, good evaluation skills, and good treatment skills. The emergency action plan has 18 parts that will make caregivers more effective. Once the plan is designed, it is critical to practice it. Practice will prepare the caregivers and help them foresee many problems. The student assistant can help by being trained to fill a role in the crisis team and by obtaining first aid and CPR training.

Key Terms

Define the following terms found in this chapter:

- emergency action plan
- pandemic
- sports medicine team
- triage

You are the AT at a cross country meet held at a local golf course. There are 10 teams in the event. What personnel, supplies, and equipment would you need to ensure this is a safe event? Describe your planning needs and explain how you will implement appropriate care throughout the entire course.

To access supplementary material for this chapter, including the Understanding Check worksheet, vocabulary quizzes, extension activities, and chapter-specific resources and forms, visit the web resource: http://ancillaries.humankinetics.com/FundamentalsOfAthleticTrainingAndSportsMedicine5E

chapter 25

Primary and Secondary Emergency Procedures

Objectives

After completing this chapter, the student will be able to do the following:

- Explain the difference between primary and secondary assessment.
- Explain the difference between signs and symptoms.
- Explain the CABs of a life-threatening emergency.
- Define the procedure used to restart breathing once it has stopped.
- Explain the types of illnesses or injuries that cause breathing and the heart to stop.
- Explain when CPR is used.
- Explain how external bleeding is controlled.
- Explain what precautions can be taken to prevent communicable diseases.
- Ask the basic questions for obtaining the history of an injury or illness.
- List the common vital signs and explain how they help identify an injury or illness.
- Determine whether an injury can cause shock.
- Describe interventions to treat shock.
- Describe the procedures that the AT uses when testing an athlete's injury.

Athletes who become injured or ill trust the AT, coach, team physician, and student assistant to render appropriate care, which is called *first aid*. In this chapter, we discuss how to conduct a primary and secondary assessment and provide first aid for life-threatening and non-life-threatening injuries. Various life-threatening injuries and conditions are listed in the sidebar. Previous chapters cover many routine athletic injuries and their care.

An AT can begin emergency procedures only after determining the problem. Taking care of an athlete who is injured or ill is like putting together the pieces of a puzzle. The AT takes the pieces of information gathered during an assessment—the mechanism of injury, history, primary assessment, secondary assessment, and vital signs—and completes the puzzle to determine what is going on with the athlete.

In the unusual case that the AT is working with athletes they are not familiar with, the AT should begin with an introduction. Next, it is important to ask permission to treat the athlete, although in most cases the athletes are teenagers and cannot refuse treatment because of the policies that many school districts and states have about who can refuse treatment. In addition, it is customary for parents to sign waivers to allow treatment in their absence. However, when a parent of an injured teenager has refused permission to treat, no treatment should be given. In that case, the AT should document the refusal of permission to treat by having the athlete sign the refusal in front of a witness. Refusal of treatment is rare but must be followed.

In emergency situations, the person with the most experience takes the lead. It is critical that everyone works as a team and knows their responsibility as part of the emergency action plan. If you need to review the emergency action plan, see chapter 24.

When investigating an athlete's injuries, the AT will ask questions and observe the athlete for signs and symptoms. A **sign** is objective evidence that can be measured or sensed, such as sweating, breath odor, temperature, blood pressure, breathing rate, and heart rate. A **symptom** cannot be seen, smelled, or heard; it is subjective evidence of what the athlete feels. Examples of symptoms are pain, nausea, and anxiety. Many signs and symptoms prompt an AT to activate EMS (i.e., call 911), and the Red Flags sidebar identifies the most common signs and symptoms requiring emergency action. The AT must talk to the athlete throughout the assessment process as a way of reassuring them. The last sense to be impaired by unconsciousness is hearing, so the AT should continue talking to the athlete. Even if the athlete is unconscious, talking to them is helpful.

PRIMARY ASSESSMENT

Injury assessment is divided into two categories: primary and secondary. The **primary assessment** deals with injuries that are life-threatening, that is, injuries involving the **ABCs**—**a**irway, **b**reathing,

LIFE-THREATENING INJURIES

1. Cardiac arrest (heart has stopped)
2. Respiratory arrest (breathing has stopped)
3. Internal bleeding
4. Shock
5. Burns
6. Heat-related illness
7. Cold-related illness
8. Asthma attack
9. Diabetic emergency
10. Drowning
11. Electrocution
12. Falls from height
13. Poisoning
14. Severe bleeding
15. Anything else that causes breathing or cardiac impairment

Adapted from NHS (2022). Available: www.nhs.uk.; American Red Cross (2021); and British Heart Foundation (2019).

and **c**irculation. The secondary assessment involves all non-life-threatening injuries. Luckily, most athletic injuries are not life-threatening.

The order in which the assessment is done can be crucial to ensuring that life-threatening injuries will be cared for first. Current American Heart Association guidelines stress that **c**ompressions come first, and then you focus on the **a**irway and **b**reathing (CAB). The primary assessment is done in the following order:

1. Check the scene to determine that you can approach the athlete safely.
2. Assess responsiveness by lightly tapping or shaking (not so hard that the neck gets twisted or jostled) and talking to the athlete.
3. Recognize that lack of responsiveness, no breathing, or abnormal breathing indicates a cardiac emergency.
4. Call 911 and obtain an AED if available.
5. Start CPR by initiating chest compressions.
6. Open the airway and provide two breaths.
7. Check for severe bleeding.

Conducting 30 compressions should take 18 seconds. The student assistant should become certified in first aid and **cardiopulmonary resuscitation (CPR)** so that when an emergency happens, they will be better prepared to help.

Most of the time, checking for an airway and breathing of an unconscious person simply involves watching the chest rise and fall and listening for breathing. When an athlete is face down, checking for breathing is more challenging. The tendency is to roll the athlete over, but this is not appropriate because it can cause further harm from the injury that just occurred. Because breathing is the priority, the AT can watch for the athlete's back to rise and fall, place a hand near their mouth and feel for breathing, or place a mirror near their mouth (the mirror will steam up if the athlete is breathing) before determining if the athlete needs to be moved or not.

Checking the Scene

The first step is to prevent any more injuries than already exist, which includes making sure you do not get hurt. Approach an athlete only when the scene appears safe. If, for example, an athlete goes down during a football play, you will need to make sure the play has stopped so you do not step onto the field and accidentally get hit by a player.

RED FLAGS

The following signs and symptoms require EMS:

- Athlete is unconscious at any time.
- Athlete is having trouble breathing or has stopped breathing.
- Athlete is dizzy or lightheaded.
- Athlete has bleeding that will not stop.
- Athlete has pain or pressure in the abdomen.
- Athlete vomits, passes out, or coughs blood.
- Athlete has fallen from a great height.
- Athlete has possible head, neck, or back injuries.
- Athlete has lost sensation or cannot move extremities.
- Athlete has seizures, regardless of history.
- Athlete has been poisoned.
- Athlete has chest pain or no heartbeat.
- The amount of care required is beyond the AT's ability.
- Athlete has broken bones, false movement, or crepitus.
- Athlete has slurred speech.
- Athlete has difficulty remembering things.
- Athlete has no pulse in an extremity.
- Athlete is in shock.

Adapted from Anderson and Barnum (2022) and American Red Cross (2021).

Determining Responsiveness

The initial task here is to determine whether an athlete is conscious and able to respond. To check responsiveness, the AT will gently talk to and tap the athlete.

An unconscious athlete may be able to hear the AT and may be able to respond to a voice if they do not have a severe head injury. The response may be no more than a squeeze of a hand, but even such a feeble sign is an indication that the athlete is hearing and reacting. No one near the athlete should speak negatively about the athlete when they are unconscious because they may be able to hear. Reasons for unconsciousness include poisoning, respiratory arrest, cardiac arrest, hemorrhaging, diabetic illness, heat-related illness, cold-related illness, and head injury.

If an athlete is able to respond clearly and logically to the responsiveness check, the AT will know that the airway, breathing, and circulation are okay. At that point in the primary assessment, the AT can skip the CABs (steps 3-7 in the primary assessment) and proceed to check for severe bleeding. It is important to recognize, however, that if the athlete does not respond, the AT must check the CABs. If other rescuers are present, they should be directed to call 911 and obtain an AED if one is available.

Initializing the CAB Sequence

If the respiratory or circulation system is impaired, the athlete's life is in danger, and the AT must respond quickly to give the athlete the best chance for survival (see figure 25.1). Quick action and early chest compressions without interruption are recommended.

- ***Circulation.*** Rescuers should start CPR immediately in the event of cardiac arrest. It is no longer recommended that pulse or breathing detection be performed first, because early chest compressions are critical for survival. There may be spurting blood; a steady, heavy flow of blood; or blood pooling. This type of bleeding is severe and is an emergency that requires immediate attention from the AT.

- ***Airway.*** An untrained or solo rescuer should provide hands-only CPR and not interrupt compressions to check the airway or breathing. A trained rescuer, or second rescuer who is able, should make sure the airway is open. To do so, the AT will place one hand on the athlete's forehead and two fingers of the other hand under the athlete's chin.

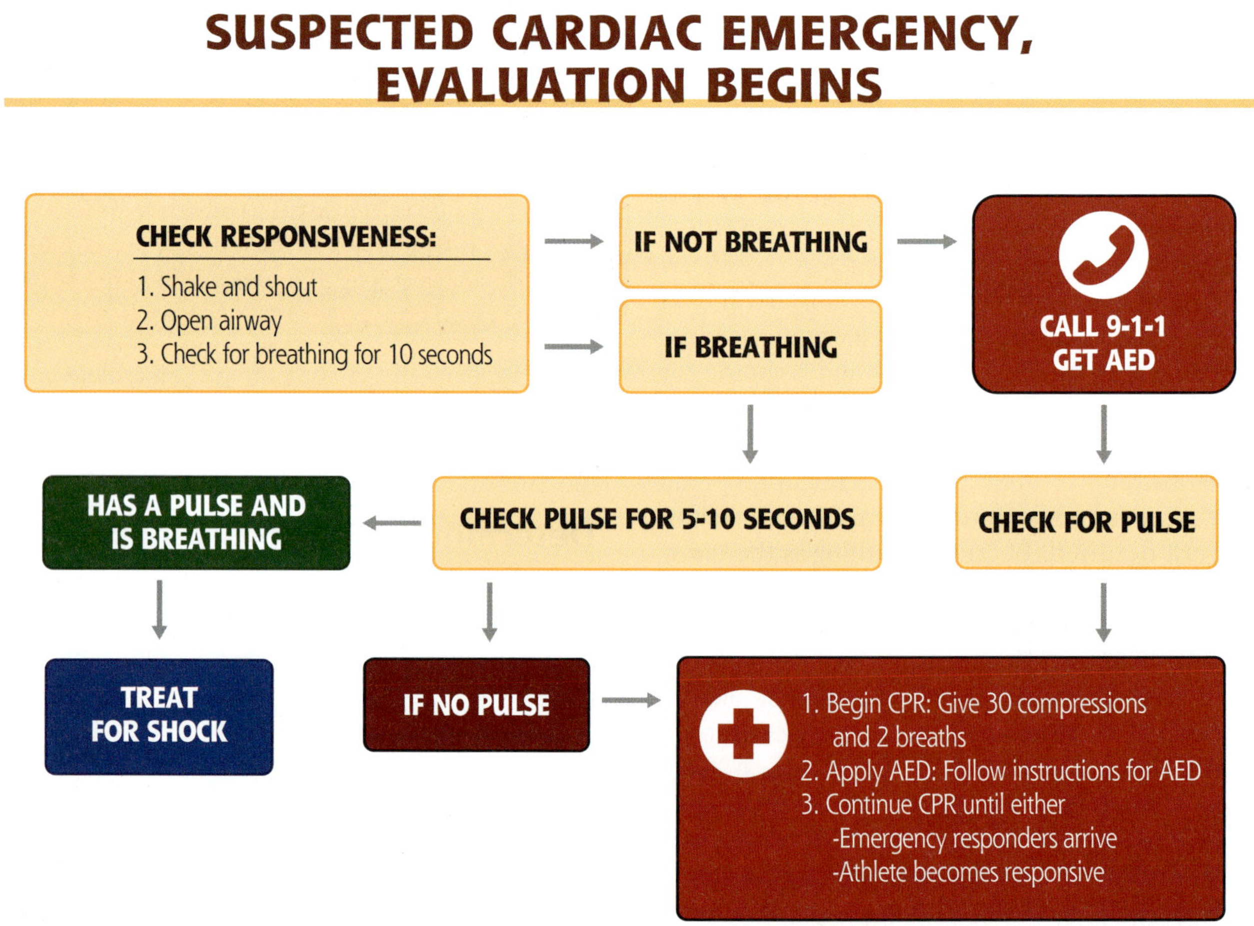

Figure 25.1 Cardiac emergency response.

Simultaneously lifting the chin while controlling the head will open the airway by pulling the tongue away from the back of the throat. This is called the *head-tilt chin-lift procedure*.

- ***Breathing.*** To check breathing, the AT will use a technique called *look, listen, and feel*. The AT will *look* at the chest and watch for the chest to rise and fall, *listen* for breathing by placing an ear close to the mouth, and *feel* for hot breath on their cheek. Checking for breathing should take about 10 seconds and should be done by a trained rescuer. The look, listen, and feel step has been removed for lay rescuers.

> **FYI**
>
> **Conscious**
>
> A conscious athlete is one who quickly responds to outside stimuli such as talking, tapping, or shouting and is aware of their environment.
>
> **Respiratory Arrest**
>
> An athlete in respiratory arrest has stopped breathing.
>
> **Diabetic Illness**
>
> Diabetes is a disease in which sugar is not metabolized properly. The chemical insulin, which helps break down sugar, may be lacking, or the tissues may have a resistance to the insulin that is present.

BREATHING EMERGENCIES

Any situation in which breathing has stopped or is compromised is considered life-threatening. Breathing emergencies can involve any part of the respiratory system, and the compromise of any part of the respiratory system can cause death. Direct traumas, such as diaphragm rupture, punctured lungs, anaphylaxis, or an illness like asthma can cause a breathing emergency. Drowning, suffocation, or an airway obstruction can also cause an athlete to stop breathing. If the brain does not receive oxygen, cells begin to die. The longer the brain goes without oxygen, the greater the number of cells that die; eventually whole portions of the brain die until the death of the athlete results. As little as 4 minutes without oxygen can cause permanent brain damage. The sooner lifesaving efforts begin, the better the chances are that the athlete will survive without brain injury. Most often, EMS will have a response team to the location in 4 to 10 minutes. If proper care begins immediately, the chances of survival are 98%. If care is delayed by 4 minutes after breathing has stopped, the chances of survival are significantly reduced.

Illnesses such as asthma that cause a breathing emergency can most often be dealt with by elevating the athlete's head and, when appropriate, helping the athlete take their medication. A punctured lung must be cared for in a different manner (see chapter 11).

The AT may use an oropharyngeal airway or a nasal cannula to protect or open the athlete's airway. The oropharyngeal airway is inserted into the mouth and keeps the tongue from relaxing and falling backward into the athlete's throat. The nasal cannula is used for rescue breathing when an athlete has a significant mouth injury. The AT will insert the tube into the nose and breathe through it.

Cardiopulmonary Resuscitation

If an AT determines that an athlete is not breathing when the primary survey is performed, mouth-to-mouth rescue breaths may be initiated. For mouth-to-mouth breathing, which is also known as rescue breathing and CPR, the AT places a protective barrier over the athlete's mouth and exhales into the athlete's lungs, causing the chest to rise. Initially, two rescue breaths are given.

Pediatric Cardiopulmonary Resuscitation

Pediatric cardiac arrest occurs primarily from asphyxia, or respiratory inefficiency, so the American Heart Association continues to support rescue breathing and chest compressions if the victim is a child. With pediatric victims, the AT will still use the CAB sequence and provide rescue breaths along with the chest compressions. If there is a pulse and no breathing, then mouth-to-mouth breathing is performed. Rescue breaths last 1 to 1.5 seconds, and one breath is given every 3 seconds (one breath every 5 seconds for an adult). After giving a breath,

What Would You Do If . . .

You are a spectator at a soccer game. The temperature is cool. A parent who is recording the game is pale and sweating. The man's wife, who knows that you are a student assistant, asks you to take a look at her husband. You check his pulse, and it's so rapid that you cannot count that fast. The man insists there is nothing wrong with him. The AT is on the sideline, watching the game.

the AT will always look at the athlete's chest. This not only helps the AT see if the athlete has begun to breathe but also slows things down so that the AT does not hyperventilate. Placing one's mouth on another's mouth or nose can transmit diseases, and several devices are available that act as a barrier between the AT and the injured person. At least one of these devices should be a part of every emergency kit.

The AT will start chest compressions after the initial rescue breaths and after checking for a pulse. Thirty chest compressions are given, followed by two rescue breaths. This procedure is continued until the athlete begins breathing or the AED arrives and is ready to be applied to the victim. The compressions are given at a rate of about 100 per minute at a depth of at least 2 inches (5 cm). The AT may need to use only one hand to get the necessary depth for a child.

Adult Cardiopulmonary Resuscitation

If the victim is an adult, the AT will start chest compressions if CPR is warranted. Thirty chest compressions are given, followed by two rescue breaths. This procedure is continued until the athlete begins breathing or the AED arrives and is ready to be applied to the victim.

To do a chest compression, overlap your hands, placing the heel of one hand on the victim's sternum and quickly compressing the chest down at least 2 inches (5 cm) for an adult. Compressions and breaths should be given at a 30:2 ratio. The rate of compressions should allow for 100 chest compressions in a minute.

The number of compressions and breaths has been updated from a previous ratio of 15:2. If there are two rescuers, the ratio of 15:2 can be done, but this is a more advanced skill. We recommend obtaining CPR certification for the professional rescuer, or basic life support, for the AT so you are capable of performing both single- and two-person CPR.

FYI

Diaphragm

The diaphragm is the muscle that separates the chest and abdominal cavities and assists in breathing.

Asthma

In asthma, the air passages narrow in response to an allergen such as pollen, dust, or mold. Exercise may also trigger an attack. The air passage may close entirely.

Anaphylaxis

Anaphylaxis is an allergic reaction in which the air passages narrow in response to a foreign protein, such as bee venom, or to a drug, such as medication to which the person has been sensitized.

Blood Pressure

Blood pressure is the pressure that the blood exerts against the walls of the vessels as it moves through them. The blood pressure of an average teenager is less than 120 systolic (when the heart beats) and less than 80 diastolic (between beats) (Fowler 2023).

Hyperventilation

Hyperventilation is rapid and deep breathing consisting of 24 breaths or more per minute.

Please note that CPR guidelines change frequently. Visit the American Red Cross, American Heart Association, and National Safety Council websites to learn when the parameters are updated. *It is your responsibility to use the most current and approved techniques for lifesaving skills.*

Obstructed Airway

An athlete's airway can become obstructed in several ways, but the tongue is the number one airway obstructer. In an unconscious athlete, especially one lying on their back, the tongue likely will relax and obstruct the air passage. Other possible obstructions are food, gum, mouth guards, broken teeth, blood, vomit, and chewing tobacco. (To prevent airway obstruction, we recommend barring food, gum, and chewing tobacco from practices and games.) A conscious athlete with an obstructed airway will grab at their throat—the **universal choking sign**—as an indication that he has a problem with the air passage (see figure 25.2). If the athlete is unconscious, the AT will have to open their airway, check breathing, and begin giving breaths before discovering that there is an airway obstruction. An airway obstruction may be partial or total.

A **partial airway obstruction** occurs when an object covers the air passage but still allows some air to flow in and out of the lungs. The athlete will grab their throat. To determine if this obstruction is partial or total, the AT will ask if they can speak, cough, or breathe. If they can, there is a partial airway obstruction. An athlete who has a high-pitched whistling noise coming from their throat has a total airway obstruction.

A **total airway obstruction** occurs when an object blocks the entire air passage and does not allow enough air to flow into the lungs for the athlete to take a breath. Under such conditions, the athlete may have a high-pitched whistling noise coming from their throat, which is caused by a small amount of air pushing past the object in the throat. A conscious athlete will give the universal choking sign. Their face will be red and their eyes will water. If an athlete is conscious but has a total airway obstruction, the AT will lean the athlete forward and perform five back blows by slapping the person between the scapulae. After five back blows, abdominal thrusts are performed. Abdominal thrusts are performed by standing behind the athlete and placing one fist against the abdomen, just above the navel. The AT reaches around with the other hand, placing it over their fist. Once the AT's hands are in place, inward and upward thrusts are performed to dislodge the object. If an athlete is unconscious and an AT determines that the airway is blocked, the athlete is evaluated as an unconscious victim and CPR may need to be performed, as described previously.

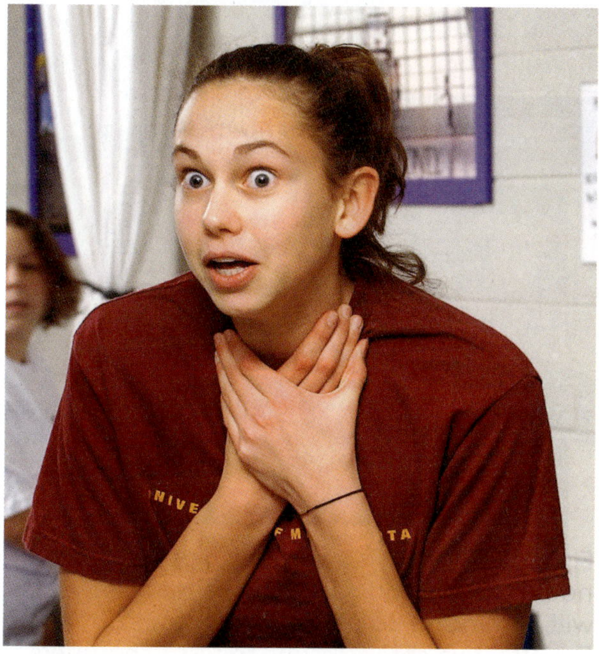

Figure 25.2 The universal choking sign.

> **? What Would You Do If . . .**
>
> In the cafeteria, a student tells a joke and another begins to cough forcefully just after laughing. The student continues to cough, and their face is turning red and tears are rolling down their cheeks. The athletes next to you say, "She's choking. Do something!"

CARDIOPULMONARY EMERGENCIES

Two cardiopulmonary emergencies concern the AT: heart attack and cardiac arrest. Both are life-threatening emergencies that must be dealt with immediately.

Heart Attack

A **heart attack** is also called an *acute myocardial infarction* and occurs when the heart muscle is damaged by a blockage of a vessel to the heart, a clot, stress, or an injury to the heart muscle that does not allow the heart to receive the blood it needs to function. A student assistant may think, "I'm going to work with healthy young athletes, so I probably won't have to know much about heart attacks." However, consider the people in the stands

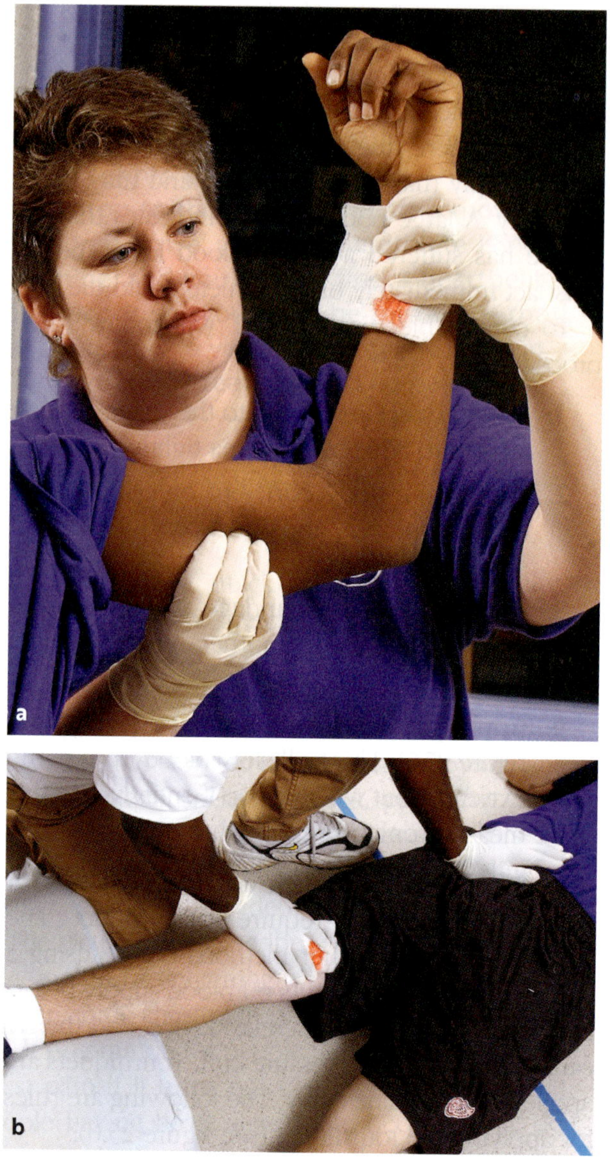

Figure 25.5 The pressure points at the *(a)* brachial and *(b)* femoral arteries.

mine if sutures (stitches), adhesive strips, adhesive, or staples are needed. Sutures will be needed if the wound is deep and the edges are gaping. When an athlete needs to be sutured, they must receive the sutures within 12 hours of the incident. In this instance, the wound should be covered with a nonstick sterile dressing and covered with a bandage to keep the dressing in place.

If sutures are not needed, proper wound care steps should be followed. The AT will first take precautions to prevent disease transmission (see the next section) by wearing gloves. Once preventive measures are in place, the wound should be cleaned.

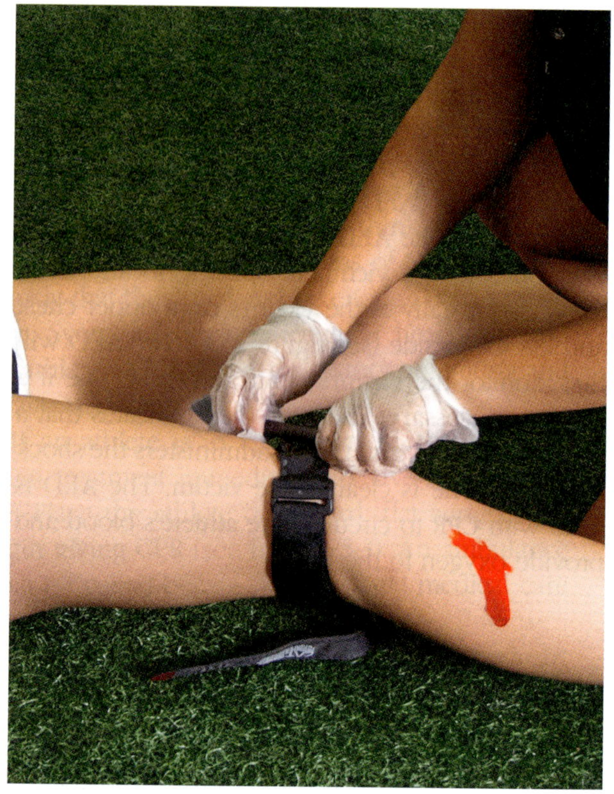

Figure 25.6 Tourniquet.

The athlete should be instructed to first wash the wound with antimicrobial soap and water. Once washed, the wound should be cleaned again with a 10% Betadine solution. If debris is present in the wound, irrigation with sterile saline can dislodge the particles. The saline should be squirted at a slight angle onto the wound and should drain away from the wound.

An antibiotic cream should be applied to prevent infection. The antibiotic cream should be applied to a sterile dressing and then the dressing applied to the wound.

Debridement

If a wound needs to be cleaned or debrided, it must be done before bandaging or wound closure. Flushing the wound with sterile water or saline can clean a simple wound without dirt or grass in it. After flushing, the need for wound debridement will become apparent. Debridement requires personal protection, a scalpel, scissors, bright light, a magnifying headset, and tweezers.

If there is dead tissue that has no blood supply, it can be removed. The AT can utilize the sterile instruments to remove pebbles, grass, dirt, or turf. Once the wound is cleaned, the AT can determine the need for bandaging or if more advanced wound closure is necessary.

Adhesive Strips, Adhesive, Suture, or Staples

If the AT determines that a wound requires closure, several options are available. Adhesive strips can be used in areas with little skin tension. A small amount of adhesion is applied to the skin on both sides of the wound. The adhesive strips are cut to size and then applied with slight tension while the wound is being held closed by a hand. The strips continue to be applied until the entire wound is closed.

Adhesive glue is in a thin-walled plastic container, which must be squeezed to release the glue. The glue comes through the tip of the container. The AT holds the wound together with one hand while applying glue over the top of the wound. Once the glue is applied, the AT should hold the skin together for about 1 minute to ensure good adherence.

Suturing should be done with an anesthetic. A wound that is under tension or is deep should be sutured. Deep wounds may need internal sutures. The AT will need to select a suture that is either absorbable or nonabsorbable. Absorbable sutures do not have to be removed. Nonabsorbable sutures are removed based on their location, between 4 and 21 days; see table 25.1 (Heritage Urgent and Primary Care n.d.; Seattle Children's 2022; Ratner 2020).

A simple suture technique is called *interrupted.* The needle is inserted starting at one end of the laceration across the wound and out the other side. Once the needle is out the other side, a surgical knot is tied. This process is repeated the length of the laceration.

A skin stapler can be used to close a wound. The AT needs to make sure the skin edges are approximated together and then add the staple. The number of staples will depend on the length of the wound. See table 25.1 for a time frame in which staples can be removed.

Infection Monitoring

There may be times when, no matter how hard the AT tries, the body part becomes infected. The infection may be noted with swelling, redness, and pus, and the athlete may have a temperature. It is important to monitor the infection daily to determine its size. The monitoring can be done by marking the skin with a marker to see if it is spreading. See figure 25.7 to see the markup of a foot that has an infection.

Draining a Hematoma

When the nailbed of a finger or toe has a subungual hematoma, it can be very painful and lift the nail away from the underlying tissue. Relief can be found from draining the hematoma. The process of relieving the hematoma requires a sterile field and instruments. Use a hot trephination to burn a hole through the nail. Blood will likely spurt out as the pressure releases. Some ATs may use a paper clip that is heated or even a nail drill that creates a hole in the nail.

Table 25.1 Suture or Staple Removal Time Frame

Suture or staple site	Removal time frame
Scalp	7-10 days
Face	4-7 days
Neck	7 days
Chest, abdomen, or back	7-14 days
Arms and back of hands	7-14 days
Legs and top of feet	10-21 days
Palms, soles, fingers, or toes	12-14 days
Crossing a joint	12-14 days

Adapted from Heritage Urgent and Primary Care (n.d.); Seattle Children's (2022); Ratner (2020).

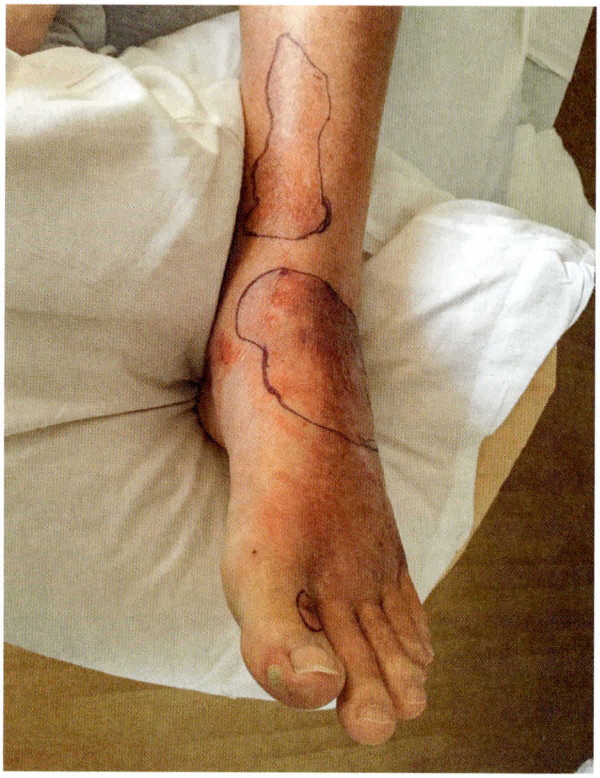

Figure 25.7 Infection monitoring.
Photo: Lorin A. Cartwright.

Ring Removal

Sometimes an athlete will forget to remove a ring, and during competition sprains or fractures that finger. This can cause rapid swelling and make it impossible to remove the ring. The AT needs to use a ring cutter to create enough space so the ring can be removed. The figure 25.8 shows an example of a ring cutter. Failure to remove the ring will cut off circulation to the finger.

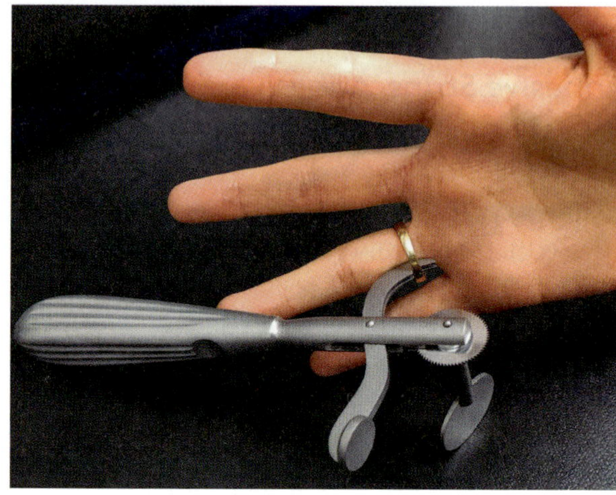

Figure 25.8 Ring cutter.
Photo: Lorin A. Cartwright.

FYI

Elevate

Elevate means to lift above the level of the heart.

Bandage

A bandage is a strip of cloth used to hold a dressing in place.

The Real World

I was sitting in the training room doing some paperwork with a senior student assistant when I looked up to see a football player being helped through the doorway. He was staggering, and he was a bloody mess—he had fallen into a glass door. I immediately dialed 911, and I told him to lie down and elevate his legs because I could see that he was showing signs of shock and hysteria. He was holding his wrists, each of which had a deep cut down to the tendons. He had a third severe laceration, a 2.5-inch (6 cm) gash across his forehead. I put on gloves and grabbed a pole of gauze. I applied direct pressure to the forehead and the worst of the two wrist lacerations.

Then things got complicated. I literally had my hands full, so my student assistant (a first responder) gloved up to help me. I thought, "This will be a great experience for her." As she was standing next to me, putting on her gloves, she said, "I'm going to faint." Before I could tell her to sit down, she did faint, striking her head on the floor, and she had a petit mal seizure caused by the bump. I could see she was breathing, so I kept my pressure on the wounds, kept an eye on her, and waited for the police and paramedics to arrive. It was quite the scene. The other athletes in the area were freaked out. Everything turned out okay, though. We got the bloody football player bandaged and off to the emergency room, where they stitched him up. My embarrassed assistant just ended up icing the large lump on the back of her head.

Steve Marti, ATC

PREVENTING COMMUNICABLE DISEASE TRANSMISSION

When dealing with bleeding wounds, the AT must protect themselves and the athlete from infection. We tend to assume that athletes are free from communicable diseases because they look and act healthy, but this is not necessarily true.

An athlete may hide certain medical conditions to avoid discrimination. If an athlete chooses to reveal such a condition, it should be noted on the records from the physical.

Communicable diseases are transmitted, either directly or indirectly, by contact with an infected person. Although most viruses and bacteria cannot live long in the absence of a host, the AT and the athletes should take sensible precautions against possible infections. They should make it a habit not to share drinking glasses or towels, and they should try to avoid people who are contagious, such as someone who is sneezing a great deal from a cold. Some viruses, namely HIV and HBV (the viruses that cause AIDS and hepatitis B, respectively), may be present in bodily fluids from oozing wounds or needles. Thus, the athletic training team should take precautions when handling body fluids or when handling cloth, paper, or surfaces that have been soaked with body fluids (e.g., blood, urine).

Special precautions must be taken against the spread of HIV and HBV, which may be present in blood or other bodily fluids. Both athletic staff and every staff member of the school should be trained in **universal precautions** and follow procedures set forth by the Occupational Safety and Health Administration (OSHA) to prevent the spread of blood-borne diseases. A person with HIV or hepatitis B may show no signs or symptoms of the disease and may not even know they have it, yet the disease may be transmitted through contact with their blood. Therefore, universal precautions must be used every time bodily fluid is present. To take universal precautions, five simple rules must be observed:

1. Carefully wash your hands after any contact with an injured athlete.
2. Use rubber gloves to create a barrier between you and the athlete. Figure 25.9 illustrates how to properly remove gloves.

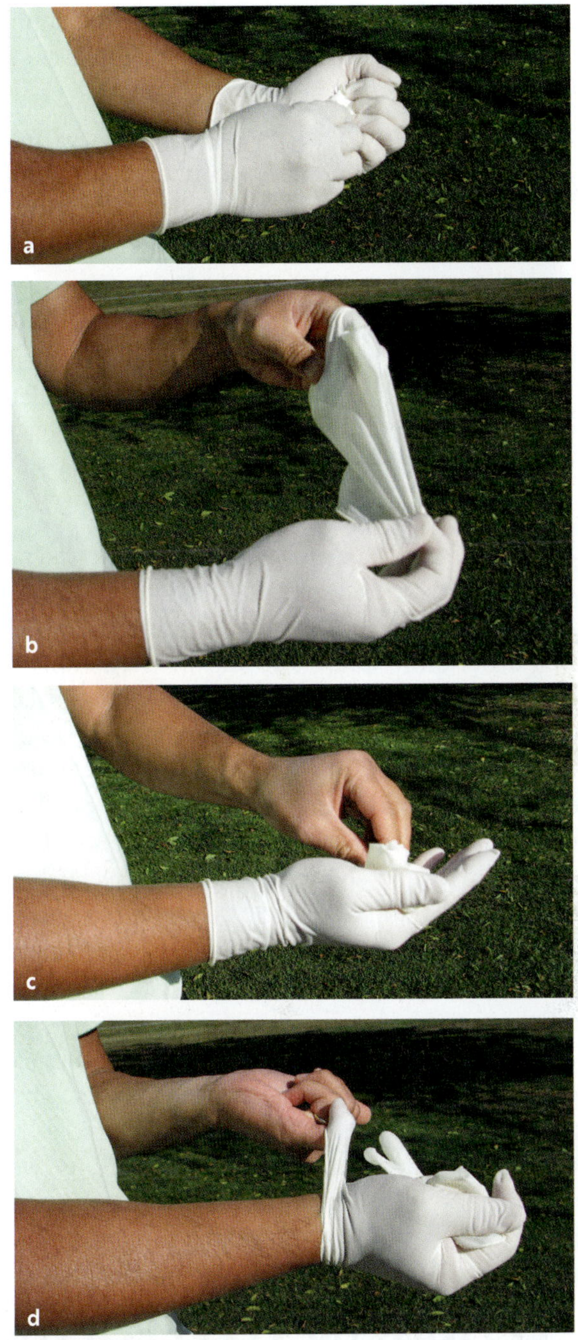

Figure 25.9 When removing latex gloves, *(a)* place all waste in one hand, and with the opposite, pinch the latex near the wrist; *(b)* pull the first glove off with the waste inside the glove; *(c)* place the first glove into the second hand; *(d)* slide a finger under the inside edge of the second glove; and pull the glove off. Discard the gloves in a biohazard container.

3. Thoroughly clean any tables, counters, or playing surfaces in an athletic training room or court with a disinfectant such as a 1:10 solution of bleach and water.

4. Deposit in a red biohazard bag any contaminated material, including clothes, gloves, or gauze pads.
5. Dispose any used needles or syringes in a specially made sharps container. If an AT is contaminated by body fluids, they must document the incident and report it to the supervisor as soon as possible.
6. When providing resuscitation, the AT will use a one-way valve mask so that air enters the airway of the athlete but does not exit back to the AT. Another option is using a bag mask, where a large bulbous container is squeezed and air enters the athlete's airway.

Athletes should observe other standard precautions, which, for example, will help to prevent the spread of common cold and flu viruses. The AT should not allow players to dip their cups into a team cooler to get water; this practice allows saliva to be mixed into the cooler. Every athlete should drink from their own glass or squeeze bottle. Athletes should avoid tasting each other's food, borrowing utensils, and sharing drinking glasses. They should also avoid sharing personal items such as combs, towels, and clothes, and they should shower after each practice. Teams must also be prepared to replace uniforms that are potentially soiled with a pathogen.

In addition to taking universal precautions, ATs can be vaccinated against certain diseases. They can be vaccinated against HBV, for example, by receiving a series of three vaccine injections over a seven-month period. The HBV vaccine is 90% effective in preventing infection.

SECONDARY ASSESSMENT

The secondary assessment is an evaluation of injuries that are not life-threatening. The AT performs a secondary assessment after they have completed the primary survey and taken care of any life-threatening injuries. In the secondary assessment, the AT will check the following in order: history, head, vital signs, arms, chest, abdomen, hips, and legs. During the secondary assessment, if the airway, breathing, or circulation changes, the AT will immediately give care and abandon the secondary assessment.

HIT

Most of the time, an AT is dealing with a specific complaint, such as "My thumb hurts." When assessing a specific body area, the AT uses the **HIT** technique (see figure 25.10). The acronym *HIT* stands for **h**istory, **i**nspection, and **t**esting. The trainer takes a history to gather information about the situation and the injury. Inspection is a visual examination of the body part, and testing includes touching, specific evaluations, checking the range of motion, and neurological testing. We will refer to the HIT technique throughout this text.

H	**History**—Take a history by asking questions and checking vital signs.
I	**Inspection**—Observe the surroundings and injured body part.
T	**Testing**—Do specific testing to determine the severity of the injury.

Figure 25.10 Athletic injury assessment follows a predictable sequence: taking a history, inspecting the area, and testing.

History

Taking a history includes both asking questions and checking vital signs. In taking a history, the AT will obtain information about what is happening and about the athlete's previous injuries and illnesses because they may play a role in the present problem (see the sidebar). If the athlete is unconscious, reviewing records of their physical and talking to other athletes who saw the injury may be helpful.

The AT will check the athlete for a medical alert tag and the records from the physical for information that may help determine the cause of the cur-

What Would You Do If . . .

The AT is doing an evaluation. Every time the AT touches a body part, the athlete responds by saying, "That hurts!" The AT tells you to get a backboard and call 911.

rent condition. The same questions can be used to take a history for any injury and illness. We refer to the questions for history of injury in the following chapters, so copy the list and keep it handy. Questions that apply to a specific body area will be listed in the appropriate chapter.

The **vital signs** checked in the secondary assessment are body temperature, skin color, breathing rate, heart rate, response to pain, pupillary reaction, ability to move, and capillary refill. The AT can also assess breath sounds and blood pressure if a stethoscope and blood pressure cuff are available. Table 25.2 outlines abnormal vital signs.

Heart Rate

Heart rate is measured at **pulse points**, where an artery lies close to the skin (see figure 25.11). The pulse points of the carotid artery and the radial artery are used most often. The carotid artery can be found by placing two fingers on the Adam's apple and then sliding them toward the shoulder until the fingers go into a depression in the neck. The radial artery is located on the volar aspect (palm side) on the thumb side of the wrist. Once the pulse is found, the AT will count the number of times the heart beats in a minute—this is the

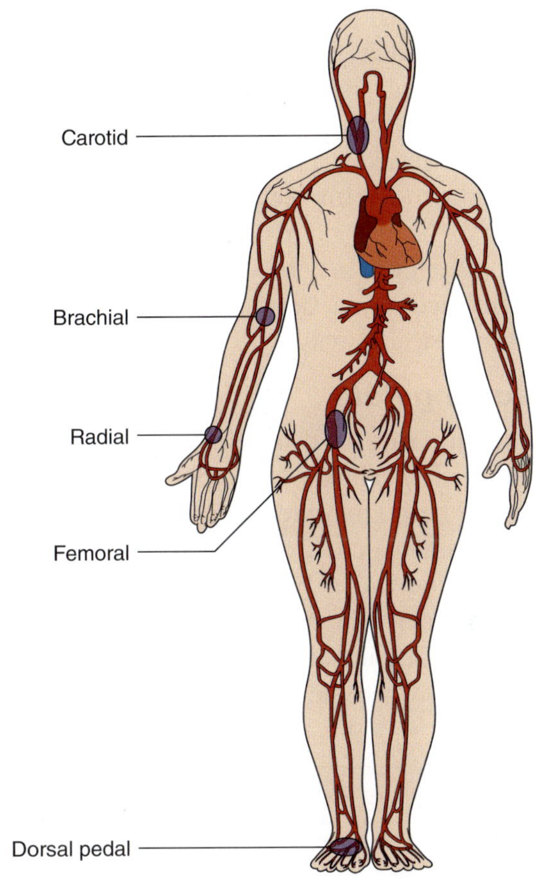

Figure 25.11 Pulse points.

Table 25.2 Abnormal Vital Signs

Vital signs	Abnormality	Indication
Pupils	Constricted Unequal Dilated	Drug or medication overdose or bright light Head injury or illness Drug or medication overdose, death, shock, heatstroke, or darkness
Pulse	Rapid and weak Rapid and strong No pulse Slow pulse	Shock, internal bleeding, diabetic coma, or heat exhaustion Heatstroke, anxiousness, or physical exercise Blocked artery or cardiac arrest Heart problem, drugs, or medications Heatstroke, inflammation, or diabetic coma
Skin color	Red White Blue	Shock, heat exhaustion, insulin shock, or low blood pressure Cardiac arrest or breathing difficulty
Body temperature	Hot and dry Cool and moist Chills Hot and moist	Heatstroke Heat exhaustion Cold exposure or illness Fever
Breathing	No breathing Decreased breathing rate Increased breathing rate	Cardiac arrest, respiratory arrest, or head injury Chest trauma or head injury Drugs or medication, shock, heart injury, or anxiety

pulse rate. The normal pulse rate for an average teenager or adult is between 60 and 80 beats per minute. A highly trained athlete, however, may have a pulse rate as low as 40 beats per minute and still be perfectly healthy. A person may also have a pulse rate below the norm because of medication (legal or illegal), heart abnormalities, or internal injuries. Rapid pulse rates may be due to shock, hyperventilation, medication (legal or illegal), anxiety, or recent physical activity.

Breathing Rate

Breathing rate is determined by counting the number of times the chest rises and falls in a minute. The normal breathing rate for a teenager or adult is between 12 and 20 breaths per minute. Breathing rates can be slower than normal due to a head injury, lung injury, medication (legal or illegal), shock, and diabetes. Breathing rates that are rapid may be the result of shock, medication

FYI

Breath Sounds

Breath sounds are heard through the chest wall with a stethoscope. No breath sounds means that the athlete is not breathing or the lungs are seriously injured.

Cystic Fibrosis

Cystic fibrosis, a disease that affects the pancreas and lungs, is inherited.

Shock

Shock is a condition in which inadequate oxygen is reaching the tissues of the body because of insufficient blood flow.

Pneumonia

Pneumonia is an inflammation of the lungs caused by an infection or irritant.

QUESTIONS FOR HISTORY OF INJURY

The following questions should be asked as part of the history:

1. What happened?
2. When did it happen?
3. Has this happened before?
4. Where was the pain initially?
5. Did you hear or feel a pop, snap, crack, slip, or give?
6. Were you able to continue participating?
7. How soon did it swell?
8. Does it feel unstable?
9. What relieves the pain?
10. How severe is the pain?
11. What does the pain feel like?
12. What treatment was applied immediately? Later?
13. Have you had a previous injury to this body part?

If the problem relates to an illness rather than an injury, ask the following questions:

1. Are you allergic to any medications?
2. What have you eaten today?
3. Are you allergic to anything else?
4. Have you had anything to drink today?
5. What events led to this situation?

(legal or illegal), anxiety, heat-related illnesses, or recent physical activity. Athletes may also have **dyspnea**, or difficulty breathing. This is common among athletes with asthma, cystic fibrosis, shock, pneumonia, lung injuries, allergic reactions, airway obstructions, or upper-respiratory illnesses (colds or flu). The AT will not tell the athlete when they are checking breathing rate because it is often hard for a person to breathe naturally if they know they are being watched. The athlete may hold his breath or breathe faster, invalidating the count. The AT will check the pulse and, while pretending to take the athlete's pulse, count the breathing rate. **Apnea** is the temporary cessation of breathing, and it is a serious symptom in an athlete because it may indicate a head injury. An athlete who has an unusual breath odor should be checked for possible poisoning, intoxication, or diabetes.

When the AT uses a stethoscope to listen to the lungs, they will listen to each side of the chest for one cycle of breathing and compare them. Then they will listen to the lower lung portions for one cycle to ensure that there are no immediate problems with the lungs.

Blood Pressure

The heart pumps blood to move blood cells, nutrients, and oxygen throughout the body. Blood pressure is the pressure that the blood exerts against the walls of the blood vessels, especially the arteries. **Systolic pressure** is the pressure when the heart is contracting, and **diastolic pressure** is the pressure when the heart is relaxed between beats. **Pulse pressure** is the difference between the diastolic and systolic pressures. The blood pressure of an average teenager is less than 120 mmHg (milliliters of mercury) systolic and less than 80 mmHg diastolic (Fowler 2023). Blood pressure can increase because of a head injury, recent activity, medication (legal or illegal), and illnesses. Blood pressure will drop because of heart failure, hemorrhage, shock, certain medications (legal or illegal), and illnesses.

Blood pressure is measured with a stethoscope and a blood pressure cuff, which is sized in proportion to the athlete's arm (see figure 25.12). The cuff is placed on the upper arm and pressurized until no blood can flow through the superficial arteries. As the pressure in the cuff is slowly released, the person listens through the stethoscope, which has been placed on the inside of the elbow, and watches the dial on the cuff. The first time a sound is heard, the person reads the dial; that is the systolic pressure. When the sounds stop, the dial is read again; that is the diastolic pressure. If a stethoscope is not available, systolic blood pressure can be taken by feeling (palpating) for a radial pulse, although this method is less accurate. As the blood pressure cuff is released, the person reads the dial when they feel the radial pulse, and that will be the systolic pressure. When taking a blood pressure reading, bear in mind that an athlete who has just finished exercising will have a higher than normal blood pressure, as will an athlete who is upset. If the AT is having trouble getting a blood pressure reading,

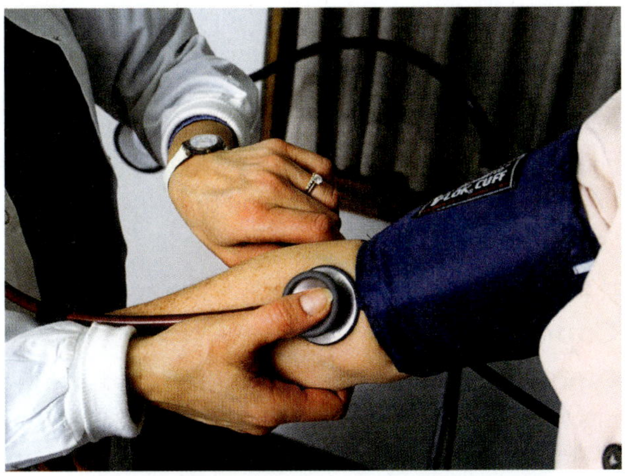

Figure 25.12 Place the stethoscope over the artery and listen as the pressure is released from the blood pressure cuff. The systolic pressure is read from the dial when the first pumping sound is heard. The diastolic pressure is read when the last pumping sound is heard.
Photodisc

What Would You Do If . . .

Two athletes collide at a soccer game. After a brief evaluation, both players are able to continue play. At the start of the second half, you notice that one of the players is on the ground. After talking with him, you notice that his wrists are flexing, and he says he has a headache.

they will check the athlete for the following:

- A heartbeat
- Shock
- Placement of the stethoscope
- Blockage of the artery

Body Temperature

Normal **body temperature** is 98.6 °F (37 °C). An athlete's body temperature can rise if they have an infection or heatstroke, and it may drop if they are in shock or exposed to cold. Electronic temperature-measuring devices, which are quick and accurate, are now available. The temperature can be taken with an oral thermometer, which is left in place for three minutes. It is also possible, although unreliable, to take a temperature by placing a thermometer in the armpit for 10 minutes. It is not possible to measure a person's temperature or even tell if they have a fever by feeling the forehead, but the AT may feel an athlete's forehead to determine if they are hot, cold, sweaty, or dry.

Skin Color

Skin color can give information about what illness or injury may have occurred. Four color changes are significant: cherry red is an indication of heatstroke or carbon monoxide poisoning, a bluish tinge is an indication of poor oxygen supply, yellow is an indication of liver illness, and a lack of color or a paleness of the nail beds and lips is an indication of shock or lack of circulation. The AT will also check for color changes in the whites of the eyes (sclera), the inside of the lip, and the fingernail and toenail beds, especially if the athlete has a dark complexion.

Capillary Refill

Capillary refill is an indication that blood is flowing to the fingertips and toes (see figure 25.13). It is determined by pressing on the nail and measuring how long it takes the color to return to normal (approximately one second). When the AT is checking capillary refill, they will check both arms or both legs at the same time. That way, the AT can tell if there is a difference between them, which may indicate a fracture or a blood clot in one of the body parts.

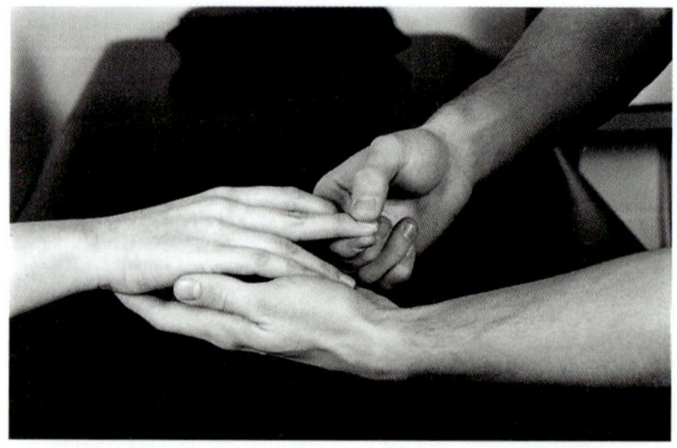

Figure 25.13 How quickly blood returns to the tip of a finger or toe after pressing on the nail bed and then releasing pressure is a measure of the blood supply to the finger. Poor capillary refill can mean restricted blood vessels or poor blood supply.

Understanding Diversity

It may be difficult to evaluate pallor or jaundice in people with darker skin. The AT may use nail beds, the sclera of the eye, or the inside of the lip to determine skin color changes (Purnell and Fenkl 2019).

Pupil Response

The eye pupils change size in response to light. When light shines into the eye, the pupils **constrict**, or get smaller, to decrease the amount of light entering the eye. In the dark, the pupils enlarge, or **dilate**, to allow more light into the eye. When the eyes do not respond normally to light changes, a serious problem is indicated. If the pupils dilate

What Would You Do If . . .

An athlete has been kept out of basketball practice because of ankle pain. She has not been able to walk but has no swelling or discoloration. During the week, she has been going to rehabilitation and has received other forms of therapy. While driving past her house, you see her playing basketball with several other people, and she has no problem running or jumping. Noticing you, she says, "Don't tell anyone. I just don't like to run."

when light shines into them, the athlete may have been poisoned or medicated, or they may even be dead. Pupils that constrict when there is darkness are an indication of heatstroke or poisoning. If the pupils are unequal in size (one is large and one is small), the AT will suspect a head injury, although a small percentage of people normally have unequal pupils. Blind people may or may not have pupillary response, depending on the origin of the blindness. Figure 25.14 illustrates pupil responses.

Ability to Move

It is important to find out if the athlete can still move. This helps determine what injury may have occurred and how to treat the athlete. **Paralysis**, the inability to move, is caused by an injury to the brain or spinal cord. The inability of an athlete to move one side of the body is known as **hemiplegia**, which is an indication of a head injury on the side opposite to the paralyzed side of the body. The extent of the paralysis depends on the location of the injury—the higher in the spine the injury occurs, the greater the extent of limb impairment. The inability to move the legs is called paraplegia, and the inability to move the arms and legs is called quadriplegia. Paralysis may be temporary; regardless, a physician must care for the athlete.

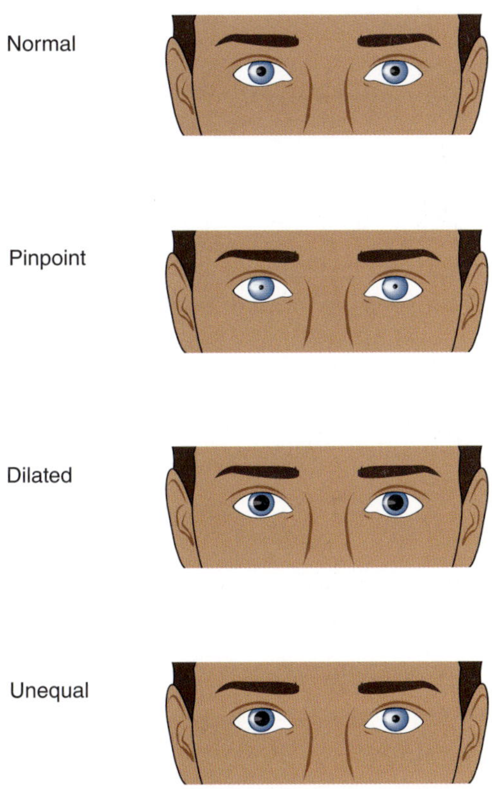

Figure 25.14 In response to light, the pupils normally get smaller. Pupils that dilate in response to light indicate a serious head injury, using medication, or death. Pinpoint pupils are an indication of medication. Unequal pupils indicate a head injury on the same side as the enlarged pupil.

Response to Pain

People respond differently to being injured. Pain cannot be used to determine the severity of an injury, because people have different tolerances for pain and will respond to the pain of an injury in different ways. Paralysis, medication, and shock can also disguise pain reactions. In addition, injuries to internal organs tend to refer pain to specific areas of the body. For example, an injury to the spleen may result in pain around the athlete's left shoulder. See figure 25.15*a* and 25.15*b* for referred pain sites from internal organs.

The Real World

One day, I arrived at work just as a fellow employee pulled into the parking lot, so we walked together across the street to the hospital. We saw a casually dressed man lying in the grass between the curb and the sidewalk, apparently unconscious. As we approached him to check his breathing, he opened his eyes and said loudly, "Please don't call an ambulance. Just let me lie here." I wondered why we shouldn't call for help, but we couldn't just leave him there, so I stayed with the man while my colleague went to the emergency room, just inside the nearest building, to report the problem. The man's skin felt cool and clammy to the touch, and when I checked his pulse, I noticed an alert tag on his wrist, which said he had epilepsy. He must have had a seizure and fallen on the grass. He said he was very tired, and his speech was slurred. EMS arrived in only a few minutes and took him to the emergency room. When I went to check on him later that morning, he had been released to his family's care. What a way to start the morning! It just goes to show that you must always be prepared for anything.

Bill Pitney, EdD, ATC

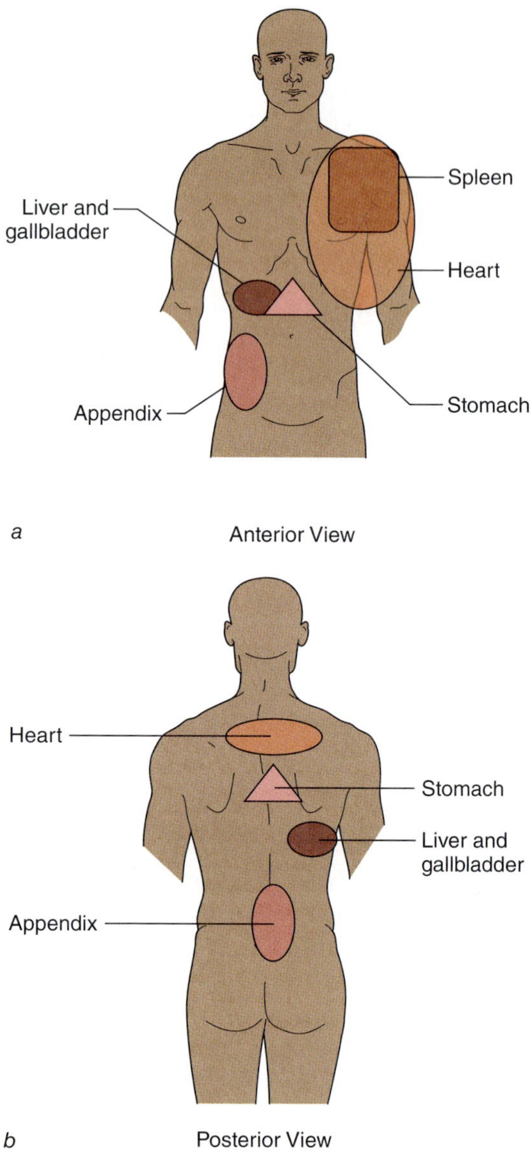

Figure 25.15 *(a)* Anterior view and *(b)* posterior view of referred pain sites from internal organs.

Inspection

The AT will observe the athlete's body and surroundings for clues as to what may have happened, which will suggest treatment options. If a chair has been tipped over, it is possible that the athlete fell out of it. Think about the injuries that could occur from a fall while sitting on a chair. Now think about the injuries that could occur if the athlete fell while standing on the chair. Are they the same? An empty bottle should raise red flags. Is this a poisoning, or was the athlete taking medication for an illness? An arm that bends where it never did before means what? The questions that are the hardest to answer are the ones on which the AT will concentrate. An even greater problem will be trying to get other athletes to talk about how the injury occurred. Some athletes may not want to help because they do not want to be involved, they fear lawsuits, or they just do not care.

Testing

Most often an AT will do the primary survey quickly, and during the history portion of the assessment, the athlete will indicate what happened. At that point, the AT can assess the body part involved. They can do specific tests to determine the severity of injury before swelling and muscular contractions occur, which will cause the body part to become immobile and make it difficult to determine the extent of the injury. The tests will also help determine how the athlete should be moved, if they should be splinted, or if medical help is immediately necessary. Testing should be stopped if the swelling is exceedingly rapid, if crepitus is felt, or if there is deformity or excessive pain.

Palpation

During palpation, the AT will examine the athlete by touch, feeling for depressions, fluid leakage, bumps, crepitus, and things that are not symmetrical. The AT will look for signs of pain on the athlete's face, decreased strength, decreased sensation, and false movement. Crepitus and excessive pain are reasons to stop palpation and splint the body part before moving the athlete. Palpation is done in the following order:

1. Head
2. Chest and thorax
3. Abdomen
4. Upper extremities
5. Lower extremities
6. Special tests

Listening to the Heart

Listening to the heart and obtaining useful information requires a lot of practice. For most ATs, listening to the heart will be limited to establishing that there is a heartbeat and determining a heart rate.

Range-of-Motion Testing

Range of motion must be tested at the injured segment as well as at the joints above and below the injury. The testing should be performed both actively and passively (see figure 25.16). That is, the injured athlete moves the injured segment if they are able (active) and the AT also attempts to move it (passive).

An athlete with a suspected broken bone, a bone with deformity, or a spinal cord injury should not be put through range-of-motion testing. Suspected broken bones should be splinted before an injured athlete is moved.

Range of motion should be measured from the anatomical position with a **goniometer** (see figure 25.17). When documenting test results, the AT should note the position the athlete was in when they took the measurements. For example, the report should state that the athlete was supine (lying on their back) or prone (face down). This allows the AT to make follow-up measurements with the athlete in the same position, thus making the measurements more consistent. It is vital that the range of motion of an injured limb be compared with that of the healthy limb.

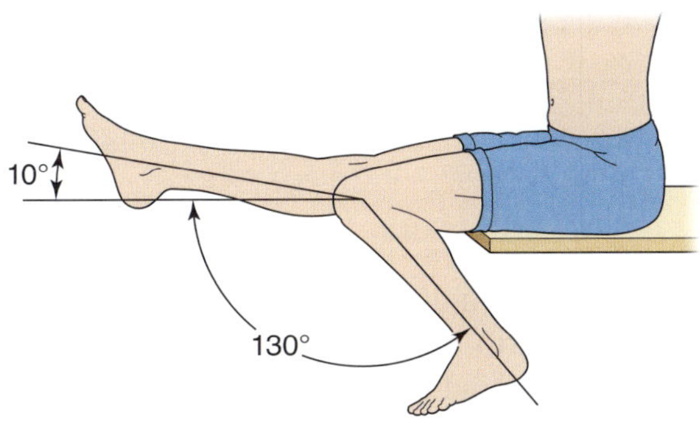

Figure 25.16 Anterior–posterior range of motion.

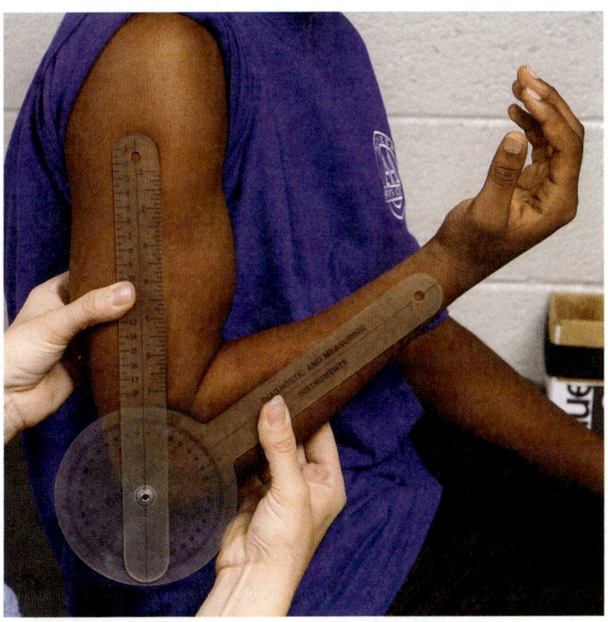

Figure 25.17 Goniometer use.

Strength Testing

Resistive range-of-motion testing helps to measure the strength of an area of the body. Muscular strength testing is often done with a technique called *manual muscle testing* (MMT), which is an objective way to determine the level of a person's strength. It is based on a grading system of zero to normal. A grade of *zero* indicates an inability to even twitch a muscle. *Trace* means an ability to perform a muscle twitch. A grade of *poor* indicates that an athlete can move a segment through full range of motion only if gravity is eliminated. *Fair* means the athlete can move a segment through full range of motion against gravity but with no other resistance. *Good* means that the athlete can move the segment through full range of motion, against gravity, and with some resistance applied by the AT. A grade of *normal* indicates that the athlete can move the segment through full range of motion, against gravity, and with full resistance from the AT. Some ATs use MMT without grading by simply comparing the resistive range of motion of an extremity with that of the extremity on the opposite side. The MMT strength-grading system allows ATs and other health care providers to document strength consistently and thus communicate the athlete's condition efficiently and effectively. The MMT strength-grading system can be found in table 25.3.

FYI

Crepitus

Crepitus is a crackling feeling under the skin.

False Movement

False movement is movement where there normally is none, such as in the middle of the forearm.

Table 25.3 Manual Muscle Testing to Determine Strength Level

Strength classifications (number or grade)	Description	
>5	Normal	The athlete can move the joint through a full range of motion against gravity and against full resistance from the AT.
4+	Good+	The athlete can move the joint through a full range of motion against gravity and against a significant amount of resistance from the AT.
4	Good	The athlete can move the joint though a full range of motion against gravity and against some resistance from the AT.
3+	Fair+	The athlete can move the joint through a full range of motion against gravity and against minimal resistance from the AT.
3	Fair	The athlete can move the joint through a full range of motion against gravity with no applied resistance from the AT. If any resistance is applied, full range of motion is not achieved.
2	Poor	The athlete can move the joint through a full range of motion only if gravity is eliminated or against gravity with assistance from the AT.
1	Trace	When asked to move the joint, the athlete will not be able to do so. However, a muscle contraction should be observable.
0	Zero	When asked to move the joint, the athlete will not be able to do so. Moreover, a muscle contraction will not be visible.

Data obtained from Anderson and Barnum (2022); Reiman (2016).

Testing to Rule Out Neurological Problems

Once strength and range of motion have been assessed, the injured athlete can be evaluated for neurological problems, which might include an inability to feel or move a body part. Each nerve that exits the spinal column is responsible for sensation and movement at a particular area of the body. By exposing these specific areas to a light touch or pricking stimulus and by asking the athlete to try to move the area, an AT can determine if a specific nerve may be involved in the injury. If a spinal cord injury is suspected, the athlete must be backboarded before being moved.

SPECIFIC CONDITIONS

Specific conditions that must be considered during a secondary assessment include shock and fractures. Here, we discuss the common signs and symptoms and the necessary care of each.

Recognizing Shock

Shock is a condition in which inadequate blood and oxygen are supplied to vital organs. The body has five organs that must always receive an adequate blood supply to maintain life: the brain, heart, lungs, liver, and kidneys. When an athlete becomes seriously injured, the body tries to protect the vital organs by increasing blood flow to the organs while decreasing blood flow to the arms and legs. The three reasons a body goes into shock are the following:

1. The blood vessels in the head, chest, and abdomen enlarge, getting ready to carry more blood. If the blood vessels in the arms and legs constrict and do not move blood into the vessels of the head, chest, and abdomen, blood pressure in these vessels decreases because the vessels have enlarged while the volume of blood has not increased. This means that the supply of oxygen to the vital organs is reduced.
2. The body will go into shock if the heart stops. Obviously, if the heart stops, no blood is flowing to the vital organs. When this happens, restarting the heart, not shock, is the first concern.
3. The body goes into shock from significant blood loss. If blood is leaking from the vessels, there is a smaller amount of blood to pump. If too much blood is lost, the organs will not get enough

oxygen and nutrients to sustain life, they will shut down, and the athlete will die.

If shock is not recognized early and treated rapidly, it can cause death. Signs of shock include agitation (usually the first sign); rapid, weak pulse; decreased blood pressure (100 mmHg or lower); cold, clammy skin; sweating; cyanosis; increasing unconsciousness; and pale skin. Symptoms are nausea, thirst, anxiety, and dizziness. Table 25.4 describes the kinds of shock and what causes each.

Treating Shock

To treat shock, treat the original injury; keep the athlete warm; if the arms and legs are not broken, elevate them 10 to 12 inches (25-30 cm) above the heart; measure breathing and pulse rate every 5 minutes; do not give anything to eat or drink; if vomiting occurs, turn the victim on their side and clear the airway; and get the victim to the hospital as soon as possible.

Pulse Oximeter

A pulse oximeter measures the amount of oxygen saturation in the blood. During an illness or injury, oxygen saturation may be too low, and it gives the AT an opportunity to supplement it (see table 25.5). Pulse oximeters can be used on fingers or toes, but fingernail polish can inhibit accuracy (see figure 25.18). Table 25.5 shows oxygen saturation levels and what it means for supplementing with oxygen.

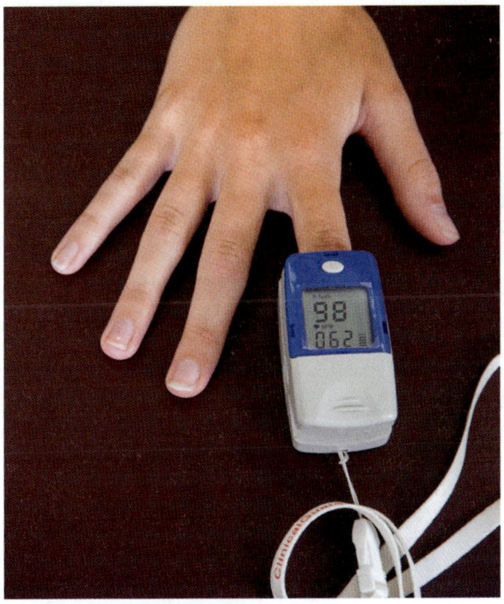

Figure 25.18 Pulse oximeter.

Table 25.4 Types of Shock

Type of shock	Characteristics
Psychogenic (fainting)	Temporary loss of nervous function, causing blood vessels to dilate
Septic	General infection, causing circulatory failure
Neurological	Loss of control over the nervous system, causing blood vessels to dilate (spinal cord injury)
Cardiogenic	Cessation of heartbeat (cardiac arrest)
Hemorrhagic or hypovolemic	Loss of blood (internal bleeding)
Metabolic	Loss of fluids through vomiting, diarrhea, or urination (diabetics)
Respiratory	Cessation of breathing, causing a change in oxygen supply in the blood, which causes organs to shut down because of oxygen loss (asthma)
Anaphylactic	Cessation of breathing caused by a toxin (bee venom or drug) in the system, causing changes to the oxygen supply within the body, which causes the organs to shut down

Table 25.5 Pulse Oximetry and Supplemental Oxygen Needed

Range	Saturation level	Oxygen needed
95%-100%	Normal levels	None
91%-94%	Mild hypoxia	1-6 L/min
90% or less	Mild to moderate hypoxia	6-10 L/min
80%-85%	Moderate hypoxia	10-15 L/min
67% or below	Cyanosis	15 L/min and higher

Adapted from Cleary and Flanagan (2020).

Oxygen Therapy

Supplemental oxygen is necessary whenever the lungs or breathing is compromised. It is important to treat the initial injury or illness while providing oxygen. Make sure the airway is open before providing oxygen. In table 25.6, the various types of delivery devices and the flow rates are listed.

Oxygen is one form of treatment that can be used when someone is in shock. The AT should check their oxygen tank weekly to ensure proper pressures and the amount of oxygen in the tank.

Intravenous Therapy (IV)

Intravenous therapy is part of therapy for patients who are in shock from fluid loss. Adding fluid will increase blood volume and its oxygen-carrying capacity, depending on the type of shock. The IV solution comes in a sterile bag with two ports, one for medication administration and one for delivering the IV fluid into the body. The AT will have to determine the best catheter and the best entry point (arm, hand, or hip). The area must have a sterile field, and the AT must protect themselves from coming into contact with bodily fluids.

Use a constricting band above the site of insertion. The IV catheter is inserted into a vein and the IV tubing is secured in place. Properly dispose of any sharps. The rate of IV flow is determined based on the need of the athlete's condition. A vein collapse, hematoma, or irritation of the vein can be complications of IV therapy.

If the athlete has head or neck injuries and is in shock, they must be placed on a backboard and sent to the hospital for care. The athlete can be covered with a blanket to maintain body heat but should be kept lying flat. An athlete with respiratory injury can have their head elevated if there are no head or neck injuries; this will make it easier for them to breathe.

FYI

Cyanosis

Cyanosis is a blue coloration of the skin caused by lack of oxygen.

Backboards

Backboards are platforms that extend from the head to the toes. An athlete is secured to a backboard (backboarded) when a spinal cord injury is suspected.

Assessing and Managing a Fracture

When assessing an athlete with a possible fracture, the AT must check capillary refill, pulse rate in the extremity, and sensation of the body part. The athlete should never be asked to use the body part because this could cause further injury. If the trainer finds poor circulation, lack of sensation, or decreased capillary refill, the athlete may have seriously injured the nerve or vessels to that body part and requires immediate attention by the team physician. If the trainer cannot tell for sure whether the part is fractured, they should splint the area to be safe.

Assessing and Managing a Subluxation or Dislocation

When the bones of a joint disarticulate, this is known as a dislocation. If the bones are partially out of alignment, this is a subluxation. The diagnosis of a dislocation is distinguished from a fracture by the following indicators:

1. Occurs at a joint
2. Difficult to move
3. Disfigurement at the site

Table 25.6 Oxygen Flow Rates

Administration type	Flow rate (L/min)	Percent of supplemental oxygen delivered
Nasal cannula	1-6	24-50
Resuscitation mask	5-15	30-60
Nonrebreather mask	8-15	80-95
Bag value mask	10-15	40-100

Adapted from Pollack (2022); Cleary and Flanagan (2020); Weekley and Bland (2022).

Complications of a dislocation include damage to the articular surface of the joint. There can be damage to muscles, nerves, and ligaments of the joint. Loss of circulation distal to the site is an emergency. A posterior dislocation of the sternoclavicular joint is an emergency because the clavicle presses on the trachea. Immobilization of a dislocation is the same as it is for a fracture.

Types of Splints

Several types of splints can be used to manage fractures and dislocations. A traction splint is used when the femur has been fractured, because the muscles in the thigh are so strong that they can cause the limb to shorten if proper splinting is not used. The traction splint pulls the bone ends apart and into alignment, which causes muscle tissue to relax, thus decreasing the pain. A rigid splint, which is made of a stiff material, is applied to the side, front, or back of an extremity. The splint must be padded and bandaged securely to the limb to hold the fracture in position. Examples of rigid splints are box splints, boards, and aluminum splints.

A semirigid splint is a moldable splint that hardens in place to hold a fracture; an example is a vacuum splint. Soft splints remain soft after the splint is applied to a fracture; examples include pillows, slings and swathes, and air splints. The trainer must check his supply of air splints regularly—they get holes and may not be usable in an emergency. Figure 25.19 illustrates various splints.

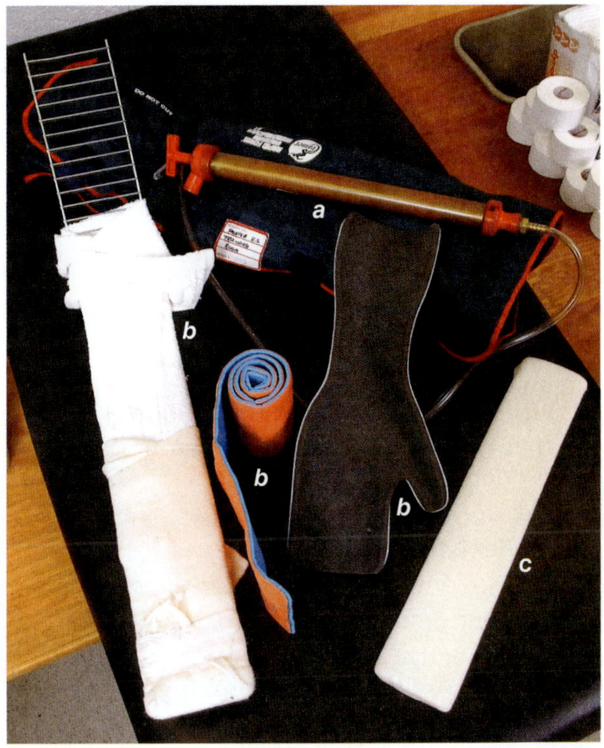

Figure 25.19 *(a)* A vacuum splint is applied and then air is withdrawn from it to mold it to a suspected fracture. *(b)* Aluminum splints are padded and molded to a specific body part. *(c)* Economical board splints are also padded.

Moving After Splinting

Once a body part is splinted, the athlete can be moved (assuming they have no other major problems) and body parts can be elevated for shock. On the way to the hospital, the AT must make sure the athlete is as comfortable as possible and prevent the splinted fracture from bouncing around in the transport vehicle. A fractured arm can be placed in a sling with a pillow between the arm and the athlete's lap. A fractured leg can be wrapped in blankets, which act as a comfort barrier, and strapped to the other leg.

PRICES METHOD

Most sprains, strains, and splinted fractures can be cared for with the **PRICES** method—**p**rotection, **r**est, **i**ce, **c**ompression, **e**levation, and **s**upport. The body part must be protected from further injury, and rest allows the body to heal. Ice, compression, and elevation reduce the swelling, and external support restricts movement at the site.

Protection and rest are necessary to prevent further injury. Protection involves splinting or padding an area. Rest is self-explanatory. The athlete should avoid being active on the injured area.

Ice is applied for no longer than 30 minutes at a time because longer applications can cause frostbite. There should be at least 40 minutes between ice applications. Essentially, time between icings should be twice the time of ice application. An acute injury should be iced no more than three times a day. For an acute injury, the ice should be crushed and placed in a plastic bag or should be a solid chunk in an ice cup. When applying ice to a body part, the athlete may experience pain and the sensation of extra pressure before the body part becomes numb.

The Real World

Our college was hosting a cross country meet about 5 miles (8 km) from campus. We were also hosting a women's soccer game on campus at the same time. I sent a senior AT student and my team physician to the cross country meet, and I stayed on campus and covered football practice and the soccer game. Midway through the first half of the soccer game, my student called me on the radio.

Here's how the conversation went:

Student: Can you send someone out here with some bee sting kits?

Me: What do you mean, kits? How many do you need?

Student: About 30 would do the trick.

Me: What?! What happened?

Student: One of the runners stepped on a yellow jacket hive in the ground, and now every runner that comes down the path is getting stung. We've had about 30 runners get stung so far, and some runners have crossed the finish line with live bees still attached to their bodies.

Me: Do you or the doctor have any bee sting kits or adrenaline?

Student: No.

Me: Has anyone developed an allergic reaction?

Student: Four runners are in trouble and 10 more are questionable.

Me: I'm activating EMS. I'm going to send at least two ambulances and have the fire and rescue squad come as well. Get the victims together in one place and triage them. Treat them all for shock.

Four runners ended up in the emergency room and were released a few hours later. Fifteen runners had localized reactions not requiring further care. Even if we had been better prepared with a bee sting kit or two, I'm not sure that we wouldn't have had significant problems, given the circumstances. It was an interesting day.

Anonymous

Compression is pressure applied to the injured body part to prevent swelling. It is achieved with pads and snug application of elastic wraps or tape. Before elevating the body part, the student assistant or AT should arrange sufficient blankets, towels, or padding to lift the body part 10 to 12 inches (25-30 cm) above the heart. The body part can then be gently lifted while the support is slid underneath.

Support relates to providing necessary ambulatory aids such as crutches, canes, or walkers. With less severe injuries, support may be a brace to allow ambulation with some stability to the area, such as a foot or ankle.

Another way to view appropriate steps of care is doing **No HARM** to an injured athlete. No HARM means that during the first 48 to 72 hours after an injury, the athlete should have **no h**eat applied to the injured area because this can cause more bleeding and swelling, no **a**lcohol ingested because this can cause more swelling, no **r**unning or activity because this may cause further injury, and no **m**assage to the area because this also can increase swelling.

Summary

An injured athlete must be assessed immediately so that prudent care can begin. The AT will assess the athlete for life-threatening injuries first: They will check the ABCs, or the athlete's airway, breathing, and circulation. An athlete who has no ABCs needs immediate care and emergency medical assistance. Everyone, including the AT, coach, and student assistant, needs to observe universal precautions when working with bodily fluids. When determining the nature and severity of an injury, the AT will conduct a complete assessment of the athlete. The secondary assessment begins with HIT. Some injuries may cause the athlete to go into shock, which can be fatal. Treatment for shock depends on its cause. Sprains, strains, dislocations, and splinted fractures are usually treated with PRICES.

Key Terms

Define the following terms found in this chapter:

- ABCs
- angina pectoris
- apnea
- body temperature
- breathing rate
- capillary refill
- cardiac arrest
- cardiopulmonary resuscitation (CPR)
- constrict
- diastolic pressure
- dilate
- direct pressure
- dyspnea
- goniometer
- heart attack
- heart rate
- hemiplegia
- HIT
- intravenous therapy
- No HARM
- paralysis
- partial airway obstruction
- pressure point
- PRICES
- primary assessment
- pulse points
- pulse pressure
- pulse rate
- sign
- symptom
- syncope
- systolic pressure
- total airway obstruction
- tourniquet
- universal choking sign
- universal precautions
- vital signs

An athlete suddenly falls ill during a cheerleading event. She is pale, dizzy, and has a rapid pulse. She reports that she has not eaten all day, and it is currently late afternoon. How do you perform the secondary survey in order to rule out a serious medical condition? What key factors would you emphasize during this initial evaluation? What are the key questions that are important to ask this athlete?

To access supplementary material for this chapter, including the Understanding Check worksheet, vocabulary quizzes, extension activities, and chapter-specific resources and forms, visit the web resource: http://ancillaries.humankinetics.com/FundamentalsOfAthleticTrainingAndSportsMedicine5E

chapter 26

Environmental Situations and Injuries

Objectives

After completing this chapter, the student will be able to do the following:

- Explain how to care for heat-related illnesses.
- Describe how the body gets rid of excessive heat.
- Explain how heat-related illnesses can be prevented.
- Describe the person who is more prone to cold- and heat-related injuries.
- Explain the treatment of cold- and heat-related injuries.
- Explain how to prevent bites from insects and snakes.

We live in a changing environment. Some days are rainy, and others are clear and sunny. Athletes like to practice in the same environment in which they will perform on game day. But sometimes they are surprised with weather they are not accustomed to, such as uncommonly high temperatures in October, which may cause problems for heat-sensitive athletes. In addition, an insect bite can lead to a life-threatening illness for some athletes. In this chapter, we discuss the first aid necessary to care for an athlete who becomes ill due to environmental factors.

HEAT-RELATED PROBLEMS

Hyperthermia is an exceptional rise in body temperature. Body temperature rises when the athlete is exercising, the environmental temperature is excessive, the athlete has an infection, or the body's temperature-regulation system has failed. The body regulates temperature via the hypothalamus gland, which is in the brain. As blood flows through the hypothalamus, heat receptors indicate a need to increase or decrease body temperature to maintain the body's core temperature at a constant 98.6 °F (37 °C), which is the temperature at which the body's systems normally function. The hypothalamus helps the body maintain a delicate balance in temperature, attempting to cool the body if heat production causes body temperature to rise or to conserve body heat if body temperature is decreasing. When body cooling exceeds heat production, the blood vessels in the arms and legs constrict, reducing the flow of blood passing close to the surface, where it would lose heat more rapidly. If body temperature begins to rise, the blood vessels in the extremities dilate so that more blood flows close to the surface in an attempt to rid the body of excess heat.

Heat-related illnesses range from mild heat cramps to severe heatstroke, which is considered a medical emergency. Heat exhaustion is considered a moderate illness.

Heat Cramps

Heat cramps are involuntary muscle contractions caused by dehydration and a loss of sodium from profuse sweating. A poor daily diet may also contribute to the problem. The calf and abdominal muscles are most likely to be involved. Heat cramps should be treated by having the athlete drink water, stretch the involved muscle, and apply ice to the muscle to alleviate pain.

Heat Syncope

Heat syncope is a brief period of fainting and dizziness that occurs during exposure to high temperatures, especially when athletes must stand for a long time or immediately following activity in the heat. Heat syncope is more likely to occur during the first few days of practicing in hot environments. If heat syncope occurs, the athlete should move to a cool environment, elevate their feet, and rehydrate by drinking cool fluids.

Heat Exhaustion

Heat exhaustion is caused by prolonged exercise in a hot, humid environment to the point of severe dehydration. Symptoms of heat exhaustion include fatigue, dizziness, nausea, headache, muscle cramps, shortness of breath, and distorted vision. Signs of heat exhaustion are excessive sweating; rapid, weak pulse; decreased blood pressure; skin that is cold and pale; and normal body temperature. To treat heat exhaustion, cool the athlete by removing them from the hot environment (get them into the shade), face a fan toward them, and apply cold, wet towels. Encourage them to sip water if they can. If they lose consciousness or the case is severe, refer them to a physician—if prompt medical attention is not given, the athlete's condition may progress to heatstroke.

The Real World

I was working on paperwork in the training room during football season when our placekicker entered the room, writhing in pain and screaming that something had bitten him on his hand. When I asked him if he knew what had bitten him, he didn't know, but it was obvious from the swelling and red marks on his middle finger that something had. I asked him what he had been doing when the bite occurred, and he said that he was retrieving his practice balls and had gone into a shrubbery bed to get one of them. Because the ball was in an odd location, he had put his hand on the trunk of a large tree to balance himself. He said he felt an immediate sting and then excruciating pain in his finger and hand. Then he came straight to the training room.

I radioed my college intern on the field and asked him to go to the tree and see if he could identify what had bitten the kicker. A few minutes later, the intern radioed back that the tree was covered with furry caterpillars. Because the kicker was starting to exhibit the signs and symptoms of anaphylaxis, I decided to contact his parents and send him to the emergency room. I also radioed out to the field and asked my intern to capture one of the bugs in a cup and bring it inside so that it could be transported to the hospital.

An hour or so later, the athlete returned from the hospital after being treated for the bite. The physicians in the emergency room had identified the culprit as the poisonous puss caterpillar. Our kicker was careful to watch where he placed his hands the rest of the season, and our staff learned something new about the little creatures our athletes sometimes run into.

Jim Berry, ATC

> **What Would You Do If . . .**
>
> The wrestling team practices in a facility where there is no direct fresh air. The temperature substantially increases by the end of practice.

Fluid Replacement

When an athlete exercises, they lose bodily fluids through sweat and evaporation. Athletes will have performance impairment if they lose 2% or more of their starting weight before exercise (Affiliated Community Medical Centers, n.d.). The AT may require athletes to weigh in before and after practice to determine the amount of fluid that needs to be replenished. Generally, 1 pound (.5 kg) of weight loss equals 23 ounces (680 mL) of water that needs to be consumed. An athlete who loses more than 2% of body weight must prehydrate using the same calculation of 1 pound equaling 23 ounces.

Heatstroke

Heatstroke is a dangerous condition where the body can no longer control its temperature. This hypothalamus dysfunction can result from exercising in a hot, humid environment; severe dehydration; excessive weight loss; obesity; or untreated heat exhaustion. Symptoms of impending heatstroke are feeling extremely hot, feeling confused, having a headache, and experiencing dizziness. Signs of heatstroke are little or no sweating; hot, dry skin; a core body temperature higher than 104 °F (40 °C); low blood pressure; rapid, weak pulse; rapid breathing rate; dilated pupils; and unconsciousness. A comparison between heatstroke and heat exhaustion is found in the Signs of Heatstroke and Heat Exhaustion sidebar.

When heatstroke is suspected, the AT should call 911 for emergency assistance and begin cooling the body as quickly as possible. According to the NATA position statement on exertional heat illnesses (Casa et al. 2015), the best way to reduce the athlete's core body temperature is to take any equipment and clothes off the athlete and immerse the athlete in a cold bath. The athlete should be immersed up to their neck in a tub with the water temperature between 35 °F and 59 °F (1-15 °C), with cold, wet towels applied to the neck, armpits, feet, and groin (see figure 26.1). Elevating the legs will help prevent shock. If the athlete is not treated immediately, death or irreversible brain damage will occur.

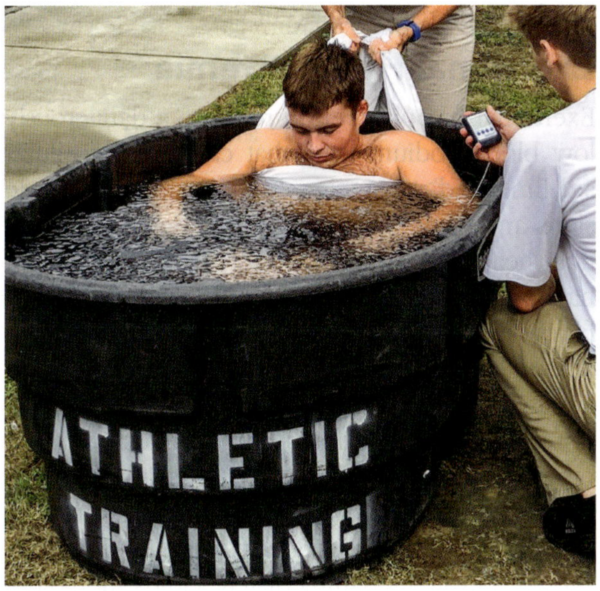

Figure 26.1 Cold-water immersion for heatstroke.

Courtesy of Katie Walsh Flanagan.

SIGNS OF HEATSTROKE AND HEAT EXHAUSTION

Heatstroke

- Unconsciousness
- Shallow breathing
- No sweating
- Red, dry skin
- Rapid bounding pulse
- High body temperature

Heat Exhaustion

- The person is conscious
- Rapid, shallow breathing
- Profuse sweating
- Pale, clammy skin
- Rapid weak pulse
- Normal body temperature

Understanding Diversity

Tips for Working With Mental Health and Culture

1. Instead of saying "mental illness," talk about it as a "biological illness."
2. Use the terms *stress* or *sadness* to ask about mental health issues—these may be more acceptable terms.
3. Have a health care provider who speaks the patient's language if necessary.
4. Ask about cultural beliefs around mental illness.
5. Ask about religious beliefs around mental illness.
6. Do not make assumptions about the patient's beliefs or religion.

Adapted from Quality Interactions (2019). Available: www.quality-interactions.com/blog/6-culturally-sensitive-ways-to-approach-mental-health.

Symptoms include headache, a feeling of cold, numbness, dizziness, and slowed breathing and heart rates. Using a rectal thermometer is the best way to determine body temperature. An athlete may be vulnerable to cold exposure if they have cardiovascular disease, alcoholism, or asthma; had previous bouts of hypothermia; have poor nutrition; are exposed to water or rain; have inadequate protective clothing; or are fatigued.

An athlete who is not treated for hypothermia is at risk of death. Hypothermia is treated by getting the athlete near a heat source, such as placing them in a warm room and removing wet clothing. Warm the athlete with a dry blanket. Be careful not to place them too close to an open flame or a heater; this may cause the blood vessels to dilate rapidly, which causes ruptures. Remember that another person is a source of heat, so getting into a sleeping bag or a blanket with the chilled athlete will help to warm them. The AT will call 911—the athlete must be seen by a physician.

Risk Factors for Cold-Related Injuries

Athletes who have had a previous cold injury, sweat, do not move, wear tight clothing, have poor nutrition, or are dehydrated are most likely to fall victim to cold injuries. Athletes with diabetes, sickle cell anemia, anemia, hypotension, or atherosclerosis are more susceptible to cold weather injuries (Army Public Health Center n.d.).

SEVERE WEATHER

Severe weather conditions increase the risk of injury to people who get caught outdoors. Thankfully, many cities support an early-warning weather system. When a severe storm is about to hit an area, a television and radio warning goes out, which may include a storm watch, storm warning, tornado watch, or tornado warning. The term *watch* indicates that conditions are right for severe weather or a tornado. A *warning* means that a storm or tornado has been sighted. In many communities, a tornado warning will activate sirens, telling people to take cover. During the severe weather season, the AT should have a battery-operated radio ready so that weather reports can be heard. The early-warning storm system will indicate when the storm has passed. Don't mess with Mother Nature. Take cover—she can be fierce!

Tornadoes

When there is a tornado warning, athletes must move to safety immediately. The safest area during a tornado is a low, reinforced area such as a basement. If protection is not available indoors, the athletes should find a ditch or low-lying area and lie as flat as possible, which will allow the tornado to pass over and will protect them from flying debris. People should not seek shelter in a car or bus—although these vehicles appear to be safe, they are easily moved by a tornado.

Thunder and Lightning

The presence of thunder or lightning means that it is time to take cover inside. A lightning detector helps the AT determine whether there is lightning in the area (see figure 26.6). Many people either are not aware of the danger or do not want to appear to be afraid, so they stay outside in severe weather, sometimes with tragic consequences. Some years ago, a group of people in Michigan were walking to a high school football game when they felt their

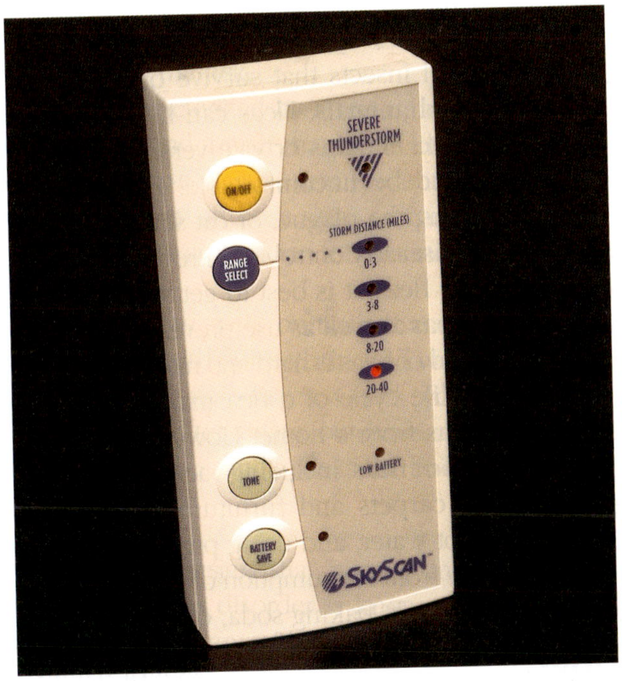

Figure 26.6 Lightning detector.

hair stand on end, which is a sign that lightning is about to strike. They were hit and knocked to the ground, and many had no heartbeat. Luckily, several ATs were attending the game and administered CPR, and all the injured survived. In another incident, three recreational soccer players tried waiting out a storm under a tree, hoping to resume a game. A bolt of lightning hit and traveled down the tree, knocking them to the ground. One of the players died when he could not be revived. Because these incidents are not unusual, NATA created a position statement for lightning safety. The following suggestions are based on this policy statement.

Each school should have an established chain of command and make a well-trained and informed person responsible for stopping play and removing athletes, coaches, and spectators from the area. This person should be informed by a designated weather watcher who monitors signs of threatening weather. Lightning-safe locations close to each field should be identified.

The best policy regarding thunder and lightning is to take cover indoors immediately. The National Weather Service (n.d.) recommends that when you hear thunder, go indoors. Safe shelters are indoors or in cars with windows closed.

If a team is caught in a sudden storm, consider the following precautions:

- Go inside.
- Stay away from all metal objects.
- Avoid electrical devices, including telephones.
- Avoid taking showers.
- Do not stand under a tree or near a flagpole or light pole.
- Do not stand on a hilltop or near the highest point of a field.
- Remove all metal objects from your body (cleats, chains, money clips).
- Assume the lightning-safe position (crouching with legs and arms together).

If an athlete has been struck by lightning, the AT must be prepared to give CPR. An electrical charge may cause the heart to stop.

The facility you choose for shelter is important. Select a substantial structure that has indoor plumbing and a phone. A concrete structure with a basement will protect you quite well.

> **What Would You Do If . . .**
>
> There is a lightning storm, and you tell the lacrosse coach that you have been sent to ask the team to leave the field. The lacrosse coach responds, "We have a practice to get through today, and I'll decide what's in the best interest of this team."

BITES AND STINGS

We share our environment with an enormous number and variety of insects and snakes. Their bites may contain harmful venom, diseases, or bacteria.

Insects

For most people, being stung by a bee or being bitten by some other insect is painful but not life-threatening. However, a few people are so sensitive

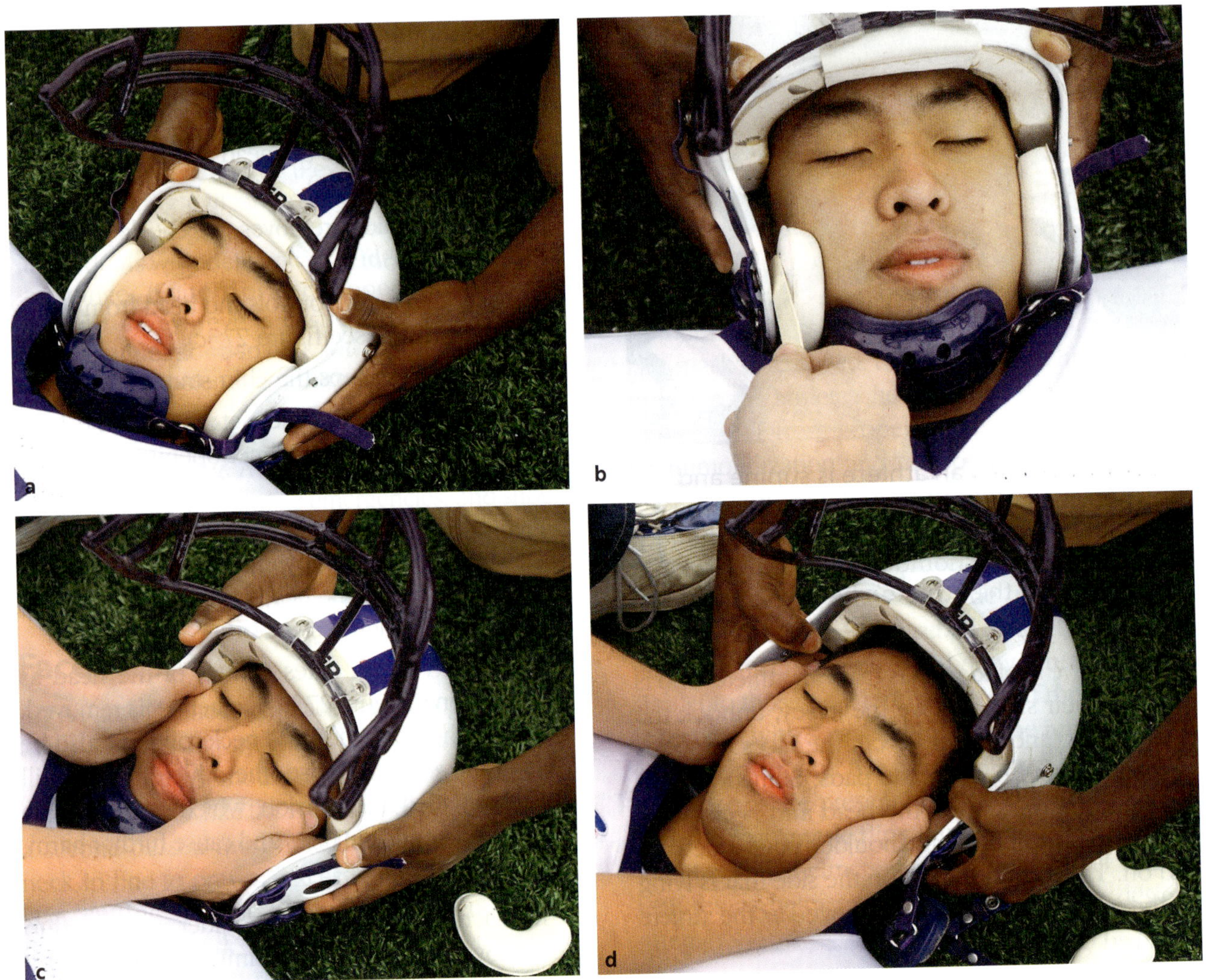

Figure 27.3 Football helmet removal. *(a)* The AT holds the exterior of the helmet, and *(b)* the cheek pads are loosened and removed. *(c)* The second rescuer controls the athlete's head from inside the helmet, and *(d)* from the top of the athlete's head, the AT grabs the helmet by the ear holes, widens the helmet as much as possible, and pulls it off.

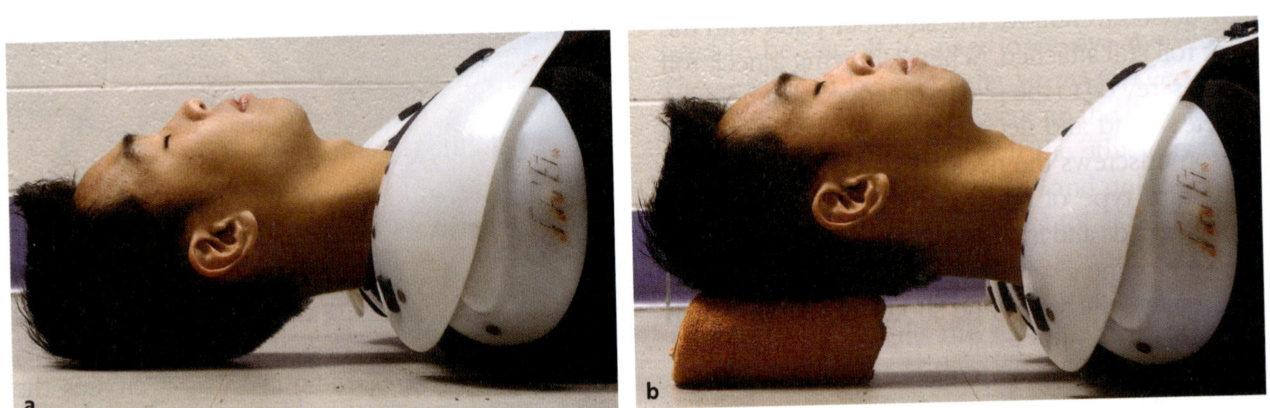

Figure 27.4 *(a)* If the helmet is removed while the shoulder pads are still on, the head will tip back to the floor at an angle. *(b)* Placing padding under the head or removing the shoulder pads maintains proper alignment of the head and neck with the body.

8. The AT fills the gap between the head and the ground with towels or other conforming cloth to keep the head and neck in line with the back.
9. The AT again takes control of the head while the second AT does a full-body assessment for injuries and treatment.

Ice hockey presents a significant issue: ice! It can be difficult because ice is cold and slippery, and the AT must plan to overcome these in the event of injury. If the helmet and shoulder pads need to be removed, follow this process listed:

1. The AT controls the head and keeps it in line.
2. The second rescuer can undo the two straps that hold the face mask in place. This will give the AT access to the airway.
3. The second rescuer cuts off the uniform to get access to the shoulder pads.
4. The second rescuer unbuckles the straps that hold the shoulder pads in place; there are at least two.
5. The second rescuer controls the head from underneath the shoulder pads inside the helmet if possible.
6. The AT unsnaps the chin strap and pulls the helmet up over the head while pulling the helmet opening apart as it crosses the athletes' ears.
7. The AT then removes the shoulder pads over the athlete's head.
8. The AT fills the gap between the head and the ground with towels or other conforming cloth to keep the head and neck in line with the back.
9. The AT again takes control of the head while the second AT does a full-body assessment for injuries and treatment.

Uniform and Padding

If the AT needs to assess a nonserious injury, the athlete can remove their own uniform if they can do it without further harm. If the injured part is a limb, first remove the uniform from the noninjured extremity. This will allow more room to manipulate the uniform around the injured body part. A sock can be removed from an injured leg or foot by widening the diameter of the sock while removing it. If that creates pain, cut the sock off.

Padding around an injured body part should be cut off—cautiously—to keep the injured body part from moving and causing unnecessary pain. Padding on the rest of the body can be removed in the normal fashion.

LIFTING AND MOVING AN ATHLETE

Once an athlete has been assessed, the AT will decide how they should be removed from the field. If the injury is minor, the athlete may be able to walk off on their own or with minimal help. However, if the injury is more serious, the AT can use devices such as straps, stretchers, and backboards to move the athlete from one location to another. When lifting an athlete, as when lifting any heavy weight, the AT must have a good base of support, keep their feet shoulder-width apart, and always look up before and during the lifting. Once the athlete has been secured to a stretcher or backboard, they should be moved feetfirst rather than sideways so that they are less likely to become nauseated.

RED FLAGS

The AT needs to intervene if any of the following occur:

- The helmet is loose and there is a spinal cord injury. (The helmet should be removed.)
- The neck hyperextends once the helmet is removed.
- The athlete is having difficulty breathing and is wearing a face mask.
- Athlete has a suspected spinal cord injury.
- Athlete has a suspected spinal cord injury and is seated.

What Would You Do If . . .

At the football game, a player has injured his knee, which has been splinted. The AT indicates that they need the golf cart to carry the injured player from the field. You try several times, but the golf cart will not start.

Under normal circumstances, injured athletes are splinted and cared for before they are moved. However, in extreme emergencies, an athlete may have to be moved before they can be splinted. If, for example, a wall is about to fall on the athlete, the AT must move them to prevent their death. If the athlete is not splinted, move them lengthwise to keep their bones aligned (see figure 27.5).

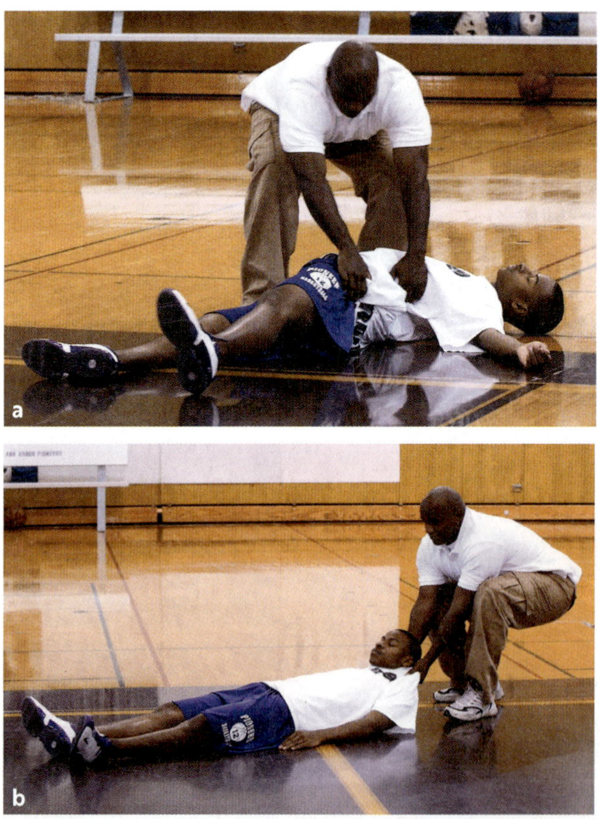

Figure 27.5 Emergency movement. *(a)* Moving an athlete sideways causes the extremities to move away from the direction of force. *(b)* Lengthwise movement is less likely to further injure the athlete. The AT must keep looking up to prevent personal back injury while lifting.

Ambulatory Movement

Ideally, an athlete will be able to walk from the field without support; the athlete is **ambulatory**. However, an athlete should not be allowed to get up and walk around before the AT or team physician has determined the extent of the injury. A serious injury should be immobilized before extrication, and an athlete with a suspected serious lower-extremity injury should not be allowed to walk without support. If two students are giving ambulatory aid, the athlete can place one arm over each assistant's shoulders, and the assistants can grasp the athlete's back or pants to give support. The athlete should not be allowed to apply pressure on the injured body part. If only one assistant is available to give aid, the assistant should be on the same side as the injury. The athlete's arm should be over the assistant's shoulder while the assistant holds the athlete's hip or pants (see figure 27.6).

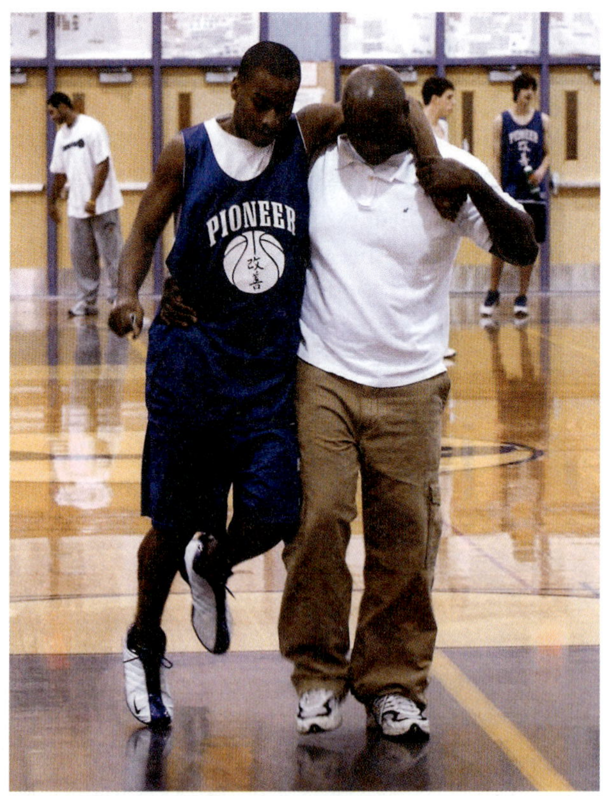

Figure 27.6 A one-person carry is used when the athlete is ill and needs support or when an injured lower extremity can support limited pressure. The injured lower extremity must be next to the rescuer.

An athlete who is not seriously injured and can cooperate may also be removed from the field using a seated carry. To perform the removal, two people face each other and lock their arms together as illustrated in figure 27.7. The athlete sits on one set of the locked arms, while the other set supports their upper back. The athlete puts their arms around the shoulders of the assistants. The athlete is carried off in the direction they are facing (see figure 27.8).

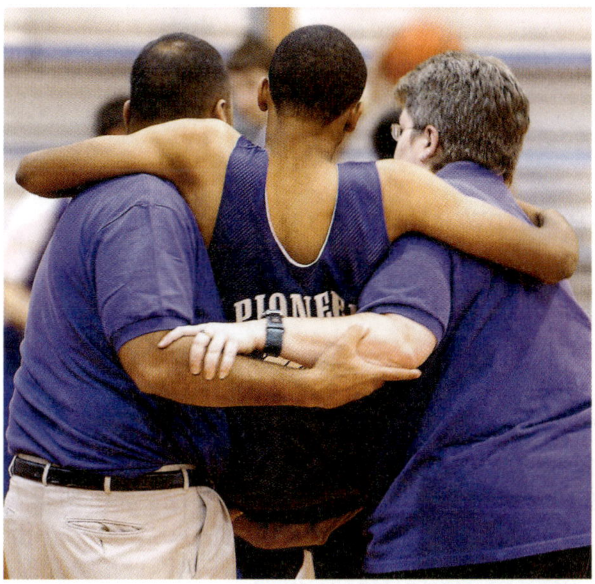

Figure 27.7 The arm lock is performed with the hand of one rescuer grasping the forearm of the other. If the hand slips off the forearm, there is still a hand to grasp, whereas if a hand-to-hand grip slips, nothing is left to hold on to.

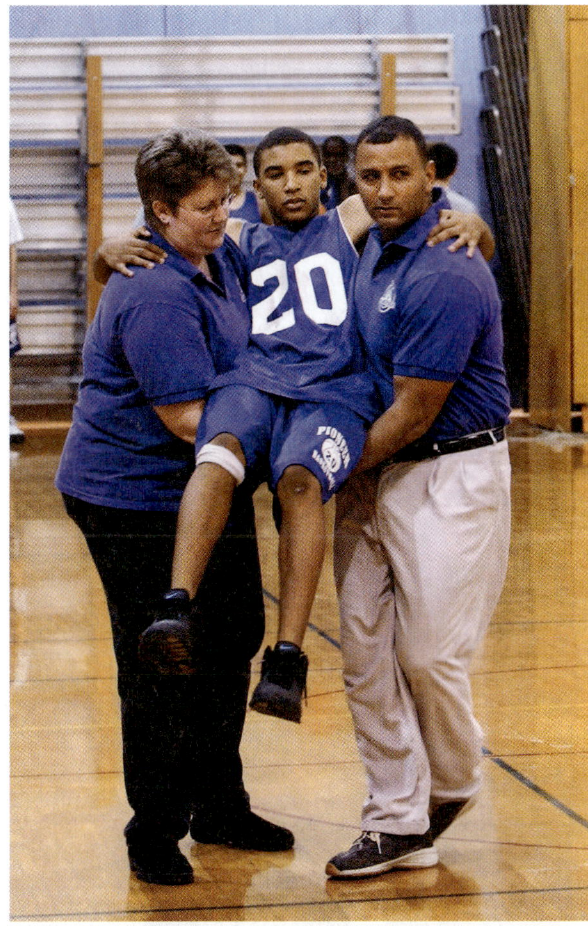

Figure 27.8 The two-person carry is used when the injured athlete cannot get off the field without help. It should not apply pressure to the injured body part. All splinting should be done before moving the athlete.

The Real World

One of the basic rules in football is to keep your head up. When the athlete has their head up, they can see better, and the neck is in a position where an impact is less likely to be harmful.

The running back was handed the ball; he dipped his head and was immediately hit by several opposing team players. He didn't get up at the end of the play. The AT assessed the player and asked him questions. The evaluation revealed that the player had a tingling sensation in both arms and legs. The AT decided not to move the player and called EMS. The paramedics evaluated the athlete and determined that he had suffered a life-threatening cervical spine injury. They called for a helicopter evacuation. It was a scary, sobering moment when the helicopter landed in the middle of the football field and evacuated the player to a local hospital.

Thankfully, the young man had suffered only muscle strains on both sides of his neck. He was kept overnight for observation and then sent home. His doctor ordered him to wear a neck brace and strengthen his neck muscles to rehabilitate the muscle strains before returning to football the following season.

His injury changed the behavior of every player on the team—they all paid more attention to their posture after that.

Anonymous

Nonambulatory Movement

In some instances, the AT will not be able to remove an athlete without additional support, such as a stretcher or backboard. The following section and the algorithm in figure 27.9 explain the modalities for nonambulatory movement.

Stretcher

A stretcher and a backboard are two different things. A backboard is rigid and is used to immobilize spinal injuries, whereas a stretcher is made of canvas and is used to transport an athlete without spinal injuries.

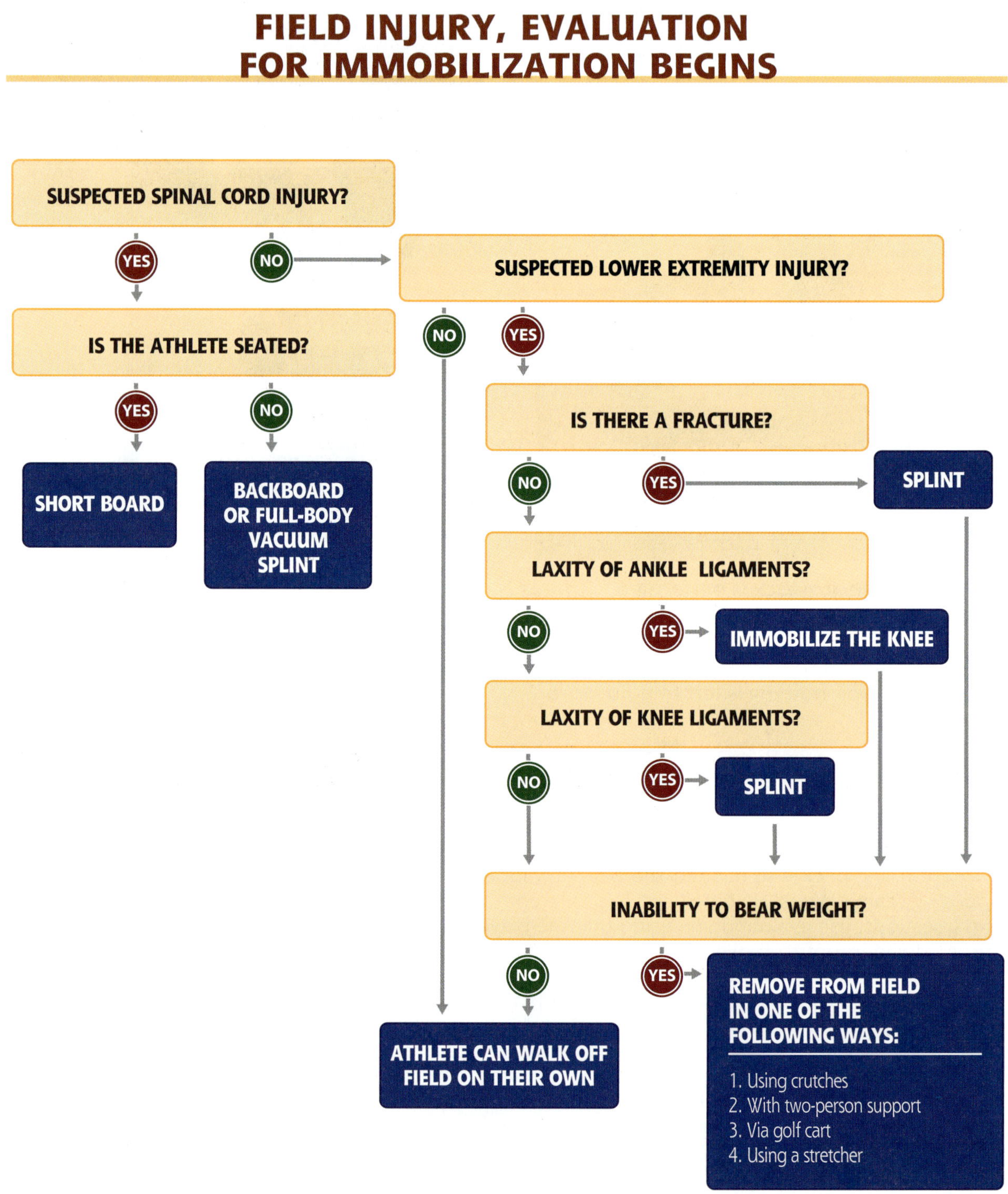

Figure 27.9 Determining which immobilization is best.

A stretcher is used for an athlete suffering from a knee injury, an asthma attack, dizziness, a diabetic crisis, and so forth. After assessing the athlete and caring for all injuries, the AT will logroll the athlete onto the stretcher and secure them in place with three straps, one each at the chest, hips, and feet. The athlete may be able to slide onto the stretcher, which is fine as long as no pressure is placed on the injured body part.

As with a backboard, it takes at least four people to carry the stretcher—one on each end and two in the middle. The athlete should be moved feetfirst or headfirst.

Scoop Stretcher

The scoop stretcher is made of metal and can be separated into two parts. One part provides a thin metal structure that slides under the athlete, and the two parts are reattached at the head and feet (see figure 27.10). Presto, the athlete is on the stretcher and has not been rolled or lifted. Athletes have one complaint about the scoop stretcher: On a cool night, the metal is cold to the touch.

Short Board

Short boards are used when an athlete reports spinal pain but is in a seated position. They should be used only by highly trained emergency personnel and ATs. Place an athlete on a short board (figure 27.11) according to the following procedure, with

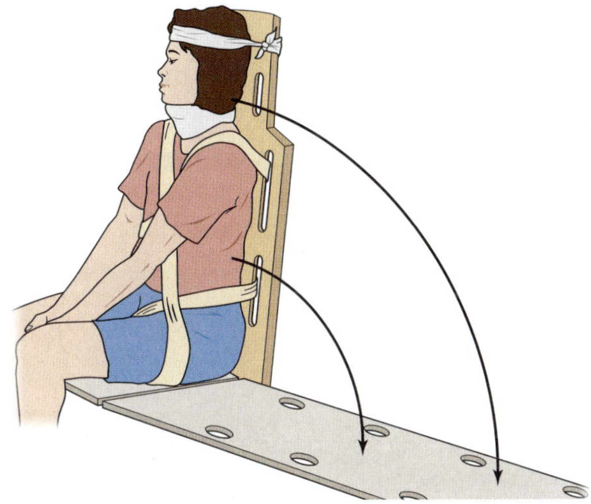

Figure 27.11 Short board. The injured person will be rotated onto their back on the long backboard.

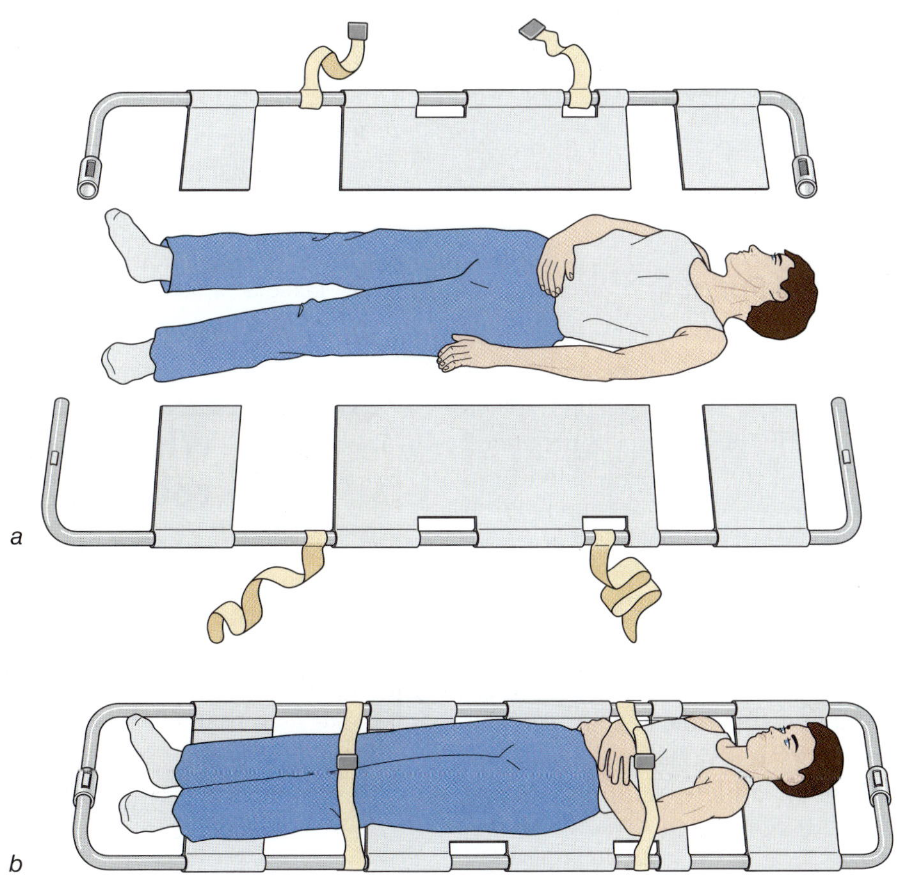

Figure 27.10 Scoop stretcher.

the person in charge controlling the head and neck of the injured person:

1. Call 911.
2. Control the head from behind.
3. Place a cervical collar on the injured athlete.
4. Prepare the short board:
    - Make sure all straps are in place.
    - Match the straps, buckle, and clip (usually these are color coded to avoid confusion).
5. With the person in charge maintaining tension on the head and neck, wedge the short board between the athlete and the chair.
6. Put the chest straps in place.
7. Control the head from the front and strap the head to the board.
8. Strap the legs with the hips flexed.
9. Place a long backboard perpendicular to the athlete's chair.
10. Rotate the athlete onto the long backboard, keeping the knees drawn up toward the chest.
11. Release the leg straps so that the legs can lie flat on the backboard.
12. Place a strap across the chest (but not over the heart area).
13. Place a hip strap.
14. Place a foot strap.

Full-Body Vacuum Splint

More recently, full-body vacuum splints have been used to stabilize an athlete with a spine injury. This splint is simply a larger version of the vacuum splints described in chapter 25. The athlete is surrounded by the nylon splint and the air is evacuated from it, creating a rigid encasement around the body.

Backboard

After an injured athlete receives an assessment and care, use a backboard for any spinal or back injury, when the extent of injuries cannot be determined, or when there is not enough time to splint obvious fractures and the injury is serious.

Backboarding an athlete requires several trained emergency personnel and ATs. One person will be in charge and direct the others. Backboard an athlete according to the following procedure, with the person in charge controlling the head throughout the operation:

1. Call 911.
2. Control the head.
3. Place a cervical collar on the injured athlete to immobilize the spine.
4. Prepare the backboard:
    - Make sure all straps are in place.
    - Match the straps, buckle, and clip (usually these are color coded to avoid confusion).
    - Remove the head block (or sandbags or rolled blanket) and keep it ready for placement.
5. Under the direction of the person in control of the head, roll the athlete 90° and position the board by sliding it just behind them; once the board is in position, roll the athlete back onto the backboard so that their head is at the top, and they are centered on the board.
6. Place both cross-chest straps over the collarbones and tighten.
7. Put the head block (or sandbags or rolled blanket) in place.
8. Tape the head to the board, with one strip over the forehead and another over the chin. (Local EMS may or may not require a chin strap.)
9. Place a hip strap.
10. Place a foot strap.

? What Would You Do If . . .

After a wrestler is safely on the backboard, it is discovered that two of the straps are crossed and are not buckled to themselves but to another strap. The straps are then switched and buckled correctly. The AT directs you to make sure that the buckles and the clips are easily identified when backboarding.

At least four people are needed to carry the backboard—one on each end and two in the middle. An alternative method for backboarding an athlete is the lift-and-slide technique. This technique requires five or more people and is used for an athlete who is already supine. As with the traditional logroll technique, the person controlling the athlete's head is in charge of the following procedure:

1. A cervical collar stabilizes the head, and the person directing the technique controls the head and neck.
2. The backboard is prepared the same as in the traditional spine-board technique explained earlier.
3. One assistant straddles the victim, facing the head, and is in charge of lifting the athlete's pelvis.
4. Two assistants are positioned on each side of the victim and are responsible for lifting his torso.
5. A fourth assistant straddles the victim and is responsible for lifting the athlete's legs. Under the direction of the person in control of the head, the team lifts the athlete, and a fifth assistant slides the spine board into position directly under the athlete.
6. On the leader's command, the team lowers the athlete onto the spine board.
7. As with the traditional logroll technique, the athlete is secured and strapped to the spine board.

After backboarding an athlete with a cervical spine injury, the head should be immobilized using foam blocks.

What Would You Do If . . .

An athlete goes down on the field. The AT has asked you to run out with her during such incidents today, but you are wearing clogs.

Summary

When an injured athlete must be examined or removed from the field, it is crucial that the injured body part be disturbed as little as possible. Movement of the body part causes pain and aggravation, and it may cause further injury. Athletes who are ambulatory may still need assistance. The AT must not be rushed into moving an athlete off the field before they are properly splinted or backboarded.

Key Terms

Define the following terms found in this chapter:

ambulatory
backboarding
extrication
neck roll

A lacrosse player is hit from behind, resulting in a penalty as the player falls forward and lands holding their low back in pain. They are complaining of tingling in their feet and severe low-back pain, and they are reluctant to move from their position. What is the proper stabilization and field removal strategy the AT would use and why? What general considerations are associated with a player in lacrosse gear with a suspected spine injury?

To access supplementary material for this chapter, including the Understanding Check worksheet, vocabulary quizzes, extension activities, and chapter-specific resources and forms, visit the web resource: http://ancillaries.humankinetics.com/FundamentalsOfAthleticTrainingAndSportsMedicine5E

Unit VIII

Reducing Risk of Athletic Injuries

wonder about the number of closure strips pictured. Applying closure strips is not the time to try to save tape; the AT must be certain that their taping will not fail when the athlete needs it most.

Turf Toe

The goal when taping for turf toe is to restrict the extension movement of the great toe. First, place anchor strips of linen tape around the foot and around the base of the great toe (see figure 28.4*a*). Then place a minimum of three strips of 1-inch (2.5 cm) linen tape from the plantar aspect of the toe anchor strip to the plantar aspect of the arch on the anchor strip (see figure 28.4*b*). Apply closure strips over the loose ends to secure these strips in place (see figure 28.4*c*). Elastic tape may also be used for this procedure. Elastic tape is especially useful around the foot because it allows the foot to expand during the weight-bearing portion of the stride without binding the foot.

Bunion

A bunion can result in discomfort because of excess pressure on the medial aspect of the shoe. To alleviate the pressure, a bunion can be taped. First, place an anchor strip around the great toe, just as with turf toe. The toe is moved in line with the first metatarsal, and strips are placed from the anchor strip along the medial aspect of the foot. Once in place, the medial strips are secured (see figure 28.5).

Longitudinal Arch

The purpose of the longitudinal arch procedure is to keep the medial foot from flattening. Start with

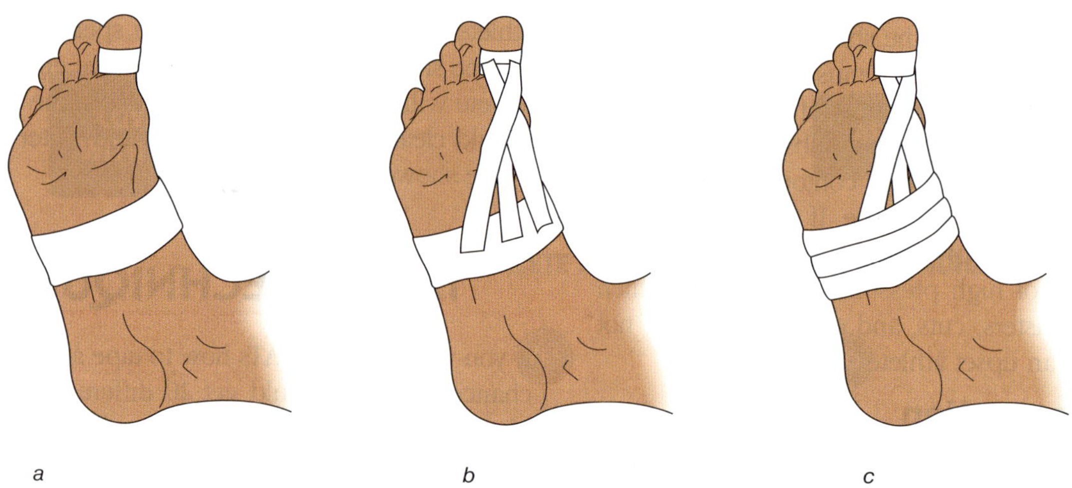

Figure 28.4 Turf toe. *(a)* Apply anchors to the foot and great toe, *(b)* apply three strips of linen tape on the bottom of the foot between the anchor strips, and *(c)* cover the ends with closure strips.

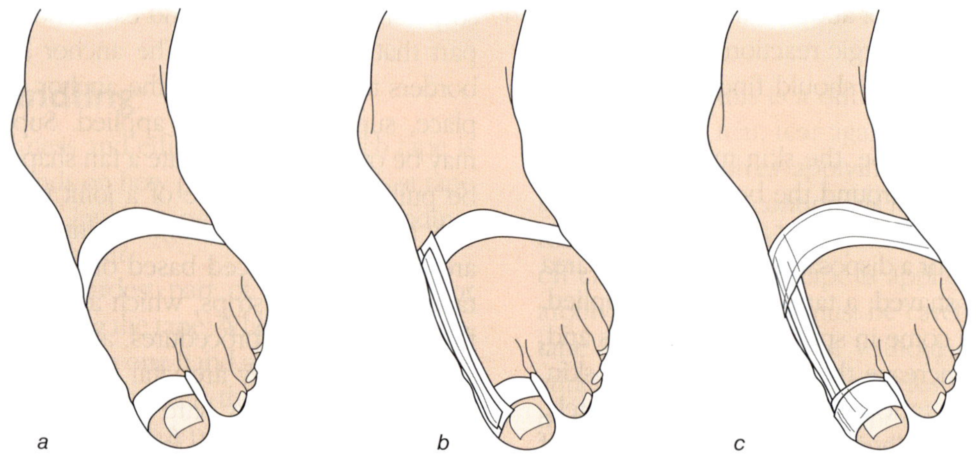

Figure 28.5 Bunion taping. *(a)* Place an anchor strip at the arch and toenail. *(b)* Place three tape strips medially on the toe. *(c)* Lock all tape in place with anchor strips.

one to three anchor strips around the ball of the foot. Start the first strip of 1-inch (2.5 cm) linen tape at the medial side of the anchor and go back toward and around the heel to the starting point at the anchor (see figure 28.6*a*). Start the second strip at the lateral side of the anchor, take it around the heel, and return to the starting point (see figure 28.6*b*). Overlap the strips until four to six strips have been placed. Cover the loose ends with closure strips (see figure 28.6*c*). Many variations of this taping procedure exist, one of which includes taping the arch with padding to support the area (see figure 28.7).

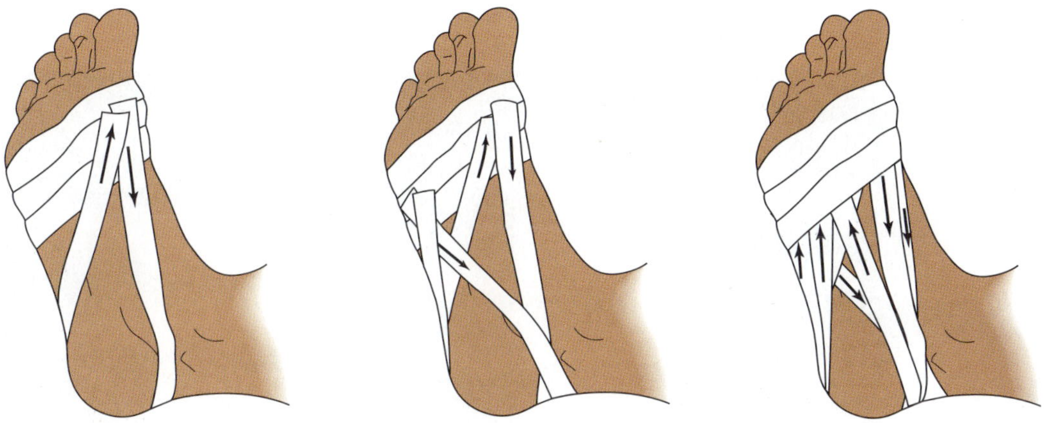

a *b* *c*

Figure 28.6 Longitudinal arch. *(a)* When taping an arch, begin with an anchor strip. Place the first strip of linen tape from the anchor back toward the heel and around to the other end of the strip at the anchor. *(b)* Place the second strip at the lateral side of the anchor, around the heel, and back to the starting point. *(c)* Once the arch strips are situated, close the loose ends with closure strips.

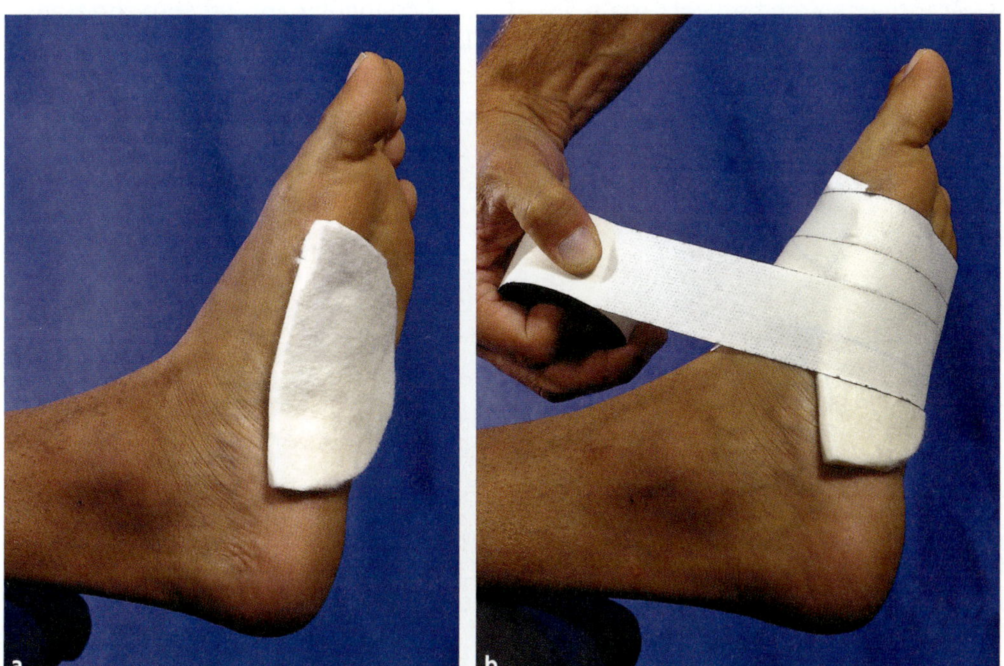

Figure 28.7 Longitudinal arch with padding. *(a)* The ankle is placed in neutral; cut a pad to fit the length and width of the longitudinal arch. The edge closest to the fifth metatarsal may need to be beveled. *(b)* Encircle the pad and the arch with tape.

Transverse Arch

The transverse arch is located at the distal end of the metatarsals. There is a slight arching of the foot in that area. The nerves for the phalanges traverse this area and can become inflamed, causing shooting pain and a thickening of the tissue in the area. This injury is known as Morton's neuroma. The AT can make a triangular pad and tape it to the transverse arch to help alleviate the symptoms (see figure 28.8).

Heel Taping

Heel taping is done when there is a contusion of the calcaneus. The application of the tape over the heel compresses the tissue together so it does not flatten as much during impact. For many athletes, this is enough to create comfort (see figure 28.9).

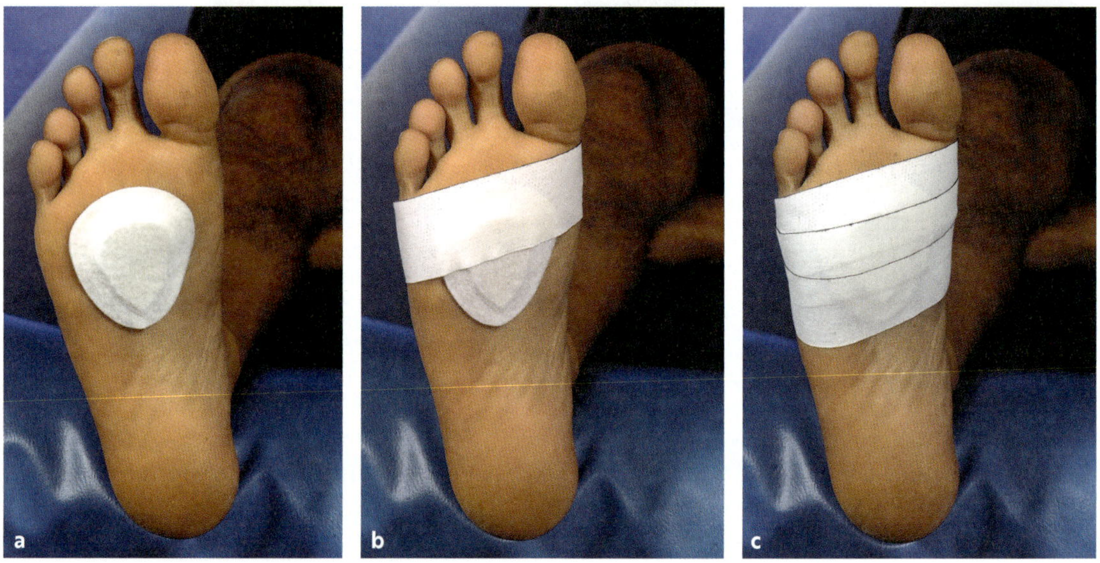

Figure 28.8 Transverse arch pad. *(a)* Create a pad that is triangular and fits into the transverse arch; it will likely need to be beveled to fit properly. *(b-c)* Tape the pad in place.

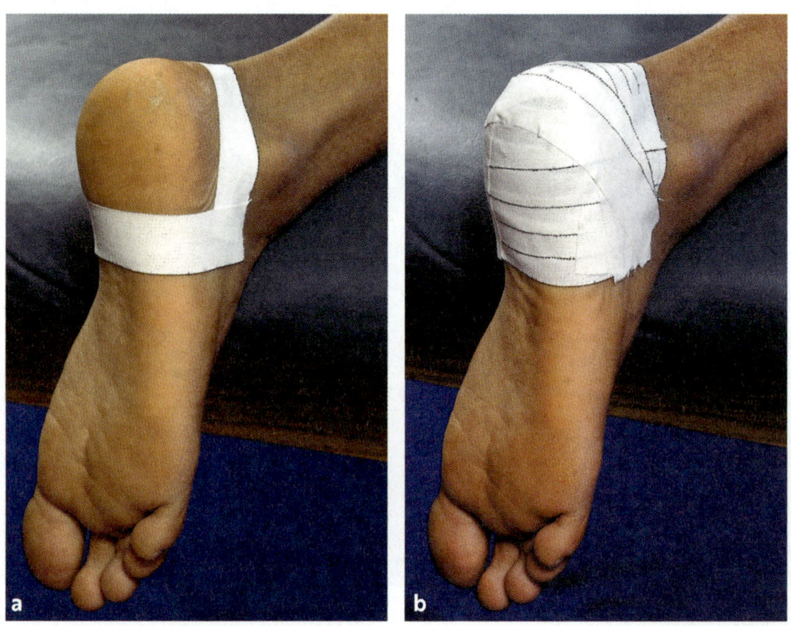

Figure 28.9 Heel taping. *(a)* Heel taping is done by alternating strips of tape starting just above the heel to each malleoli. Apply tape from metatarsal arch to the previous strip of tape. *(b)* Repeat this process until the entire heel is enclosed.

Closed Basket Weave

The closed basket weave is used mostly to give support and help prevent inversion ankle sprains. Begin the closed basket weave with one anchor strip at the lower leg just below the bulky portion of the calf muscle and one at midfoot. With the anchors in place, begin placing support strips called *stirrups* and *horseshoes* on the ankle. The first stirrup is applied to the anchor strip on the medial aspect of the leg, pulled under the foot, and pulled up to the anchor strip on the lateral aspect of the leg (see figure 28.10*a*). Once a stirrup is applied, place a horseshoe strip at the distal aspect of the lower leg (around the ankle) from the lateral aspect to the medial aspect (see figure 28.10*b*). Apply these strips alternately, overlapping them until a minimum of three stirrups and three horseshoes have been applied (see figure 28.10*c*).

Once this is completed, apply a figure eight around the ankle. Start the figure eight at the outer anklebone (lateral malleolus) and guide the tape across the top of the ankle down to the medial aspect of the foot. The figure-eight strip will then come up the lateral side of the foot just in front of the lateral malleolus and run a course to the medial malleolus and then around to the back of the lower leg, stopping at the lateral malleolus (see figure 28.10*d*). Once the figure-eight strip is in place, apply two heel locks (one forward and one reverse). Start one heel lock just above the inside anklebone (medial malleolus) and angle the strip downward so that it crosses the outer aspect of the heel. Then the tape runs a course across the bottom of the foot and upward on the inside aspect, angling toward the outer anklebone (lateral malleolus), where it stops (see figure 28.10*e*). Start the next heel lock just

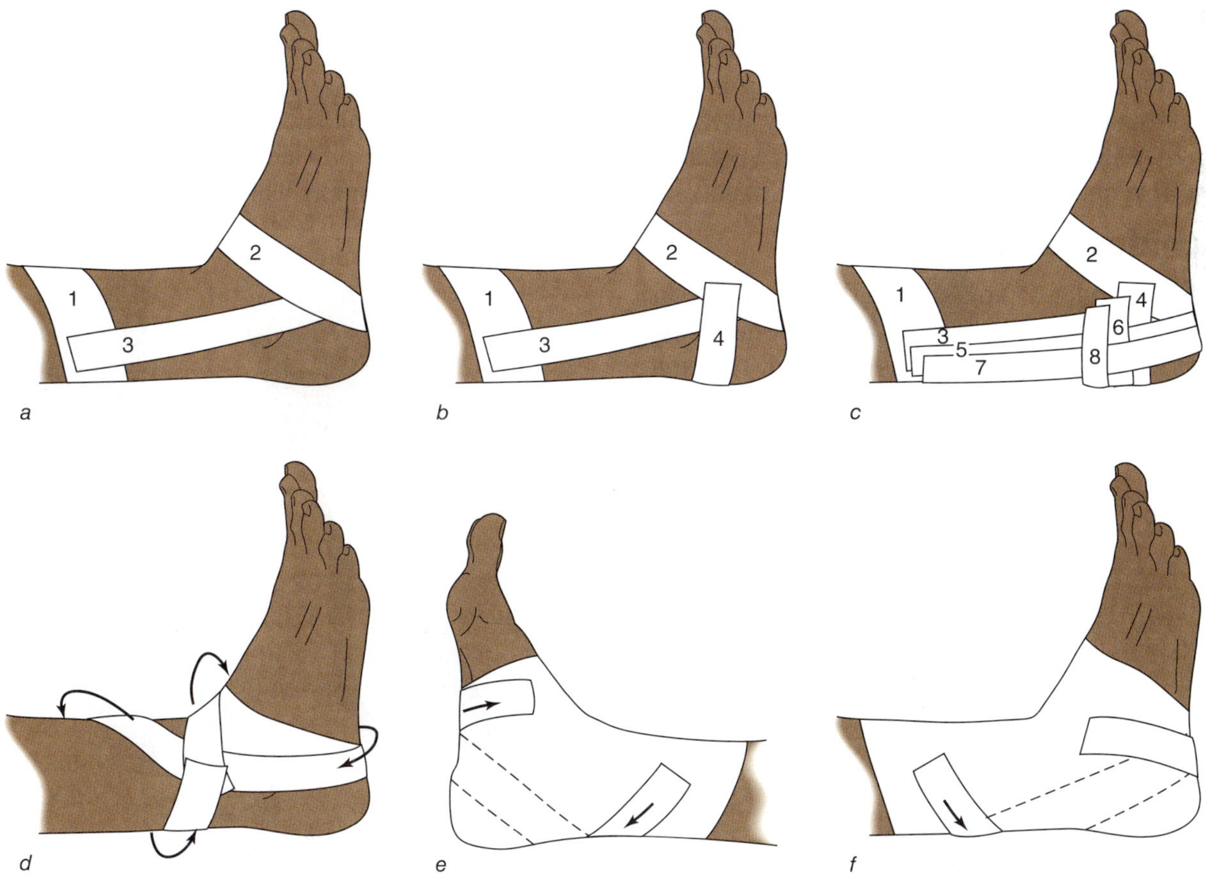

Figure 28.10 Closed basket weave. *(a)* Once the anchors are in place (1 and 2), a stirrup is applied (3), *(b)* and a horseshoe strip is applied (4). *(c)* Stirrup and horseshoe strips are applied in alternating fashion (5-8), *(d)* followed by the figure-eight strip. *(e-f)* Heel locks are applied after the figure eight from above the ankle, wrapping under the heel.

in a fan shape between the anchors across the back of the knee (see figure 28.15*b*). Finish by placing closure strips across all tape ends (figure 28.15*c*).

In figure 28.16, flexible tape is used for a knee hyperextension. The benefit of this type of taping is that it can be left on for several days.

Patellofemoral Taping

Several patellar tracking problems can cause pain. Problems may be patellar tilt, patellar rotation, and patellar glide. The McConnell taping techniques use rigid tape to correct these types of concerns. In figure 28.17, a patellar glide issue is being corrected.

An alternative to rigid taping of anterior knee problems can be done utilizing kinesiology taping. The concept of improving the patellar track is part of this taping (see figure 28.18).

Elbow Hyperextension

One of the most common ways elbows are injured is from falling on an outstretched arm, which makes the elbow vulnerable to hyperextension injuries.

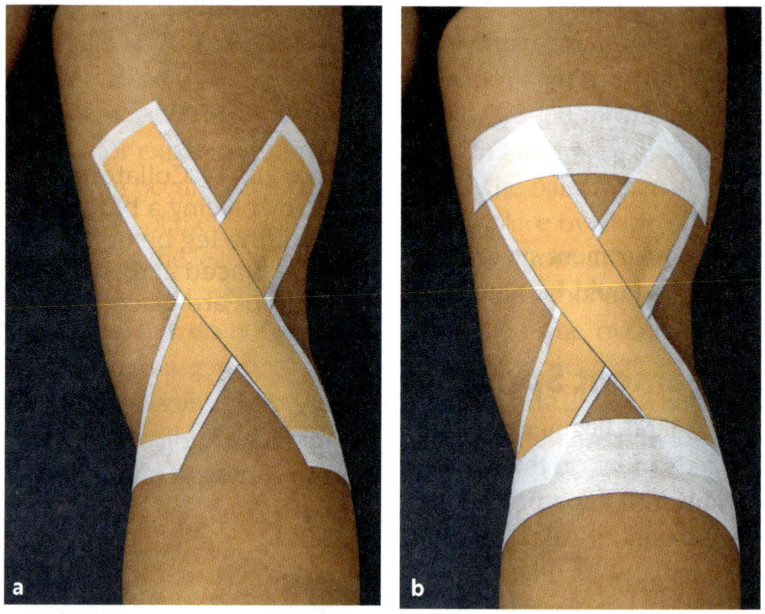

Figure 28.16 Knee hyperextension taping with flexible tape.

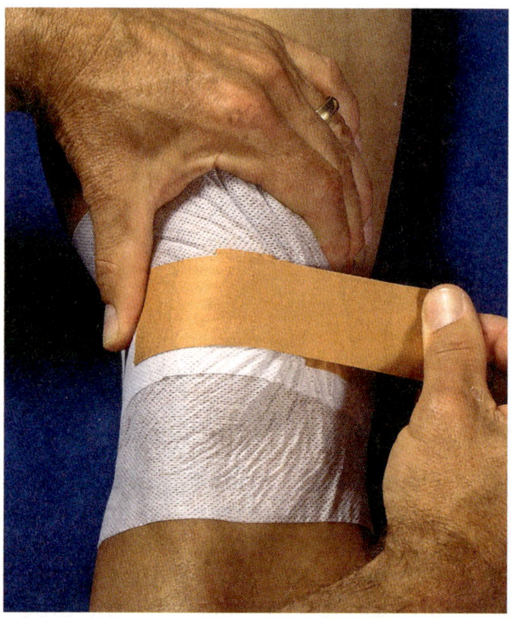

Figure 28.17 Patellar glide taping.

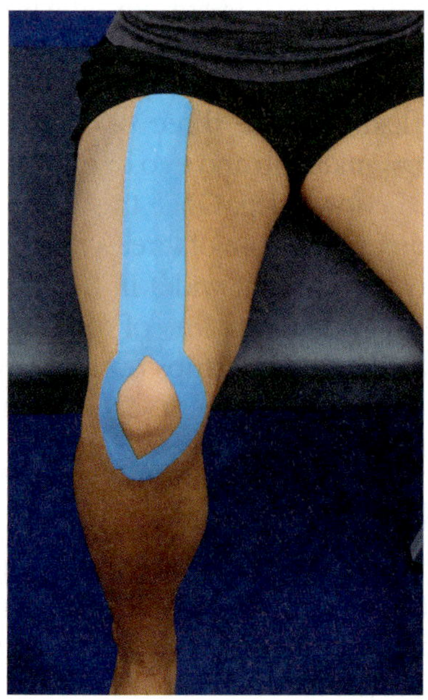

Figure 28.18 Kinesiology taping of anterior knee.

The goal of taping for an elbow hyperextension injury is to limit extension. Before taping, first place the elbow in a slight amount of flexion. Place anchor strips at the top of the biceps of the upper arm and at the mid- to lower forearm. Before applying the anchor strips, make sure the athlete is making the biceps muscle tight. When the anchor strips are in position, place three to five strips in a fan shape across the front of the elbow, running from anchor to anchor (see figure 28.19*a*). Elastic tape is preferred for these strips, but linen tape is also acceptable. Apply closure strips over the anchors at the upper arm and forearm to cover all tape ends (see figure 28.19*b*).

An alternative to linen taping of an elbow hyperextension is kinesiology taping. The concept of the taping is the same (see figure 28.20).

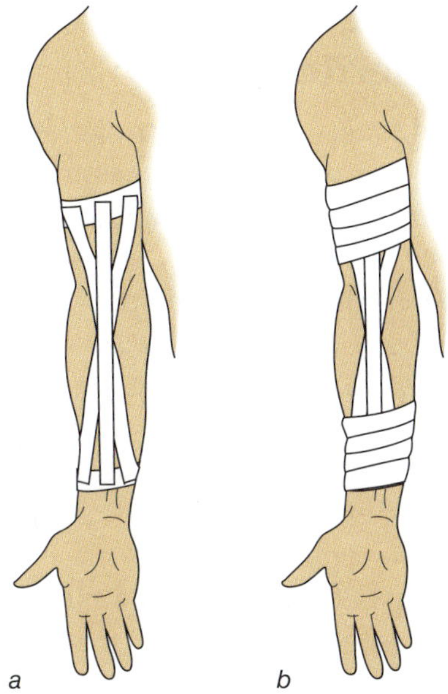

Figure 28.19 Elbow hyperextension taping procedure. *(a)* Elbow hyperextension anchor strips are applied and tape placed in a fan shape over them. *(b)* The tape job is finished with closure strips.

Lateral Collateral Ligament Sprain

Sprains of the collateral ligament occur with overuse or valgus or varus stress. Taping the ligament can provide extra support. Figure 28.21 shows an anchor above and below the elbow joint with overlapping fanning of tape.

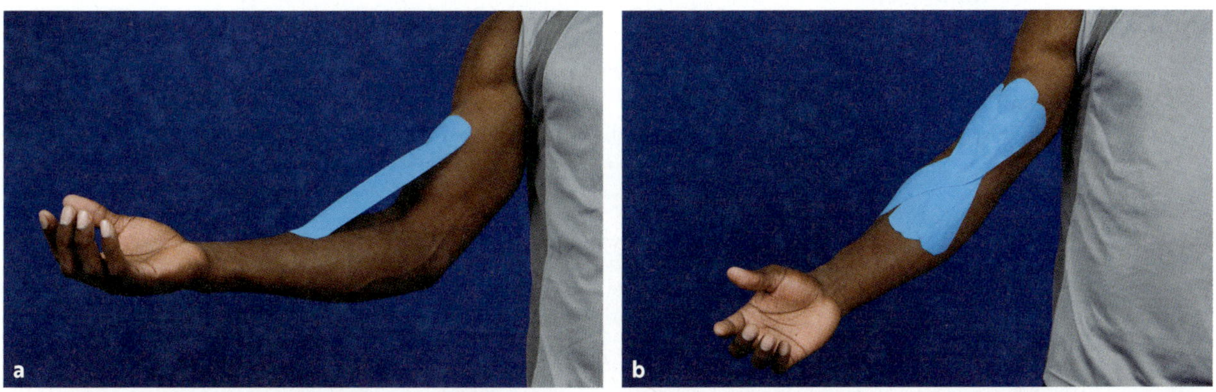

Figure 28.20 Kinesiology taping of elbow hyperextension.

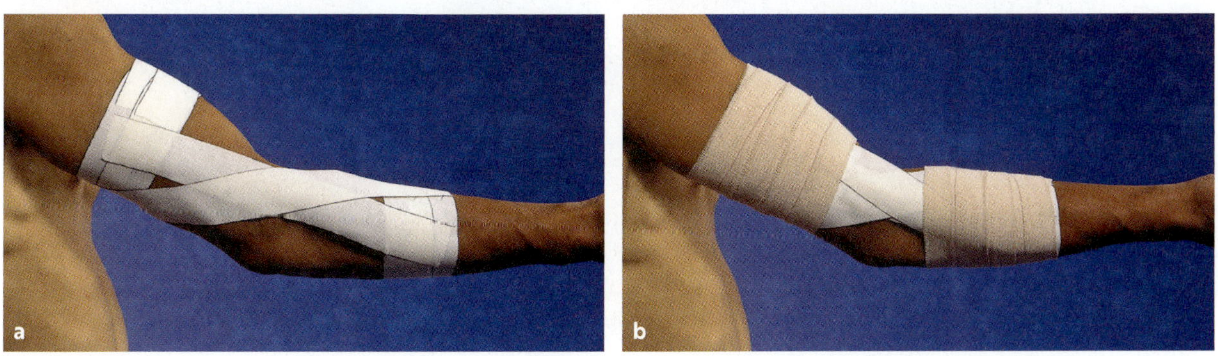

Figure 28.21 Lateral collateral ligament taping.

Wrist Hyperextension and Hyperflexion

Sprains and strains are common injuries to the wrist. Hyperflexion and hyperextension mechanisms cause most wrist sprains; therefore, the goal for wrist taping is usually to prevent excessive flexion or extension. Most wrist injuries are caused by hyperextension.

To prevent wrist hyperextension, start by placing an anchor strip around the distal aspect of the forearm and another around the hand just above the knuckles. With the anchors in place, position the wrist into slight flexion and place a minimum of three strips of linen tape in a fan shape across the palmar aspect of the wrist (see figure 28.22*a*). Closure strips are placed over the tape ends to secure them (see figure 28.22*b*).

Thumb Hyperextension

Begin taping for a thumb hyperextension injury by placing anchors around the wrist, around the hand, and around the top of the thumb, just above the nail. The thumb is then positioned into slight flexion, and strips of 1-inch (2.5 cm) linen tape are applied over the back of the thumb in a fan shape between the anchors on the thumb and wrist (see figure 28.23*a*). Once these are in place, a tape wrap called a *spica* can be wound around the joint. Beginning at the palmar aspect of the wrist, guide the 1-inch (2.5 cm) tape toward the back aspect of the thumb, loop it around the thumb, and then guide the tape toward the dorsal aspect of the wrist and tear the tape (see figure 28.23*b*). Repeat this spica one more time and then apply closure strips around the wrist and around the hand to cover all tape ends. Also, to keep the thumb stable, a **checkrein** (see figure 28.23*c*) can be used to connect the index finger and the thumb.

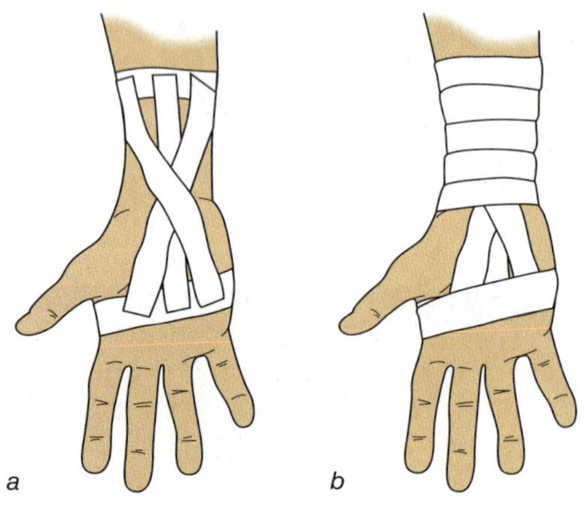

Figure 28.22 Wrist hyperextension tape procedure. *(a)* Wrist hyperextension anchor strips and fan strips and *(b)* closure strips.

> **FYI**
>
> **Spica**
>
> A spica is a taping or wrapping procedure applied to joints such as the thumb, shoulder, or hip. It is a figure eight applied to an area so that the tape or wrap encircles the joint and gives support.

Finger Sprain

Finger sprains are commonly treated using buddy taping; that is, the sprained finger is moved toward an adjacent noninjured finger and either the first and second or third and fourth fingers are taped together. Tape is applied between the joints of the fingers; rarely is it applied across the joint itself (see figure 28.24).

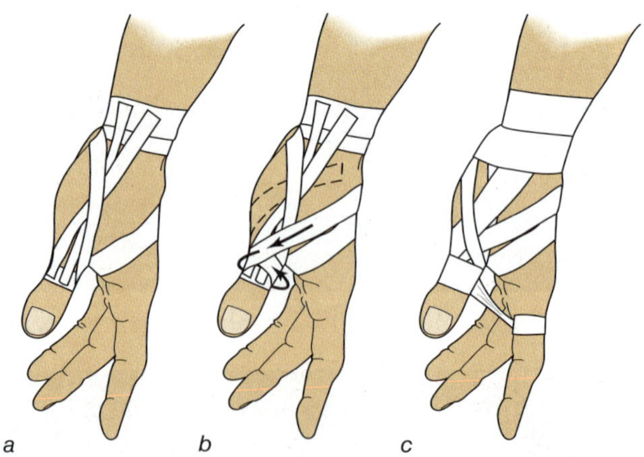

Figure 28.23 Thumb hyperextension procedure. *(a)* Thumb hyperextension taping begins with anchors on the wrist, hand, and thumb and fan strips of tape on the dorsal aspect of the thumb, and continues with *(b)* thumb taping complete with spica and *(c)* checkrein.

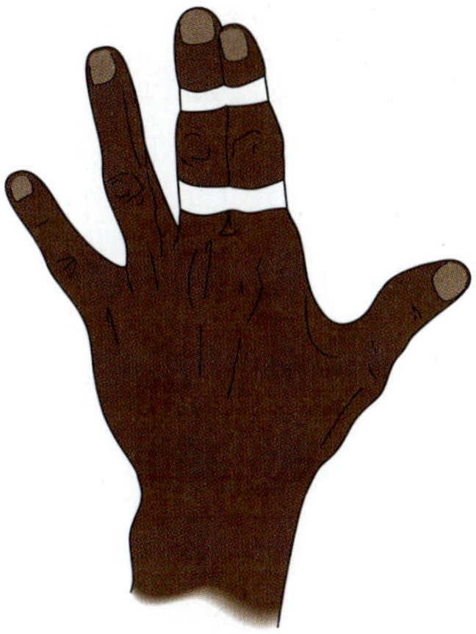

Figure 28.24 Buddy taping for a finger sprain.

ELASTIC WRAPPING TECHNIQUES

When an athlete suffers an injury, **elastic wraps** can apply compression and support the area. Elastic wraps come in various widths and lengths and are used for many musculoskeletal injuries, such as sprains and strains. Because elastic wraps can be washed and reused, they are less expensive than tape. Similar to tape, elastic wraps come in a variety of sizes. Common widths include 2, 3, 4, and 6 inches (5, 8, 10, and 15 cm). Two- and 3-inch (5 and 8 cm) elastic wraps are often used around the wrist or hand, 4-inch (10 cm) wraps are commonly used around the foot or ankle, and 6-inch (15 cm) elastic wraps are used around the thigh, hip, or shoulder.

Ankle Sprain or Strain

When applying an elastic wrap, leave the toes exposed so you can check circulation (see figure 28.25). Begin at the bottom of the foot, close to the toes, and wrap to above the ankle. Overlap the wrap by one-half of the width each time while working up over the ankle, and use a wrap at least 4 inches (10 cm) wide so that the finished wrap does not roll up on the edges and become too restrictive. Begin with moderate pressure, and as the wrap is applied toward and above the ankle, decrease the amount of pressure. Always check the athlete's circulation after the wrap has been applied.

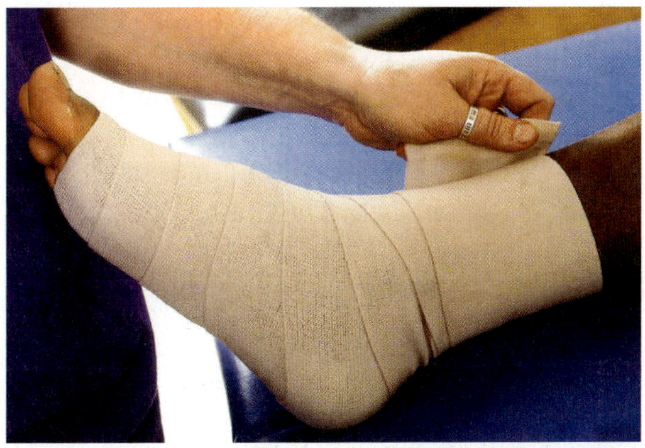

Figure 28.25 Elastic wraps are applied to joints to prevent swelling.

REMOVING TAPES

Here are various techniques for removing tape:

- Remove each layer in reverse order of application.
- To decrease pain, pull the tape at a 45° angle while gently pulling the skin in the opposite direction.
- Use taping scissors (those with a blunt end on the bottom blade of the scissor) to cut the tape from the proximal to distal ends, avoiding the area of injury.
- Use a tape cutter to cut from proximal to distal, avoiding the area of injury.
- Apply adhesive tape remover between the body part and the tape.
- After any tape has been removed, inspect the skin for any blisters, wounds, or reactions to tape and then care for the athlete accordingly.

The Real World

I worked with an athlete who had once sprained his finger, and he liked to have his fingers buddy taped. He also felt that elastic tape was better for him than linen, so I used elastic tape. On one occasion during practice, the athlete ran to the sideline and asked me to tape his fingers. He had a late class that day so he had not been taped before practice. I had some 1-inch (2.5 cm) elastic tape, and I began applying it to his hand, taping his fingers together. He was in a hurry to get back to practice and was practically dancing with impatience. He kept looking behind him to watch practice, and his hand was moving all around. Although I warned him several times to keep his hand still while I cut the tape, he continued to fidget. Sure enough, when I was cutting the tape he moved his hand toward the scissors, and I snipped the webbing of skin between his fingers. Although the wound was minor, I felt bad. The moral of the story is this: Precut the lengths of elastic tape before applying them to the body unless you are in a controlled setting, such as the athletic training room.

Anonymous

Thigh Injury

When wrapping the thigh for hamstring or quadriceps injuries, use a double-length 6-inch (15 cm) elastic wrap and begin just above the knee. Overlap the wrap as it is applied upward toward the hip. While applying the wrap in a spiral around the leg, use subtle upward and downward angles to contour the wrap appropriately. The finished product will look as though there are *X*s up the front of the wrap. Secure the wrap in place with elastic tape (see figure 28.26).

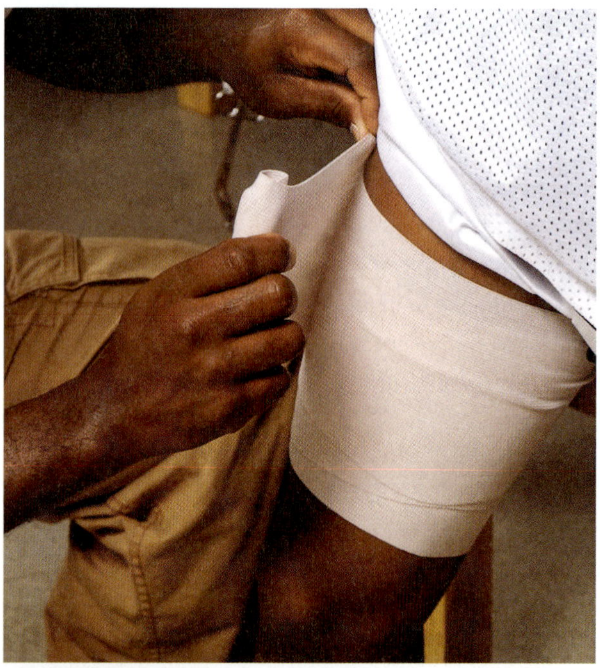

Figure 28.26 Thigh wrap. Wrap the thigh from above the knee toward the hip.

Groin (Adductor) Strain

Begin by having the athlete put on compression shorts, spandex shorts, or other shorts over which the wrap can be applied comfortably. When wrapping adductor strains, place the hip in a slight amount of flexion and adduction by placing a small block of wood under the heel or using a small step. Secure the wrap around the proximal thigh, continue by moving the wrap around the waist above the iliac crest and then down around the upper thigh, and repeat. Secure the wrap with elastic tape (see figure 28.27).

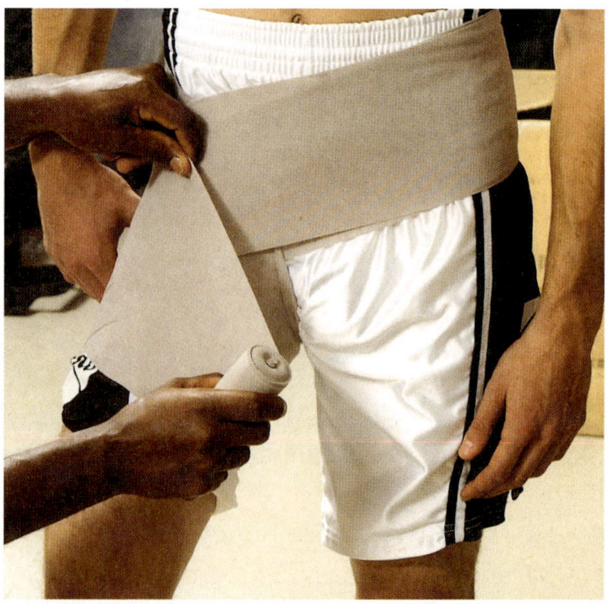

Figure 28.27 Adductor strain wrap. Note the slightly flexed and adducted position of the thigh.

Hip Flexor Strain

Begin by having the athlete put on compression shorts, spandex shorts, or other shorts over which the wrap can be applied comfortably. When wrapping hip flexor strains, place the hip into flexion and slight adduction by using a small block or step under the heel. Secure the wrap around the proximal thigh and apply the wrap in a counterclockwise direction. Progress by moving the wrap around the waist above the iliac crest and down around the upper thigh, and then repeat. Secure the wrap in place by taping over it with elastic tape (see figure 28.28).

Shoulder Dislocation

Elastic wraps are often applied to the shoulder to restrict motion that causes shoulder dislocations (see figure 28.29). To begin, have the athlete place the arm to be wrapped on the hip and the other arm straight out, like a teapot. Secure the wrap around the upper arm, applying the wrap in a clockwise direction. Once the wrap is secured to the upper arm, pull the wrap from the posterior aspect of the shoulder around the front of the chest, under the opposite arm, and across the back to the shoulder. Loop the wrap around the upper arm (clockwise) and repeat. Secure the wrap by taping over it with elastic tape. This wrapping of the shoulder is known as a spica.

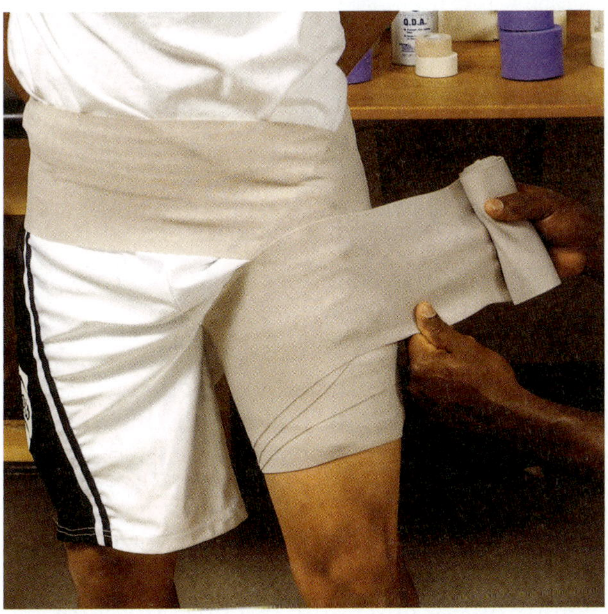

Figure 28.28 Hip flexor strain wrap. Note the flexed position of the hip and leg.

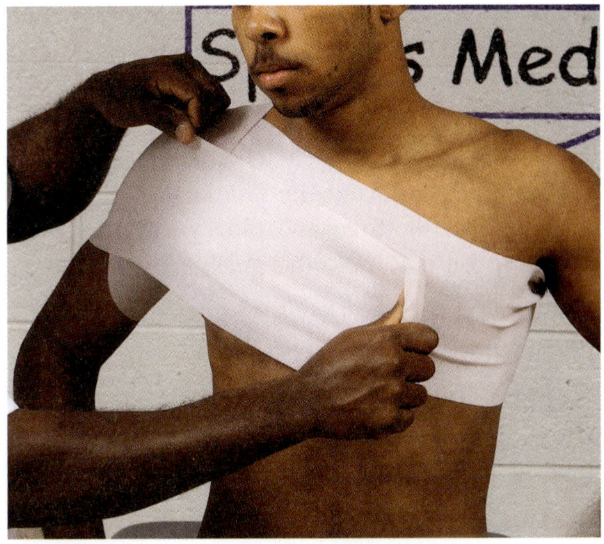

Figure 28.29 Shoulder spica. The athlete's arm is on the hip with the shoulder spica applied using an elastic wrap. This position puts the upper arm in an internally rotated position.

BANDAGES AND THEIR USE

A bandage is a cloth strip that is used to cover a wound over a sterile dressing or to immobilize a body part. The three forms of bandages are tubular, roller, and triangular.

Tubular

A tubular bandage is used on extremities to cover wounds or as a precursor to a cast. Fingertips and toes are difficult to keep clean, so a tubular bandage may be a good choice. Figure 28.30 shows a slip-on tubular dressing that may need to be cut to size for

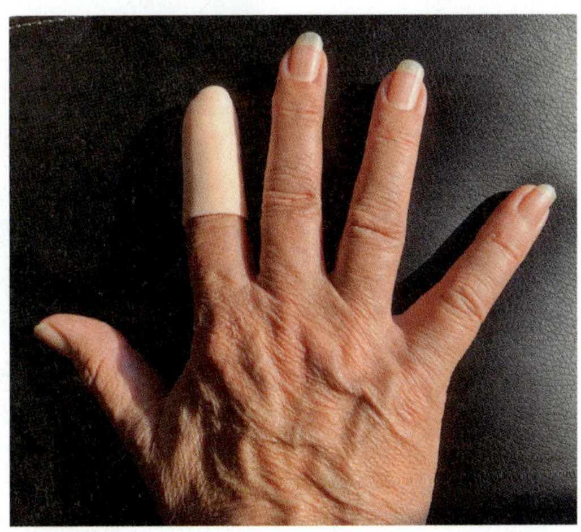

Figure 28.30 Commercial tubular bandage.
Photo: Lorin A. Cartwright.

length. Figure 28.31 shows a tubular dressing using a tubular gauze cage and stockinette.

Roller

Roller bandages are used when there is a large wound area to cover. The bandage starts at the distal end of the area and moves proximal. The sole purpose is to hold the sterile gauze in place, not necessarily to put compression on it.

Triangular Bandage

A triangular bandage can be used in multiple ways: as a sling, to cover a wound, or to help immobilize a body part. Using the triangular bandage as a simple sling, the short side of the bandage points at the athlete's elbow. The two long ends of the triangular bandage go around the athlete's neck and tie in the back. To finalize the sling, a knot is tied behind the elbow.

To cover a wound, fold the bandage into a 2-inch (5 cm) cloth. Place the midsection of the cloth underneath the wound and encircle it, tying the final knot on top of the wound.

A triangular bandage folded into a 2-inch (5 cm) cloth can be used to hold a splint at varying spacing for immobilization. It can be used with a windlass to become a tourniquet.

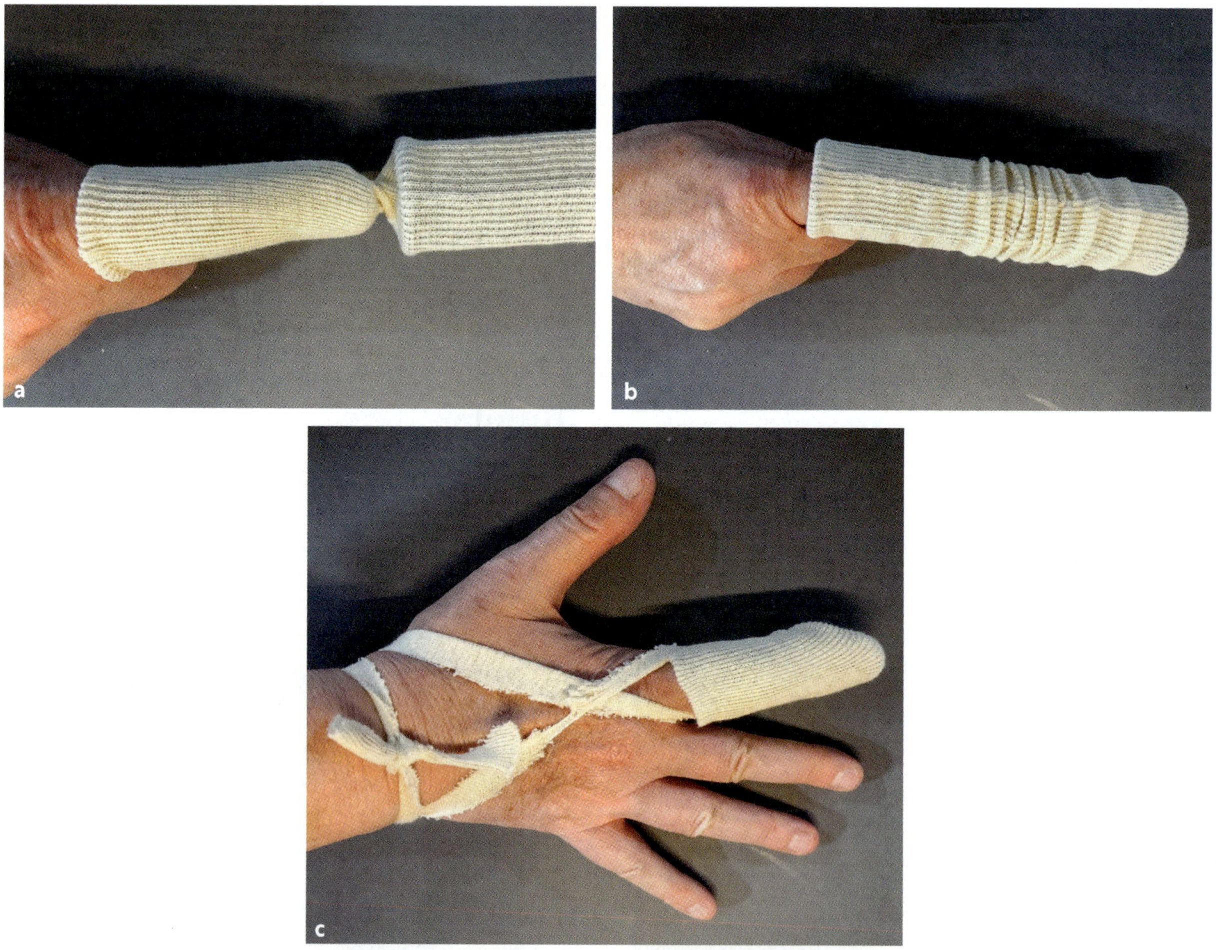

Figure 28.31 Tubular gauze cage. *(a)* Place the stockinette over the tubular cage, place the cage over the finger, and rotate the cage at the base of the finger, *(b)* pull the cage to the distal end of the finger and rotate the cage at the tip of the finger, repeating *(a)* and *(b)* a couple of times. *(c)* When at the base of the finger, split the stockinette and wrap around the athlete's hand.

Photos: Lorin A. Cartwright.

CASTING

Casting is used when the body part involved is unstable, such as with a displaced fracture. Casting can be done once the physician has set the fracture. The advantage of casting is that it provides complete immobilization and protection.

The casting material is either plaster or fiberglass. Fiberglass comes in a variety of colors, and an athlete may select a cast color to show school pride. The advantages of fiberglass are that it is lighter and does not deteriorate in water. Some companies offer customized casts (see figure 28.32). The physician may determine which type of cast is best for the athlete. The extremity being casted is covered with stockinette and padding.

Circular Casting of a Forearm

In this application, there is a simple uncomplicated fracture of the ulna or radius. After the fracture is reduced and swelling has reduced, the forearm is prepped for casting. Apply the stockinette from the elbow to the tips of the fingers. Cut a hole for the thumb. Next, apply the padding the over the same area as the stockinette, overlapping the padding by 50%. Ultimately, the cast will be two finger-widths from the elbow and two finger-widths from the metacarpal phalangeal joint. Using room temperature warm water, place the plaster into the water. Starting at the palm, use a circular motion that overlaps on itself to the elbow and then back toward the wrist. Fold over the excess stockinette and padding. A second plaster bandage material is placed in the same way, incorporating the stockinette and padding. There should be eight layers of plaster bandage. Check the athlete's range of motion in fingers, thumb, and elbow. There should not be any binding. The cast will be solid after 36 hours.

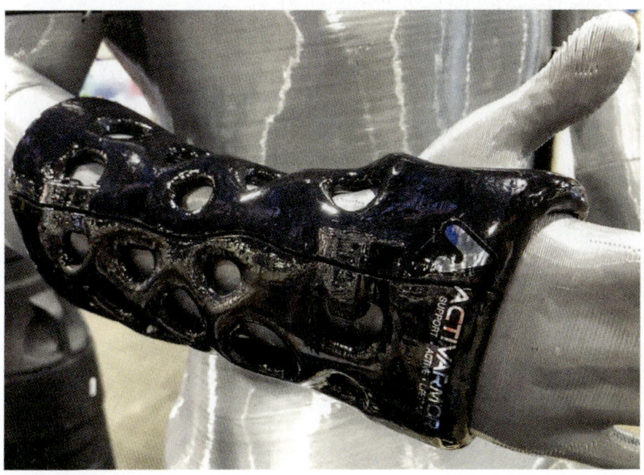

Figure 28.32 A customized cast.
Photo: Lorin A. Cartwright.

Lower-Leg Casting

The foot should be placed at a 90-degree angle. In this scenario, fiberglass casting material will be used. The lower-leg casting technique is similar to the forearm technique. Stockinette is placed over the lower leg from beyond the toes and proximal to the knee. Padding is placed over the entire area, same as the stockinette, overlapping the padding by 50% each pass. There may additional padding needed over the lateral and medial malleoli. Place the first roll of fiberglass casting material in water and squeeze out the excess. Starting just distal to the knee joint, roll the casting material distally while overlapping by 50% on itself. Once the roll gets to the foot, make sure there is at least two finger-widths from the metatarsal phalangeal joint. The length of the roll will allow you to return proximally to the knee. Fold over the stockinette and padding at the toes and knee. Incorporate the stockinette and padding into the next roll of fiberglass casting. The cast will be solid after about 30 minutes. Some athletes prefer the fiberglass casting material because it comes in various colors that can match the school of their choice.

Protecting a Cast

If a plaster cast gets wet, it degrades and can become ineffective. When a fiberglass cast gets wet, it does not degrade; however, the stockinette and padding will take a long time to dry. This can cause an irritation for the athlete. In any case, it is best to keep the cast dry. Cast covers will allow the athlete to shower as long as high-pressure water does not beat on the edge of the cast cover. An athlete cannot use the cast cover to swim.

Removing a Cast

To remove a cast requires a cast-cutting tool, a cast spreader, and medical scissors (see figure 28.33). This is where the cutting tool will traverse the

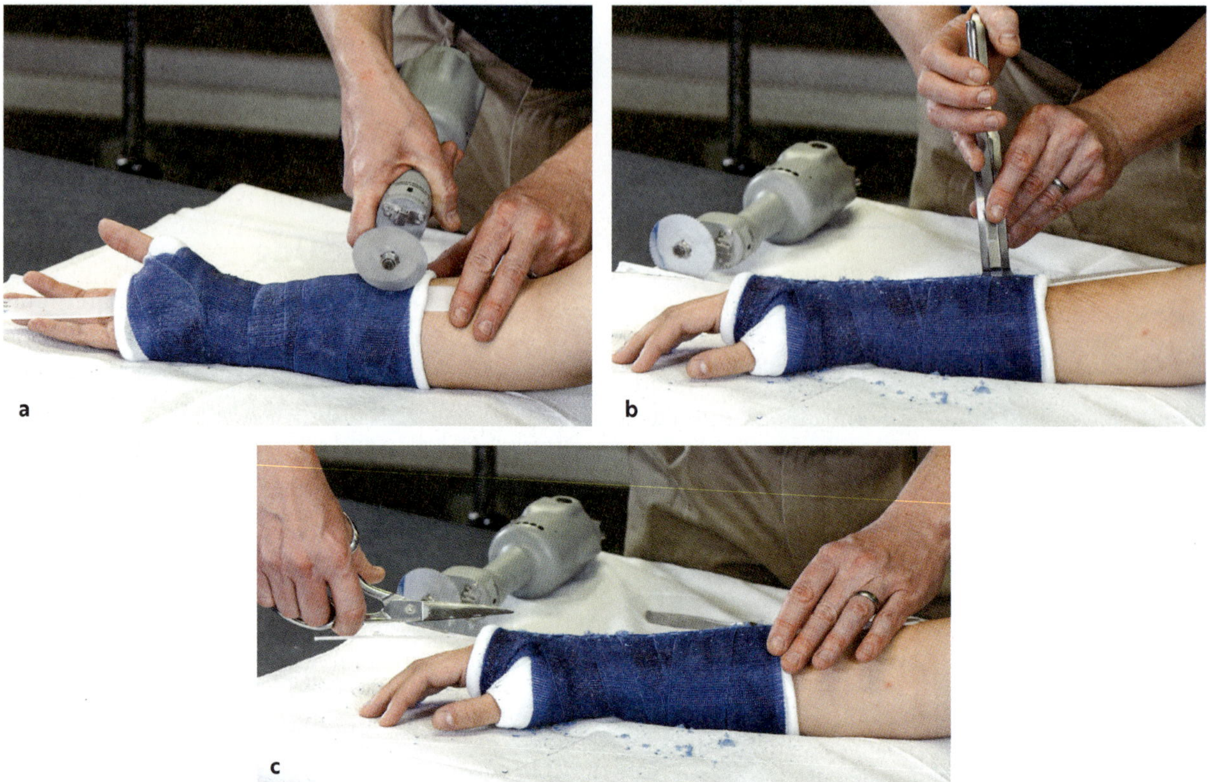

Figure 28.33 Cast removal. *(a)* Cut cast with cast saw the length of the cast. *(b)* Use a cast spreader to open up the cast. *(c)* Use medical scissors to cut through the stockinette and padding.

length of the cast. For simple arm casts, one opening with the cutting tool is all that is needed. For longer casts, two openings will be needed, one on each side of the cast. Use the cast spreader to open the cast and the medical scissors to cut through the stockinette and padding. Open the cast and the extremity is free again.

RED FLAGS

When has taping or wrapping become a problem?

- Edema distal to the taping or wrapping
- No pulse distal to the taping or wrapping
- Rubbing of the tape on the skin causing blisters or wounds
- A rash over the taped or wrapped area

Summary

Taping and wrapping have become essential skills for any AT. Tape and wraps are commonly used for immediate injury care, such as to secure a dressing, pad, or ice, as well as for injury prevention. Tape application relies on understanding tape selection, tape handling, skin preparation, and taping techniques. Linen, elastic, and hybrid tape are used for different reasons, and a variety of application techniques exist.

Key Terms

Define the following terms found in this chapter:

- checkrein
- elastic tape
- elastic wraps
- hybrid tape
- kinesiology tape
- linen tape
- moleskin
- rigid tape

An athlete reports to the athletic training room with pain along the medial portion of the bottom of the foot. The AT identifies that the athlete has a medial arch strain and, after treatment, provides a tape job to help support that region. What tape job should the AT select for this injury and why? What instructions do you suspect the AT will give this athlete?

To access supplementary material for this chapter, including the Understanding Check worksheet, vocabulary quizzes, extension activities, and chapter-specific resources and forms, visit the web resource: http://ancillaries.humankinetics.com/FundamentalsOfAthleticTrainingAndSportsMedicine5E

chapter 29

Protective Equipment and Durable Medical Equipment Used in Athletics

Objectives

After completing this chapter, the student will be able to do the following:

- Explain the principles of protection.
- Describe guidelines of protective equipment use.
- Explain what protective equipment is necessary for various sports.
- Describe proper equipment application.
- Explain the best durable medical equipment for a particular situation.

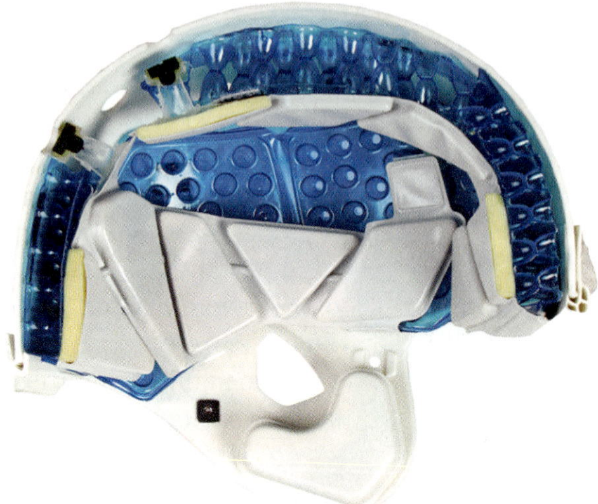

Figure 29.4 Football helmet interior of Schutt F7 2.0.

Photo courtesy of Certor Sports (Parent Company of Schutt Sports).

helmets have specialty plates that allow impacts to be disbursed over the entire helmet, and there is a liner layer that prevents forces from reaching the head (Schutt 2023). The Riddell SpeedFlex helmet has a patented side-impact protection, a five-point custom inflation liner, a ratcheted chin strap, and strategically placed padding with a liner to protect the head (Riddell 2014).

What Would You Do If . . .

A lacrosse player has a laceration on the bridge of his nose. You notice blood inside the front of the helmet. When you ask the athlete how the injury occurred, he says, "Some guy hit me, and the helmet shifted down." You tell him you would like to have the equipment manager look at the helmet. He says, "This happens every year. I just get stitches and that's it."

Ice Hockey

Ice hockey helmets are manufactured by several companies, but each one is tested and must meet CSA standards. They do not, however, need to be retested annually. The helmet interior is made of foam that conforms to the helmet shell. A hockey helmet should fit snugly. If it is too loose, it will not protect the head under significant impact. The last helmetless professional hockey player retired in 1997. Now all players in the National Hockey League wear helmets. Ice hockey helmets are also used in sports such as lacrosse and field hockey. Goalkeepers in many sports wear ice hockey helmets because they are lightweight yet effective (see figure 29.7*a*).

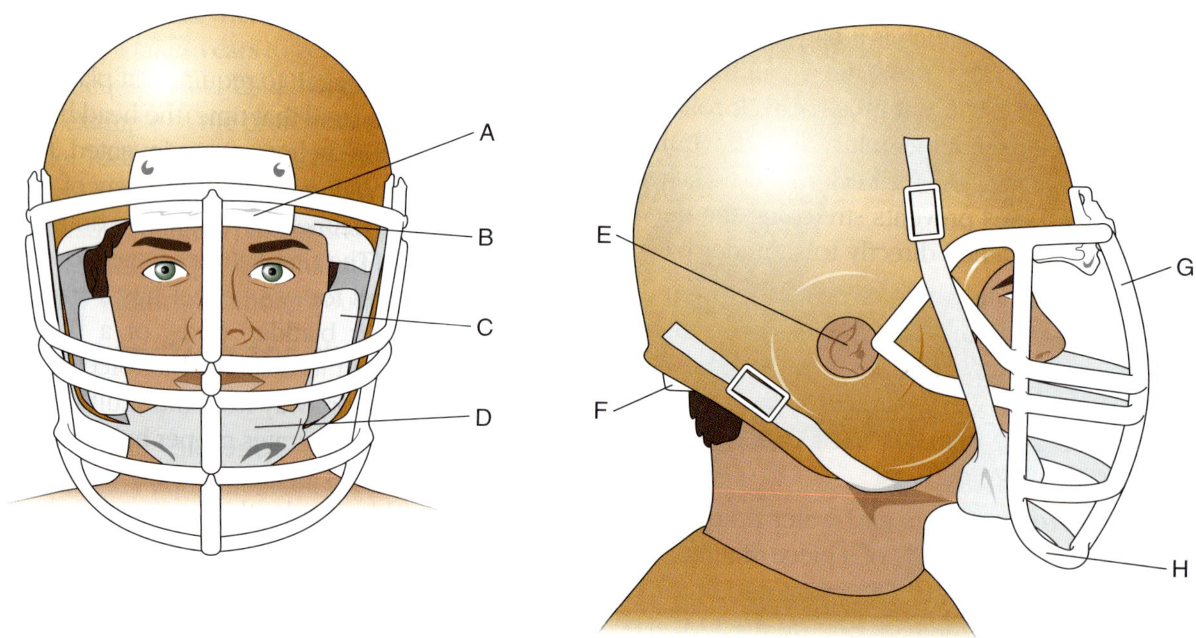

Figure 29.5 *(a)* The interior of the helmet must be one finger-width above the eyebrow, *(b)* the forehead pad must fit snugly against the forehead, *(c)* the cheek pads must fit snugly against the cheeks, *(d)* the chin strap must be snug and square on the chin, *(e)* the ear hole must line up with the ear canal, *(f)* the neck pad must be snug to the head, *(g)* the face mask must be three finger-widths from the nose, and *(h)* the face mask must be lower than the chin.

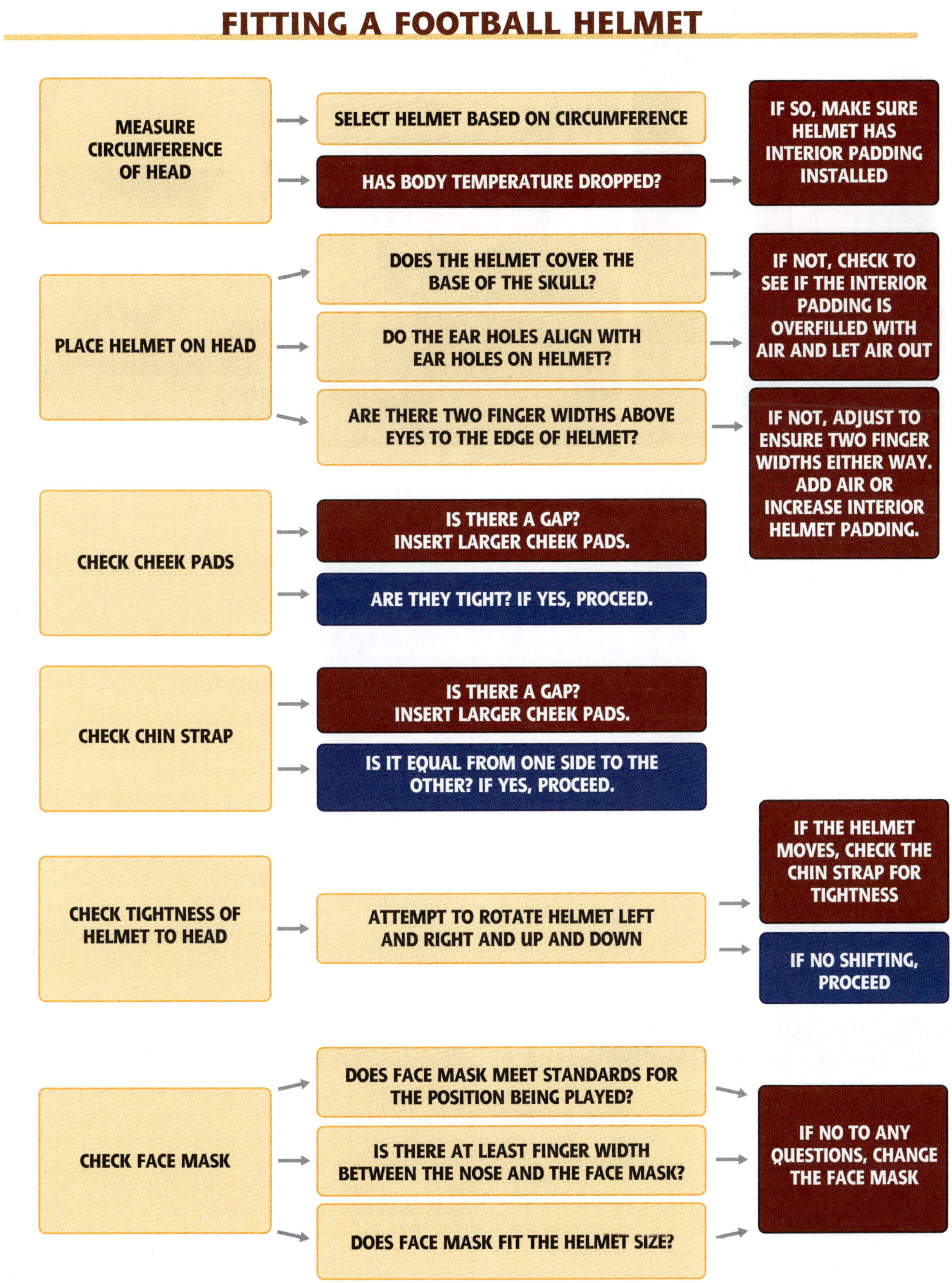

Figure 29.6 Fitting a football helmet.

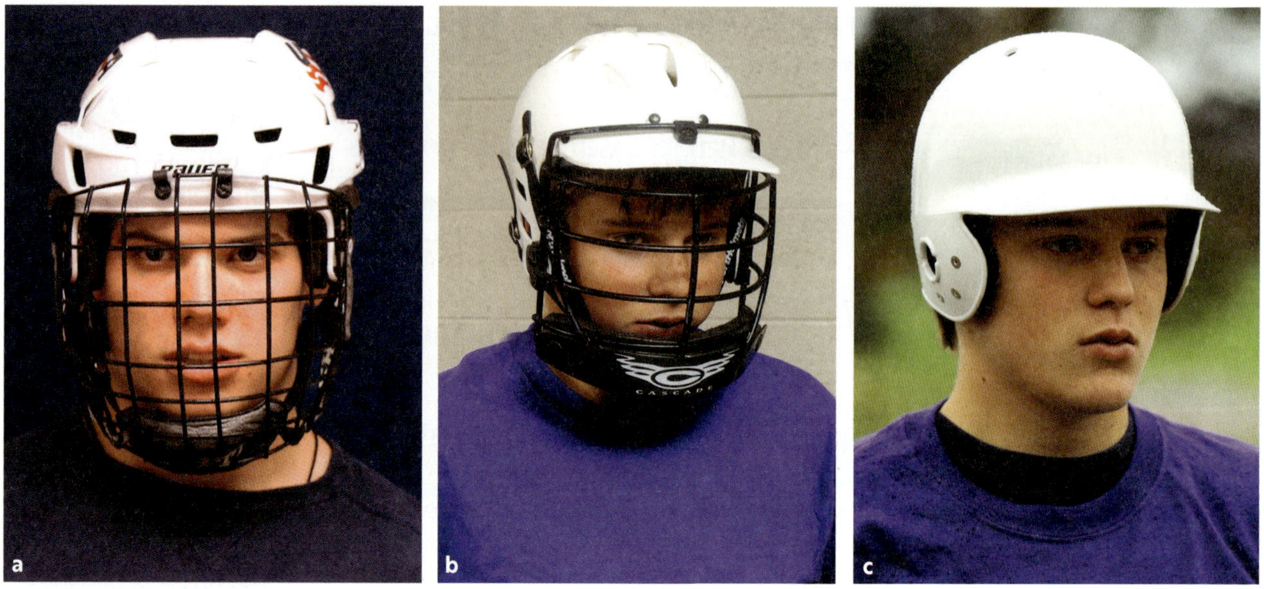

Figure 29.7 *(a)* Ice hockey helmet, *(b)* lacrosse helmet, and *(c)* batting helmet.

Lacrosse

Similar to hockey helmets, lacrosse helmets have a protective plastic shell with interior foam. The helmet has a four-point chin strap to stabilize it on the head. Lacrosse helmets are required for male players and must meet NOCSAE standards (see figure 29.7*b*). Only the goalie wears a helmet in women's lacrosse.

Cycling

Cycling helmets are tested by ASTM and the Consumers Product Safety Commission (CPSC). Those in competitive cycling are not required to have their helmets tested after purchase. The Consumers Product Safety Commission (n.d.) suggests that if a cyclist crashes and hits their head, a new helmet is warranted. If a cyclist has worn the same helmet and it shows wear and tear, such as cracks or degradation of the interior liner or straps, it should be replaced. A helmet should be replaced regardless of condition after 5 to 10 years of purchase (Consumers Product Safety Commission n.d.).

Skiing or Snowboarding

The ASTM, Snell, or CEN are the certifying groups that put labels on the helmet certifying the helmet has been tested and passed rigid standards. Helmets for downhill skiing or slalom should include a chin guard as a part of the helmet. Whenever there is an impact to the head, the helmet should be replaced, even if there are no visible cracks (Canadian Ski Council 2018). Helmets should be replaced every 3 to 5 years, regardless of impact (EVO 2020-2021).

The Real World

I fit all freshman, junior varsity, and varsity football players' helmets for the season. As I was walking behind the quarterback on the sideline before the start of a game, I noticed a white cloth sticking out the back of his helmet. Investigating further, I discovered that the player had stuffed a sock in place of the posterior pad. I asked him why he had altered his helmet. He replied, "I lost the other pad, and I know if the coach finds out, he'll be upset and not play me." "Okay," I said, "Come here. Put your helmet on with the sock in place of the pad." I did all the usual stress tests, and the results convinced him that this was a bad idea. I took him to the helmet repair kit and found a new posterior pad. The coach never found out—it was our little secret.

Suzy Heinzman, ATC

When fitting a skiing or snowboarding helmet, make sure the hair is at the length one would typically have. There should be no adornments. Put the skiing goggles on. The helmet should sit two fingers above the eyebrows. Put on the chinstrap, and make sure there is no space between the face, forehead, and the back of the neck. When the athlete shakes their head, the helmet should not move. Adjust the padding for thickness to create a snug fit (Centers for Disease Control and Prevention n.d.).

Baseball and Softball

All batting helmets are required to have the NOCSAE inspection seal, but they need not be tested annually. Batting helmets for players from Little League through college are required to have earflaps on both sides (see figure 29.7c). Professional baseball players are required to wear helmets, but earflaps are not required. However, most professionals wear a helmet with an earflap on the side closest to the pitcher when they are batting. The helmet interior is lined with hard foam, which distorts slightly on impact. Depending on the league, a chin strap or even a face mask might be required. Batting helmets with face masks are required for all fielders in Little League games.

Face Guards

Many sports involve a great deal of contact and ball movement that put an athlete at risk for facial injuries. Several sports have implemented the use of face guards to protect an athlete's face from contusions and lacerations.

Football

In football, the face mask is made either of rubber-covered metal or plastic. The face mask must be appropriate for the position the athlete will be playing. Quarterbacks and receivers wear face masks without a center bar so that they can see better. Running backs and defensive backs wear face masks with center bars. Linemen, defensive ends, and linebackers wear extended masks with center bars to keep fingers away from their face and throat. Properly fitted, the face mask must be three finger-widths from the nose.

Ice Hockey

There are three types of face masks for hockey helmets: full wire, full plastic (see figure 29.8), and half plastic. The wire face mask has small (1 in. or 2.5 cm) square openings that prevent a puck or stick from entering. The full plastic face mask is clear, but sometimes the mask gets foggy during play. College-aged and younger athletes are required to wear full face masks, either wire or plastic. Referees and professional hockey players use the half mask.

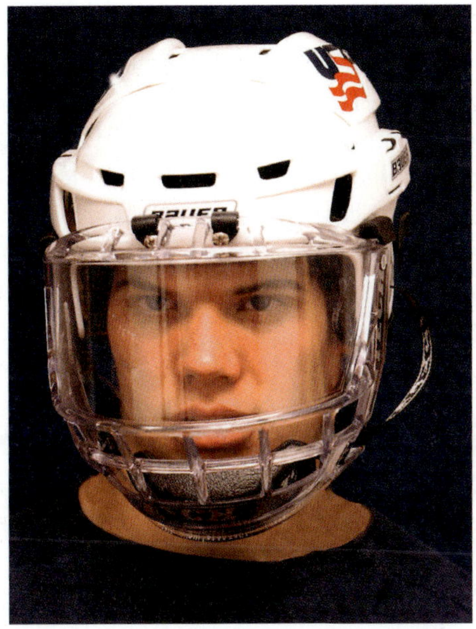

Figure 29.8 Ice hockey helmet with a clear face shield.

One of the scariest things in ice hockey is a laceration of the throat. An ice skate cutting the jugular vein or carotid artery can cause death in a short amount of time. Many players opt to wear a cut-resistant neck guard.

Lacrosse

Men's lacrosse face masks are connected to the helmet and provide full face wire protection. The wire mask has small openings to prevent a stick or ball from entering. A large, thick chin pad is placed at the base of the face mask to protect the athlete's chin. Lacrosse goalies are required to attach throat protectors to their face masks. A properly fitting lacrosse helmet will not shift positions when the athlete rotates their head.

Women's lacrosse players, like field hockey players, wear an eye mask. The eye mask protects the eyes from contact with a stick or ball and is attached with an elastic strap that fits around the back of the head.

Baseball and Softball

A catcher wears a face mask that attaches to a protective helmet. The face mask has a padded interior surface that rests against the face and elastic straps to hold it in place. It allows the catcher to see while protecting the face from errant balls. Many states require softball players to wear a face mask when hitting. Face masks for softball are attached to the batting helmet.

PROTECTIVE EQUIPMENT FOR THE UPPER BODY

Protective equipment for the upper body must allow the athlete to move yet also absorb shock. Designers are challenged to make devices that can take impact in a variety of positions. Most equipment is made of a hard exterior plastic shell with padding close to the body.

Shoulder and Upper Arm

Shoulder pads are the main protection for the shoulders in hockey, football, and lacrosse. All shoulder pads are designed similarly—a plastic exterior with soft padding next to the skin.

Football shoulder pads are designed for the position the athlete plays (see figure 29.9*a*). Regular shoulder pads cover the chest and shoulders. A quarterback wears pads that are smaller and allow for more shoulder movement; a lineman's pads are larger and longer. The pads lace in the front and have straps that run from the back and lock in the front. The soft padding is covered with a sweat-resistant material.

Compared with football pads, ice hockey and lacrosse shoulder pads are made of thin padding (see figure 29.9*b*). They lace and have a hook-and-loop closure in the front so that they are easily removed. These pads can be cleaned in a regular washing machine.

Shoulder lifts are thin (.5 in. or 1 cm) pieces of padding that are worn under shoulder pads. Lifts provide additional padding, and they are sometimes used after an injury. The lifts lace in the front and have underarm straps from back to front. Athletes who hit or who get hit the most often wear lifts—these include quarterbacks, running backs, and

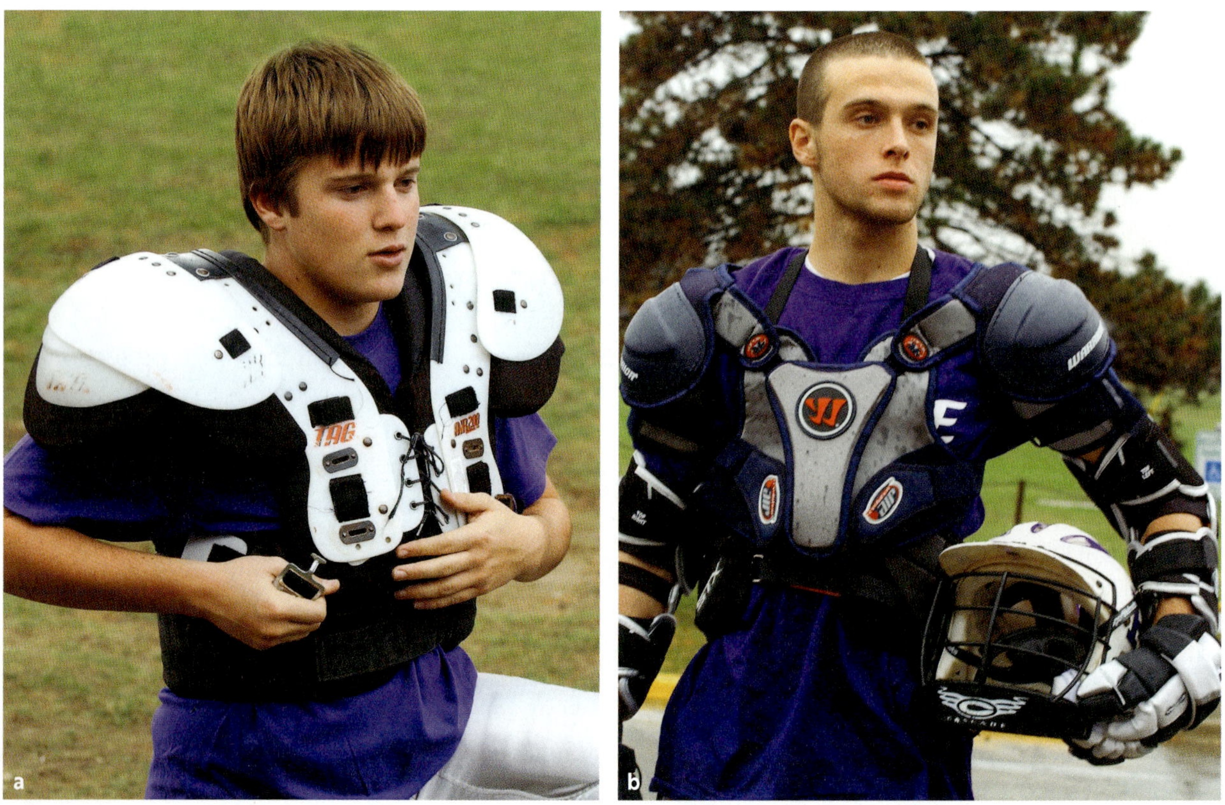

Figure 29.9 *(a)* Football shoulder pads and *(b)* lacrosse shoulder pads.

RED FLAGS

Get rid of helmets in the following conditions:

- Cracked
- Missing parts
- Has been altered
- 10 years or older
- Cannot be sanitized
- Not certified by the proper agency
- Being used improperly

linebackers (see figure 29.10). An athlete, whether they play football, lacrosse, or ice hockey, can have a customized compression shirt or pants with pads designed for them. In figure 29.11, one can see the padding attached to the compression garment.

A restrictive harness for the glenohumeral joint is worn when an athlete has had a shoulder joint dislocation or subluxation. The harness is tightened to keep the arm from being lifted up and abducted, because this is the position in which the shoulder is injured. The harness is made of straps that can be adjusted to limit motion (see figure 29.12).

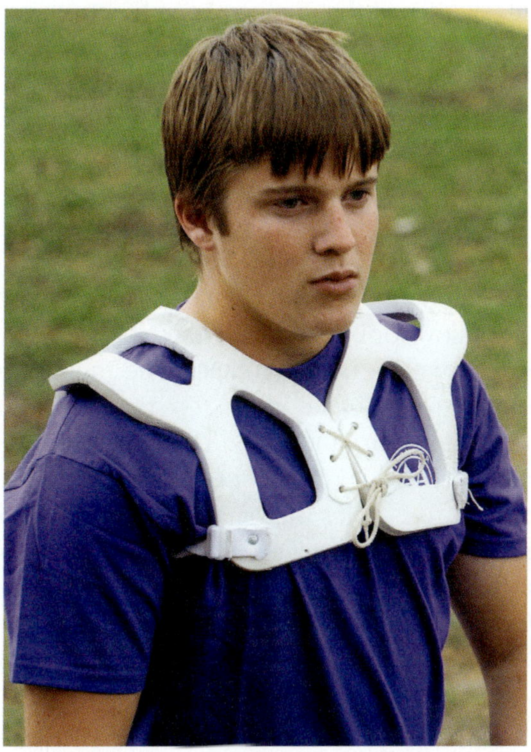

Figure 29.10 Shoulder lifts.

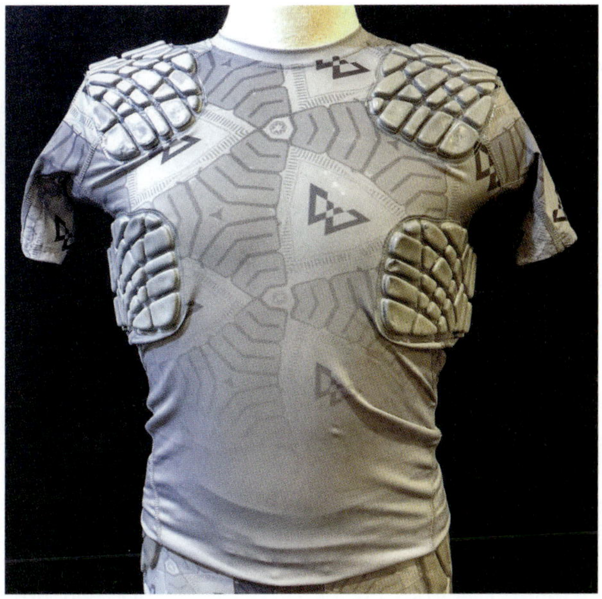

Figure 29.11 Shoulder and rib protection.

Photo: Lorin A. Cartwright.

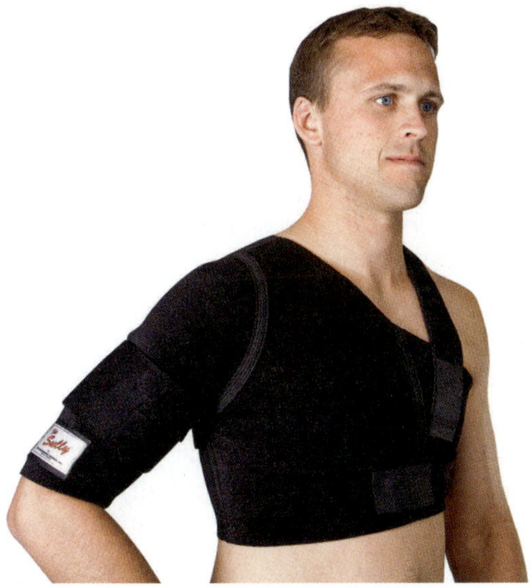

Figure 29.12 DonJoy Sully shoulder brace.

Courtesy of Enovis Corporation

Elbow, Wrist, and Hand

Of all athletes, football and ice hockey players wear elbow pads most often (see figure 29.13*a*). Football players wear pull-on elbow pads, which are soft pads enclosed in elastic material. Hockey players wear pads with plastic exteriors that are fastened in place with hook-and-loop closures. The newest hockey pads are made of thick, soft padding covered with sweat-resistant material. An elbow sleeve

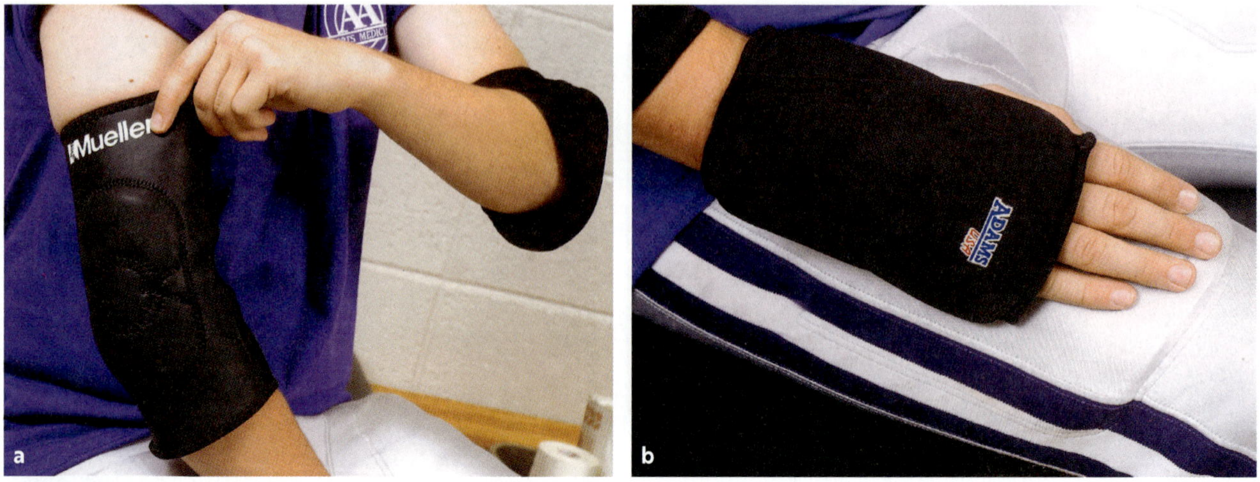

Figure 29.13 *(a)* Two types of elbow pads and *(b)* a pull-on hand pad.

is made of either elastic or neoprene for warmth. The sleeve lacks padding so it does not offer protection from impact, but it is supportive and can prevent abrasions.

An elbow hyperextension brace can be utilized in any sport. An athlete who has hyperextended their elbow can utilize this type of brace to prevent further injury to the joint.

Soccer, ice hockey, football, field hockey, and lacrosse players use gloves. The glove style varies by sport. Soccer goalies wear a glove that has a tacky leather palm. A field hockey goalkeeper wears a leather glove that is padded on both sides for protection because she is not allowed to use a closed hand on the ball. Field hockey players and some women lacrosse players wear gloves to protect them from contusions caused by balls and sticks.

Ice hockey goalies wear a different glove on each hand. The glove that is used to catch pucks consists of a large leather mitt that is strapped tightly around the hand and extends up to the middle of the forearm. The other hand has a glove attached to a large pad called a *blocker*. It has a leather palm and a big chunk of padding over the top of the hand and fingers. A football lineman wears a fingerless glove with padding for the back of the hand, which is used during blocking. As an alternative to the glove, the lineman may wear a pad that can be pulled on over the back of the hand to protect it (see figure 29.13*b*). Wide receivers use gloves made of neoprene, which is tacky and good for catching the ball, to protect the hands from cold and abrasions.

Baseball and softball players wear mitts designed based on their defensive positions. The leather mitt is heavily padded on the fingertips and thumb. Most players catch a ball in the web of the glove, but sometimes they catch one in the palm portion. The palm of the glove is not padded well, and a ball caught in the palm can cause bruising. Protection against a bruised palm is to wear a palm pad that has a loop. The loop is put over one of the fingers and the pad then lays over the palm. The pad is relatively thin so that the hand can fit into the mitt.

Wrist braces are typically made of cloth with metal inserts or stays that are covered. Players need this brace when they have an injury such as a sprain or strain. The brace may have laces or Velcro that allow for better comfort or support.

A protective thumb spica brace can be used when there has been an injury to the thumb or wrist that needs immobilization (see figure 29.14). Some sports do not allow for braces below the elbow if there is the potential for bodily contact. The thumb spica brace may have metal inserts or stays covered by cloth, with Velcro and laces. This brace can allow participation while protecting the area of injury.

Skiers use poles that have hand protection against hitting slalom gates. They also wear forearm guards that protect against contusions and lacerations when going around the gates. Both are made from high-impact plastic, with the forearm guard held in place by straps.

Baseball and softball players like to protect their hands and fingers while on the basepaths. In some instances, the player will hold dirt in their hands, keeping the fingers tucked in to avoid being stepped

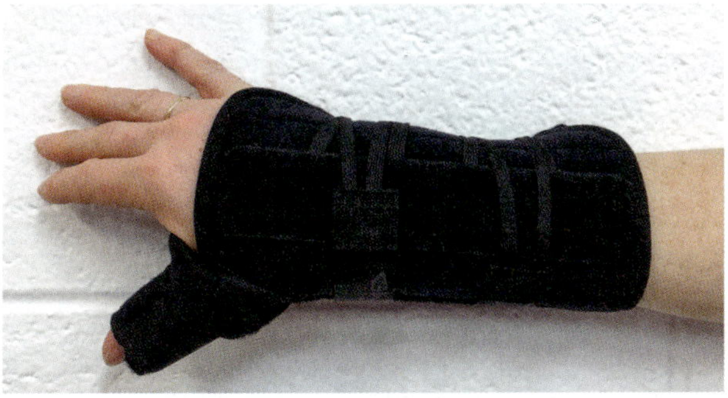

Figure 29.14 Thumb spica brace.
Photo: Lorin A. Cartwright.

on. A sliding mitt has solid plates on both sides of the mitt to prevent injury. The mitt is fastened to the wrist with straps (see figure 29.15). Some athletes try to protect their throwing hands. Some may slide with one hand as the lead hand into a base, which puts it more at risk. The mitt may be worn on the lead hand for protection.

A batter's elbow shield is used by baseball and softball players to prevent bruises. The shield is hard and is worn on the upper arm at the elbow, on the arm closest to the pitcher. When a ball is thrown, the elbow is one of the more prominent areas of impact (see figure 29.16).

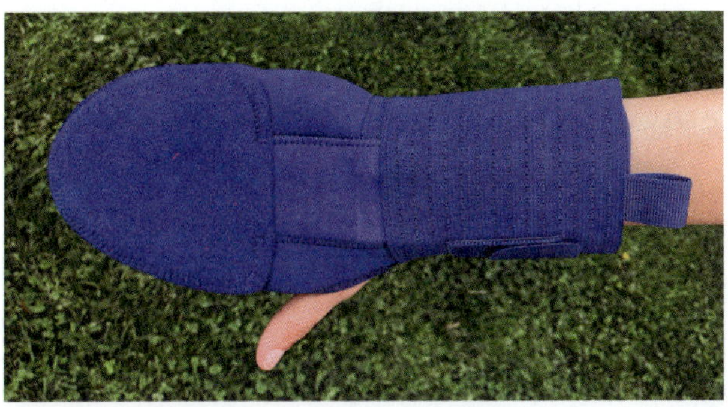

Figure 29.15 Sliding mitt.
Photo: Lorin A. Cartwright.

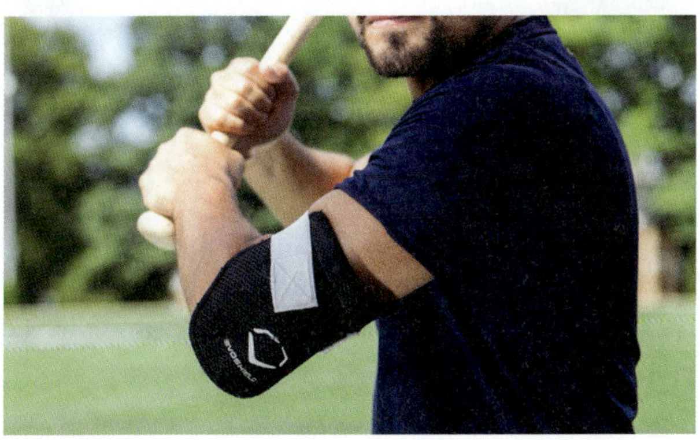

Figure 29.16 Elbow shield.

Some bowlers wear a wrist support with a metal insert. The purpose of the support is to maintain correct hand position throughout the release. The consistent position of the wrist at release helps the bowler with the rotation of the ball.

Tennis players and golfers who may suffer with epicondylitis can use a compression brace. Within the brace is a compression pad that is placed over the affected tendon. The compression changes the point of stress, allowing pain relief.

Ribs, Sternum, and Abdomen

Football shoulder pads offer some chest protection but only for the uppermost ribs and the sternum, and a specific pad is often necessary to protect the ribs (see figure 29.17). No other shoulder pads offer chest protection. Football equipment manufacturers have also designed a sternum protection pad that is not standard equipment but can be worn if an athlete requires extra protection.

Specific equipment has been designed to protect the chest and abdomen in various sport activities. Chest protectors, for example, protect both the abdomen and the chest.

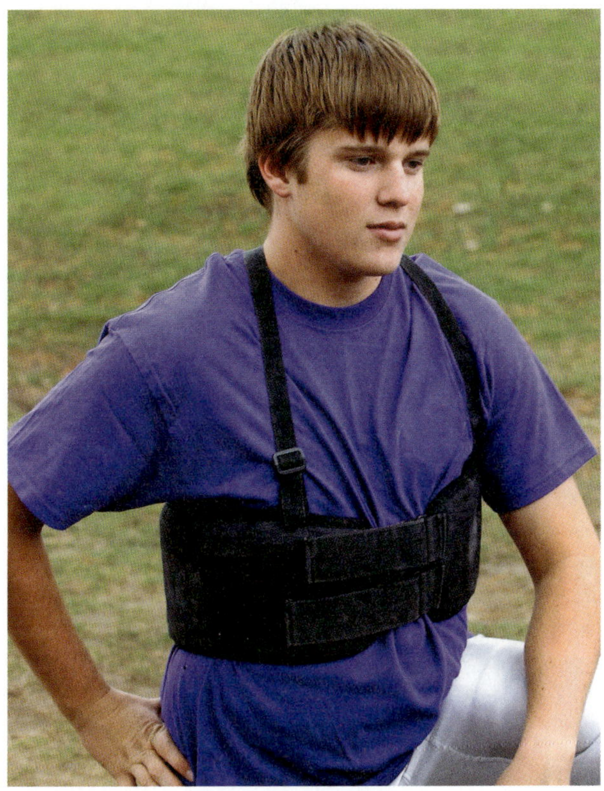

Figure 29.17 Rib protector.

In field hockey, baseball, and women's lacrosse, players wear a standard chest protector designed specifically for baseball and softball. It is made of soft padding inside a durable cloth cover and uses elastic straps to hold it tightly against the body. Little League baseball players use a similar type of chest protector while batting. A word of caution: Chest protectors are not safety rated. This means anyone can design a chest protector and claim that it works.

A catcher wears a chest protector that is 0.75 inch (2 cm) thick to prevent baseball impacts against the body. The protector is made of padding that covers the chest and abdominal areas. It is big and cumbersome yet effective in preventing injury as well as deadening the ball (see figure 29.18).

Athletes who have been or are likely to be injured and those who receive the most impacts, such as quarterbacks, running backs, and wide receivers in football, are equipped with rib protectors. Participants in impact sports such as men's lacrosse, football, and ice hockey are likely to need this equipment.

Downhill and slalom skiers may wear a vest with chest and back protection. This vest acts like a form of body armor needed in the event of a crash to reduce injury. These vests are not mandatory items.

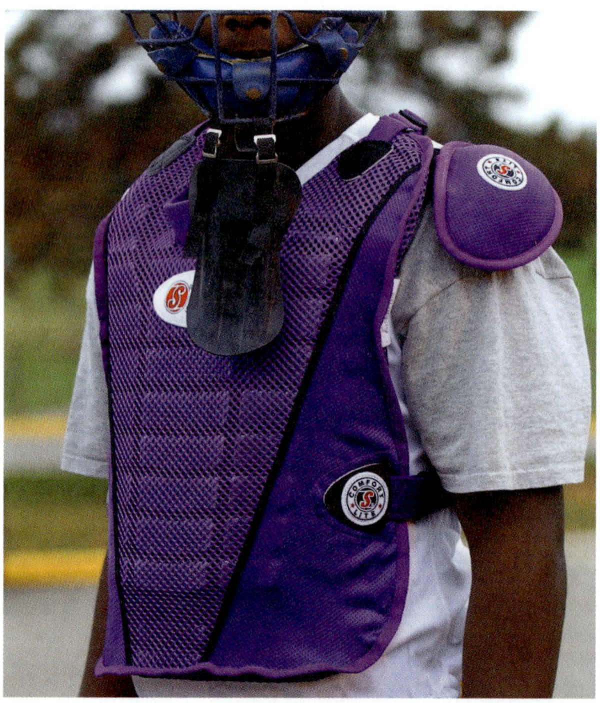

Figure 29.18 Chest protector for baseball.

Skiers may opt to use stealth-impact padded tops, which fit under a racing suit. These tops have padding on the forearms, shoulders, and along the lateral portion of the back. This top provides mobility along with protection from contusions.

Low Back

Back braces are designed to keep the athlete warm and to limit motion. Most back braces are made of neoprene or elastic and are fastened tightly in the front with a hook-and-loop closure. Back braces have small metal wires inside to provide a more stable brace (see figure 29.19).

PROTECTIVE EQUIPMENT FOR THE LOWER BODY

Lower-body protection must not hinder the athlete's movement. If you watch professional football, you will notice that many players do not wear all the pads or standard-sized pads required by the rules in high school or college. Players at the professional level are paid to play and be fast; they believe that lower-body protective padding slows them down and may cost them their jobs.

Thigh, Hip, and Tailbone

Thigh pads are used in four sports: football, field hockey, women's lacrosse, and ice hockey. Thigh pads must be big enough to cover the quadriceps musculature. They must fit properly, and the pants that cover them must be snug. Football and hockey pants are designed to hold the pads tight against

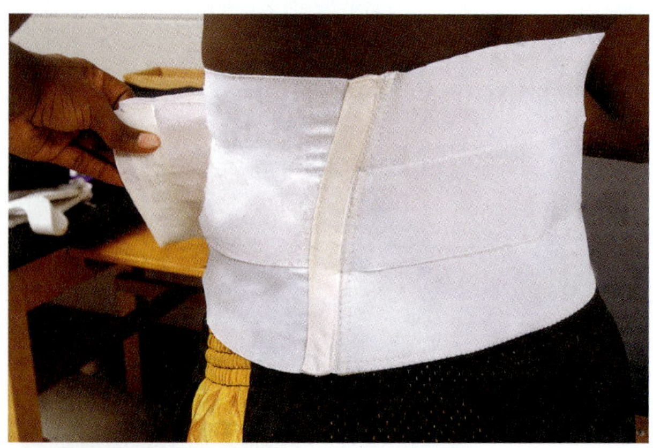

Figure 29.19 Back brace.

the bony areas they protect (see figure 29.20). Ice hockey pads go inside a pair of fitted shorts. These shorts hold thigh, hip, and lower-abdomen pads and lace up in the front. Ice hockey pads are effective, and field hockey and women's lacrosse goalkeepers wear them for protection.

Many athletes use lower-extremity compression clothing to gain a competitive edge. For runners, it has shown some benefit by increasing endurance and potentially reducing muscle pain and inflammation (Engel et al. 2016). Hettchen and colleagues (2019) found that there was benefit for wearing compression tights for improving recovery after intense exercise.

Soccer goalkeepers wear shorts or long pants with hip pads in them. The padding is lightweight to allow maximum movement and provides limited protection. Compression shorts were originally designed to hold football pads in place over the muscles, but they are now used to provide support and warmth to the muscles without padding. In baseball and softball, a thin fiber pad that covers the hip is added to prevent sliding abrasions.

Protective cups are made from a hard plastic and carbon fiber, and some have metal inserts. Protective cups are used to protect genitals. Contact sports typically require wearing a cup: rugby, ice hockey, baseball, boxing, mixed martial arts, lacrosse, and

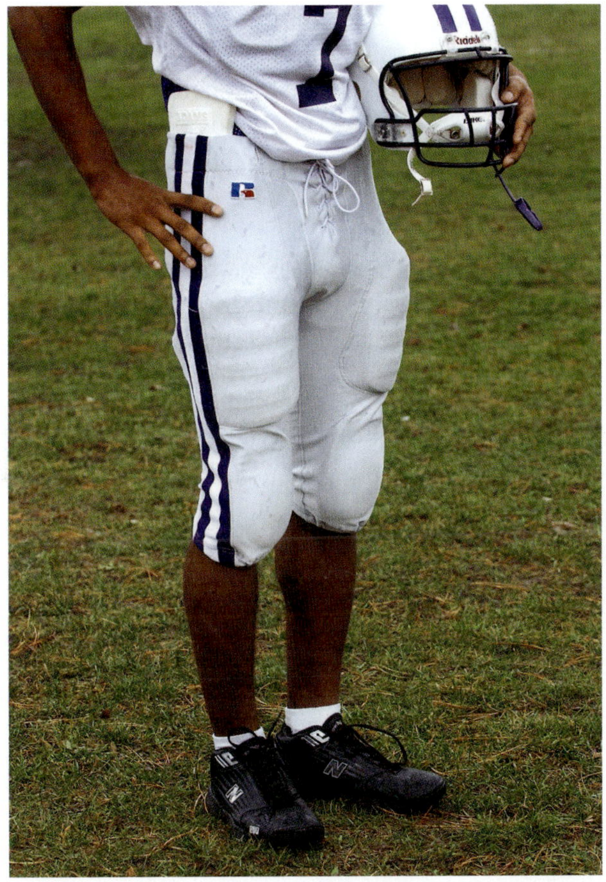

Figure 29.20 Football pants are designed to hold a variety of pads in place to protect the thigh, iliac crest, and knee.

Understanding Diversity

Differences Between Male and Female Skeletons

	Male	Female
Height	Taller	9% shorter
Bone density	50% more	Less density
Pairs of ribs	12	12
Leg length	Longer	Shorter
Arm length	Longer	Shorter
Finger length	4th finger longer than 2nd finger	
Torso		Longer
Joint mobility		Greater mobility
Pelvis width	Narrower	Wider
Skulls		10% thicker
Vision	Better long-distance focus	Better peripheral vision and better color perception
Hearing		Hear better in high-frequency range
Voice	Deeper	

Adapted from Fair Play for Women (2017)

football. Young women may use a similar product, but it is referred to as a protective guard. In sports where there is the potential for a hard ball traveling at a high speed, a guard could be used. Female ice hockey and softball are sports where the guard is most often used.

Athletes have found benefits when wearing compression shorts. These types of shorts are made of elastic and polyester material. Compression shorts may have a pocket for the insertion of a protective cup or guard.

Knee

Repetitive bruises to the knee can limit an athlete's ability to play. Thus, knee pads are designed to cover the anterior aspect of the knee. The pads, which are made of foam and covered with an elastic material, are sewn into an elastic sleeve that is pulled on over the foot and up to the knee.

A variety of neoprene sleeves provide warmth and support, including patellar and shin sleeves, hinged sleeves, and sleeves with stays. A patella brace has a horseshoe-shaped pad that fits around the patella to prevent it from slipping out of alignment.

A football player may wear a hinged knee brace, which is a metal or plastic bar with a hinge that protects the joint but allows flexion and extension of the knee (see figure 29.21). Some players, especially linemen and quarterbacks, think the brace prevents knee sprains. The braces are worn laterally because most blows come from that side and stretch the medial ligament. Athletes claim that these braces slow them down, but the effect is insignificant. An athlete who has bowlegs or knock-knees should not wear this type of brace because it tends to straighten the knee and cause soreness. Instead, that athlete should have their knees taped, even though taping takes more time. Currently there is conflicting research on the effectiveness of wearing the brace, so the athlete's parents should decide if their child will use it.

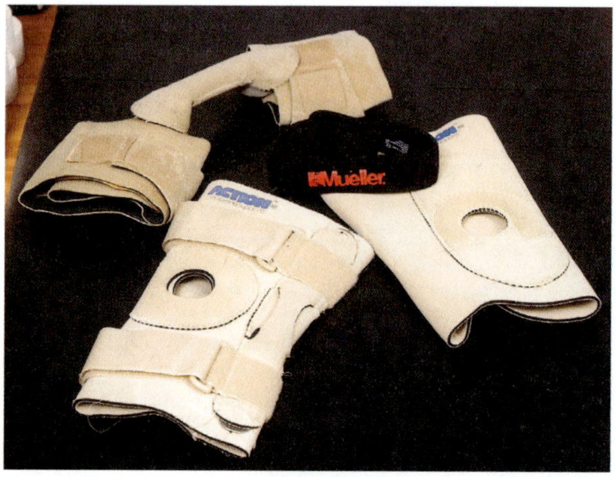

Figure 29.21 Knee braces.

Lower Leg

In some sports, a shin guard and knee pad are combined into one protective pad, which is usually a hard outer plastic shell with a padded interior. A catcher in baseball or softball and ice hockey players wear such protection. Straps hold the shin guard in place (see figure 29.22).

A catcher's shin guard has an extension that covers the ankle. In ice hockey, field hockey, and soccer, the ankle is not covered and is vulnerable to injury from blows. For ice hockey, a special pad that covers both malleoli and the front part of the

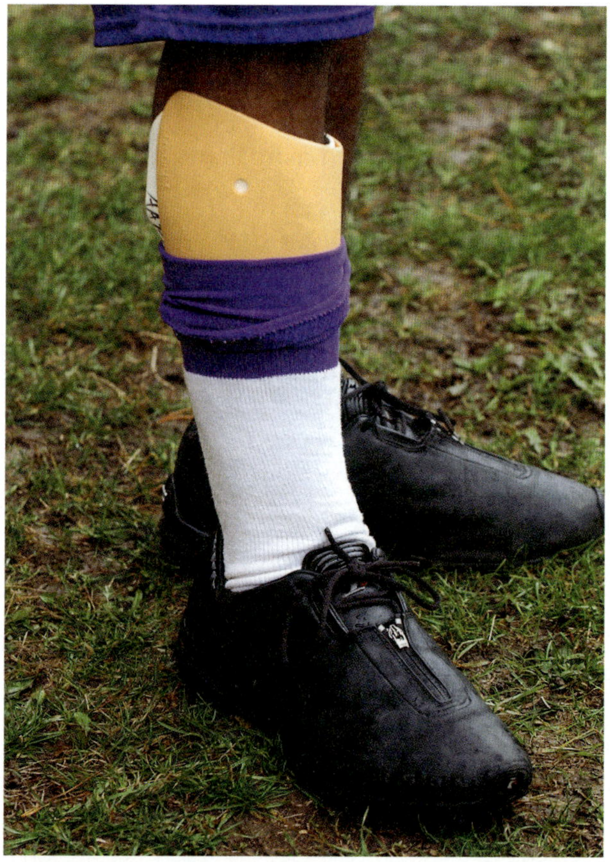

Figure 29.22 Shin guard.

ankle is used only after a player has suffered a contusion of the anterior ankle.

Field hockey and ice hockey goalkeepers wear pads that cover the foot, shin, thigh, and knee. The thick padding is made of foam, cotton, and plastic and is covered with canvas or leather, with flaps around the sides of the legs and the feet. The pads are designed for protection and for deadening the ball on impact. The pads come in various sizes based on the distance between the instep and the groin (the inseam) to ensure proper fit. They are held in place with buckled straps. The goalie pads are effective for preventing injury.

Baseball and softball players who foul balls off their feet or lower legs may choose to wear a batter's guard. The distal portion of the guard covers the anterior aspect of the longitudinal arch. The proximal portion of the guard covers the anterior aspect of the lower leg. The guard prevents bruises and the pain from being hit. It is removed once the player gets on base.

Slalom skiers wear a high-impact plastic shin guard to protect them from the impact of gate poles. The shin guards are held in place with Velcro strapping.

Foot and Ankle

In many sports, athletes' feet are stepped on and injured. The top of the foot can swell so much that the athlete is unable to wear a shoe. The AT may have to design a special pad to protect the top of the foot when an injury occurs.

Heel cups are designed to prevent heel bruises. There are two types of cups: a rubberized padded cup and a rigid plastic cup (see figure 29.23). The rubberized cup has an elevated heel that can compress downward so that the heel never makes contact with the interior of the shoe. This type of heel cup is good for athletes who have been injured. A plastic heel cup fits snugly and does not allow the fat tissue to flatten, thus protecting the heel.

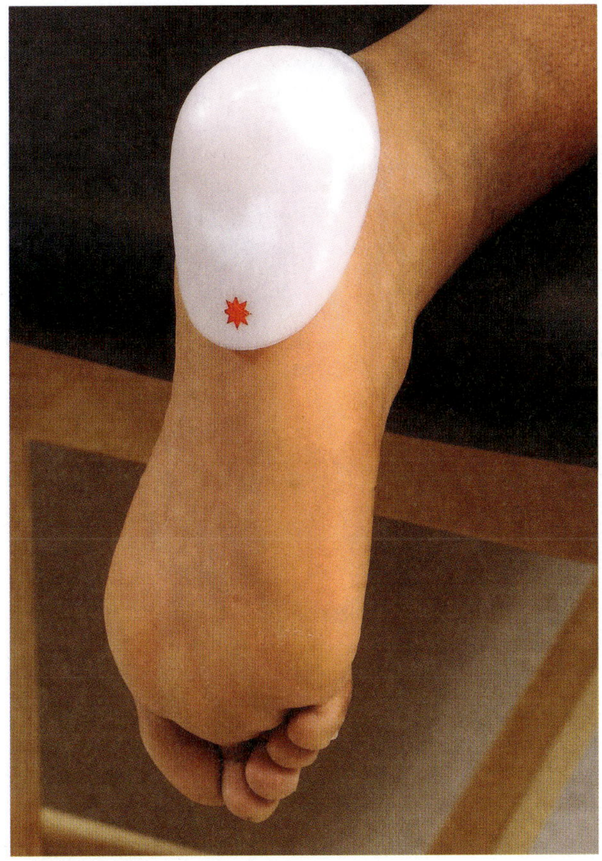

Figure 29.23 Heel cup.

A heel pad is a soft cushion made of rubber, foam, or felt and is placed between the heel and the shoe. Heel pads are used to prevent bruises and to equalize the length of an athlete's legs if they are different. Unless it is being used to lengthen one leg, a pad should be used in each shoe.

Arch supports are soft foam, rubber, or leather pieces. The foot flattens during every step, and an arch support keeps the foot from flattening too much. Most athletic shoes have built-in arch supports. The athlete must purchase a shoe with an arch support that fits their foot.

Ankle braces come in elastic, lace-up, and hinged versions. The elastic pull-on ankle brace provides only minimal support; however, it does give the athlete an awareness of their ankle, thus possibly preventing an injury. The lace-up ankle brace is similar to a shoe without a toe (see figure 29.24).

? What Would You Do If . . .

The best baseball player on your team slides into second base and sprains an ankle. You notice that there is not enough tape to apply a protective support. Thinking quickly, you remember that one of the bench sitters has an ankle brace.

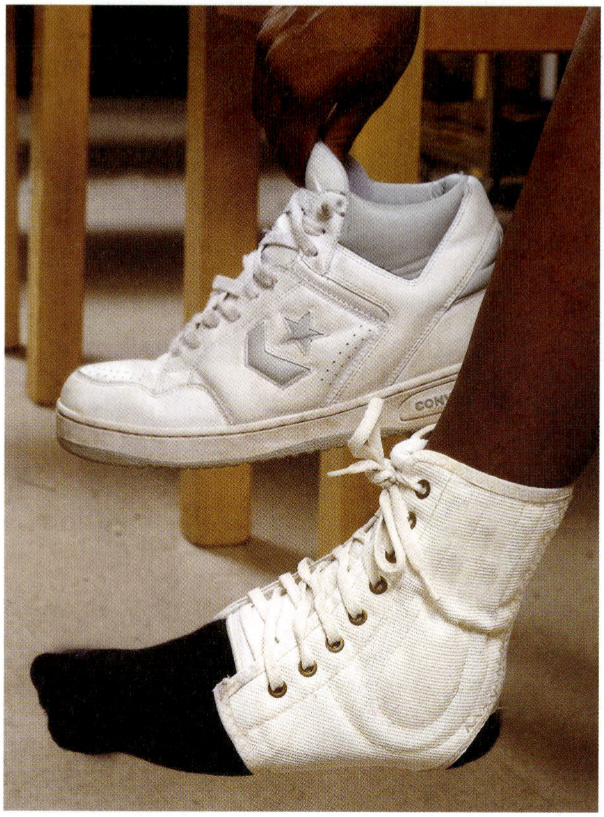

Figure 29.24 Ankle brace.

The brace is laced up tightly, especially over the ankle, to limit movement. Some lace-up braces have pockets in which to insert plastic pieces that prevent inversion and eversion. In other lace-up braces, a figure-eight elastic strip can be pulled tightly around the ankle to prevent inversion or eversion.

ATs have become accustomed to designing special equipment to meet athletes' needs. In some cases, foam and plastic pads provide needed protection, and other times taping and supportive wrapping will be the most effective. Padding and equipment are the first line of protection from impact. Before the start of a game, the officials will ask to inspect and approve braces, soft casts, and anything with metal hinges. Equipment that lacks approval cannot be used.

DURABLE MEDICAL EQUIPMENT

Durable medical equipment are items that can be used repeatedly. Examples of durable medical equipment include oxygen, canes, walkers, kneelers, wheelchairs, and crutches.

Oxygen

Those who need oxygen therapy can use several forms. On the sideline of an athletic contest, the AT may have small emergency tanks capable of oxygen administration for a short time (see figure 29.25). Large tanks of oxygen can be attached to wheelchairs or used at home, and they last a long time, depending on the rate of flow. There are also oxygen concentrators. An oxygen concentrator can take air and concentrate it into medical-grade oxygen. Concentrators can be as large as a suitcase or as small as a purse.

Tanks or concentrators need a regulator. The regulator is attached to the top of the tank, and it is set to the proper flow rate of oxygen for the patient's condition. For those who need oxygen for long periods of time, a humidifier is added between the tank and the face mask. A humidifier increases moisture and prevents nosebleeds and membranes from drying out.

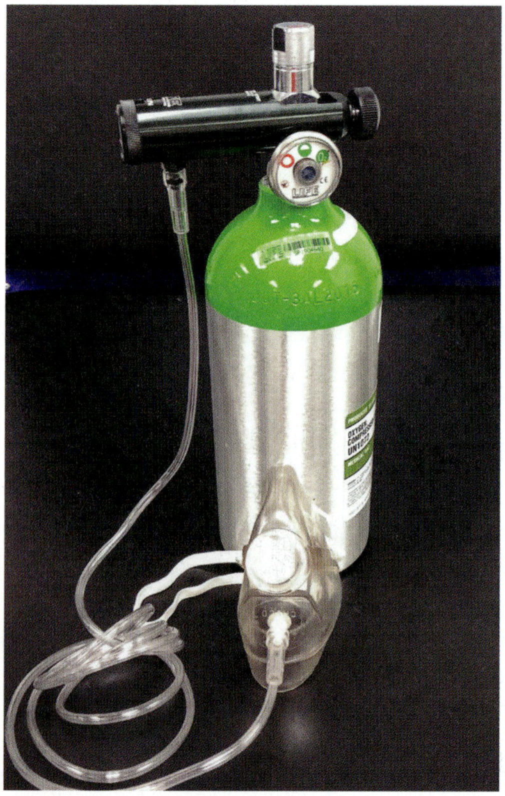

Figure 29.25 Oxygen tank.

Photo: Lorin A. Cartwright.

Canes

When an athlete needs mild balance support, a cane is a good option. Canes can be made of wood, aluminum, or carbon fiber material. The cane is fitted as the athlete stands, their arm dangling at the side. The top of the cane should be high enough so that it is level with the wrist. The cane is held in the hand opposite the injured lower extremity. Canes have a single tip or a quad tip. A quad tip is used when more stability is needed.

Walkers

Several types of walkers are used to provide support. When a person is standing in the walker, there are four legs, each with tips: two on the anterior aspect and two on the posterior aspect of the body. When the athlete stands, the top of the walker meets the wrist with the arm in full extension. When fitted properly, the elbow will be bent to allow pressure on the hands and upper extremity and not on the injured lower extremity. For those who require support but have more mobility, a three-legged walker or one with wheels may be the best fit.

Upright walkers allow pressure to be taken on the forearms instead of the hands. This type of walker allows the athlete to stand more upright, which may prevent thoracic and cervical pain.

Some walkers have brakes to hold the walker still when necessary. Walkers may also come with a seat to allow respite in the event of fatigue.

Knee Walker

A knee walker has four wheels, a padded platform, and handle bars with brakes (see figure 29.26). A knee walker is an alternative for crutches. The knee walker allows the athlete to keep pressure off the lower leg, ankle, and foot. The knee walker is adjusted to the height of the athlete so when they kneel on it, they are upright with hands on the handlebars. The uninjured leg pushes the walker, and it moves while the handlebars can be turned to change direction.

The positive aspect of the knee walker is the ease of use and the ability to take pressure off the upper extremities, and it does not require great strength to use it. The negative is that it cannot be used when there are stairs, so crutches still need to be utilized.

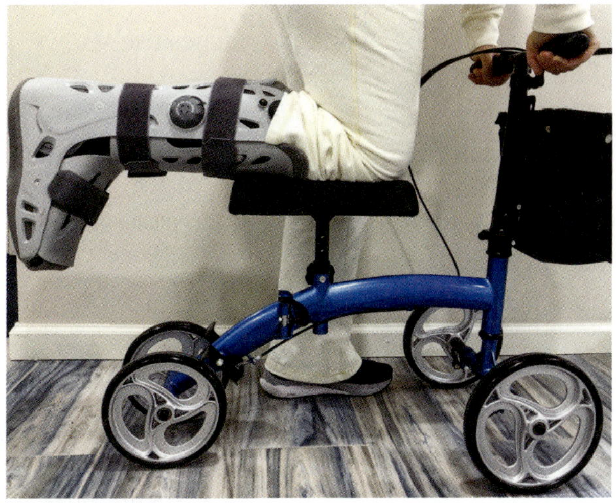

Figure 29.26 Knee walker.
Photo: Lorin A. Cartwright.

Wheelchairs

Wheelchairs can be used to move an ill individual who cannot walk or who has a lower-extremity injury. Standard wheelchairs have two large wheels that assist the user in propelling it forward and two smaller wheels in the front that allow for mobility. The rear tires have manual hand brakes to prevent the chair from moving when the athlete is getting in or out. The chair has two adjustable leg rests that can be elevated or removed should they not be needed.

A caregiver can push the wheelchair with the handles on the back of the chair. An athlete may choose to push on the large wheels and maneuver the chair themselves. Wheelchairs can be folded and put in a vehicle for transport to a destination. Lightweight wheelchairs are much easier to transport. Lightweight wheelchairs are usually equipped with hand brakes and four smaller wheels. The lightweight chair has to be pushed by a caregiver.

Crutches

Crutches are typically constructed from wood and aluminum. Foam arm covers and foam hand covers take off the pressure from those areas. When an athlete has an injured lower extremity and pressure must be taken off the injury, crutches are an option. The tip of the crutch and the hand grips adjust to fit an athlete according to their height. Aluminum crutches tend to have spring-loaded buttons that allow for easy fitting. Wooden crutches use screws and nuts for fitting these crutches.

When fitting crutches, the athlete stands with the shoes they intend to wear. There should be 2 inches (5 cm) between the armpit and the arm cover. The elbows should be bent at 30° when the hands are on the grips.

> **? What Would You Do If . . .**
>
> You are taping an athlete's ankle. Your nail scratches her shin, causing a minimal amount of bleeding. You notice that your nails are about 0.75 inch (2 cm) long. You just had an expensive manicure.

Summary

Equipment protects athletes from injury when they are participating in sport. Athletes must be educated about the purpose and use of equipment because, although no equipment will totally prevent injury, it can decrease the severity of injury. Properly fitted and certified equipment is essential—old or noncertified equipment should be discarded.

Key Terms

Define the following terms found in this chapter:

- Canadian Standards Association (CSA)
- National Operating Committee on Standards for Athletic Equipment (NOCSAE)

A wrestler recently sprained his anterior cruciate ligament. He is required to wear an anti-rotation brace to stabilize the knee. Will he be allowed to wear this type of brace during competition? What modifications might be required to allow his participation? What are the regulations in high school regarding these devices in this sport?

To access supplementary material for this chapter, including the Understanding Check worksheet, vocabulary quizzes, extension activities, and chapter-specific resources and forms, visit the web resource: http://ancillaries.humankinetics.com/FundamentalsOfAthleticTrainingAndSportsMedicine5E

chapter 30

Basic Diagnostic Imaging and Testing

Objectives

After completing this chapter, the student will be able to do the following:

- Understand the importance of diagnostic imaging and testing to complete the clinical evaluation in certain injuries and conditions.
- Differentiate between basic imaging and testing procedures.
- Understand the role of the health care provider in referring patients for diagnostic imaging and testing.
- Appreciate the scope of selected diagnostic imaging and testing procedures as tools for health care providers.

Diagnostic imaging and testing can provide information needed to formulate a comprehensive clinical picture. Although many injuries and conditions can be diagnosed without testing, some require more extensive tests to fully reveal their severity or cause. The many diagnostic imaging and testing procedures used today are beyond the scope of this text; however, in this chapter, we focus on the most commonly prescribed tests in sports medicine. These tests are typically ordered by physicians and read by specialists. Those who interpret radiological tests are called radiologists. Testing is conducted by medical specialists called pathologists or medical technicians.

ATs are faced with many decisions regarding the care of their athletes. Although our clinical evaluation skills are strong, sometimes we need to determine whether further testing is needed. Physicians rely on ATs to do preliminary evaluations to assess the need, if any, for referral for diagnostic imaging or testing, which can be expensive but are necessary in certain cases. Understanding the role of referral and requests for testing and imaging is a huge responsibility. Knowing the fundamental concepts of each test and its scope helps ATs serve as that vital link in the sports medicine team.

Diagnostic testing comes in many forms. Diagnostic imaging is used quite frequently in athletic training and sports medicine. ATs and other health care professionals work closely with physicians to facilitate diagnostic testing and interpretation. Although many allied health care professionals are practiced at reading basic diagnostic images, only a **radiologist** is credentialed to formally read many of the tests in this chapter. The following sections provide an overview of common diagnostic imaging procedures and tests.

X-RAYS

Unlike the X-ray machines used at the airport to determine if you are trying to bring aboard illegal devices, X-rays in sports medicine are used to detect fractures and other bone issues. Musculoskeletal injuries are quite common in sports medicine. X-rays are one of the most commonly prescribed tests. It requires special X-ray equipment and a trained professional called an X-ray technician to administer it. X-rays highlight the bone tissue, making it appear whiter than other tissues and effective for diagnosing fractures, arthritis, and bone tumors. X-rays can be used on all body parts and can also be performed with stress to help determine if there is damage to the ligaments that connect the bones together (see figure 30.1). These tests typically take only a few minutes to perform. Images are usually taken from more than one angle so that the bone is seen from multiple perspectives. Often, the doctor can do a preliminary read on the X-ray to determine the degree of injury, even though most X-rays are sent out to radiologists for a formal reading. X-rays are a simple, relatively inexpensive way to get a good look at bony tissue without exposure to high radiation levels, making it a valuable tool for sports medicine professionals.

BONE SCANS

A **bone scan** is another radiological test used to focus on injuries and conditions of bony tissue. This test typically takes about 30 to 60 minutes to perform and requires the patient to lie still throughout the procedure. A bone scan is a nuclear imaging procedure because the patient receives an injection containing low-level radioactive tracers that are attracted to areas of injury. Patients usually receive the injection, drink two glasses of water, and then get the actual scan done about two hours later to allow time for the tracers to collect in the injured areas and create what doctors call an area of increased uptake. These "hot" areas in the tissue can indicate fractures and stress fractures, tumors, arthritis, avascular necrosis (area of decreased blood flow), or infection. A bone scan creates an image that looks a lot like the skeleton itself and can detect problems with the bone about 6 to 12 months earlier than a standard X-ray (see figure 30.2). This procedure is safe for adults and children, although

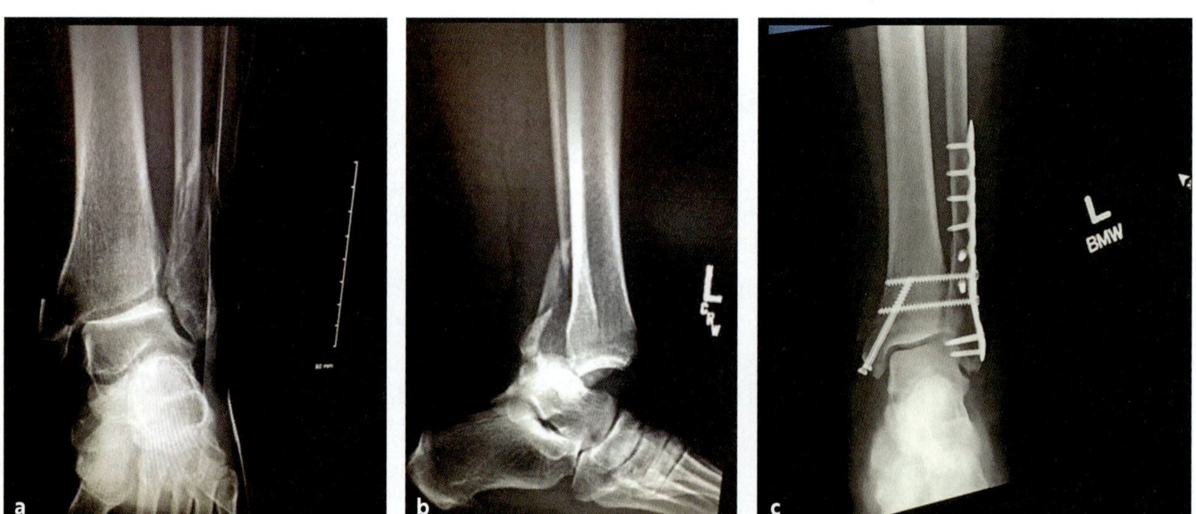

Figure 30.1 X-rays showing a foot injury with *(a)* anterior view, *(b)* lateral view, and *(c)* medical hardware in place to repair an injury.

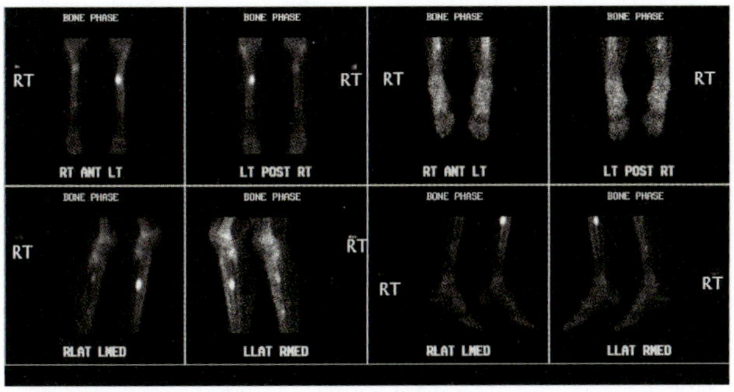

Figure 30.2 Bone scan.

special considerations are needed for kids to help them remain still for the duration of the test. Special equipment is needed to administer this test, so the cost tends to be higher than for most other tests.

CT SCANS

Computerized tomography (CT) scans are commonly referred to as "CAT scans" but are actually CT scans. They are widely used in sports medicine. CT scans use X-ray technology to produce images of slices of tissue. These images create a map and allow the doctor to see different tissue types. CT scans are used commonly with injuries to the joints and dural tissue (brain and surrounding linings). However, CT scans can also be used to detect complex fractures, intra-articular lesions, and loose bodies in a joint (see figure 30.3). This test typically takes about 10 to 20 minutes to perform and requires that the patient remain very still so that clear images can be obtained. Since CT scans require costly equipment housed in a large space, they are expensive to administer and require a trained professional to run the examination. Like other tests, a radiologist performs the final reading and determines the official outcome of this test. The CT scanner is a tube, so obese patients and pregnant women typically cannot safely or comfortably complete this exam. In these cases, the physician can prescribe alternative testing procedures. Some CT scans are administered with a contrast dye that is injected through an intravenous line. The dye helps the physician to differentiate between tissue types and highlights certain tissues more intensely.

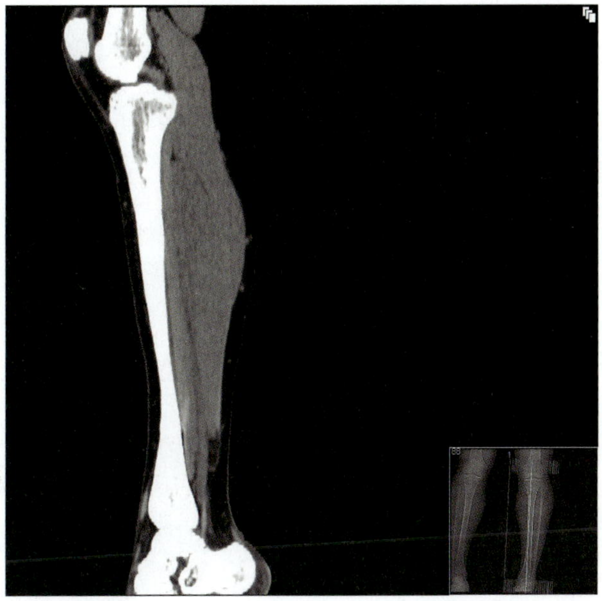

Figure 30.3 CT scan.

MRI

Magnetic resonance imaging (MRI) is another diagnostic imaging test that is costly to perform but provides good distinction between different tissue types, which is helpful in diagnosing medical issues. MRI uses a magnetic field to align protons to create a picture of the tissues in the body, primarily bone, fluid, muscle, and fat. It is standard for this test to take about 20 to 60 minutes to perform. Due to the mechanism of the machine, a series of loud noises usually requires using earplugs or headphones during the procedure. In sports medicine, MRIs are commonly used for conditions such as stress fractures, malignancies (cancer), and bone marrow diseases (see figure 30.4). Although many physicians prefer this test, the cost of administering it and of the equipment is quite high. Due to the size of the machine and the strong magnetic pull used to perform the test, it needs a dedicated space that is secure and private. Two types of MRI machines are commonly used: open and closed MRI. As with the CT scan, the tubular shape of the machine often causes problems for obese or claustrophobic patients. The open MRI was created to accommodate those who may struggle with these conditions. Other limitations to MRI technology and

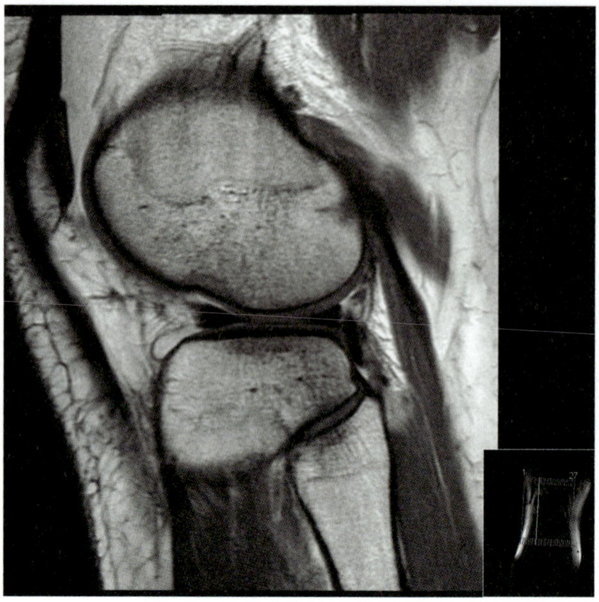

Figure 30.4 MRI image.

testing include blurry images if the patient moves as well as limitations for those with pacemakers and metal implants.

ULTRASOUND

When most people hear the term ultrasound, they think about imaging a fetus during pregnancy. Although this is a common use for this diagnostic test, it serves a slightly different purpose for musculoskeletal conditions. Ultrasonography is performed by an ultrasound technologist who has trained specifically to perform all types of ultrasound imaging. Many sonographers (people who administer ultrasounds) continue to get additional training to perform more advanced ultrasound diagnostic testing. As with all diagnostic imaging tests and procedures, a radiologist typically reads the results for a formal diagnosis since they are trained specifically for this task. To perform the test, an aqueous gel is squirted onto the skin to create a good environment for the sound waves generated by the machine to travel. These high-frequency sound waves create images as they bounce off various tissues, including small tendons and ligaments. This noninvasive procedure can be performed in about 15 minutes, depending on the diagnosis. A specialized ultrasound called the Doppler can even detect blood flow to reveal dangerous clots. Although the test is relatively simple to perform, it is costly to administer and must be done by trained professionals.

As a side note, sports medicine professionals also use therapeutic ultrasound as a modality to treat certain conditions and injuries such as bursitis and tendinitis. Although the equipment may look similar, it is used to create thermal and nonthermal therapy to promote healing rather than as a diagnostic tool.

DEXA SCANS

Another valuable test used for diagnostic imaging in sports medicine and health care overall is a bone densitometry. The bone densitometer, called the **dual-energy X-ray absorptiometry (DEXA) scan**, detects bone loss in areas such as the hips and lower spine. For this test, invisible X-rays reflect off bone and soft tissue, creating a clinical picture of bone health in general. This simple, noninvasive test is quick and easy to perform and is important in detecting osteoporosis, which can lead to fractures. Osteoporosis results in a gradual loss of bone tissue, causing the bones to be more fragile, thinner, and more likely to break. Specific populations are vulnerable to osteoporosis, such as postmenopausal women, smokers, alcoholics, diabetics, and those with other clinical conditions. An X-ray technician performs this test as the patient lies on the table and a scanner moves slowly over their body. Although standard results are widely available on the Internet in the format of T-scores to estimate the risk of developing a fracture and in Z-scores reflecting the patient's bone health compared to others in their age, size, and gender group, a doctor must read the test results and provide recommendations for treatment or care if needed. This test uses only one-tenth of the radiation of a standard X-ray, and it is convenient and simple to use.

PET SCANS

A specialized test, the **positron emission tomography (PET) scan** is commonly used in neurology (study of the brain and nervous system), oncology (study of cancers), and cardiology (study of the heart). The PET scan is a nuclear medicine test,

RED FLAGS

Contraindications to radiation tests include the following:

- If a radiation detection badge reads positive
- If the athlete is pregnant (must wear protective apron)
- If the athlete has metal implants or foreign bodies
- Some contact lenses
- If the athlete has an insulin pump
- Any other health condition as determined by physician

like the bone scan, but this test focuses on the metabolism of specific tissues or organs. Although often used alone as a diagnostic tool, it can be used with a CT and MRI to get a more complete clinical picture. Again, specialized scanning equipment is needed. This scan creates an image to be interpreted by a radiologist.

BLOOD TESTING

Blood tests can detect many conditions in the human body and are used extensively and frequently in health care. After the blood is collected and stored properly, it is sent to a laboratory to be processed for the specific test the doctor ordered. The most common blood work ordered is the **complete blood count (CBC)**, which can detect conditions such as anemia (low iron count), infections, clotting problems, and other disorders. The CBC looks at the counts of **red blood cells (RBC)**, which reflect oxygen-carrying capacity; **white blood cells (WBC)**, which fight infection; platelets, which detect clotting issues; hemoglobin, which detects iron content; hematocrit, which detects how much space the RBCs take up; and mean corpuscle volume, which detects the size of the RBCs. See table 30.1 for standard ranges for the complete blood cell count.

Metabolic tests are also commonly ordered to detect the chemicals in the blood that indicate

Table 30.1 Standard Ranges for Complete Blood Cell Count, Basic Metabolic Panel, and Lipoprotein Panel

Complete Blood Count (CBC)	Standard range
White blood cell count	3.4-9.6 billion/L
Red blood cell count	Males: 4.35-5.65 trillion/L Females: 3.92-5.13 trillion/L
Hemoglobin (Hgb)	Males: 13.2-16.6 g/dL Females: 11.6-15 g/dL
Hematocrit (Hct)	Males: 38.3%-48.6% Females: 35.5%-44.9%
Platelet count	Males: 135-317 billion/L Females: 157-371 billion/L
Basic metabolic panel	**Standard range**
Sodium	136-144 mEq/L
Potassium	3.7-5.2 mEq/L
Glucose	64-100 mg/dl
Calcium	8.5-10.2 mg/dl
Creatine	0.8-1.2 mg/dl
Lipid panel	**Standard range**
LDL	<100 mg/dl
HDL	>60 mg/dl
Triglycerides	<150 mg/dl

Complete blood count adapted from Mayo Clinic (2023). Basic metabolic panel adapted from MedlinePlus (2021). Lipid panel adapted from Cleveland Clinic (2021).

the health of the muscles, including the heart and other vital organs such as the kidneys and liver. A basic metabolic panel measures blood glucose (sugar), calcium, and electrolytes to help doctors determine the health and function of the body as a whole. See table 30.1 for standard ranges for the basic metabolic panel chemistry. Other common blood tests to detect heart conditions and health are called lipoprotein panels. A lipoprotein panel provides information about total cholesterol, LDL (bad) cholesterol, HDL (good cholesterol), and triglycerides. See table 30.1 for standard ranges for the lipoprotein panel. These specific tests are important to understand and manage, especially as one ages, to ensure heart health. Although a physician may order many more blood tests, these tests are the most common. Blood tests provide valuable information for the doctor to consider and a ground for referral to specialists if abnormalities are found. A hematologist is a doctor who deals with disorders of the blood. Depending on the condition found, other specialists may get involved as well.

Understanding Diversity

Common Blood Types by Ethnicity

Ethnicity	O positive %	A positive %	B positive %	AB positive %
African American	47	24	18	4
Asian	39	27	25	7
Latin American	53	29	9	2
White	37	33	9	3

Adapted from Medical News Today (2023); Statista (2023).

Summary

Diagnostic testing and imaging procedures are important in sports medicine. Being aware of the different types of tests and the purpose of each one helps the AT communicate effectively with the physicians as diagnoses are made. Also, as the frontline provider in most situations, having accurate information helps the AT educate the patient on what to expect and why the test is being prescribed. Working together to assist the patient is a critical role for health care providers and understanding the basics of each of these procedures makes the AT a valuable asset for the health care team.

Key Terms

Define the following terms found in this chapter:

- bone scan
- complete blood count (CBC)
- computerized tomography (CT) scan
- dual-energy X-ray absorptiometry (DEXA) scan
- positron emission tomography (PET) scan
- radiologist
- red blood cells (RBC)
- white blood cells (WBC)

A young athlete reports to the athletic training room after visiting their general practice physician. The doctor ordered a DEXA scan, and the athlete has no idea what this scan is for or why they had to have one. The athlete indicated that they had an eating disorder for nearly 5 years and are now recovered. What can the AT tell the athlete about this scan and why it might be needed after a long-term nutritional deficiency caused by eating disorders?

To access supplementary material for this chapter, including the Understanding Check worksheet, vocabulary quizzes, extension activities, and chapter-specific resources and forms, visit the web resource: http://ancillaries.humankinetics.com/FundamentalsOfAthleticTrainingAndSportsMedicine5E

Unit IX

Other Athletic Conditions and Concerns

chapter 31

Systemic Conditions

Objectives

After completing this chapter, the student will be able to do the following:

- Describe conditions that cause illnesses.
- Understand how to prevent conditions and illnesses from occurring.
- Know that many signs and symptoms are similar among conditions.
- Describe various conditions that affect athletes.

An athlete may have a preexisting condition that can reduce the ability to perform normally. The AT and team physician will attempt to discover all such conditions during the preparticipation physical. Knowing of a condition and preparing to care for it before a crisis occurs can make everyone more comfortable, and some conditions require limited activity. In this chapter, we discuss respiratory, vascular, lymphatic, immune, and gastrointestinal conditions as well as diabetes, epilepsy, arthritis, thyroid disorders, the female athlete triad, and rhabdomyolysis.

RESPIRATORY CONDITIONS

Respiratory tract conditions generally affect the lungs. Any condition that reduces an athlete's ability to get air into the body will make it difficult to perform at a high level. The most common respiratory condition is asthma.

In bronchial **asthma**, certain triggers may cause the air passages (bronchial tubes) to narrow, obstructing breathing. The triggers vary from person to person but include allergies, emotional distress, exercise, and body chemistry responses. In some cases, there may be a genetic component. An athlete with bronchial asthma describes it as running the 100-yard (91 m) dash and then trying to catch your breath while breathing through a straw. Coughing that does not bring up phlegm is common. The athlete will wheeze on exhalation and will be in obvious respiratory distress. Asthmatic athletes will have medication, often in the form of an inhaler, to open the air passage; this use obviously should be permitted.

In 2023, Morris produced guidelines for asthma management in athletes (see sidebar, Asthma in

Athletes). According to Morris, the major signs and symptoms for asthma include the following:

- Tightness in the chest
- Coughing or wheezing
- Shortness of breath or lack of full breath
- Diminished physical ability due to breathing difficulty

An asthma attack can be a scary experience for the athlete and the AT. The AT needs to remain calm because exciting the athlete will only make the asthma more uncontrollable. The AT should ask the athlete to relax and breathe in through the nose and out through the mouth (see figure 31.1). By concentrating on the breathing pattern, the athlete can focus on something constructive. The athlete will be more comfortable sitting up than lying down. If the athlete is not getting better, the AT should call for an ambulance and get medical attention immediately. If the athlete stops breathing, the AT should attempt to perform mouth-to-mouth resuscitation, but that may not be successful because air cannot get to the lungs through the closed-off bronchial passages. An athlete who has had an asthma attack for the first time needs to be seen by a physician for evaluation.

Asthmatic athletes are often required to give their inhalers to their coaches before practice so the medication is available if they need it and should give them to the coach or AT to hold during practice or a game. Athletes who fail to provide an inhaler that day are not allowed to practice. As a backup measure, some ATs carry the athlete's second rescue inhaler. An athlete should not use another

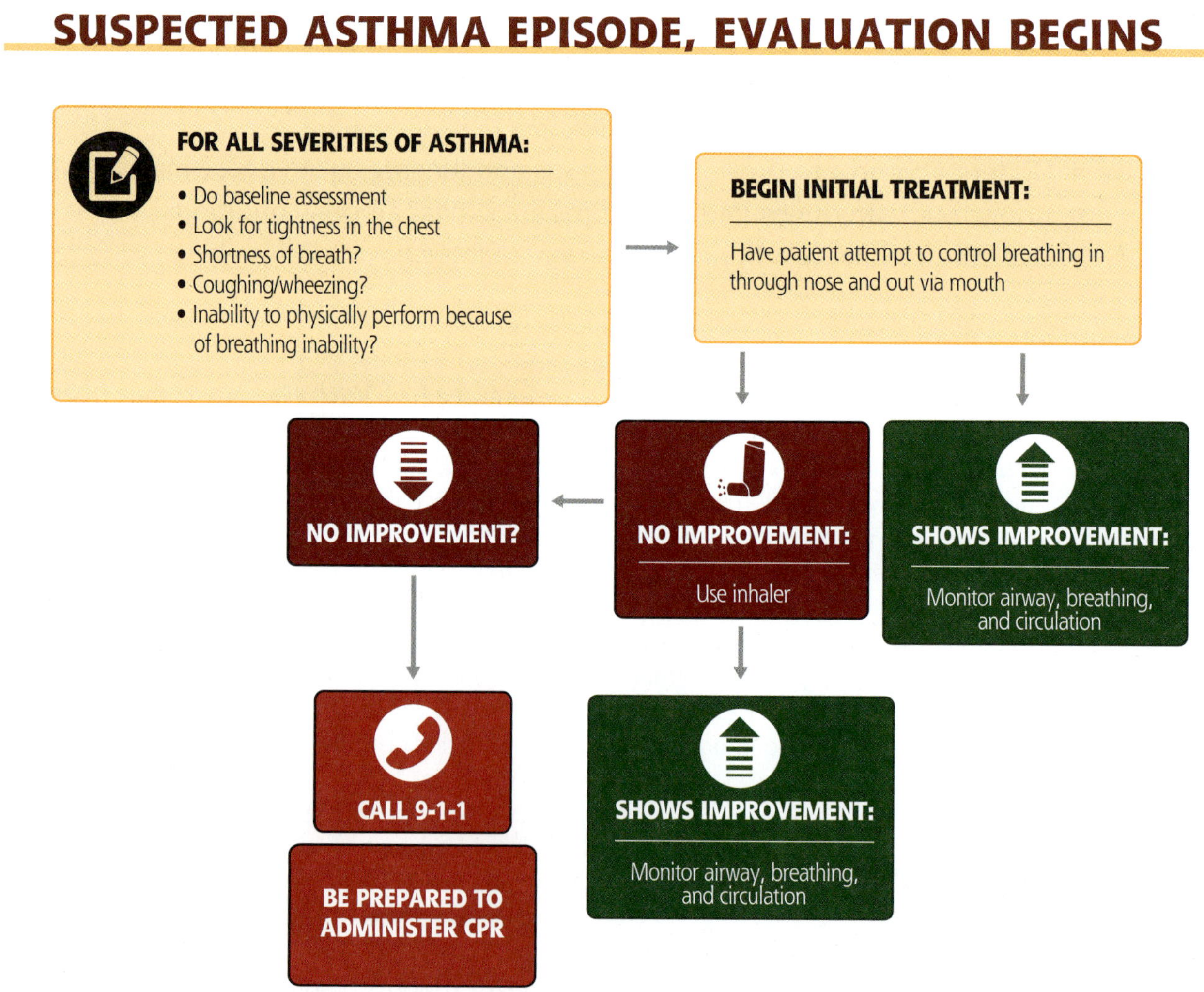

Figure 31.1 Managing asthma.

ASTHMA IN ATHLETES

The classification guidelines for the severity of asthma are as follows:

Step 1: Mild intermittent—Symptoms occur two or fewer times per week (with two or fewer nighttime symptoms per month), and the athlete has brief attacks; intensity varies.

Step 2: Mild persistent—Symptoms occur daily, and an event may negatively affect physical activity level. Nighttime symptoms occur five times or more per month.

Step 3: Moderate persistent—Symptoms occur daily, and an event will negatively affect physical activity level. Nighttime symptoms occur more than five times per month.

Step 4: Severe persistent—Continual symptoms, frequent attacks, and limited physical ability occur; nighttime symptoms are frequent.

athlete's medication because asthma medications vary. Each state and school district has rules about school personnel dispensing medication, so the AT should check the rules before handling someone else's medication.

Checking the environment for allergens can help prevent an asthma attack in athletes known to have them. The athlete and AT should access web-based resources to check the pollen level in a specific geographical area.

The American Thoracic Society (2013) recommends that those who have asthma do the following:

- Use a short-acting medication 15 minutes before exercise.
- Partake in warm-up exercise before exercising heavily.
- Those with more severe forms should use an inhaled steroid medication daily.
- Those with allergies and asthma should consider using an antihistamine.
- Use a mask when exercising in cold weather.

Understanding Diversity

A cleft lip and palate are birth defects that occur while the baby is developing. The lip and palate (roof of the mouth) do not fuse to form a closed palate or lip. The result is that the baby will need surgery to repair the area. Cleft lip and palates are more likely to be found among Asians, Native Americans, or Hispanics (Nationwide Children's Hospital 2023).

VASCULAR CONDITIONS

If there is a problem with the blood, heart, or blood vessels, an athlete can become ill. The AT should know about hypertension, hypotension, anemia, hemophilia, and Raynaud's phenomenon.

Hypertension

Hypertension is blood pressure above normal levels. (See chapter 25 for more information about blood pressure.) If blood pressure is taken on several occasions and the systolic pressure is above 130 mmHg at rest or the diastolic pressure is above 80 mmHg at rest, hypertension is present. Hypertension has several causes, including poor diet, stress, overexercising, and severe vascular damage, such as constriction, or narrowing, of the blood vessels from disease. Hypertension can also cause vascular damage. Athletes with high blood pressure may report frequent headaches. They should be referred to a physician to determine the severity of the disease and treatment. Hypertension can usually be controlled with medication.

Hypotension

Hypotension is abnormally low blood pressure. A person with hypotension is below 90 mmHg systolic and below 60 diastolic mmHg. Some medications cause hypotension, and an athlete taking such medications may pass out as blood pressure decreases. An athlete who has been bedridden may experience hypotension and may even pass out when they sit up or walk for the first time because the vascular system is no longer used to responding to changes in body position. After they move around for a few days, the hypotension subsides. An athlete who is in shock or losing blood will also experience hypotension. It is important to know the cause of hypotension so it can be treated. To get the athlete's blood pressure back to normal, the athlete may have to be treated for shock, bleeding may need to be stopped, or their medication may have to be changed.

Anemia

Anemia is the lack of red blood cells necessary to provide oxygen to the body tissues. Anemia occurs from blood loss, insufficient iron, improper functioning of cells, medication, or malfunction in the construction of cells. Anemia caused by surgery is corrected by blood transfusions. Menstrual anemia corrects itself in a couple of days.

Iron-Deficiency Anemia

Red blood cells must have iron to carry oxygen. When iron is insufficient, the condition is known as iron-deficiency anemia. The athlete may not be eating enough iron-rich foods to meet the average person's needs, or they may have an unusually high need for iron. This condition can be resolved by eating liver, beef, oysters, and iron-enriched cereals. An athlete with iron-deficiency anemia will have pale skin, fatigue, dizziness, decreased capillary refill, and tiredness. The signs and symptoms are not unlike the characteristics of cross country runners at the finish of a race. The best way to identify this type of anemia is through a blood test.

Sickle Cell Anemia

Sickle cell anemia is a chronic inherited disease. Although it is often thought of as an illness found in African Americans, it also occurs in people of other races; for example, people of Eastern European descent are also at high risk for sickle cell anemia.

The normal red blood cell is round and has a large surface area for carrying oxygen. The red blood cells of an athlete with sickle cell anemia look like sickles or crescents (see figure 31.2). The sickling of the cells causes them to hook onto the sides of blood vessels, producing a logjam of cells in the capillaries. Also, the sickle cell is not capable of carrying as much oxygen as a normal red blood cell would, so oxygen is not carried efficiently to all parts of the body. The athlete with sickle cell anemia who is in crisis may have a blue skin tone, feel nauseated and weak, and have abdominal pain. Most often the athlete can be treated with high-flow oxygen from an oxygen tank; therefore, some ATs and team physicians have oxygen tanks available. However, if signs of shock or respiratory distress are evident, the athlete should be transported to the emergency room. Athletes with sickle cell anemia have problems at high altitudes, and it may be best to restrict playing time or not allow the athlete to travel to these places. Preventing a sickle cell crisis includes taking in fluids, avoiding high altitudes (above 4,000 ft or 1,220 m), warming up well, and avoiding short bursts of activity.

Hemophilia

Hemophilia is a blood disorder that delays blood clotting, with consequent difficulty in controlling bleeding even after minor injuries. Hemophilia is a sex-linked inherited blood condition that is carried by females but occurs in males. An athlete with hemophilia may not be able to return to action after an injury, and bleeding may continue to the point that a blood transfusion is necessary. An athlete can be taught to self-administer shots to improve clotting time. Hemophilia cannot be cured, but it can be controlled. An athlete with hemophilia should play noncontact sports to help avoid unnecessary bleeding episodes.

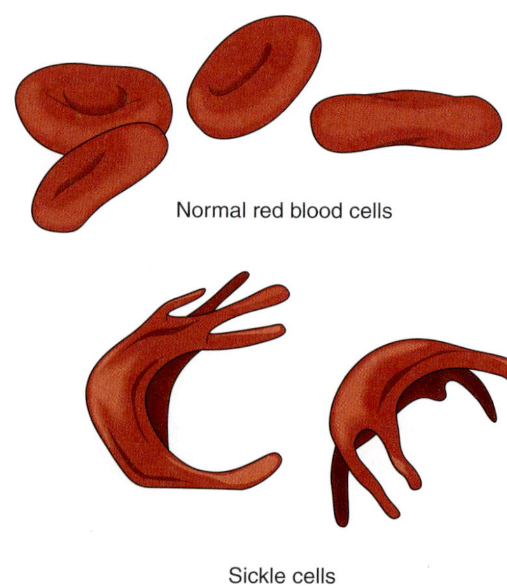

Figure 31.2 Normal red blood cells and sickle cells.

Raynaud's Phenomenon

Raynaud's phenomenon is caused by decreased blood flow to the fingers, ears, toes, and nose. The decreased blood flow is caused by a vasospasm of the arteries. The vasospasm is in response to medications, stress, or cold, and these are considered primary causes (Johns Hopkins 2022b). Secondary causes of Raynaud's include diseases such as lupus, thyroid disorders, and pulmonary hypertension (Johns Hopkins 2022b). Those with connective tissue autoimmune disorders, smokers, or injury to the area are at greater risk of Raynaud's (Johns Hopkins 2022b).

The body part involved will turn white when the vasospasm occurs. The body part may swell with warming (Johns Hopkins 2022b). If the lack of circulation is chronic, it may cause gangrene with possible amputation of the body part (Johns Hopkins 2022b). The best care for Raynaud's is to maintain constant warmth, avoid cold exposure, stop smoking, and take medication to treat other contributing conditions (Johns Hopkins 2022b).

LYMPHATIC CONDITIONS

The lymphatic system helps regulate fluid throughout the body by using lymphatic vessels. The lymph fluid carries white blood cells to protect the body from infection. The two types of white blood cells are B lymphocytes and T lymphocytes (American Cancer Society 2022). B lymphocytes make antibodies that fight bacteria and viruses, and T lymphocytes destroy germs or abnormal body cells (American Cancer Society 2022).

The lymph nodes are where white blood cells are stored. The lymph nodes are in the neck, armpits, chest, abdomen, and groin (National Cancer Institute 2022). The AT should be familiar with non-Hodgkin's lymphoma and Hodgkin's lymphoma.

Non-Hodgkin's Lymphoma

Non-Hodgkin's lymphoma is a cancer of the white blood cells. Most often, the cancer starts in B lymphocytes (American Cancer Society 2022). Though the cancer can occur at any age, those at risk include those older than 65; other risks are being male, being overweight, race (African American or Asian), a family history of lymphoma, being a smoker, or exposure to harmful chemicals (American Cancer Society 2022).

Signs and symptoms of non-Hodgkin's lymphoma include enlarged lymph nodes, fatigue, shortness of breath, frequent infections, bruising easily, chills, weight loss, swelling of the abdomen, night sweats, fever without infection, and feeling of fullness quickly after eating (American Cancer Society 2022). Treatment will be determined by the physician based on the type and severity of the cancer. Possible treatments are chemotherapy, immunotherapy, radiation, stem cell transplant, surgery, and targeted drug therapy (American Cancer Society 2022).

Hodgkin's Lymphoma

Hodgkin's lymphoma is a cancer of the white blood cells, similar to non-Hodgkin's lymphoma. The identifier that differentiates the two lymphomas is the presence of Reed-Sternberg cells. The Reed-Sternberg cells are tumor cells that are only present in Hodgkin's lymphoma. The signs and symptoms of Hodgkin's lymphoma includes swollen lymph nodes in the armpits, neck, or groin; fatigue; fever; night sweats; weight loss; and itching and painful nodes after drinking alcohol (Mayo Clinic 2022b). Risk factors include a family history of lymphoma, being male, previous Epstein-Barr infection, and HIV infection. It is most often diagnosed in people in their 20s and 30s and those 55 and older (Mayo Clinic 2022b).

The diagnosis can include removal of a lymph node for testing, a blood test, imaging, a bone marrow test, and a physical examination (Mayo Clinic 2022b). Treatment will be based on the severity of the cancer. Traditional treatment includes chemotherapy, radiation, immunotherapy, a bone marrow transplant, and targeted drug therapy (Mayo Clinic 2022b).

IMMUNE SYSTEM CONDITIONS

The immune system fights off fungi, bacteria, parasites, and viruses that can cause infections and diseases. The immune system has white blood cells, skin, mucous membranes, and organs (Cleveland Clinic 2022). The immune system learns about the germs and attacks them to protect the body. Autoimmune disorders occur when the immune system reacts to an invasion that does not exist. The immune system attacks healthy cells, causing conditions such as lupus, chronic fatigue syndrome, and fibromyalgia.

Lupus

This autoimmune disorder can attack any part of the body, but typical body parts are the heart, kidneys, skin, and joints (Lupus Foundation of America 2021). Those most at risk are women under the age of 40, those with a family history, and those who are African, Hispanic, Native American, or Asian (Johns Hopkins 2024).

Because lupus can attack so many body parts, the signs and symptoms can vary. The Lupus Foundation of America (2021) identifies a butterfly-shaped rash, fatigue, and joint pains as early warning signs. Sores in the mouth or nose, loss of hair, stiff joints, swollen joints, chest pain with breathing that lasts for more than 24 hours, a rash that occurs after exposure to sun, low blood cell counts, weight loss, and a fever are also signs and symptoms of lupus (Johns Hopkins 2022).

Lupus is not curable but needs to be managed to avoid organ damage. A physician will determine the course of treatment. Treatment will be based on which organs are being attacked or compromised. Anti-inflammatory medications and immunosuppressants are traditional treatments. With flare-ups, the treatment will likely change.

Chronic Fatigue Syndrome

Researchers have yet to define the cause of chronic fatigue syndrome (CFS). Sotzny and colleagues (2018) showed evidence of a multifaceted process that plays a role, including infection, immune response, and environmental issues. The Centers for Disease Control and Prevention (2018) identified five possible causes: infections, changes in the immune system, stress, changes in how energy is produced, and a genetic link. The result ultimately is fatigue, memory issues, headaches, enlarged lymph nodes, disturbed sleep, unexplained joint and muscle pain, dizziness, and sore throat (Mayo Clinic 2022a). The signs and symptoms will continue for six months, which leads the physician to the diagnosis (Centers for Disease Control and Prevention 2018).

Treatment will depend on the signs and symptoms and their management. Stress reduction is encouraged, as is using cognitive behavioral therapy, engaging in moderate exercise, and taking medication (Britannica 2023). CFS is a chronic condition.

GASTROINTESTINAL CONDITIONS

The gastrointestinal tract includes the organs that are involved in processing food, such as the stomach and large and small intestines. Here, we discuss common conditions that affect the gastrointestinal tract.

Indigestion

When an athlete eats a food that the body has difficulty digesting, they have indigestion. The stomach has a high acid content to break down food. When acid levels are high, the acid may go up into the esophagus, causing a burning sensation called *heartburn*. The athlete may burp, have excessive gas, feel nauseated, and even vomit. They may experience pain around the heart that mimics the sensations of a heart attack. Serious cases of indigestion cause anxiety, sweating, pale skin, and nausea. Such cases must be referred to a physician. The athlete should avoid overeating and eating foods that cause indigestion. A physician can recommend over-the-counter medications to control stomach acid. However, if used too often, these medications may mask a more serious problem. If problems persist, a physician should be consulted to rule out a more serious condition such as ulcers.

Food Poisoning (Gastroenteritis)

Food poisoning is a common cause of diarrhea or upset stomach. Recently, there have been many incidents of poisoning from foods (including fruits, meats, dairy products, and vegetables) contaminated with *E. coli* (*Escherichia coli*). Preventing food poisoning requires careful food handling and preparation—washing hands and utensils, cook-

> **What Would You Do If . . .**
>
> A good friend of yours is dying to tell you a secret, and you promise not to tell anyone. He says he is trying out for the football team and has told only you that he is a hemophiliac.

ing foods thoroughly, and bleaching countertops, dishrags, and cutting surfaces. An athlete with food poisoning will complain of abdominal pain, tiredness, vomiting, nausea, diarrhea, and possibly a high temperature. The athlete should rest, drink plenty of fluids, and be referred to a physician.

Appendicitis

An athlete with appendicitis will feel pain over the lower right quadrant of the abdomen. Common signs and symptoms include diarrhea or constipation, nausea, vomiting, and increased temperature, all in a couple of hours. The person will find that bringing the knees to the chest is the most comfortable position. The athlete needs to be referred to a physician for care because the appendix must often be surgically removed. The athlete will be sidelined for at least four weeks if it is removed. In severe cases, the appendix can rupture and spread the infection throughout the abdominal cavity, which can result in death.

DIABETES

Diabetes occurs when the pancreas does not secrete insulin effectively or when the body is resistant to insulin. Insulin is a key hormone responsible for glucose (a form of sugar) entering cells and fueling them. An athlete with untreated diabetes may lose weight, become unusually thirsty, urinate more often, get tired faster than usual, and have a high level of sugar in the blood. After a diabetic athlete eats, their blood sugar level rises, and the pancreas releases insulin so that the body can control the blood sugar. If the blood sugar level gets too high, it is called **hyperglycemia**; if it gets too low, it is called **hypoglycemia**. If a diabetic athlete who uses insulin forgets to eat, their blood sugar level may fall below normal, causing them to pass out (figure 31.3). Something similar may happen due to exercise. An exercising athlete requires energy from the bloodstream (blood glycogen). If a diabetic athlete exercises excessively, they may use additional sugar for energy, and if they also take insulin, this situation can cause dangerously low blood sugar levels.

There are four forms of diabetes: type 1, type 2, gestational, and prediabetes. With type 1 diabetes, the body simply is unable to produce insulin. With type 2 diabetes, the body produces insulin but the

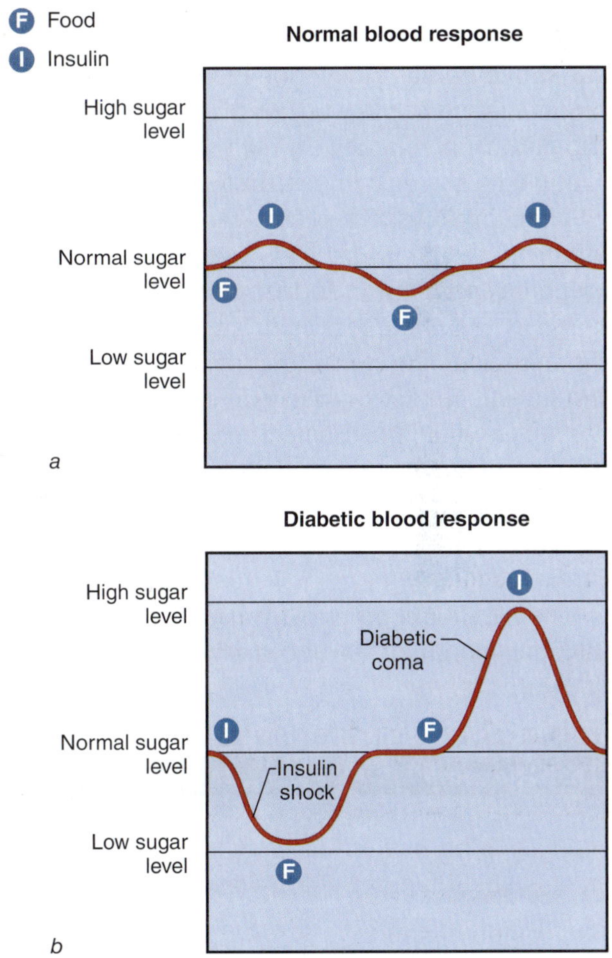

Figure 31.3 Insulin response. *(a)* An athlete with normal blood sugar response: The athlete eats food, insulin is released, and the blood sugar level returns to normal. *(b)* Insulin shock occurs in a diabetic when the blood sugar is very low. The athlete may have taken insulin but failed to eat enough food. A diabetic coma occurs when blood sugar is very high. The athlete may have forgotten to take insulin just before or after eating.

cells are resistant to it and fail to use it properly so that glucose can get into the cells. Most Americans diagnosed with diabetes have type 2. Gestational diabetes occurs in pregnant women. People with prediabetes have high blood sugar levels but not so much that they are diagnosed with type 2 diabetes.

Insulin Shock

An athlete who needs insulin injections to survive is insulin dependent. An insulin-dependent athlete usually takes insulin several times a day, especially near meals. Like anyone, an insulin-dependent athlete may not always eat regularly. If they take insulin and then fail to eat, they may go into **insulin shock** because they took medication to lower blood sugar when it was not high. Insulin shock can also happen if they eat high-sugar food that is absorbed before insulin returns to a standard level.

When insulin shock occurs, the athlete will feel lightheaded and weak and have an ashen skin tone and rapid pulse. In many cases, the athlete will appear to be intoxicated. The AT should give the conscious athlete juice or candy so that the insulin will be temporarily counteracted, and then the athlete should consume a meal to level off the insulin. Table 31.1 presents the signs and symptoms of insulin shock and diabetic coma. If the athlete is unconscious, liquid glucose (sugar) can be placed under the tongue.

The AT should never place hard candy or food into the mouth of an unconscious athlete—this action may cause an airway obstruction. Diabetics may carry a glucagon emergency kit specifically designed to bring blood sugar up into a safe range. If the AT cannot remember the treatments for diabetic emergencies, they should give the athlete glucagon—it will help the athlete in insulin shock, and it will not make a diabetic coma any worse. Whenever a diabetic athlete is unconscious, the AT should call EMS and get them to the nearest hospital.

In 2022, the Centers for Disease Control and Prevention set up a plan for managing athletes with type 1 diabetes (see the sidebar, Diabetes Care Plan). It suggests that each athlete have a diabetes care plan for all practices and games. Based on the content of this care plan, an AT must have a blood sugar monitoring kit available as well as the appropriate items to care for an athlete in the event of hyper- or hypoglycemia.

Glucose Monitoring

It is important for those who have diabetes to monitor glucose levels on a regular basis. One method is to use a lancing device that pricks the fingertip. The blood drop is placed on a testing strip. The strip is inserted into a blood glucose tester that provides the amount of glucose in the athlete's system.

A wearable blood glucose meter allows for monitoring levels every 15 minutes without pricking the skin each time. The meter is attached to the skin and the glucose level is sent by Bluetooth to the athlete's phone.

Table 31.1 Comparisons Between Diabetic Coma and Insulin Shock

Diabetic coma	Insulin shock
Conscious but confused	Unconscious
No seizures	Seizures possible
Breath smells fruity	Breath smells normal
Low blood pressure	Normal blood pressure
Thirsty	Not thirsty
Rapid breathing	Normal breathing
Dry skin	Sweating
Possible fever	Normal body temperature
No body sensations	Tingling in hands and feet
Gradual onset	Rapid onset
Normal food intake	Little food intake
No headache	Headache
No response to food	Quick response to food

HOW TO ADMINISTER GLUCAGON

1. Open the glucagon kit.
2. Wipe the top of the glucagon bottle.
3. Take the cap off the needle of the syringe.
4. Inject the fluid into the glucagon bottle, leave the needle in the bottle.
5. Rotate the bottle back and forth to mix the ingredients.
6. Tip the bottle upside down and pull the syringe plunger until the liquid is in the syringe.
7. Inject the glucagon liquid into either the person's thigh, upper arm, or buttocks.
8. Leave the needle in the skin for at least three seconds after the injection.

Adapted from Mass General for Children (2019).

The American Diabetes Association (2022) recommends the following target blood sugar levels:

- Before meals: between 80 and 130 milligrams per deciliter (mg/dL) or 4.4 to 7.2 millimoles per liter (mmol/L)
- Two hours after starting a meal: less than 180 mg/dL (10.0 mmol/L)

Diabetic Coma

A **diabetic coma** may occur when there is not enough insulin to control the amount of sugar in the blood. A diabetic coma may be preceded by an illness that alters the amount and availability of insulin. The coma comes on gradually with signs of vomiting and high temperature. The symptoms the athlete experiences are thirst, abdominal pain, nausea, and confusion. The athlete approaching a coma will present labored breathing, sweet-smelling breath, and low blood pressure. A diabetic coma may be prevented by helping the athlete administer their insulin. Athletes may carry premade insulin shots; if conscious, they can inject themselves when a shot is needed. Rush an unconscious athlete to a hospital emergency room.

RED FLAGS

Call 911 if the athlete has any of the following situations:

- A seizure
- Is unconscious or about to go unconscious
- Has slurred speech or is incoherent
- Is having difficulty breathing
- Has high or low blood pressure
- Has a fever or unexplained abdominal pain

What Would You Do If . . .

A diabetic ice hockey player has forgotten to bring his juice box with him for a snack. He tells you he can get along without a snack this time.

EPILEPSY

When the brain does not work properly, the entire body can malfunction. **Epilepsy** is the general term given to various disorders marked by disturbed electrical rhythms of the central nervous system.

The cause of epilepsy can be chemical, neurological (brain defect), infectious, or traumatic. A sign that an athlete has epilepsy can be a grand mal **seizure**—they may shake, drool, lose bladder control, or lose consciousness. The athlete who is about to have a grand mal seizure may hear a sound or see an aura, warning them to move to a safe area before the seizure begins. If the seizures are controlled by medication, exercising will not cause more problems. There is no reason to keep

DIABETES CARE PLAN

According to the Centers for Disease Control and Prevention (2022), to manage diabetes in athletes, each athlete should have a care plan that includes the following:

Every Day

- Monitor blood sugar levels and write them down each time levels are taken.
- Check feet daily for any imperfections such as sores, blisters, swelling, and so on.
- Exercise daily and write down what exercises were performed, the number of repetitions, and the amount of weight (if weights were used).
- Eat healthy and write down what the athlete ate and how much on a daily basis.
- Maintain records for the type of insulin the athlete uses as well as the dosages and adjustments.

Every Three Months If Blood Sugar Goals Are Not Being Met

- Have an A1C test.
- See your doctor.

Every Six Months

- Get your teeth cleaned and let the dentist know of your diabetic history.

Every Year

- Have kidneys tested.
- Have a cholesterol check.
- Have an eye examination.
- Have a foot check by a physician.

Centers for Disease Control and Prevention (2022).

an athlete from participating because of epilepsy. Care for an athlete having a grand mal seizure includes moving items out of their way, loosening their clothing, padding their head, and allowing the seizure to end on its own. Because the tongue may fall back and block the airway, the athlete should be monitored for breath sounds. If an athlete experiences a seizure for the first time, the AT should call EMS for immediate emergency care.

ARTHRITIS

Arthritis is the inflammation of a joint. In athletes, arthritis may result from an injury, repetitive trauma, or surgical intervention. Arthritis is a degeneration of the joint surfaces. Typical signs and symptoms are swelling, joint deformity, pain, grating during movement, and stiffness.

Gout is an inherited form of arthritis. It generally stays in one joint of the lower extremities. Uric acid buildup in the joint is the cause.

Juvenile rheumatoid arthritis may be found in some high school athletes. An overgrowth of the connective tissue occurs in a synovial joint. The extra tissue attaches to the articular surface of a joint, causing degradation of the joint surface. The most common joints for juvenile rheumatoid arthritis are in the feet and hands.

Osteoarthritis occurs with aging or after an injury to the affected joint. The articular cartilage breaks down, causing the ends of bones to be in direct contact with each other. This direct contact creates friction and continual degradation of the joint.

The Real World

One afternoon, a student-athlete rushed into the training room shouting that a student had seriously injured herself while running in the hall. I grabbed my bag and ran from one end of the school to the other. I found the injured girl lying face down and unconscious, with her glasses askew. She was breathing and had a normal heartbeat. Saliva was dribbling from her mouth, but she had no visible wounds. No one could tell me what had happened, and no one knew her name. Furthermore, she was not wearing identification or medical alert tags. Other ATs who arrived on the scene performed a head-to-toe assessment and checked for a medical alert tag while I held her head to keep her neck in alignment. Because she was unconscious, we immediately called 911. She was eventually backboarded and taken to the hospital, still unconscious. Had she accidentally run into the wall and knocked herself out because she wasn't watching where she was going? Did she have a previous condition that caused her to faint? We had no idea. The mystery was solved when it was determined that she had experienced her first seizure.

Lorin Cartwright, MS, ATC

THYROID DISORDERS

The thyroid gland produces hormones that aid in bodily functions. The gland is in the anterior aspect of the neck anterior to the trachea. It is not seen but can be palpated if the athlete swallows. Two common disorders are hypothyroidism and hyperthyroidism.

Hypothyroidism

A thyroid hormone deficiency is called hypothyroidism. Often, hypothyroidism is caused by an autoimmune disease, thyroid surgery, radiation therapy, thyroiditis, or medication (Mayo Clinic 1998-2023). In some instances, other factors such a cancer or the removal of all or part of the thyroid gland will cause hypothyroidism.

Signs and symptoms of hypothyroidism include weight gain, fatigue, dry skin, hair loss, muscle weakness, sensitivity to cold, a slowed heart rate, and being tired (Mayo Clinic 1998-2023a). The diagnosis is made by a physician utilizing a blood test and ultrasound. Medication is the course of treatment with annual monitoring of thyroid levels so adjustments can be made if necessary. For those who have cancer, other treatment will be necessary beyond medication.

Hyperthyroidism

Hyperthyroidism is the over production of thyroid hormones. The most common cause is an autoimmune disorder called Graves disease. The primary sign of Graves disease is a goiter (an enlargement of the neck). Other signs and symptoms include weight loss, anxiety, irregular heart rate, sleep problems, lack of concentration, nervousness, tremors, depression, increased hunger, fatigue, more frequent bowel movement, and an enlarged thyroid gland (Mayo Clinic Staff 1998-2023b).

There are three forms of treatment: medication, radioactive iodine, and surgery (Mayo Clinic Staff 1998-2023b). Beta blocking medications reduce tremors and heart issues (Mayo Clinic Staff 1998-2023b). Radioactive iodine oral medication treatment causes the thyroid to shrink, reducing its activity (Mayo Clinic Staff 1998-2023b).

FEMALE ATHLETE TRIAD

Disordered eating, amenorrhea, and osteoporosis are associated with one another: If a female athlete restricts caloric intake and exercises heavily, her menstrual cycle may stop and her bone health will be compromised. These three conditions are collectively known as **female athlete triad syndrome**. This triad is common among female athletes who are driven or pressured to achieve high-level sport-related goals. Prevention of the triad is critical, and athletes, parents, coaches, and administrators should be educated about the three conditions as well as preventive strategies.

Some athletes who are worried about how they look in a uniform may end up with an eating disorder as they try to attain a certain weight or look a certain way. Eating disorders often appear in sports such as swimming, cross country, track, gymnastics, and wrestling. Officials who give scores based on a look, image, or smile push athletes in the wrong direction. Athletic associations and coaches could help by being more accepting of baggy shorts, shirts, or skirts—but do not count on that happening.

Disordered eating is an umbrella term for many problematic eating behaviors. Abnormal eating behaviors include anorexia nervosa, whereby an athlete restricts food intake, and bulimia nervosa, characterized by high caloric intake followed by self-induced vomiting. Both conditions are complex and need to be treated from not only a nutrition standpoint but also psychological, sociological, and physiological standpoints. Anorexia and bulimia are most often thought of as eating disorders that occur chiefly in white women, but they also are common among men and athletes of color. Anorexia nervosa and bulimia have a death rate of 22%. The AT should check with the athlete's physician for advice on the athlete's ability to participate safely if they have an eating disorder. See the Preventing, Detecting, and Managing Disordered Eating sidebar.

Amenorrhea is a condition whereby an athlete's menstrual cycle stops or an athlete fails to have a menstrual cycle by the age of 16. Some causes of amenorrhea are low body weight; endurance activities such as distance running, cycling, or swimming; high stress levels; and disordered eating. Dysmenorrhea is a painful menstrual cycle. Both amenorrhea and dysmenorrhea can be caused by hormonal imbalances, among other things, and a full evaluation by a physician is warranted to rule out serious conditions. One key issue with both conditions is that the athlete's bone health can be compromised, leading to fractures and osteoporosis.

PREVENTING, DETECTING, AND MANAGING DISORDERED EATING

Recommendations for screening for and treating disordered eating include the following:

- Use the SCOFF questionnaire to detect eating disorders. The SCOFF questions are noted by Nolan and colleagues (2022), and the acronym is highlighted within each question:
  - Do you make yourself **S**ick (make yourself vomit) because you feel very full?
  - Do you worry that you have lost **C**ontrol over how much you eat?
  - Have you recently lost more than **O**ne stone (14 lbs or 6.3 kg) in a 3-month period of time?
  - Do you believe you are **F**at when others think you are too thin?
  - Would you say **F**ood has taken over your life?
- Use a multidisciplinary team that includes a mental health care provider, physician, family, dietitian, athletic administrator, coach, and athlete to develop goals and the rehabilitation plan for an eating disorder.
- Build a trusting relationship with all members of the multidisciplinary team.
- Use a low-intensity progression when returning the athlete to training.
- Returning the athlete is based on the following factors: The athlete is medically stable, laboratory test results are normal, the athlete is nutritionally stable and no longer practicing disordered eating, the athlete is able to handle psychological stressors, and the athlete is in compliance with the multidisciplinary team recommendations.
- Adjust exercise and activity throughout the athlete's return to activity.

Adapted from Coviser et al. (2018).

Osteoporosis is a loss of bone density. It occurs due to hormonal imbalances, poor or inadequate nutrition, and lack of exercise. Genetic factors also play a role in whether one is at risk of developing osteoporosis. A lack of bone density results in frailty and a high risk of fractures. As you might imagine, if an athlete has an eating disorder, it can put them at risk for osteoporosis.

RHABDOMYOLYSIS

Rhabdomyolysis is a serious condition caused by muscle injury. The muscle injury can be a blow to the muscle or overworking the muscle, which causes death of muscle fibers. The blood absorbs the toxins from the tissue loss and sends them to the kidneys to be excreted from the body (Stuart et al. 2024; Rawson et al. 2017). Because the tissue damage is so significant, the kidneys may not be able to remove the toxins; this can lead to kidney failure. Athletes are prone to rhabdomyolysis in two instances: They lack physical conditioning or they are well muscled and are going through extreme conditioning.

Signs and symptoms include muscle weakness, muscle pain, abdominal pain, nausea, vomiting, fever, rapid heartbeat, inability to stand, and dark-colored urine (WebMD 2016). The difficulty with diagnosing rhabdomyolysis is that muscle soreness, nausea, and weakness may be assumed to be a typical part of conditioning for a sport. It is imperative that the AT ask about urine color, check the athlete's pulse rate, and monitor body temperature. Because rhabdomyolysis can be life-threatening, the athlete needs to be referred to a physician for immediate attention.

The physician will recommend fluid hydration to improve chemical balance. It may take some time before the athlete is able to return to physical activity. Prevention is the best approach to rhabdomyolysis. This includes hydration, maintaining a level of fitness even in the off season, and gradually increasing exercise intensity over time (NCAA Sports Science Institute 2013).

Summary

Certain medical conditions affect an athlete's ability to participate in sport. The AT must be prepared to respond to emergencies because an incorrect evaluation can result in serious consequences if the athlete has a condition such as appendicitis, asthma, or diabetes. Regular physical exams can help find certain conditions early. Conditions that are not preventable, such as asthma, diabetes, or epilepsy, may be controlled by medication and careful monitoring. The AT should know if an athlete is in a high-risk category for certain conditions so they can assist the athlete in taking preventive measures, such as selecting the proper sport, using protective equipment, making sure medication is available, and knowing first aid.

Key Terms

Define the following terms found in this chapter:

- amenorrhea
- anemia
- asthma
- diabetes
- diabetic coma
- disordered eating
- epilepsy
- female athlete triad syndrome
- hemophilia
- hyperglycemia
- hypertension
- hypoglycemia
- hypotension
- insulin shock
- rhabdomyolysis
- seizure
- sickle cell anemia

An athlete recently had a physical and the doctor drew blood for testing. As the AT, you notice the lab results indicated a condition called anemia. What are the characteristics of this condition and how would the doctor know this from the blood work? What can the athlete be advised to do when dealing with this condition?

To access supplementary material for this chapter, including the Understanding Check worksheet, vocabulary quizzes, extension activities, and chapter-specific resources and forms, visit the web resource: http://ancillaries.humankinetics.com/FundamentalsOfAthleticTrainingAndSportsMedicine5E

chapter 32

Communicable and Dermatological Conditions

Objectives

After completing this chapter, the student will be able to do the following:

- Explain how a communicable disease is transmitted.
- Explain how contagious diseases affect athletic competition.
- Describe how to control and prevent contagious diseases.
- Describe the common signs and symptoms of contagious diseases.
- Understand the types of dermatological conditions and how they are transmitted.
- Understand the limiting factors of participation with a dermatological condition.

Our environment has microorganisms that cause infectious diseases. The immune system helps defend the body from foreign cells and substances, but when the immune system is low or the invader is strong, a person will become ill. Many illnesses can be transferred from one person to another through the air, bodily contact, using each other's personal items, or unsanitary conditions. The student assistant and AT will come in contact with illnesses daily. To help prevent the spread of communicable diseases, the AT (and students) can keep vaccinations current, clean the training room daily, avoid bodily fluids and sick athletes, use personal protective equipment (PPE), screen athletes during physical examinations, maintain healthy nutrition and hydration, and get enough sleep. In this chapter, we discuss various communicable diseases and dermatological conditions.

DEFENDING AGAINST MICROORGANISMS

Microorganisms are tiny. These bacteria and viruses are everywhere in the environment, including on and in everyone's body. If a microorganism is one the body has never previously encountered, it might create an infection.

Infectious microorganisms that manage to get into the body are attacked by the lymphocytes of the **immune system**. Lymphocytes are specialized leukocytes, the white blood cells that attack invaders.

When physicians draw blood, it is easy to check the number of leukocytes. Elevated numbers of leukocytes may mean the body is fighting an infection. Low numbers of leukocytes are an indication that the immune system is deficient, so the athlete may be susceptible to infectious microorganisms.

Some microorganisms are effectively fought with a **vaccination**—tiny amounts of the microorganism (sometimes live and sometimes dead) that are injected into the body. Once the body detects the microorganism, it begins to fight it and build immunity against it. There are vaccinations against many diseases, including tetanus, measles, flu, hepatitis B, mumps, and polio. Viruses cause all of these except tetanus, which is caused by bacteria.

Disease is transmitted in four ways: direct contact, indirect contact, through the air, and through a vector. When a person encounters someone carrying a communicable disease, that illness can be transferred. An example of direct contact is the spread of bodily fluids such as blood. Some organisms live on objects; when these objects are used, the disease can be transmitted. This is an example of indirect contact. Airborne transmission of disease occurs when droplets from a cough or a sneeze are propelled in the air and inhaled by another person. Wang and Bourouiba (2017) indicate that a cough or sneeze can send droplets in the air up to 26 feet (8 m). Insects, especially those that suck blood, are an example of a vector; the insect gets a disease while biting an infected person and then transmits it by biting another person.

Together with medical communities, some governments have done an outstanding job of increasing public awareness of communicable diseases.

> **? What Would You Do If . . .**
>
> You notice that thirsty athletes are unwilling to wait in line while the watercooler distributes water slowly. The athletes take the lid off the cooler and dip their cups in, drink, and dip some more.

People are more careful than they used to be around others who appear to be ill. People who are coughing and sneezing cover their mouths and wipe their noses. We can all do our part to prevent the spread of disease by getting vaccinations, washing our hands, using sterile techniques, and staying at home when early signs and symptoms of illness appear. Sharing food, water, or clothing should be avoided. Daily cleaning of clothing, training tables, and doorknobs will reduce the possibility of infection through contact with these items.

When the AT notices an athlete with cold and flu symptoms—sneezing; itchy, watery eyes; low-grade fever; runny nose; sore throat; headache; tiredness—or signs of a rash, the athlete should be referred immediately to a physician for care. Many early signs and symptoms of life-threatening illnesses mimic those of mild contagious illnesses. Neither the AT nor the athlete should risk spreading a contagious disease among teammates and classmates. There have been several outbreaks of measles (rubeola) among athletes when, unknowingly, an infected athlete was allowed to participate in a tournament—the illness can devastate every team attending. The physician should indicate when it is safe for the athlete to return to play.

See figure 32.1 for steps to control the outbreak of contagious diseases.

Viral Diseases

Many viral illnesses once caused misery and even death for millions of children, though most have become rare because of public childhood vaccination programs. They are occasionally seen in the United States in both children and adults, so ATs and their assistants should be aware of them. Of the viral diseases listed next, aseptic meningitis and plantar warts are not childhood diseases.

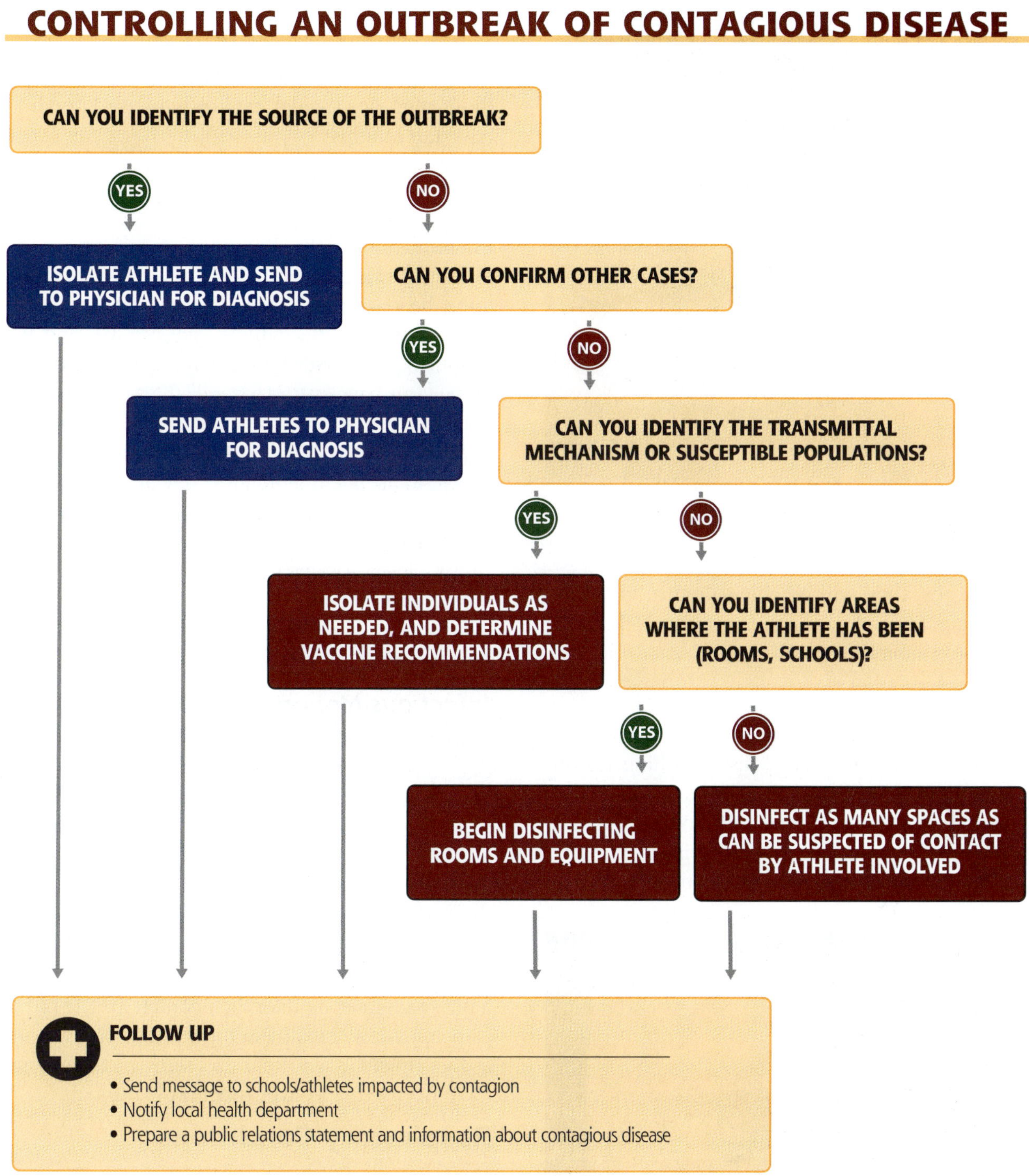

Figure 32.1 Steps to control outbreaks of contagious diseases.

Chicken Pox (Varicella)

A virus causes **chicken pox**, which is characterized by a polka-dot body rash, a low-grade fever, tiredness, itching, and headache. The rash will leave small, craterlike scars if bumps are broken open (see figure 32.2). The athlete who gets this rash is able to spread it to others on the team through nose or mouth secretions and fluids from broken blisters and needs to be referred to a physician for treatment. After about one week, when the athlete has

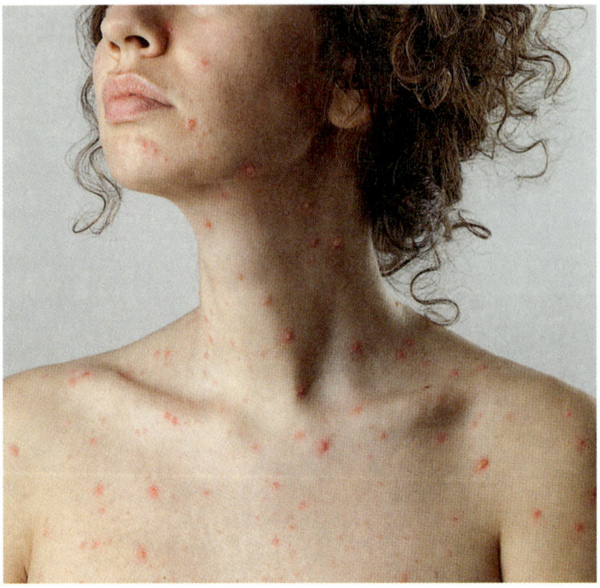

Figure 32.2 Chicken pox.
CactuSoup/E+/Getty Images

dried scabs, they will be able to return to school and competition. A vaccination against chicken pox is now available.

Mumps

A virus causes **mumps**. The athlete will feel tired and have a headache. The distinguishing feature of mumps is swelling of the glands below and in front of the ear, which causes a fullness of the face and difficulty talking and swallowing (see figure 32.3). The swelling subsides in about a week. The athlete must be referred to a physician, who will recommend isolation, rest, fluids, aspirin, and soft foods. Prevention includes vaccination or avoiding those who do not feel well or who are known to have the mumps.

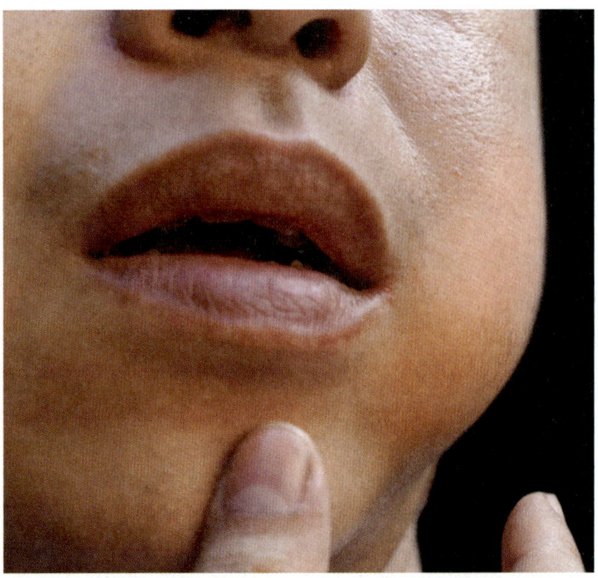

Figure 32.3 Mumps.
Zay Nyi Nyi/iStock/Getty Images

Aseptic Meningitis

Aseptic meningitis is characterized by a viral inflammation of the coverings of the brain. The virus will cause the athlete to have flu-like symptoms: headache, stiff neck, fever, and vision problems. If healthy, the athlete can survive, and the virus runs its course in about two weeks. Outbreaks of the virus have caused several athletes to be hospitalized, however, and some have even died from it.

Some ATs tolerate two practices that can contribute to aseptic meningitis: They allow players to dip cups into watercoolers, and they allow players to touch their lips to cooler spigots. Prevention is simple. Every player uses their own cup, no one dips a cup into the cooler, and no lips touch the watercooler spigot. Watercoolers and bottles must be cleaned after each use with a bleach solution.

Infectious Mononucleosis

Infectious mononucleosis is a viral infection that causes extreme fatigue, fever, body ache, and an enlarged spleen. The enlarged spleen means that athletes are at risk for splenic ruptures if they are allowed to participate with this condition. Also called *mono*, infectious mononucleosis is caused by the Epstein-Barr virus and is transmitted to others through saliva. For this reason, it is often called the *kissing disease*. An athlete with mono must rest, and a physician must monitor their condition. The physician can allow the athlete to return to play as long as their spleen is a normal size, signs and symptoms have resolved, and liver function is normal.

Respiratory Conditions

The respiratory tract includes the nose, sinuses, trachea, bronchi, and lungs, any of which can be affected by viruses or bacteria. Common respiratory tract conditions are colds, sinusitis, pneumonia, influenza, asthma, and bronchitis.

Common Cold (Coryza)

The **common cold** is caused by a virus. Signs and symptoms of a cold include a sore throat, coughing, sneezing, runny nose, loss of voice, and tiredness.

To prevent a cold, athletes must maintain a good diet, wash their hands frequently, avoid others who have colds, avoid being in crowds, and avoid sharing cups. A viral illness can be treated only symptomatically, which means treating the signs and symptoms of the illness. An athlete with a sore throat or cough may use throat lozenges, and tissues should be used to cover coughs and dab runny noses. An athlete who is tired should rest. A rundown athlete who does not treat the cold may become more susceptible to other illnesses.

Laryngitis

An inflammation of the larynx is called laryngitis. Laryngitis can be caused by an infection of the upper-respiratory tract or from talking too much or too loudly. The athlete with laryngitis will have a sore throat and no voice. The infection may also involve the rest of the body, so they may have a fever. Drinking water will help humidify the throat and keep the athlete more comfortable. They will need to refrain from talking until the infection subsides. The athlete should treat the symptoms, but if they have a fever, the athlete should see a physician.

Bronchitis

Inflammation of the bronchial passages, called **bronchitis**, can be caused by an infection or an allergy. The athlete will have a fever, sore throat, tiredness, chills, a deep cough, and even wheezing. Bronchitis mimics colds, flu, and other respiratory conditions. It is best for the AT to refer athletes to a physician if they have persistent coughing and wheezing.

Flu (Influenza)

An athlete with **influenza** will report headaches, nausea, vomiting, dizziness, tiredness, stomach upset, chills, and possibly fever. The flu is communicable, and the sick athlete should stay away from their teammates. The athlete is treated symptomatically and should get plenty of rest. A team physician cannot do much to comfort the athlete once they have the flu. Some over-the-counter medications decrease nausea, headache, and body aches. The athlete can avoid getting the flu by getting a flu shot and avoiding those who are ill. An antiviral medication can be given to those who get the flu to help remediate the illness.

Coronavirus (COVID-19)

COVID-19, a coronavirus, caused a worldwide pandemic. The **coronavirus** is spread through droplets. The droplets are released through the air when a person breathes, talks, coughs, sneezes, or sings. After exposure to the virus, it can take between 2 and 14 days for symptoms to appear. A person who is infected with the virus is contagious up to two days before their symptoms appear. According to Johns Hopkins (2022), a person will remain potentially contagious for 10 to 20 days.

Signs and symptoms of COVID include a cough, chills, shortness of breath, sore throat, headache, fatigue, and congestion (Johns Hopkins 2022). Additional symptoms may include a fever, body aches, loss of taste or smell, diarrhea, nausea, and vomiting. Long-term effects can include respiratory failure, heart conditions, lung and kidney failure, nervous system problems, and even death (Johns Hopkins 2022).

A rapid test is utilized to determine if a person has COVID. This test is done by inserting a cotton-tipped applicator into each nostril and rotating it several times. The cotton-tipped applicator is then placed in contact with the liquid provided in the kit. Wait 15 minutes and check to see if the test is positive. A positive test is an indication that the person has COVID.

Treatment of COVID-19 depends on severity. For milder COVID cases, a person may isolate, stay at home, and take medication to deal with signs and symptoms. Those with more severe cases may require hospitalization, antivirals, IV medications and fluids, supplemental oxygen, and other supportive measures.

It is best to protect oneself from the virus by improving one's immune system, eating a balanced and healthy diet, exercising, wearing an approved mask, and getting plenty of rest. A vaccination is available for COVID, and there are boosters for those who would like them.

DERMATOLOGICAL CONDITIONS

Dermatological conditions affect the skin. These conditions can cause redness, rashes, itching, sores, and pain. The conditions can be caused by an infection, it can be genetic, or it can be from coming into contact with something such as poison ivy.

Skin Infections

The skin is a primary protector against disease—it keeps microorganisms from entering the body. It is critical to wash microorganisms off the skin to prevent the spread of disease (see the sidebar). Even so, some microorganisms directly infect the skin and then enter the body (see table 32.1). As another way of preventing the spread of skin infections, high school wrestling rules require that any wrestler with open sores be kept from wrestling. A physician's note indicating that the wrestler's rash is not communicable can permit participation, but the wrestling official can overrule the note.

Some skin rashes are the result of an invader that attacks the whole body, such as measles. In other cases, the invader attacks a localized area of the skin. Some skin areas become irritated by padding or athletic equipment and then an infection occurs. It is important to recognize skin irritations early to prevent them from spreading to other athletes. A referral to a physician can keep a skin condition under control.

Skin Autoimmune Disorders

The human body can attack itself when a person has an autoimmune disorder. With skin immune disorders, the tissue affected is the skin.

Urticaria (Hives)

Urticaria or hives is a rash that can be contained in one body part or can cover the entire body. Histamine is released in the body as a result of a reaction to an irritant such as medication, something in the environment, food, stress, insect bites, or an infection (Mayo Clinic 2022a). The skin rash is raised and can be the size of a dime or as large as a saucer.

Determining the cause of hives is a process of elimination. Ask the athlete these questions: What did you eat? What medications did you take? What did you encounter? What were you doing just before getting the rash? If these questions do not lead to the answer, it's best to refer the athlete to a physician. It is possible that the hives will go away without any intervention and go undiagnosed. Traditional treatment is over-the-counter antihistamines.

A serious complication of hives is anaphylaxis. This means the allergic reaction can progress to lightheadedness, swelling about the face, hands, and feet, difficulty breathing, and unconsciousness. Anaphylaxis is a medical emergency and requires a call to 911.

! RED FLAGS

Referral to a physician is necessary in the following cases:

- There is a bruise that was not caused by direct contact.
- The athlete has an enlarged liver.
- There are flu-like symptoms.
- The AT suspects a *Staphylococcus* infection.
- The athlete has a rash of unexplained origin.
- The athlete has large amount of swelling in the glands below the ears.

Table 32.1 Types of Skin Lesions

Type	Characteristics
Crusts	Dried accumulations of pus, often thought of as scabs. Often associated with impetigo and cold sores.
Pustules	Collections of pus from infection. Often associated with wounds, folliculitis, furuncles, and acne.
Ulcers	Open weeping wounds. Often associated with burns or trauma.
Vesicles	Collections of clear fluids under the skin. The vesicles may be singular or in bunches. The contagion is in the fluid, so breaking a vesicle causes the disease to spread. Some vesicles are of no consequence, such as a blister. When vesicles break, they are prone to infection.

HAND WASHING

1. When using paper towels to dry hands, first unroll the towel from the dispenser without touching the paper towel.
2. Use the automatic liquid soap dispenser—if you do not have one, get one.
3. Turn on the water with your forearm.
4. Lather your hands and wrists, scrubbing under the fingernails and any jewelry.
5. Say your ABCs twice—this is a long enough scrubbing time.
6. Rinse your hands.
7. Tear off the paper towel and dry your hands.
8. Using the wet paper towel, dispense another clean paper towel.
9. Throw out the used wet towel.
10. Turn off the water with the clean paper towel.
11. Open the bathroom door with the same paper towel.
12. Discard the paper towel.

Dermatitis

There are three forms of dermatitis: contact dermatitis, seborrheic dermatitis, and eczema. Contact dermatitis is caused by coming in contact with something that irritates the skin, such as latex or jewelry. Seborrheic dermatitis and eczema can be caused by dry skin, infections, genetics, or problems with your immune system (Mayo Clinic 2022b). Those more inclined to have dermatitis are older, have allergies or a family history of allergies, have a family history of dermatitis, have a compromised immune system, or have contacted chemicals (Mayo Clinic 2022b).

Symptoms include a rash, itching, dry skin, flaking skin, blisters, and crusting of skin (Mayo Clinic 2022b). Treatment may require a skin biopsy to eliminate other skin conditions. Treatment for dermatitis can be as simple as removing the irritant from the skin or may require more significant treatment like corticosteroids (Mayo Clinic 2022b). Conservative management for dermatitis includes moisturizing your skin, applying a cool and wet cloth, taking a warm bath, drying the skin by patting with a towel, using medicated shampoos, avoiding chemicals, and relaxation (Mayo Clinic 2022b). Dermatitis is not contagious.

Dermographism Urticaria

Those that may be more susceptible to dermographism urticaria are athletes with diabetes, with hyperthyroid or hypothyroid conditions, who are in menopause, who are under stress, or who are pregnant (Nobles, Muse, and Schmeider 2022). The contact of the skin creates a raised wheal that lasts up to a half hour. One of the differentiating factors is that the pattern of the contact is exactly how the wheal will appear. Some people have found it fun to write a name on their skin when this condition exists. According to Nobles, Muse, and Schmeider (2022), approximately 2% to 5% of the population have this condition, and the athlete may feel itching and prickling sensations.

Antihistamines are the treatment of choice for those whose signs and symptoms do not resolve on their own. Light therapy has a short-term effect, but dermographism returns after two to three months (Nobles, Muse, and Schmeider 2022). Additional treatment includes vitamin C (Nobles, Muse, and Schmeider 2022). There are several forms of dermographism, and it is best to have the diagnosis determined by a physician. Most athletes who have flare-ups of this condition will see complete resolution between 5 and 10 years (Nobles, Muse, and Schmeider 2022).

Common Skin Conditions

In this section, some of the more common skin conditions are covered. Acne, sebaceous cysts, psoriasis, paronychia, and hidradenitis suppurativa are discussed here.

Methicillin-Resistant Staphylococcus Aureus (MRSA)

MRSA is caused by *Staphylococcus aureus* bacteria. Because this bacteria is resistant to many antibiotics, MRSA is difficult to control and resolve. According to the Centers for Disease Control and Prevention (2024a), signs and symptoms of MRSA include swelling, pain, redness, warmth, pus drainage, and a yellow or white core or center to the wound. The athlete is also likely to have a fever. In many instances, the wound will first appear as a small spider-bite lesion. Athletes suspected of having MRSA or other infections should be examined by a physician right away. Treating MRSA involves strong antibiotics along with having the wound drained by a physician.

To prevent the spread of MRSA, the AT will need to disinfect surfaces and clothing as well as any areas the athlete came in contact with. The physician will determine when it is safe for the athlete to return to activity. Athletes should change their wound dressing daily and observe for any signs of infection.

Folliculitis

Folliculitis is an inflammation of a hair follicle. The athlete will need antibiotics to cure the infection, which is caused by bacteria, but they can participate with proper covering of the follicles. Wet hot packs can open the follicle, which may look like a pus-filled sore, and help reduce the infection faster (see figure 32.6). Athletes who wear protective equipment such as shoulder pads are more prone to folliculitis. These athletes should wear an additional layer of lightweight clothing to help decrease the pressure on the follicles.

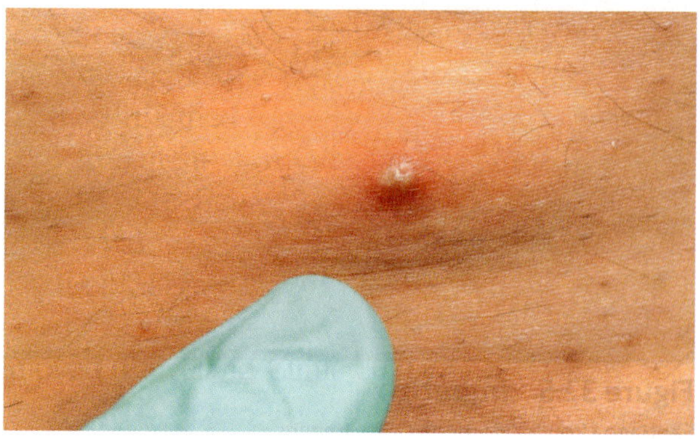

Figure 32.6 Folliculitis.
Ocskaymark/iStock/Getty Images

Boils (Furuncles)

Furuncles, or boils, are bacterial infections in skin glands. The boil will be bright red with a hard central core that is painful when touched (see figure 32.7). The furuncle will look like a large pimple, and the athlete may want to squeeze it. Instead, they should apply warm packs several times a day to draw the infection outward. The AT must use caution to prevent the bacteria from getting on the hot packs; it is helpful to assign a towel to the infected athlete that is then sent to the wash daily. All parts of the body that have contact with protective equipment are prone to this infection, and it needs to be treated by a physician.

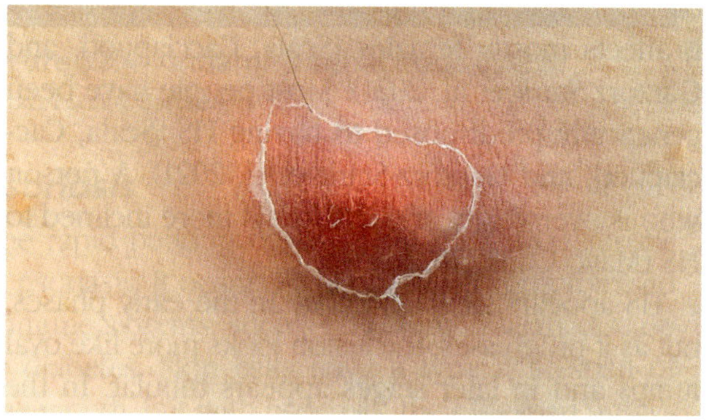

Figure 32.7 Furuncles.
AlxeyPnferov/iStock/Getty Images

Carbuncles

Carbuncles are caused by a bacterial infection. A cluster of boils on the skin is referred to as a carbuncle. As the infection enlarges, there will be pus at the head along with dead tissue (see figure 32.8). Characterizing features of a carbuncle are that they are red, swollen, and painful under the skin and have a white tip at the head. Some carbuncles will

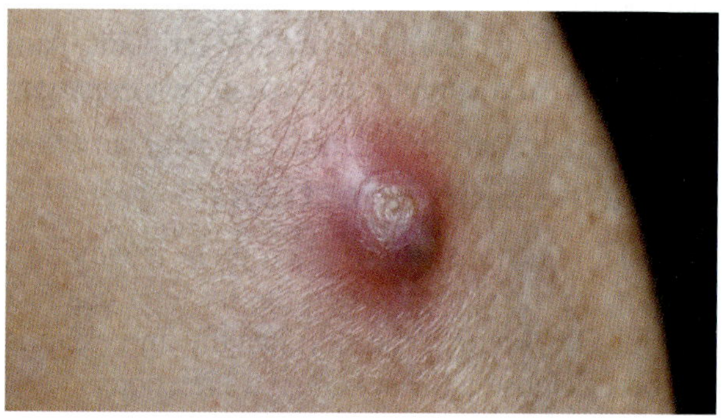

Figure 32.8 Carbuncles.
Zay Nyi Nyi/iStock/Getty Images

drain on their own—a hot compress can help—while others will need to be drained by a physician. Even with draining the carbuncle, some patients may require antibiotics.

If carbuncles cause a systemic infection, the athlete can feel malaise, have a high temperature, and feel nauseated (Mayo Clinic 1998-2023). Some infections found in carbuncles are antibiotic resistant. Prevention is the best treatment. Carbuncles should be kept clean and covered with a nonporous bandage. Other athletes who have been in contact with the infected athlete should shower. All equipment the infected athlete has touched should be sanitized with an antibacterial. Launder all towels, sheets, and clothing that has been in contact with the athlete.

Fungal Skin Infections

Fungal infections are caused by a form of fungus, usually a yeast or mold. These infections thrive in dark, moist environments. Individuals with compromised immune systems or compromised skin are also more vulnerable to fungal infections.

Athlete's Foot (Tinea Pedis)

Tinea pedis, commonly called athlete's foot, is caused by a fungal infection. Athlete's foot results in red, dry, scaly, itchy skin (see figure 32.9). Over-the-counter antifungal medication is often effective in resolving the condition. The athlete can help prevent tinea pedis by cleaning and drying their feet.

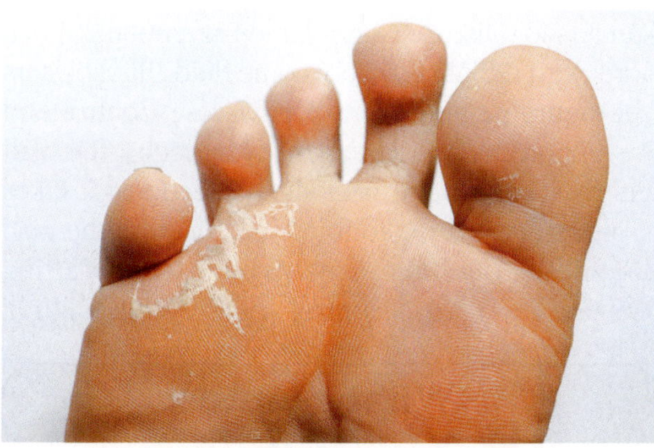

Figure 32.9 Athlete's foot fungus.
Yusuke Ide/iStock/Getty Images

Ringworm (Tinea Corporis)

Tinea corporis, commonly called *ringworm*, is caused by a fungal infection. A red, scaly, ring-shaped abnormality appears on the skin (see figure 32.10). Antifungal creams are frequently prescribed to resolve the condition. This condition is commonly spread from contact with infected clothing, equipment, or another person's body.

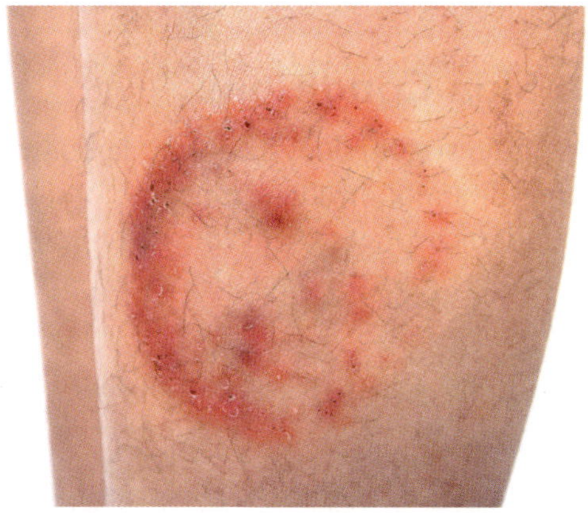

Figure 32.10 Tinea corporis.
Phanasitti/iStock/Getty Images

Jock Itch (Tinea Cruris)

Tinea cruris or jock itch is caused by a fungal infection that causes a red, itchy rash. This rash is found in moist areas of the body, such as the groin and inner thighs (see figure 32.11). It is important to prevent jock itch by not sharing towels, wearing clean clothes, staying dry, and changing wet clothes often. Jock itch is contagious by contact, so it's important to treat it, cover it, and not share equipment or towels or clothing. Treatment includes over-the-counter antifungal medication. More serious cases may require prescription medication.

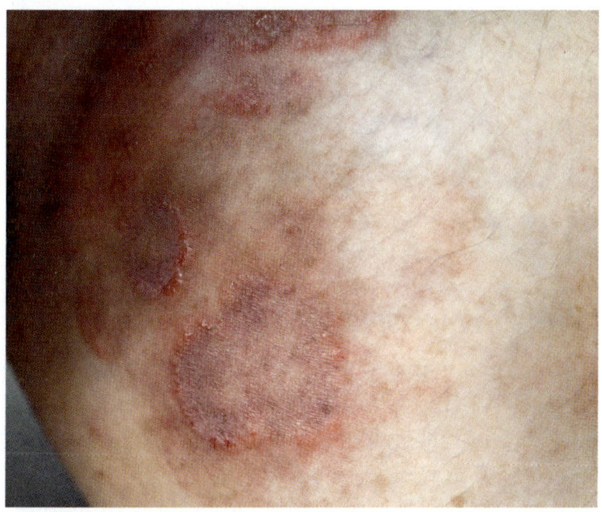

Figure 32.11 Tinea cruris (jock itch).
HengDao/iStock/Getty Images

FYI

Cold Sore

A cold sore is a group of blisters around or in the mouth caused by the herpes simplex virus.

Viral Skin Conditions

The immune system does its best to keep the body safe from different invaders. One line of defense is the skin, which prevents invaders from getting in. In the case of a virus, direct contact may be how it is transmitted.

Measles (Rubeola)

There are two types of measles: rubeola and rubella (German measles). Viruses cause both. **Rubeola** causes cold symptoms, with a cough and high temperature in the early stages. As the disease progresses, the body becomes covered with a rash, including inside the mouth (see figure 32.12). The athlete will be tired, their eyes will be sensitive to bright light, and they will have a headache. The AT should refer the athlete to a physician, who will treat the symptoms. Rubeola is prevented through vaccination.

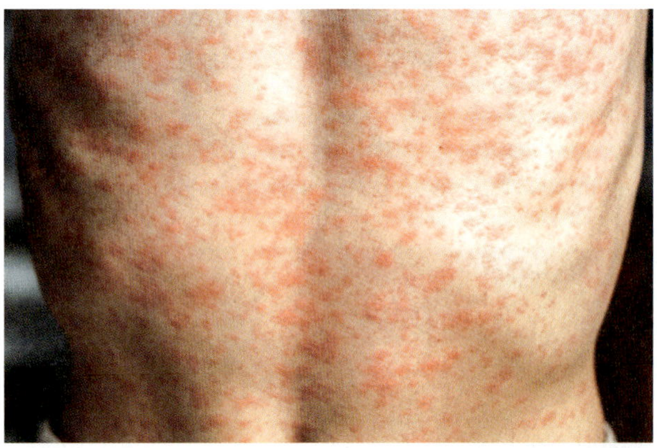

Figure 32.12 Measles.
Natalya Maisheva/iStock/Getty Images

German Measles (Rubella)

Rubella causes a rash that starts at the head and covers the body within a day's time (see figure 32.13). The rash will stay for about three days, but the athlete remains contagious for about five. They are treated for pain or itching. Rubella is prevented through vaccination.

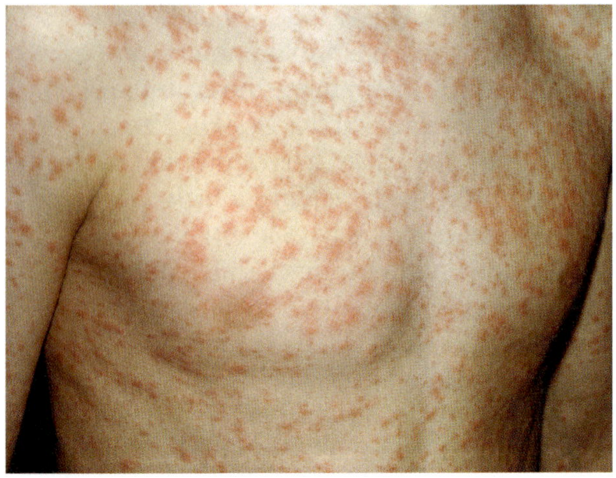

Figure 32.13 Rubella.
PR. PH. FRANCESCHINI/CNRI/Science Source

Shingles (Herpes Zoster)

According to the Centers for Disease Control and Prevention (2019), about 32% of people in the United States will develop shingles during their lifetime. Most of the people who develop shingles have previously had chickenpox.

Shingles (herpes zoster) is caused by the same virus that causes chickenpox. Once the person has the virus in their body after having chickenpox, it can remain dormant for years. The virus can reactivate later, causing shingles.

When shingles reactivates, it will do so along the dermatome where it was dormant. Some signs and symptoms include tingling, itching, burning of the skin, headache, upset stomach, fever, and chills (Centers for Disease Control and Prevention 2019). It starts with red spots that become fluid-filled blisters (see figure 32.14; Centers for Disease Control and Prevention 2019). After about two weeks, the blisters dry out and are no longer infectious. It takes approximately three to four weeks before the rash disappears, but there may be permanent scarring (Centers for Disease Control and Prevention 2019).

What Would You Do If . . .

The AT evaluates an athlete and is puzzled by the signs and symptoms of a rash. You recognize the signs and symptoms as being similar to those of measles, which you had as a child.

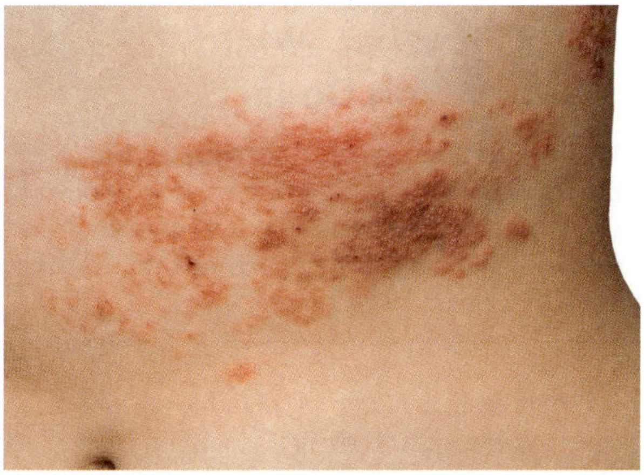

Figure 32.14 Shingles.
Franciscodiazpagador/iStock/Getty Images

Some complications that occur include pain and skin infections, and if it is around the eye, it can cause visual problems or damage to the eye. If shingles is near the ear, it can cause ear pain and vertigo and affect muscles around the face (Centers for Disease Control and Prevention 2019).

The fluid from the shingles rash can spread the virus to other people who have never had chickenpox or had the chickenpox vaccine. A person who is infected this way will develop chickenpox, not shingles. The best thing to do is to cover the rash when it is actively able to be spread.

Treatment for shingles is antiviral medication and pain relief. The earlier medication is given, the more it will reduce the severity of infection and decrease the duration of pain. Nerve pain is one of the long-term complications of shingles. For some, a vaccine is available to reduce the chance of getting shingles and it is usually given after the age of 50.

Plantar Warts (Human Papillomavirus)

Plantar warts occur when human papillomavirus (HPV) enters a small cut or lesion in the skin. At the feet, this usually occurs at pressure areas such as the balls or the heel. Plantar warts are characterized by hard, slightly raised areas with brown or black pinpoint-sized dots in the center. Plantar warts can be painful, especially as they enlarge. Athletes should see a dermatologist if the warts persist—they will likely need to be treated.

Molluscum Contagiosum

Molluscum contagiosum is caused by a virus that raises pink lumps in the area of contact (see figure 32.15). A physician removes the lumps surgically and applies a medication. They usually heal without scarring.

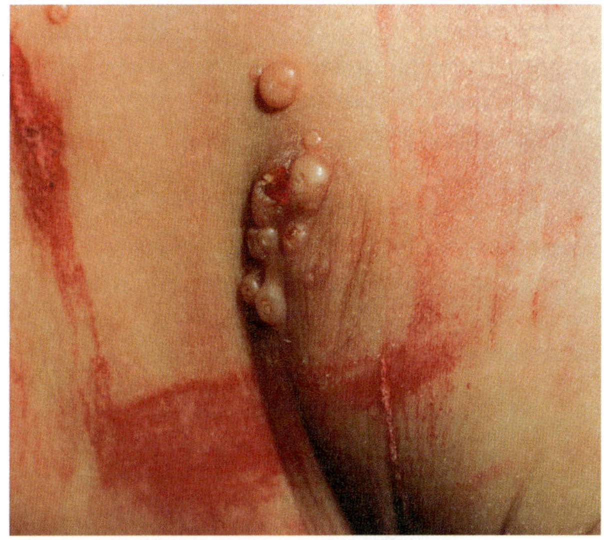

Figure 32.15 Molluscum contagiosum.
BSIP/UIG Via Getty Images

Herpes

Herpes simplex is a virus that causes an infection of the skin or mucous membranes. Herpes simplex is categorized as type 1 or type 2. The virus stays in the body, and when the immune system weakens, a cold sore can appear (see figure 32.16). The athlete needs to get enough sleep, good nutrition, and exercise to prevent outbreaks.

Signs of **herpes** include a weeping open blister with a red base and a yellow crust, swollen glands, and possibly a fever. Herpes simplex is spread by

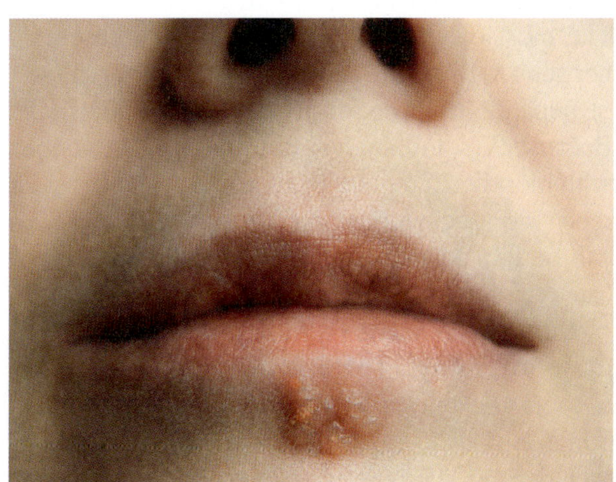

Figure 32.16 Herpes simplex.
Basak Gurbuz Derman/Moment/Getty Images

skin-to-skin contact. In sports characterized by considerable contact, such as wrestling and rugby, herpes simplex can spread rapidly. This is often referred to as *herpes gladiatorum*. Prevention involves showering after practice; covering all open wounds; excusing athletes with open wounds from practice; making sure that athletes do not share towels, toothbrushes, or clothes; and washing mats before and after each use with a bleach and water solution or commercial product. Herpes runs its course in about two weeks. Three things will help a person who is subject to cold sores: eating properly (well-balanced meals), getting enough rest, and, most important, managing stress.

BLOOD-BORNE CONDITIONS

Two contagious blood-borne diseases are HIV and hepatitis. These diseases are transmitted especially by contact with infected blood. Say an athletic trainer treating an athlete's bleeding wound gets blood in a cut on her hand. Microorganisms in the blood can easily enter the cut. Needles or razors shared by more than one athlete may also transfer blood from one person to another. The best way to prevent transmittal is to place a barrier between the infected athlete and others. The universal precautions discussed in chapter 25 should be employed in these situations.

Hepatitis A, B, C, D, and E

Hepatitis is a viral illness that affects the liver. The most commonly known of these viruses are hepatitis A, B, and C. The abbreviation for each form of hepatitis has this format: HAV, HBV, and HCV. Because ATs and student assistants are in contact with blood on a regular basis, they should consider receiving vaccinations. Exposure to this condition can be limited by observing universal precautions (see chapter 25).

Hepatitis A virus (HAV) infects the liver, causing it to enlarge. This form of hepatitis is rarely chronic and does not often cause permanent liver damage (Davis 2017). The signs and symptoms include jaundice (yellow coloring of the white part of the eyes and skin), loss of appetite, an enlarged liver, pain over the liver, potential fever, tiredness, nausea, and a rash. HAV is transmitted by contact with contaminated food, drink, blood, or feces. A blood test is the best way to diagnose HAV. Treatment includes plenty of rest, no exercise, and increased fluid intake. Affected athletes should avoid others until the infectious period passes.

> **What Would You Do If . . .**
>
> While cleaning up after an athlete who was bleeding profusely, you notice a drop of blood on a recent abrasion on your forearm. You know the athlete and trust that they do not have any communicable diseases.

Hepatitis B virus (HBV) causes an infection of the liver. The virus tends to persist in the blood of the infected athlete and can be transmitted by contact with infected blood, including dried blood. Those infected with HBV have it for life and are more prone to cirrhosis (liver disease)—they may feel tired and nauseated and experience a lack of appetite. Some infected people may be carriers of the disease but are not themselves ill. The signs and symptoms of HBV are not unlike those of a cold or flu. The athlete will have signs of jaundice—yellowing of the skin and sclera—and needs immediate medical attention to control the damage from HBV. It is possible that they will have chronic problems and may even die. The good news is that HBV is preventable through a series of shots.

Hepatitis C virus (HCV) is transmitted by direct contact with bodily fluids from an infected person. The signs and symptoms of HCV are the same as for HAV and HBV. The virus is diagnosed with a blood test. Many people infected with HCV will not show signs and symptoms until the disease has progressed, causing permanent damage to the liver. HCV may lead to death if not treated early enough. It is treated with antiviral medication and can be cured if diagnosed early in the disease process (Cox 2017). HCV can be prevented by following universal precautions and avoiding equipment that may have been used by the infected person.

Hepatitis D virus (HDV) can infect a person if they had HBV. Essentially it is a second bout of

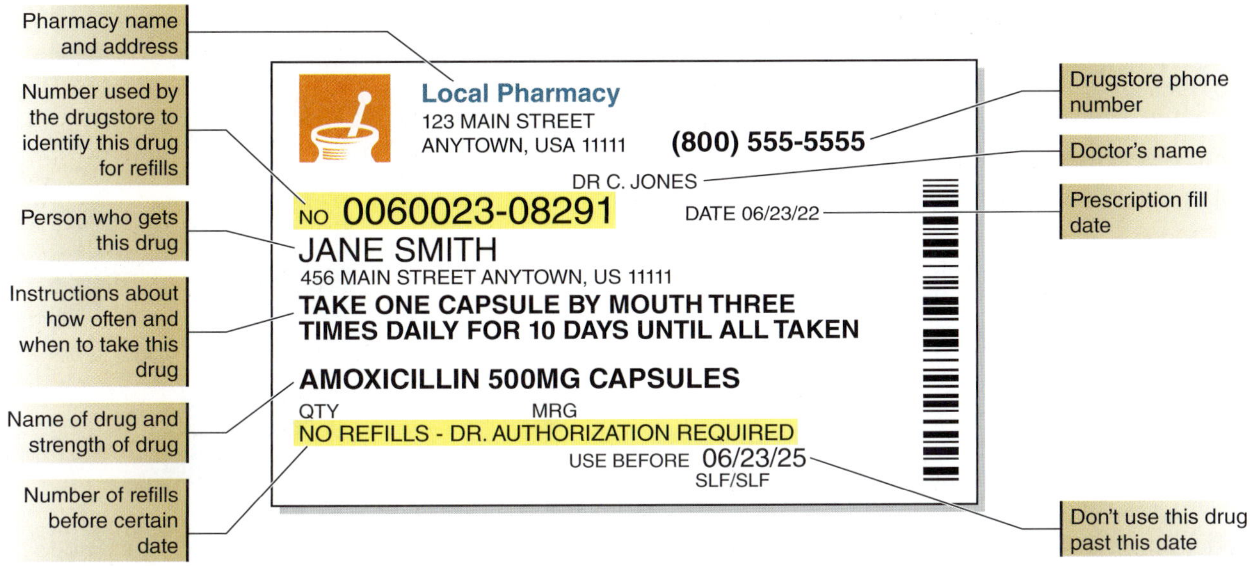

Figure 33.2 Prescription label.

Reprinted by permission from M.A. Cleary, T.E. Abdenour, and M. Pavlovich, *Clinical Pharmacology in Athletic Training* (Champaign, IL: Human Kinetics, 2022), 18.

chemical structure, and 3) same therapeutic action (Cleary, Abdenour, and Pavlovich 2022). Some drugs can be classified into more than one category. Following are typical drug classifications.

Analgesic Drugs

Drugs that are used to manage pain are known as analgesics. Analgesics can be over-the-counter or prescription. Some prescription analgesics are so powerful that if they are used improperly, they can cause addiction, overdose, or death. Examples of analgesics are aspirin, opioids, fentanyl, naloxone, oxycodone, acetaminophen, COX inhibitors, and nonsteroidal anti-inflammatory drugs (NSAIDs).

Nonsteroidal Anti-Inflammatory Drugs

Nonsteroidal anti-inflammatory drugs (NSAIDs) reduce the amount of tissue swelling after an injury. They include aspirin and ibuprofen, which are over-the-counter drugs, meaning they can be legally purchased without a prescription.

After an injury, aspirin can be used to reduce pain. Aspirin is a blood thinner and can cause more swelling in an area initially. An athlete who is anemic should avoid aspirin because of its blood-thinning ability; it will be counterproductive to resolving the anemia.

Ibuprofen reduces pain and swelling and is commonly used for strains and sprains. In large amounts, it often causes an upset stomach; therefore, it should be taken with food. Regularly taking ibuprofen in large doses can cause liver and kidney damage.

> ***Understanding Diversity***
>
> Many people find that acupuncture helps relieve numerous types of pain. Acupuncture is a component of traditional Chinese medicine that involves inserting fine needles in specific areas of the body to elicit a physical response.

Local Steroids

A **local steroid** is applied to the skin or injected in a joint to reduce swelling and pain; it should not be confused with anabolic steroids. Local steroids are used mainly for allergies, skin disorders, or joint pain. Injected local steroids can weaken tendons. The team physician prescribes them and will also monitor their use.

Beta-Adrenergic Drugs

Beta-adrenergic drugs maintain the airway during an asthma attack by controlling the release of chemicals. These medications are available by prescription only and can be administered via injections, inhalation, or pills. It is common to see athletes with inhalers. However, sometimes athletes are not allowed to use the inhaler during competition.

Of course, if the athlete needs the inhaler to save their life, they must use it, regardless of the activity. The rules regarding medication change constantly. The AT should check the rules of each sport annually to determine which drugs are acceptable. The proper use of an inhaler is found in figure 33.3.

Epinephrine

Epinephrine is used in life-threatening allergic reactions, such as an insect bite, food allergy, or a reaction to medication. Epinephrine comes in a prefilled injectable device with a needle, which gives a predetermined dose. The athlete or AT can inject the predetermined dose into the lateral aspect of the athlete's thigh. The athlete may need a second predetermined dose. An EpiPen is prescribed for the athlete who has this type of allergic reaction (see figure 33.4).

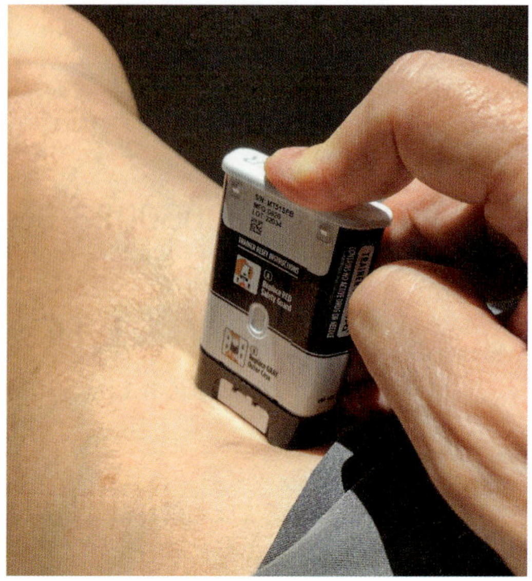

Figure 33.4 EpiPen.
Photo: Lorin A. Cartwright.

Muscle Relaxant Drugs

Muscle relaxants are prescribed for athletes in acute pain caused by muscle spasms. The medication works on the nerve to reduce pain signals being sent to the brain. Using this form of medication may cause the athlete to be tired and interfere with their athletic performance.

Antivirals

When a viral infection attacks the body, antivirals can be used to decrease symptoms and potentially decrease the length of illness. An antiviral cannot kill the virus, but it gives the body time to build immunity. According to the Cleveland Clinic (2024), an antiviral blocks the receptor so that the virus cannot attach itself to healthy cells, and it can decrease the amount of active virus within the body. These factors give the body's immune system time to build an immunity against the virus.

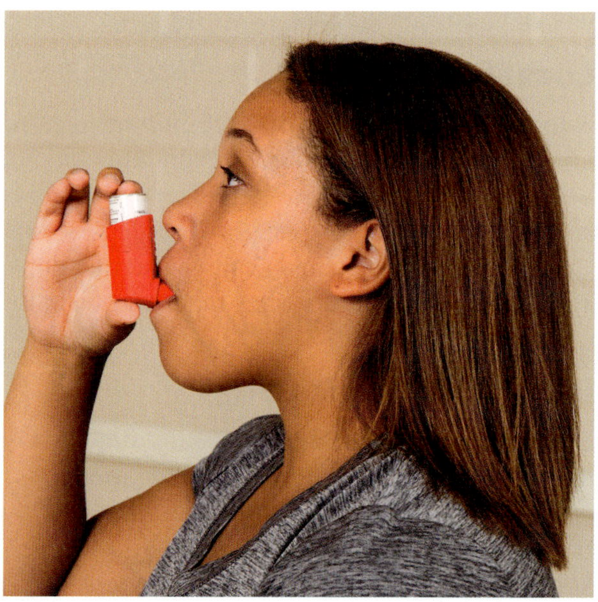

Figure 33.3 Inhaler use.

Antibiotics

A physician prescribes antibiotics for bacterial infections. There are many antibiotics, the most famous of which is penicillin and its derivatives. The drug enters the bloodstream and assists white blood cells. Using an antibiotic improperly can cause bacteria to change and become resistant to the drug; thus, the drug must be taken as prescribed and until it is gone so that the infection will not flare up again. When bacteria become resistant to antibiotics, the infection can take over.

Antifungals

Athlete's foot, toenail fungus, ringworm, jock itch, and yeast infections are treated by antifungals. Antifungals can come in the form of a spray, IV, cream, or pill. Some fungus infections are readily cleared up, while others take months. Fungus of the feet or toenails tend to take a longer time. Antifungals keep the fungus from multiplying.

Antidepressants

Antidepressants work on brain chemistry, especially those that effect an athlete's mood. For those who have depression, this is one form of treatment. The medication takes a few weeks to create a change in brain chemistry and may require dosage adjustments.

RECREATIONAL DRUGS

Drugs that people use but that have no medical purpose are called **recreational drugs**. Many recreational drugs such as alcohol and tobacco are legal for some age groups and illegal for others. Other recreational drugs, such as cocaine, are illegal for everyone. Using illegal drugs can present at least three major problems:

1. Negative side effects, ranging from lack of motivation to death.
2. Unknown impurities in the drugs, which result from the lack of legal control over their manufacture and sales and can have unexpected side effects, including death.
3. Involvement with criminal elements, which can result in legal and personal problems.

Depressants

A depressant slows down an athlete's brain and affects the ability to respond, maintain balance, or hear. An athlete can be less inhibited, and judgment can be impaired. There are a few common depressants, such as alcohol and barbiturates.

Alcohol

Alcohol is produced by fermentation, which occurs when yeast breaks down the carbohydrate in grains or fruits. Alcohol is consumed as beer, wine, and hard liquor.

> **What Would You Do If . . .**
>
> Before the start of every hockey game, the players have a ritual of inhaling from ammonia capsules. They say it makes them more aware of what's going on in the game.

The alcohol content in a can of beer, a glass of wine, and a shot of hard liquor—all of which are considered one drink—is roughly equivalent. The difference in volume is the amount of water present with the alcohol. Beer has the most water, and liquor has the least.

Alcohol causes the heart rate, breathing rate, and reaction time to slow; thus, it is a depressant. The slowing of bodily processes is not what an athlete needs during competition—imagine the runner who runs slower, loses balance, loses concentration, and forgets what they are doing. Alcohol also slows reaction time, which makes it unsafe for the drinker to drive. The body treats alcohol as a poison, and it is sent to the liver for detoxification. It takes about an hour and 20 minutes for the liver to detoxify one drink. If the body cannot remove the alcohol fast enough, the person will become intoxicated and perhaps vomit the poison from the body. If the drinking continues, the person may lose consciousness, go into a coma, or die. Loss of consciousness occurs when the blood alcohol content is 0.4%, and death occurs shortly thereafter.

Those who use alcohol persistently and excessively are prone to liver disorders, nutrition problems, illnesses, brain disorders, stomach ulcers, and early death.

When an athletic trainer is caring for an athlete with a suspected alcohol intoxication, there is one caution: Intoxication can have signs and symptoms similar to diabetic ketoacidosis (see figure 33.5).

Barbiturates

These pills are taken for relaxation to the point of sedation, euphoria, and to counteract anxiety (Drug Enforcement Agency 2022). Seizures and insomnia are traditional medical uses. For those who misuse this medication, impaired judgment similar to intoxication and confusion and staggering are characteristics (Drug Enforcement Agency 2022).

Stimulants

The primary effect of a stimulant is speeding up the body's systems. There are medical uses for stimulants, such as managing ADHD or a need for greater alertness. Familiar stimulants are caffeine and tobacco products.

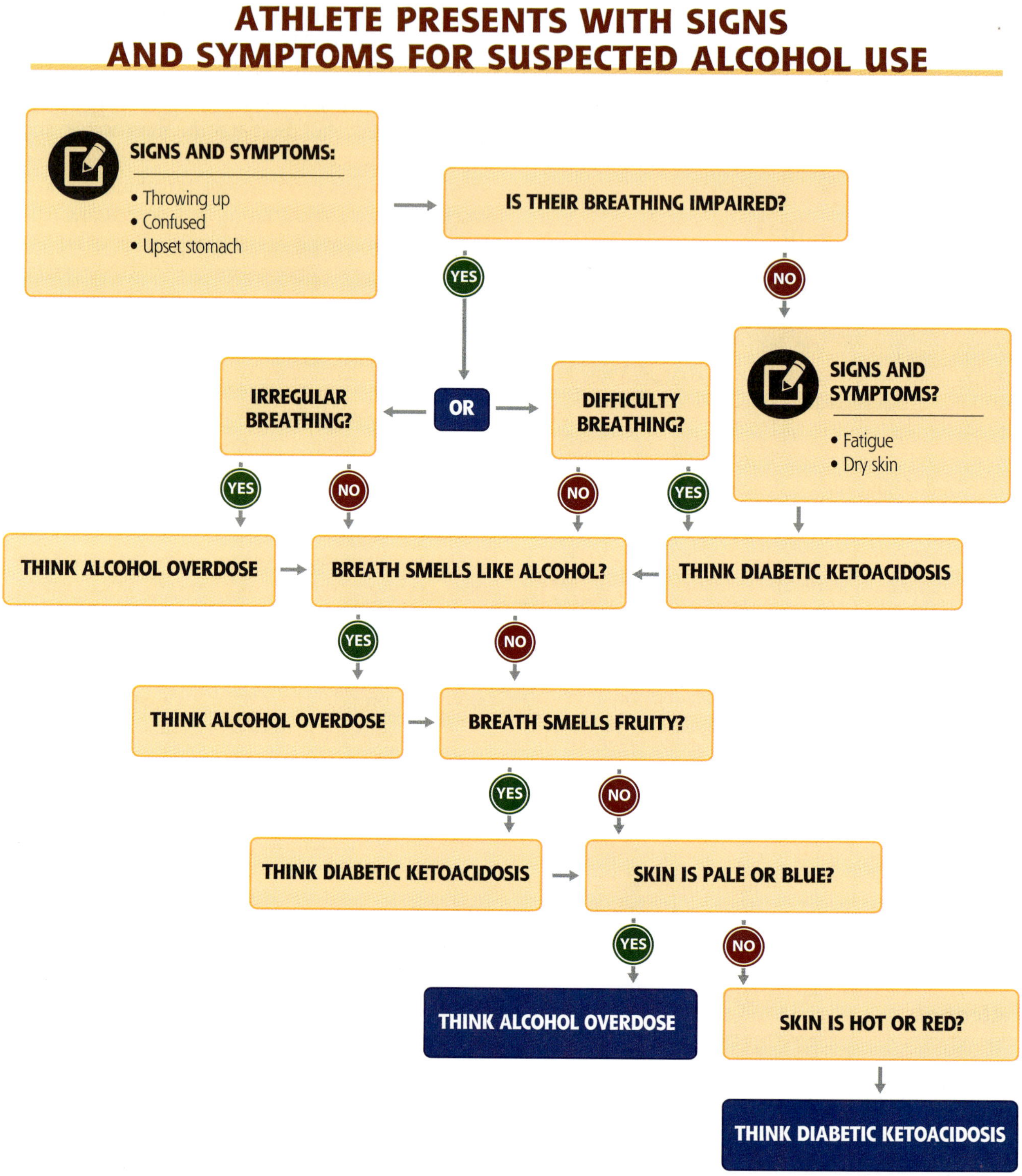

Figure 33.5 Is it alcohol overdose or diabetic ketoacidosis?

Caffeine

Caffeine is a drug found in coffee, tea, and chocolate as well as in some brands of aspirin, cold medications, weight-loss products, and soda. Caffeine is a stimulant, meaning it increases heart and breathing rates. It is also a diuretic, meaning it flushes fluids from the body. Some athletes in endurance events such as marathons have used caffeine because they thought it would improve their endurance, but since you cannot take bathroom breaks when you're running a marathon, it is better to avoid caffeine.

> **What Would You Do If . . .**
>
> The golf team has just won the state title. You are invited to a party at a local hotel. At the hotel, the entire team is drinking and smoking cigars. Your ride home stumbles up to you and says it's time to go.

The amount of caffeine in products varies. Athletes may have difficulty sleeping after ingesting caffeine. An athlete with a headache may take an aspirin to help the pain without checking to see if it contains caffeine and then lie awake all night. Athletes who become addicted to caffeine may have headaches, nausea, and tiredness when they go through withdrawal.

Tobacco

Tobacco may be used in two forms: smoked and smokeless. Tobacco is smoked in cigarettes, cigars, or pipes. Cigarette smoking is highly addictive. It lowers stamina and has many negative long-term side effects. It greatly increases a person's chances of developing lung cancer, heart disease, emphysema and other breathing disorders, and blindness from macular degeneration. Some people think that cigar and pipe smoking are not as damaging as cigarettes, but this idea is incorrect.

Smokeless tobacco—snuff or chewing tobacco—is placed against the gums, and nicotine is absorbed into the bloodstream. Athletes use this form of tobacco because they have seen professional athletes use it, especially baseball players. Nicotine increases heart and breathing rates. All forms of smokeless tobacco contain cancer-causing substances.

Smokeless tobacco is regulated by the laws applying to all tobacco, so sale to a minor is illegal. High school and college association regulations state that smokeless tobacco is not to be used. In professional ranks, use of smokeless tobacco is currently not regulated.

E-cigarettes create an aerosol out of nicotine for inhalation. Vaping may lead to asthma, lung disease, and cardiovascular disease (Johns Hopkins 2022). E-cigarettes contain nicotine and are addictive. Much more research needs to be done to determine the long-term consequences and the chemicals involved (Johns Hopkins 2022). Popcorn lung is an inflammation of the lung that may lead to scarring of the airways (Johns Hopkins 2023). A flavoring, diacetyl, is added to the liquid in e-cigarettes, and it causes lung inflammation and scarring (Johns Hopkins 2023).

People who use smokeless tobacco can develop precancerous cells of the cheek, tongue, and gum within two years of use. These cells, called **leukoplakia**, develop quickly because of the frequency with which the smokeless tobacco is held in the cheek. The precancerous cells are white and may have blisters. If a cancerous growth occurs, surgery may involve removing the jaw and possibly the tongue. If the cancer has spread throughout the body and the warning signs are overlooked, the athlete may die. In addition, smokeless tobacco can cause serious dental complications—gum disease, bad breath, and cavities are more common among smokeless tobacco users than among others.

Tobacco candy and tobacco mints, another form of smokeless tobacco, have become a popular way to obtain nicotine. This type of smokeless tobacco takes the form of dissolvable strips or pellets that are flavored and packaged to look like candy. Smokeless tobacco is nicotine with the same health hazards, including addiction, heart disease, cancer, dental disease, and risks for unborn babies.

> **What Would You Do If . . .**
>
> A baseball player pulls back his lip and asks you what the blisters on the inside of his cheek and gum indicate. He reveals that he chews tobacco when his family is not around.

> **FYI**
>
> **Emphysema**
>
> Emphysema is an incurable lung disease characterized by the inability to breathe deeply. It is progressive and will eventually destroy the sufferer's ability to take in enough oxygen to sustain life.

Cocaine

Cocaine is a white powder that can be inhaled to give the user a feeling of euphoria—a feeling of well-being. The euphoric effects are short in duration. The more a person uses cocaine, the greater their tolerance, and the more of it they will require to achieve the same euphoric state. Users will exhibit restlessness after use.

Side effects of cocaine use include death from heart problems, suppression of the immune system, poor nutrition, and cocaine bugs—the hallucination that insects are crawling under the skin. There are no benefits to be derived from using cocaine.

Methamphetamines (Meth)

Meth is made from products that contain pseudoephedrine. Common over-the-counter products like antihistamines and pain medications contain pseudoephedrine. The products are kept behind the counter at a pharmacy so that the amount sold is controlled.

Meth can be a pill, powder, or rocks (crystal meth) in appearance (Drug Enforcement Agency 2022). The drug is snorted, sniffed, injected, or smoked. Ultimately the user feels awake and excited, with increased breathing rate, heart rate, blood pressure, and body temperature (Substance Abuse and Mental Health Services Administration 2018). Long-term use of meth can lead to stroke, heart attack, or organ injury (Substance Abuse and Mental Health Services Administration 2018).

Narcotics

Narcotics are made from the poppy plant. They have a legitimate therapeutic need in the instance of pain. When used appropriately and controlled, the medication works effectively. Some people use opioids and can become addicted.

Oxycodone

Oxycodone is a prescription painkiller that can produce feelings of euphoria and relaxation. The tablet form is taken orally, or it can be crushed and sniffed, heated, and inhaled (Drug Enforcement Agency 2022). The overdose of this drug can be remediated by using naloxone, or Narcan (see figure 33.6).

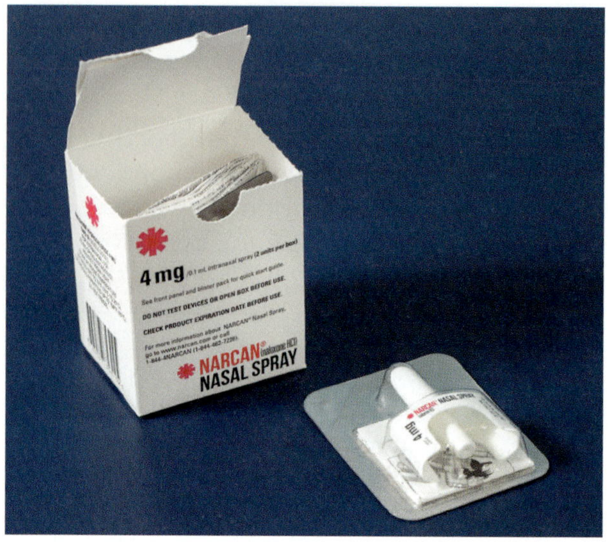

Figure 33.6 Naloxone.

Opium

Opium is derived from the poppy plant. Users report euphoria followed by relaxation (Drug Enforcement Agency 2022). An overdose of opioids can cause the person to have respiratory distress. Pinpoint pupils; vomiting; pale, purple lips and finger nailbeds; and unresponsiveness may also accompany an overdose.

It is imperative to call 911 to initiate an emergency response, begin CPR as dictated, and administer Narcan (naloxone) if you have it available. Narcan is a nasal spray or can be injected.

Marijuana or Cannabis

The *Cannabis sativa* plant is grown for personal use, but some is grown for distribution. Marijuana is legal in some states and in certain formulations. The leaves, stems, and seeds of the plant are dried and crushed. A marijuana cigarette is rolled and smoked. Marijuana's active ingredient is THC. The effect on the body is relaxation, with slow motor and response time.

CBD (Cannabidiol)

CBD is made from the *Cannabis sativa* plant and its use is for medical benefit. CBD is legal as long as the THC level remains low. For athletes, CBD may be legal in some instances while prohibited in others.

CBD has been used for the relief of pain, anxiety, seizure disorders, Parkinson's disease, and Crohn's disease (WebMD 2005-2022). CBD is ingested, applied to the skin, or taken sublingually.

Hallucinogens

Hallucinogens are drugs that alter an athlete's perception or mood. Hallucinogens are made from plants, fungi, or synthetically (Drug Enforcement Agency 2022). Some of the more common street drugs are MDMA, LSD, mushrooms, and salvia.

MDMA

MDMA is short for methylenedioxymethamphetamine and goes by the slang term *ecstasy*. This drug can enhance sensory perception, mental stimulation, and physical energy. It is addictive for some people and can cause muscle cramping, blurred vision, nausea, and chills (National Institute on Drug Abuse 2020).

LSD

LSD is a hallucinogenic drug that has no medical use. LSD is ingested. A sugar cube, a tablet, or a small piece of paper are ways that LSD is distributed. This hallucinogenic drug distorts space and time. An athlete who has used LSD can have flashbacks several months after not taking it (Drug Enforcement Agency 2020a).

Mushrooms

Mushroom is the street name for a hallucinogenic drug made from psilocybin-bearing mushrooms. The mushrooms are dried and eaten, causing the effect. An athlete can hallucinate or have a reaction like panic and psychosis.

Salvia

According to the Drug Enforcement Agency (2020b), salvia is an herb that is abused for its hallucinogenic effects. It can be chewed, smoked, or vaporized. Psychic effects, body distortions, object distortions, panic, laughter, paranoia, and hallucinations are some experiences of salvia use.

Designer Drugs

A designer drug is one in which the formulation of the synthetic ingredients create a potent substance (Anderson 2022). These drugs mimic the effect of illegal drugs, but their formulation changes frequently; thus, they are difficult to regulate (Anderson 2022).

Bath Salts

Bath salts is a designer drug made of synthetic cathinone. Cathinones are stimulates made from the khat plant. This drug inhibits neurotransmitters in the brain. The drug is inhaled, injected, smoked, swallowed, or used rectally (Puckey 2022). Effects of bath salts on one's mood can include lots of talking, increased sex drive, a rush, euphoria, increased wakefulness, hallucinations, and more empathy (Puckey 2022).

Side effects of use can include seizures, rapid heart rate, chest pain, diaphoresis (profuse sweating), high blood pressure, increased temperature, decreased appetite, and muscle spasms (Puckey 2022). High doses of bath salts can lead to psychiatric issues and violent behavior (Puckey 2022).

Spice

Spice or K2 is a designer drug that is a synthetic cannabinoid. The Drug Enforcement Agency (2022) says that most spice is made in Asia and smuggled to the United States. It is sold as incense. Spice is smoked or vaped or laced into other items for use. Short-term effects include rapid heart rate, increased blood pressure, hallucinations, anxiety, tingling, tremors, seizures, and unconsciousness. Long-term effects can include heart attacks and kidney injury.

Krokodil

This is synthetic opioid, so it causes sedation and pain relief. Krokodil is an injectable illegal drug (Drug Enforcement Agency 2019). Those who abuse it long-term may end up with skin appearing like that of a crocodile. Along with skin damage to blood vessels, thrombosis, blood clots, and amputations have been noted (Drug Enforcement Agency 2019).

PERFORMANCE-ENHANCING DRUGS

A performance-enhancing drug is one that an athlete believes will make them play better. An athlete may choose to use alcohol to calm down before a game. Some athletes may use cocaine to get fired up. Other athletes use steroids to increase muscle bulk. Regardless of the drug used to improve performance, its use is illegal. Most often, drugs do not enhance performance and may even cause death.

DMSO

After research on animals showed that **dimethyl sulfoxide (DMSO)** decreased healing time and wound swelling, veterinarians began using it as an anti-inflammatory agent. Some athletes have considered using DMSO to speed their return to participation after an injury. DMSO is absorbed quickly through the skin and leaves a garlicky taste in the mouth. It has never been approved for human use, but athletes have found ways of obtaining it. No human studies show that DMSO works, and the long-term side effects are unknown.

Ephedra

Ephedra was used for quite some time as a weight-loss drug. In sports where thinness and body weight needed to be controlled, athletes sometimes used it. Ephedra can cause health problems such as high blood pressure, heart attack, and strokes. In 2004, the Food and Drug Administration (FDA) banned the sale of supplements containing the drug.

Blood Doping

An athlete participating in an endurance event can benefit from having extra oxygen-carrying blood cells, and the more red blood cells they have, the better their oxygen-carrying ability. Based on that theory, an athlete may have blood drawn and stored while the body replaces the lost blood cells. They then inject the stored blood just before the event so that they have more red blood cells than usual. However, placing additional blood into an athlete's system can result in shock.

Anabolic Steroids

Anabolic steroids are hormones such as testosterone, the male hormone that is responsible for creating and maintaining male secondary sex characteristics. Physicians prescribe anabolic steroids to treat asthma, severe muscle injuries, and arthritis. Steroids have been used to combat the side effects of cancer, which may cause the whole body to atrophy. Athletes use anabolic steroids to build muscle.

? What Would You Do If . . .

Just before the start of an all-day wrestling tournament, a wrestler shows you a new product from the health food store—the latest fad. He drinks the green frothy substance before you have a chance to ask him what it is.

Androstenedione, often referred to as *andro*, is a steroid hormone that is used by some athletes looking for a competitive edge. Androstenedione increases testosterone production in men over a short time, usually an eight-hour period.

When athletes discovered that greater muscle mass could be obtained artificially, they began taking steroids to increase strength. Steroids are injected and ingested by a method called *stacking*, which means the athlete uses a combination of pills and injections to try to avoid the side effects caused by taking a single high dose all at once. However, side effects cannot be avoided. A man using anabolic steroids will experience the following side effects: acne, decreased testicular output, heart problems, cancer, addiction, enlarged breast tissue, mental illness, hair loss, weakened ligaments, decreased growth, violent behavior (roid rage), vascular problems, and impotence. In women who use anabolic steroids, side effects include deepening of the voice, addiction, cessation of the menstrual cycle, increased body and facial hair, and decreased body fat.

Steroid use is illegal in all competitions, including professional and Olympic competitions. Gold medals have been taken away from athletes who have used steroids. Asthmatics are allowed to use their inhalers, but drug testing boards regulate the amount of steroids allowed.

Human growth hormone (HGH) is a protein-based hormone used to facilitate muscle growth. HGH is sometimes prescribed by physicians when a child has a growth disorder. Sport organizations have banned HGH.

Gamma hydroxybutyrate (GHB) is often referred to as a *club drug* because it is a central nervous system depressant. When used with alcohol, it can incapacitate victims and prevent them from resisting sexual assault. Anabolic effects are associated with GHB because it can help synthesize protein and thus facilitate muscle building. A side effect of GHB use is seizure or coma (National Institute on Drug Abuse 2020).

Beta Blockers

Beta blockers can enhance an athlete's performance, especially in shooting sports. Being able to hold a gun steady is a clear advantage that these drugs bring. These have been banned for shooters.

Bromantan

Being mentally and physically sharp is a distinct advantage for any athlete. Bromantan is a stimulant that can provide this type of advantage. This drug was banned for competitors in 1997 (Gill 2017).

DRUG TESTING

As competition to be the best in sport increases, athletes and others are more susceptible to the lure of using drugs to enhance their performance. Drug testing is used widely by many athletic organizations, including the National Collegiate Athletic Association (NCAA), the Olympic Committee, and the NFL, who have listed specific banned substances. Drug testing is also used in the workplace of many health care facilities. It typically involves a urine test. Commonly tested drugs include steroids, stimulants, depressants, and marijuana.

As a member of the health care team, it is important to work collaboratively with physicians to understand the potential tests that will be prescribed. The algorithm in figure 33.7 presents the basic flow of screening tests that are typically performed in sports medicine. Although these tests are commonly used, far more specific tests will be prescribed based on the preliminary findings of the more familiar tests. Understanding the type of test and the reason it is being prescribed helps ATs communicate with the physician and patient more effectively.

Cleary, Abdenour, and Pavlovich (2022) explained the process involved in drug testing. The school or organization needs to decide which drug testing method will be used. There are five methods: urine, blood, hair, saliva, and sweat. Each method has advantages and disadvantages, so determine which one best meets the requirements for the organization. Urine testing is easy to do, but the specimen has to be taken in the presence of an eyewitness so that no masking agent or introduction of other fluids occurs. The NCAA and U.S. professional sports use urine testing as their method of choice.

The person collecting the specimen has to be trained in those procedures. The area where the specimen is collected has to be clean and inspected. The beaker for specimen collection is selected at random by the athlete. The urine is divided into two vials for testing. The athlete, the person who collects the specimen, and the witness must sign and document the collection and chain of custody. The specimen must be secured, sealed, and shipped to an approved laboratory (see table 33.2 for specimen protocol).

At-home drug tests can be purchased in a local pharmacy, and they test urine for illegal or prescription medications. The AT may use them if they need to monitor athletes who they believe are using illegal or prescription medications. A positive test requires that the sample be sealed and sent to a laboratory for confirmation.

Masking Agents

Some athletes may try to use a masking agent to cover up an illegal substance in their specimen. Examples of masking agents are probenecid, finasteride, diuretics, and ketoconazole (Cleary, Abdenour, and Pavlovich 2022).

Testing Results

When a drug test comes back positive for a banned substance, the athlete has a consequence. There is a progressive disciplinary plan for those who continually fail a drug test. Ultimately, the athlete will be removed from competition.

OVER-THE-COUNTER (OTC) DRUGS

Over-the-counter (OTC) drugs can be purchased at a store without a prescription. The forms of

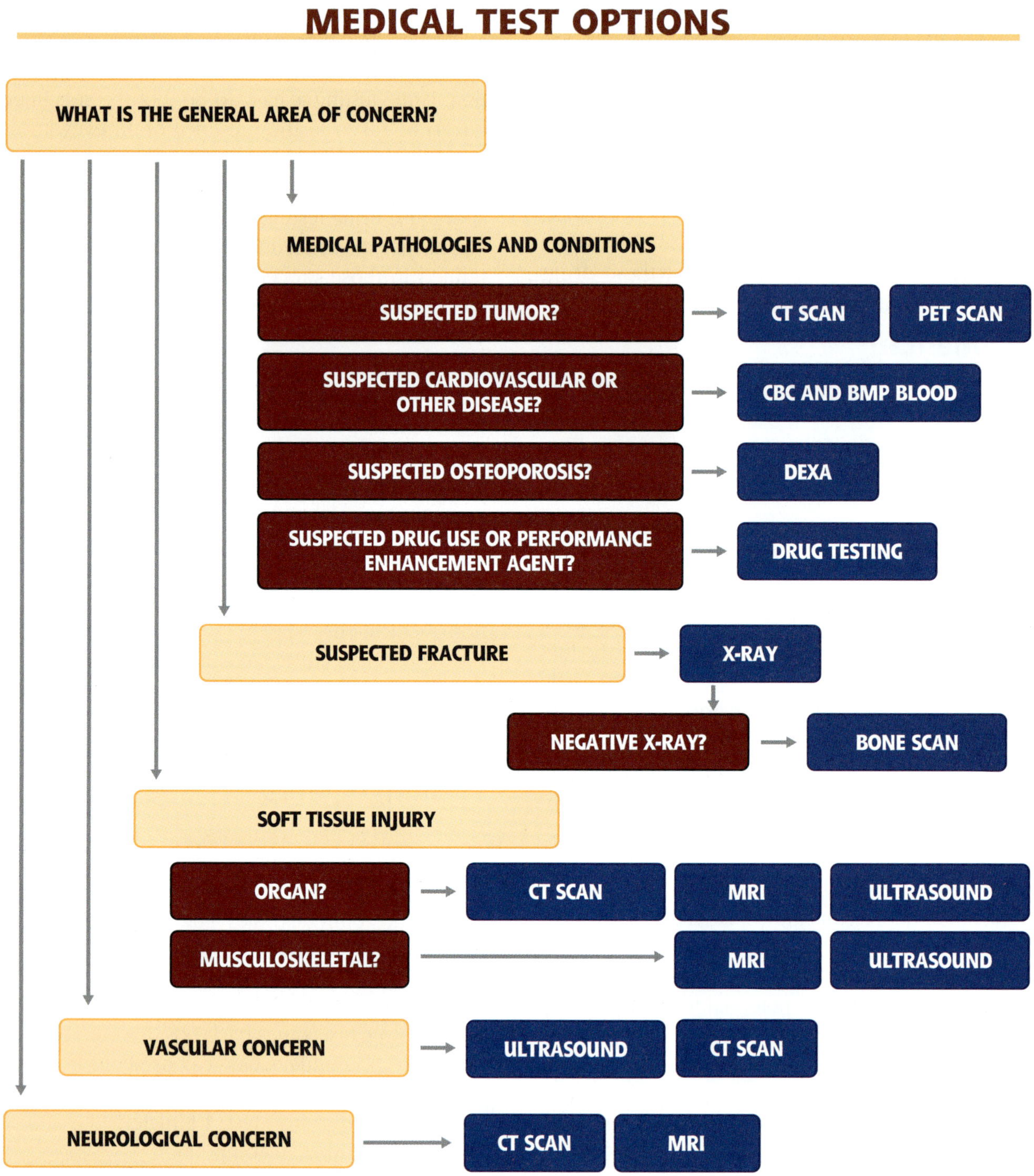

Figure 33.7 Medical test options.

medication include laxatives, aspirin, cold medications, vitamins, eye drops, antifungals, first aid cream, allergy medications, and medications for upset stomach. Many of these drugs required a prescription at first, but over time proved to be safe enough to be made readily available. This does not mean that OTC drugs are safe for any use, since they can cause illness when used improperly. It is imperative to follow the instructions on the label for safe and effective use of OTC drugs.

Table 33.2 Specimen Protocol

Phase of the protocol	Description of phase
Collection station	Use of the exclusive marshalling area and restroom for specimen collection is limited to the collector, institutional representative, and selected athletes. Only food or drink provided by the institution is allowed in the area.
Specimen beaker	The athlete reports to the testing area with photo identification, signs in, selects a random beaker, and applies a specific barcode to the container.
Specimen collection	The collector must witness the athlete urinating in the specimen beaker. The use of the restroom must be exclusive to the testing area at all times during the testing process.
Viability of the specimen	To ensure that the specimen concentration has not been tampered with, a normal urine specimen should have the following characteristics: • Specific gravity ≥1.005; samples <1.005 are not sent for analysis. • Temperature: 90 °F to 100 °F (32 °C to 37.7 °C) within 4 min of voiding. • pH: 4.5-8.0 • Urinary creatine ≥20 mg/dL
Dividing the sample	A viable specimen is split into A and B samples and poured into separate vials by the collector. It is then secured for shipping. The athlete witnesses the process of dividing the specimen and preparing the samples for shipment. If a specimen is unacceptable, the athlete must remain in the approved testing area until she provides a viable specimen.
Chain of custody	The chain of custody is maintained by providing the athlete with documentation regarding the testing logistics, including the specimen identification number and the DCO's name.
Shipment of sample	Signatures from athlete, collector, and the institutional witness certify the accuracy of the collection process. Samples are shipped to an approved laboratory for testing.

Reprinted by permission from M.A. Cleary, T.E. Abdenour, and M. Pavlovich, *Clinical Pharmacology in Athletic Training* (Champaign, IL: Human Kinetics, 2022), 18.

DRUG ABUSE

People are living longer, partly because of the medications available now. Unfortunately, many people have the false notion that medication can solve any problem. Physicians are prescribing more medications, and recreational drugs are readily available. Some athletes choose to use drugs because they think their athletic performance will improve. Students pressure other students to use so they are not alone, and many students and athletes see professionals or their parents using drugs and copy that behavior. Athletes who use drugs may appear to enjoy themselves and seem more relaxed because the drugs reduce inhibitions. Ultimately, however, people who use drugs can develop short- and long-term health problems. Remember, more students and athletes choose not to use drugs than those who do, and the benefits of abstaining are greater than any benefits to athletic performance.

The Real World

I was working with an impressionable athlete who made a habit of jumping from fad to fad, looking for the most up-to-date methods for improving his fitness. He indicated that he had constant diarrhea but could not pinpoint a reason. I had him write down everything that he ate and all the supplements that he took. I compared all the foods and supplements and found that he was overdosing on vitamin C. Once he stopped taking large doses, his diarrhea went away. I recommended that he see a dietitian to help him develop a proper diet, but unfortunately, he did not heed my advice. He decided to simply try another new dietary fad.

Anonymous

For high school athletics, the banned drugs may differ, but prohibition tends to revolve around the following classifications:

1. Stimulants to heighten alertness and enhance reaction time
2. Anabolic agents (anabolic steroids) to build muscle
3. Diuretics to excrete fluids to lose weight
4. Peptide hormones to gain strength and build muscle

These drug classifications are banned because they give one athlete an unfair advantage over another or because of negative health-related side effects. Usually, they are banned for both these reasons.

An athlete should check the banned substance list before taking any medication, even over-the-counter ones. The NCAA, the World Anti-Doping Agency, and the U.S. Anti-Doping Agency have banned substances lists that can be found on their websites.

SAFETY IN DISTRIBUTION OF MEDICATIONS

A physician prescribes drugs based on a person's weight, sex, age, pregnancy status, known organ health, and known allergies. It is imperative that those who take medications follow through by taking medications as prescribed, reporting any side effects, and not saving medications for the next illness. Because drugs are specific to the individual, sharing drugs can cause an overdose or other side effects.

The AT will be designated to give medications prescribed by a physician while the student is at practice or an event. The school should have a distribution policy, which should be followed to protect both the athletes and the AT. A typical policy includes a prescription, permission to administer, rules for storing the medication, directions for how to administer it, and directions for how to receive new medication as it runs low.

The AT needs to see a copy of the prescription to ensure that it is properly used and that the precautions are fully understood. If the athlete is a minor, the parent of the athlete must provide written permission for the AT to dispense the medication. This permission must be given annually. All medications must be stored in a locked cabinet so that only the AT has access to them. The medication must be clearly labeled for the particular athlete. The container where the medication is to be stored must have a lock. Many schools require that the AT document the administration of the medication, which will include time, amount given, a witness, the AT's signature, and the date. Finally, the plan will include contacting the parent when there is a week's worth of medication left so new medication will arrive in a timely fashion.

When traveling into another state or country with prescription medications, the AT must know the law. In the AT's home state, they may be able to distribute medication, but in another state they may be restricted. In other countries, it is especially important to know the rules. Having CBD oil, like Britney Greiner did in 2022, could place the athlete or the AT in jail. Before traveling overseas, check with the Department of Homeland Security, the U.S. Department of State, and the U.S. Food and Drug Administration for more detail about which medications are permitted.

PROPER DISPOSAL OF MEDICATIONS

When medications are no longer needed, it is necessary to dispose of them. The simplest solution might appear to be to flush medications down the toilet, but this practice may contaminate our lakes and streams. The FDA has recommended that certain medications can be safely flushed. Go to the FDA website and check out the list of medications that can be flushed.

Some medications can be disposed of in the regular trash (see figure 33.8). The U.S. Food and Drug Administration (2018a) recommends the following four steps:

1. Remove the medication from its original container and place it in dirt, coffee grounds, or cat litter.
2. Place all the material into a sealed bag or container.
3. Throw the bag or container in the trash.
4. Scratch out all personal information on the prescription bottle before discarding it.

For additional information on how to dispose of medications, speak directly with a pharmacist or someone at your local police station.

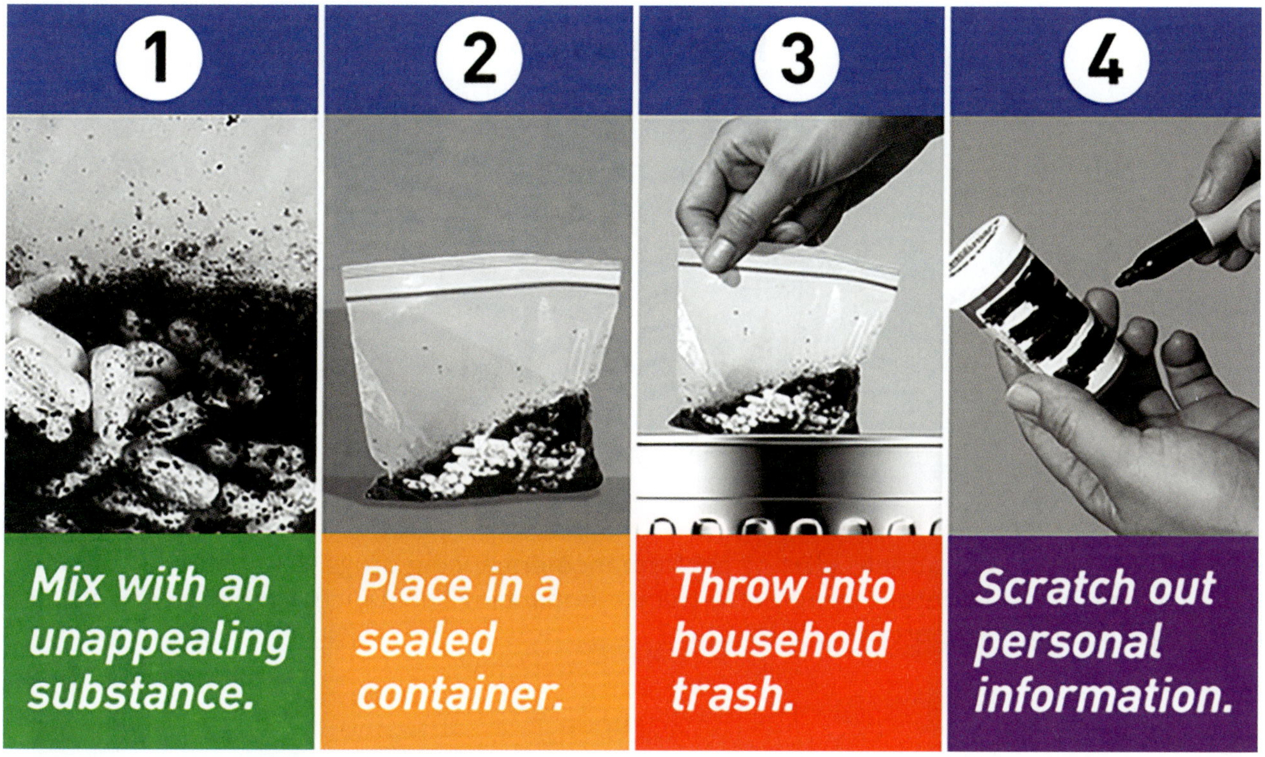
1
Mix with an unappealing substance.
2
Place in a sealed container.
3
Throw into household trash.
4
Scratch out personal information.

Figure 33.8 How to dispose of medication properly.
Reprinted from U.S. Food & Drug Administration (2018).

Summary

Athletes use drugs, which may be therapeutic or recreational, for a variety of reasons. Therapeutic drugs assist an athlete returning from an injury or recovering from an illness or to prevent illness during competition. Over-the-counter drugs can be purchased to treat problems such as headaches and colds. Recreational drugs have no real health value—they are used during social occasions and for the feelings they create.

Some athletes use a drug to improve their performance, only to find out that the improvement is a myth. Caffeine, anabolic steroids, and oxygen are commonly used as performance-enhancing substances. Athletes who use performance-enhancing drugs may see an improvement in their performance, but the side effects and long-term problems outweigh any benefits.

The side effects of all drugs must be considered. The team physician should be consulted to determine proper use and dosage of a drug. Drugs can become habit forming, and addiction can be dealt with through various programs depending on the type of drug involved. Drug testing is commonplace among elite athletes. Olympic and international competitors are tested for banned drugs on a regular basis.

Key Terms

Define the following terms found in this chapter:

- anabolic steroids
- androstenedione
- beta-adrenergic drugs
- dimethyl sulfoxide (DMSO)
- drug
- effective dose
- ephedra
- gamma hydroxybutyrate (GHB)
- generic name drug
- half-life
- human growth hormone (HGH)
- leukoplakia
- local steroid
- nonsteroidal anti-inflammatory drug (NSAID)
- over-the-counter (OTC) drug
- recreational drug
- steady state
- therapeutic drug
- trade name

As an AT, you suspect an athlete is using performance-enhancing drugs. What steps must you take if you realize an athlete is using performance-enhancing substances? What guidelines or policies require you to report this use of drugs?

To access supplementary material for this chapter, including the Understanding Check worksheet, vocabulary quizzes, extension activities, and chapter-specific resources and forms, visit the web resource: http://ancillaries.humankinetics.com/FundamentalsOfAthleticTrainingAndSportsMedicine5E

chapter 34

Nutrition and Weight Management

Objectives

After completing this chapter, the student will be able to do the following:

- Understand metabolism.
- Understand the basic food groups.
- Understand the role that nutrition plays in a healthy body.
- Design a diet for an athlete.
- Understand how to read a food label.
- Understand that food misconceptions are common among athletes.

The body's fuel is food, and its energy system is known as **metabolism**. Food that can be broken down by the body for use consists mainly of carbohydrates, protein, and fat. Other nutrients include vitamins, minerals, and water. The heat-producing, or energy-producing, value of food is measured in calories, and if the body does not require all the metabolized calories for growth, maintenance, or heat, it stores them, yielding weight gain. If the number of calories brought in is less than what the body needs, the athlete will lose weight. When the body needs energy, it uses carbohydrates first, then fat, and then protein or the body's muscles—people who are starving lose muscle because the body needs it for fuel.

Metabolism is the sum of the chemical changes that take place as the body functions. The body's metabolism can change depending on activity level and sex. Men and teenagers normally have higher metabolisms, as do people who exercise. An athlete's metabolism slows as they get older.

The basal metabolic rate (BMR) is the number of calories needed to maintain current body weight when the body is at rest. A body at rest burns calories for breathing, circulation, cell production, and digestion (Garnet Health 2016). The BMR is calculated based on age, height, weight, and gender.

MAJOR NUTRIENTS

Nutrients are substances that the body uses in metabolism. They include water, vitamins, minerals, carbohydrate, fat, and protein.

Water

Water is an essential component of the diet and makes up about 57% of total body weight. Water is necessary for proper body functioning. It is beneficial to kidney function, excretion, chemical reactions throughout the body, sweating, blood flow, and joint lubrication. Water comes from the faucet, in bottles, or in various products such as soda, sport drinks, juice drinks, coffee, and tea. When an athlete is competing, the AT must remember that most athletes do not drink enough water to replace what they lose in sweat. Also, an athlete's thirst level is a poor indicator of how much water is needed to replace sweat.

When an athlete fails to replace the fluids lost through sweating or other normal body processes, they can become dehydrated. Signs and symptoms of dehydration include headache, dry mouth, dizziness, fatigue, and thirst. Another indicator that a person is dehydrated is the color of urine (see figure 34.1). The urine should be clear; a bright-yellow color indicates dehydration. Mild dehydration occurs when an athlete loses 2% or more of body weight.

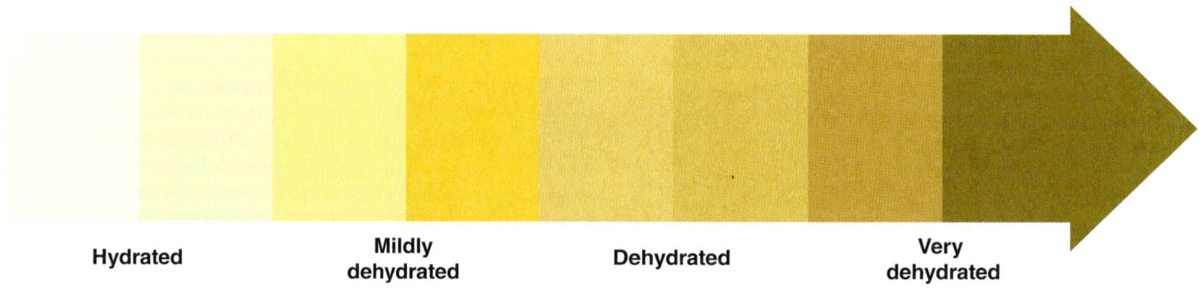

Figure 34.1 Urine color test.

Adapted from CDC (2017); NSW Health (2024).

FLUID REPLACEMENT

According to the 2019 Korey Stringer Institute (KSI) statement for exercise and fluid replacements, the AT needs to determine sweat rates for athletes. This involves the following:

- Check the hydration level of the athlete preexercise using a urine color chart.
- Weigh the athlete nude before exercise.
- Have the athlete exercise for one hour at the same or similar intensity level and conditions for a typical practice.
- The athlete is to refrain from drinking fluids during this workout.
- Weigh the athlete nude after this exercise.
- Calculate the difference before and after the workout.
- Every 2.2 pounds lost equals one liter of sweat loss.
- The calculation is: preexercise body weight − postexercise body weight = weight loss
- Weight loss/2.2 = L/hour
- The athlete should drink that amount of water during their workout to prevent dehydration.
- Rehydration should occur within two hours of exercise completion.

Adapted from Korey Stringer Institute (2019).

Even this small amount of dehydration can result in poor athletic performance.

Wrestlers are notorious for cutting weight to get into a particular weight class. Unfortunately, they usually cut the weight over a short time, losing only water weight and becoming dehydrated. This restriction of water and the water-weight loss will cause the wrestler to be fatigued and much less effective. Wrestlers who want to lose weight need to be supervised by a dietitian, and they must still drink eight glasses of water per day.

Vitamins

Vitamins help the body perform specific functions by regulating metabolic processes. Vitamins are found in all foods, so people who eat a balanced diet get all the vitamins they need (see table 34.1). An athlete who eats improperly, however, will need to obtain vitamins through supplements to meet the daily needs for proper body functioning.

Vitamins are either fat soluble or water soluble. Fat-soluble vitamins include A, D, E, and K. Water-soluble vitamins include B complex (B_1, B_2, B_{12}) and C. Fat-soluble vitamins dissolve in fat before being used by the body, whereas water-soluble vitamins dissolve in water before being used by the body. Excess fat-soluble vitamins are stored in the liver, and excess water-soluble vitamins are urinated out of the body.

What Would You Do If . . .

You are hauling a 10-gallon (38 L) watercooler out to football practice. The head coach stops you, removes the lid, and pours in a container of creatine. You are shocked. The coach responds by saying, "If we are going to win a state title, we need a little extra advantage." He insists that you bring him the watercoolers every day.

Minerals

Minerals are inorganic chemical elements necessary for building bones and muscles, conducting nerve impulses, and maintaining normal metabolism and heart function. Minerals are found in all foods, and the athlete does not require a supplement unless their diet is unbalanced. The incidence of some diseases has been reduced after scientists added minerals to commonly used products. For example, fluoride is added to water to prevent tooth decay, and calcium is added to orange juice to help bolster its intake for those who do not like dairy products. Bone strength is improved by the added calcium for growing athletes as well as the prevention of osteoporosis as athletes age. See table 34.2 for a list of common minerals and their sources.

Table 34.1 Vitamin Overview

Vitamin	Type	Food source	Deficiency
A	Fat soluble	Butter, cheese, carrots, green leafy vegetables	Impaired vision, eye inflammation, blindness
B_1	Water soluble	Whole grains, legumes, meat products	Weakness, confusion, muscle atrophy
B_2	Water soluble	Green vegetables, milk, eggs, whole grains	Dry, cracking skin; skin irritation
B_6	Water soluble	Meat, whole grains, legumes, green leafy vegetables	Dry, cracking skin; skin irritation; anemia
B_{12}	Water soluble	Meat, fish, eggs, milk	Anemia, neurological disorders
C	Water soluble	Fruits, green vegetables, potatoes, tomatoes	Immune system deficiencies, bleeding gums, dry skin
D	Fat soluble	Dairy products, fish oils, sunlight	Bone loss, rickets
E	Fat soluble	Nuts, vegetable oil, whole grains, butter, green leafy vegetables	Neurological disorders (deficiencies are very rare)
K	Fat soluble	Green leafy vegetables	Bleeding

WATER OR SPORTS DRINK?

	Beverage type	
Ingredients	**Water**	**Sports drinks**
Flavor	Lack of flavor may prevent fluid intake	A drink with a flavor preference encourages fluid intake
Carbohydrate	Lacks ability to provide energy	Helps maintain carbohydrate oxidation
Sodium	Provides no sodium	Helps maintain blood glucose levels and keeps fluids within the system
Potassium	Provides no electrolytes	Helps maintain electrolyte balance
Protein	Lacks protein so no exercise performance	May improve exercise performance

Adapted from Korey Stringer Institute (2019); Rowlands, Kopetschny, and Badenhorst (2022).

Table 34.2 Mineral Overview

Mineral	Food source	Deficiency
Calcium	Dairy products, spinach, almonds	Decreased bone density, tooth formation
Iron	Beef, eggs, broccoli	Anemia
Magnesium	Nuts, beans, seeds, legumes	Muscle weakness, fatigue, cramping
Phosphorus	Dairy products, meats	Anemia
Potassium	Raisins, bananas, peas, beef	Muscle cramping, heart problems
Selenium	Nuts (Brazil), tuna, beef, eggs	Heart disease, hypothyroidism, weakened immune system
Sodium	Salt	Hyponatremia (with endurance events over 4 hours, coupled with high volume of water intake)
Zinc	Oysters, fortified breakfast cereal, almonds, cheese	Growth retardation, loss of appetite, impaired immune function

Carbohydrate

Carbohydrate is the main fuel source for the body. Carbohydrate digestion begins in the mouth when it is mixed with saliva secreted by the salivary glands. Nutritionists recommend that carbohydrates make up 40% to 50% of the daily diet and that athletes get 55% to 60% of their calories from carbohydrates. See examples of carbohydrates in the sidebar.

Fiber is the indigestible material found in foods high in carbohydrates. Fiber stimulates the intestines, so diets high in fiber reduce constipation and colon disease. A list of high-fiber carbohydrates is found in the sidebar.

Many people, including athletes, restrict carbohydrate intake to lose weight. Many foods that are high in carbohydrate have extremely high nutritional value, and greatly reducing them in a diet may lead to other health problems. Most people get plenty of protein if they eat a balanced diet. There is speculation that decreasing the intake of carbohydrates and increasing the intake of protein and fat may increase cholesterol and the risk of heart disease.

When an athlete eats, it takes about 36 hours for the food to be processed and made into a stool and exit the body. During the transition from food to stool, nutrients and fluids are absorbed. Stool consistency has seven types according to the Bristol Stool Chart (see figure 34.2).

CARBOHYDRATES

Simple

- Honey
- Fruit
- Soda
- Sport drinks
- Candy and sweets

Complex

- Bread
- Potatoes
- Bagels
- Cereal
- Beans
- Vegetables
- Nuts and seeds
- Pasta

HIGH-FIBER CARBOHYDRATES

- Beans
- Vegetables
- Nuts and seeds
- Fruits
- Lima beans
- Peas
- Almonds
- Prunes
- Kidney beans
- Corn
- Sunflower seeds
- Apples
- Broccoli
- Bananas
- Coconuts

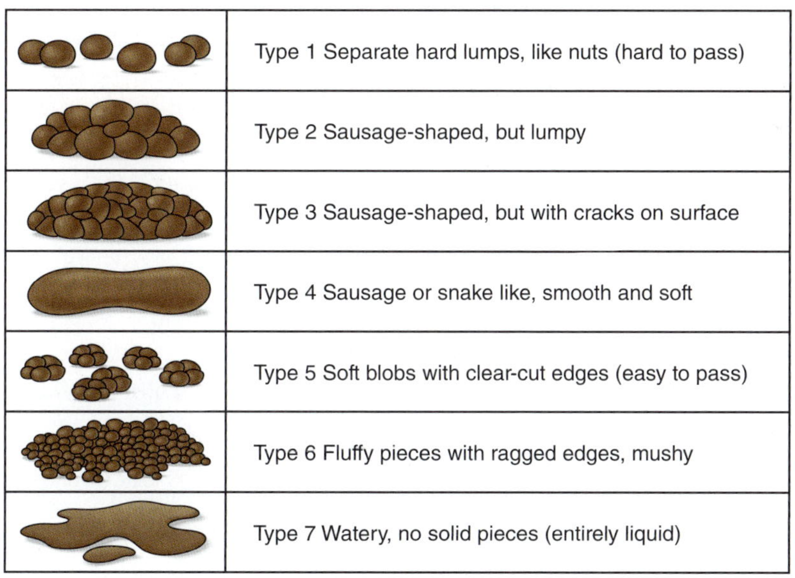

Figure 34.2 Bristol stool chart.
Adapted from WebMD.

Stool color can change depending on the athlete's diet and liquid bile. Most stools are brown, which is perfectly normal. Green is typical in those who eat a diet high in green vegetables. The color red can be associated with eating beets or eating foods with red food coloring. If a stool is bright red, it means there is an active bleed somewhere in the large intestine (WebMD 2020). Black stools can be a sign of bleeding in the stomach or small intestine. Some medications and iron supplements can also cause a black stool (WebMD 2020).

Fat

Fat is a necessary component of a healthy diet. For example, the female reproductive system cannot function properly without a certain amount of fat, and the body cannot support a pregnancy without enough body fat. In addition to being a source of energy, fat helps cells function, is required for the metabolism of some vitamins, and helps maintain normal body shape. Dietary fat can be classified as saturated or unsaturated.

> **What Would You Do If . . .**
>
> The latest fad diet is eating a single food: cabbage. The athletes mention that they can eat cabbage any way they want but nothing else is on the menu. They rave about how much weight they have lost, and you begin to think, "Maybe I should try this diet."

Saturated fat is found primarily in animal products such as meat, chicken skin, lard, milk, cheese, cream, butter, some oils (e.g., coconut), and chocolate. Unsaturated fat is generally found in plant products such as soybeans, nuts, and some oils (e.g., olive, canola, peanut). Although fat can make food taste better, too much may contribute to an unhealthy lifestyle and lead to illness. Heart disease, high blood pressure, diabetes, some cancers, and obesity have all been linked to excessive fat intake, especially saturated fat. An athlete needs to review the amount and kinds of fat they are eating and determine if they can improve their diet.

Cholesterol is a fatlike substance produced in the body to perform essential cellular functions. Some cholesterol is not essential for life and is stored in the blood vessels. Cholesterol accumulation on a vessel wall can close off the vessel over time and lead to a heart attack.

Cholesterol levels in the body increase when more saturated fat is consumed. Many people avoid foods with cholesterol as a way of decreasing cho-

EXAMPLES OF FAT

Unsaturated fat

- Fish
- Margarine
- Vegetable oil
- Olive oil
- Fish oil
- Peanut oil
- Nuts

Saturated fat

- Meat
- Chicken skin
- Lard
- Whole milk
- Cheese
- Some oils (coconut and palm)
- Chocolate
- Butter
- Processed cheese
- Ice cream
- Cream cheese
- Cocoa butter

High cholesterol

- Brains
- Kidneys
- Liver
- Egg yolk
- Cheese
- Lobster
- Dark turkey meat
- Butter
- Pork
- Ice cream
- Lamb
- Veal
- Cream
- Salmon
- Shrimp

lesterol in the blood vessels, so many food manufacturers label foods as *cholesterol-free*. Cholesterol occurs in all products containing animal fat—it is found in egg yolks, milk, cream, cheese, butter, and all red meats. See the sidebar for examples of foods that are sources of fat.

Cholesterol is divided into two types: good and bad. The bad cholesterol (low density) can clog your arteries and cause heart disease. Good cholesterol (high density) can be helpful to your body. When bad cholesterol levels are high and good cholesterols levels are low, you are at serious risk for heart conditions.

Trans fat, or trans-fatty acid, is created when hydrogen is added to vegetable oil so it is more solid. Many foods are fried in trans fat, but the consequences are harmful. Trans fat raises bad cholesterol levels and lowers good cholesterol levels. Ingesting trans fats also increases the risk of developing type 2 diabetes. There is no safe level of trans fat to ingest.

Protein

The basic components of protein are **amino acids**. The body uses amino acids to form new tissues and repair damaged ones. Teenagers are growing and must make sure they are getting enough protein so that their growth is not slowed; they require more protein than adults do. Protein is found in meat, beans, nuts, dairy products, fish, and eggs. Protein is the last source of energy used by the body. Anywhere from 15% to 20% of an athlete's daily diet should be protein. A list of protein sources is found in the sidebar, Examples of Protein.

Protein supplements are sold for those who may not get enough protein in their diet. Manufacturers of protein supplements advertise that their products build muscle. However, high amounts of protein in an athlete's diet can lead to higher body fat (because protein-bearing foods usually have a lot of fat), loss of calcium from bones, and dehydration.

HEALTHY DIET

Proper nutrition is vital to a healthy life. Many leading causes of death are related to how we eat. According to the United States Department of Agriculture (USDA) dietary guidelines (see the sidebar, Dietary Guidelines), a healthy diet emphasizes fruits, vegetables, whole grains, and fat-free or low-fat dairy products; includes lean meats, poultry, fish, beans, eggs, and nuts; and is low in saturated fat, trans fat, cholesterol, salt (sodium), and added sugar.

A balanced diet provides all the nutrients necessary to remain healthy. It should contain portions from each food group. The food groups identified by the USDA include grains, fruits, vegetables, meat and beans, milk, and oils. The quantities of the food groups are identified in MyPlate (figure 34.3 and table 34.3); note that a higher intake of grains, fruits, and vegetables is recommended. The MyPlate

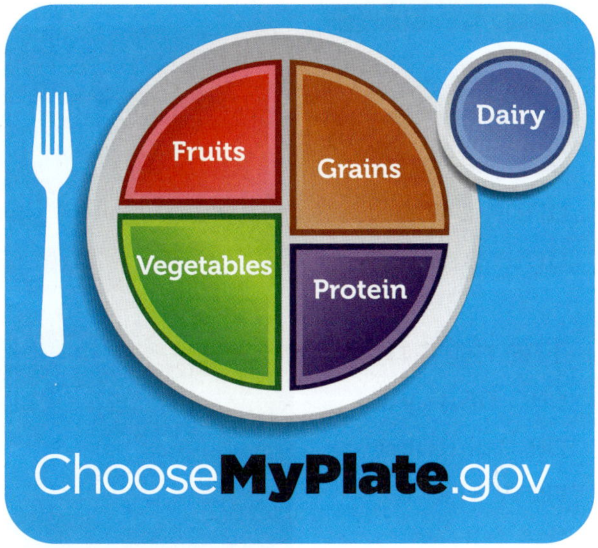

Figure 34.3 MyPlate.
USDA's Center for Nutrition Policy and Promotion.

Table 34.3 MyPlate Daily Servings for 2,000-Calorie Diet

Groups	Daily servings
Fruit group	4 servings or 2 cups
Vegetable group	5 servings or 2.5 cups
Grain group	6 oz (170 g)*
Meat and beans group	5.5 oz (156 g)
Milk group	3 cups
Oils	24 g or 6 tsp
Discretionary calories	No more than 267 calories

*3 oz (85 g) from whole grains

plan will be different based on age, height, weight, sex, and physical activity. Because different cultures place varying emphases on food intake, other food guidelines exist. The CANFIT organization has designed an example of the Native American food pyramid, which can be found online by searching that topic or visiting the Department of Agriculture website. See figure 34.4 for 10 tips to a great plate.

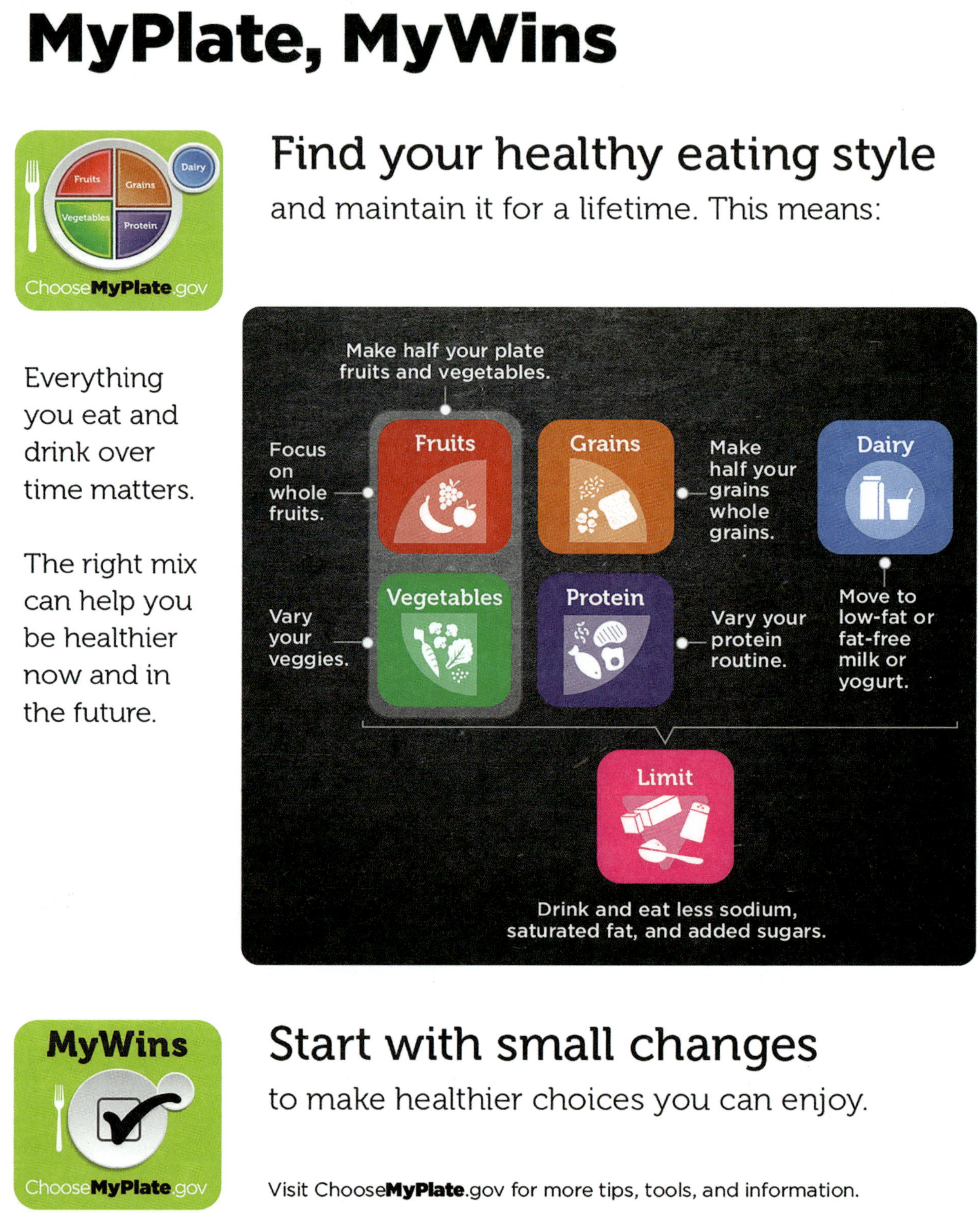

MyPlate, MyWins
Fruits
Grains
Dairy
Vegetables
Protein
ChooseMyPlate.gov
Find your healthy eating style
and maintain it for a lifetime. This means:
Everything you eat and drink over time matters.
The right mix can help you be healthier now and in the future.
Make half your plate fruits and vegetables.
Focus on whole fruits.
Fruits
Grains
Make half your grains whole grains.
Dairy
Vary your veggies.
Vegetables
Protein
Vary your protein routine.
Move to low-fat or fat-free milk or yogurt.
Limit
Drink and eat less sodium, saturated fat, and added sugars.
MyWins
ChooseMyPlate.gov
Start with small changes
to make healthier choices you can enjoy.
Visit ChooseMyPlate.gov for more tips, tools, and information.

Figure 34.4 10 tips for a great plate.

USDA's Center for Nutrition Policy and Promotion.

EXAMPLES OF PROTEIN

High protein

- Beef
- Chicken
- Fish
- Turkey
- Lamb
- Veal
- Pork

Medium protein

- Regular yogurt
- Greek yogurt
- Pinto beans
- Dried peas
- Soy nuts
- Cottage cheese
- Scallops

Low protein

- Seeds
- Nuts
- Cheese
- Milk
- Green peas
- Quinoa
- Eggs
- Lentils
- Most beans

DIETARY GUIDELINES

Key recommendations from the USDA dietary guidelines include the following for adults:

The recommended calory intake is 1,600 to 2,400 calories for females and 2,000 to 3,000 for males.

	1,600 calories	2,000 calories	2,400 calories	3,000 calories
Vegetables (cups/day)	2	2.5	3	4
Fruits (cups/day)	1.5	2	2	2.5
Grains (ounces/day)	5	6	8	10
Dairy (cups/day)	3	3	3	3
Protein (ounces/day)	5	5.5	6.5	7
Oils (grams/day)	22	27	31	44

From U.S. Department of Health and Human Services and U.S. Department of Agriculture (2020-2025).

UNDERSTANDING FOOD NUTRITION LABELS

Most people do not pay close attention to what they eat, but the Food and Drug Administration (FDA) requires nutrition labeling. The label provides a quick look at what the product contains so one can make a decision on the nutrient value. The label can be found on the back or side of the package. In 2020, the FDA made changes to the label to make it easier for consumers to understand (figure 34.5). When reading a label, it is important to understand the following items:

- Number of servings in the container
- Serving size
- Number of calories based on one serving size
- Amount of fat per serving and the percentage of it for a daily diet (based on an adult 2,000-calorie diet)

Nutrition Facts	
8 servings per container	
Serving size	**2/3 cup (55g)**
Amount per 2/3 cup	
Calories	**230**
	% Daily Value*
Total Fat 8g	**12%**
Saturated Fat 1g	**5%**
Trans Fat 0g	
Cholesterol 0mg	**0%**
Sodium 160mg	**7%**
Total Carbohydrate 37g	**12%**
Dietary Fiber 4g	**14%**
Total Sugars 1g	
Added Sugars 0g	
Protein 3g	
Vitamin D 2mcg	10%
Calcium 260mg	20%
Iron 8mg	45%
Potassium 235mg	6%

*The % Daily Value (DV) tells you how much a nutrient in a serving of food contributes to a daily diet. 2,000 calories a day is used for general nutrition advice.

Figure 34.5 The new nutrition label.
From U.S. Food and Drug Administration (2020).

- Amount of sugar added to the food per serving and the percentage of it for a daily diet
- Nutrients listed, such as vitamin D, calcium, iron, and potassium, and their percentages of the daily diet

Ideally, the athletic diet should have little or no added sugar and be low in saturated fat. Food labels make it easier for athletes to take control of what they eat.

CALORIC BALANCE

For the body to maintain a specific weight, the calories ingested should match the calories burned through daily activity and exercise. If an athlete wishes to gain or lose weight, the **caloric balance** will need to be adjusted. With weight loss, for example, the athlete will need to increase the calories burned, decrease the calories ingested, or, as suggested by the Cleveland Clinic (2022), both.

What Would You Do If . . .

In the locker room, a swimmer accidentally drops her purse. All the contents fall out onto the floor. As you politely help her pick up her things, you notice she has some opened containers of laxatives and diet pills.

Weight Loss

People who need to lose weight should follow the Centers for Disease Control and Prevention (2022) guidelines for weight loss. These guidelines state that 150 minutes per week of moderate-intensity physical activity will provide modest weight loss. It is essential that people looking to lose weight also restrict their caloric intake to a moderate level. Severe limitation of calories will not be more effective than moderate restriction. Athletes should consult with a physician before engaging in a weight-loss program.

Weight Gain

People looking to gain weight should have the goal of increasing their muscle mass; gaining more fat should not be the goal. No more than 2 pounds (1 kg) per week should be gained. To increase muscle mass, resistance training and conditioning of the muscles should be performed along with a slight increase in calorie consumption. With more resistance training, an athlete will need slightly more protein in their diet.

Obesity

Obesity is defined as an excessive level of body fat as determined by a person's body mass index (BMI). A person's BMI can be calculated using the following formula: BMI = [weight (lb) ÷ height (in.)^2] × 703. An adult who has a BMI of 30 or higher is considered obese. Obesity is a risk factor for many problems and is associated with higher cholesterol levels, hypertension, kidney disease, joint problems, diabetes, lung diseases, cancer, heart disease, and early death. Obesity is usually caused by a combination of factors, including heredity, overeating, and lack of physical activity.

A tendency toward obesity can begin at birth because of genetic factors. Moreover, a child born to obese parents is likely to pick up their habits and also become obese. Overeating means that an athlete ingests more calories than the body uses, and the additional calories are stored as fat in the body.

Many people are active in their teenage and college years. Once an athlete takes a job and starts a family, it becomes difficult to maintain the same level of physical activity. The decrease in physical activity coupled with the same eating habits yields weight gain. Exercise must be a priority for athletes who have stopped playing sports if they want to avoid gaining weight.

People are born with a certain number of fat cells. As they continue to eat and gain stored fat, the fat cells increase in size until they can hold no more, and then more fat cells are produced. Once a fat cell is produced, it does not go away. A weight-loss diet will cause the fat cells to shrink but not go away. People have undergone liposuction to have their fat cells sucked out, but eating habits do not change because of liposuction. People can come home with a body that appears new only to go back to their old eating habits, which will give them their old body back.

Fat is deposited in genetically predetermined areas. In other words, no one can control where the extra calories are deposited or where fat will be burned off with exercise. In women, fat is likely to be deposited in the hips, breasts, abdomen, and thighs. In men, it is likely to be deposited in the abdomen, chest, and thighs.

In some sports, obesity is not an issue. For instance, football requires several large players on the line. In wrestling, the various weight classes will accommodate the obese wrestler. Shot-putters, hammer throwers, and sumo wrestlers all tend to be large and sometimes obese.

! RED FLAGS

Refer the athlete to a physician in the following circumstances:

- They lose a lot of weight quickly.
- They gain a lot of weight quickly.
- They fatigue earlier than other athletes.
- You suspect an eating disorder.
- They are dizzy or lightheaded.

SPORT NUTRITION

ATs are frequently asked what types of foods an athlete should eat to be the best. The answer is simple: Eat a well-balanced meal, as suggested by MyPlate. Balanced meals provide all the nutrition requirements to be healthy and perform well. When designing a program, the AT and dietitian need to know if the athlete wants to gain, lose, or maintain weight.

The AT and dietitian can develop a plan that will ensure all nutrition needs are met based on a physical assessment. An athlete trying to gain weight will be placed on a diet in which the number of calories eaten exceeds the energy expended. An athlete trying to lose weight will be placed on a diet that supplies fewer calories than the amount of energy expended. The athlete's weight loss should not exceed an average of 2 pounds (1 kg) a week. They should never increase room temperatures, sit in a hot tub or sauna, wear rubberized clothing, or work out in high temperatures with lots of clothes to lose weight. An exercise and weight-loss plan designed by the AT and the dietitian is the only plan to follow.

Pregame Meals

Pregame meals should be high in carbohydrate and fluids. Carbohydrate is easier to digest than fat and protein, and it can be converted into energy to be used immediately. The pregame meal should be eaten three to four hours before activity. Water is the best liquid to drink, and the athlete should make sure they are well hydrated about one hour before competition.

Understanding Diversity

Ramadan is a month of fasting. It is a time for Muslims to remember the suffering of the poor and to appreciate the things that Allah has given them. Fasting occurs during the day and includes no water or food. Food is allowed after dark (*iftar*) and before sunrise (*shurooq*). If a person is ill, it is acceptable to eat during the fasting hours. A person who is taking medication that requires taking food at the same time may have an upset stomach while fasting.

Athletes who are anxious about an upcoming competition may use carbohydrate-loaded sport drinks. Sport drinks are digested quickly, which helps the anxious athlete avoid feelings of nausea.

When the AT and dietitian are considering a pregame meal, they should remember the diversity of the team. Some athletes may have specific food preferences, such as Mexican, Arabic, Greek, or Latin foods. The AT has homework to do: analyze these foods and determine what is acceptable before a game. Another consideration is religious holidays. An athlete may observe a holiday by fasting or by not eating meat. The AT and dietitian should be aware of this issue a week in advance to best prepare the athlete for the holiday diet. Vegetarians have special protein needs and should work with the AT and dietitian to make sure their food needs are met. The sidebar lists the types of vegetarians.

Some good pregame foods include pasta, fruit, plain crackers, rice cakes, cereal, vegetarian foods, potatoes, meatless lasagna, soup, rice, juice, bread, raisins, pancakes, and waffles. Besides eating foods high in carbohydrates, the athlete should eat familiar foods. The pregame meal is no time to experiment. See figure 34.6 for how water affects the body.

Postgame Meals

The team may do something to celebrate after a game, and food can be there to replenish energy. However, ATs should not use food as a reward (e.g.,

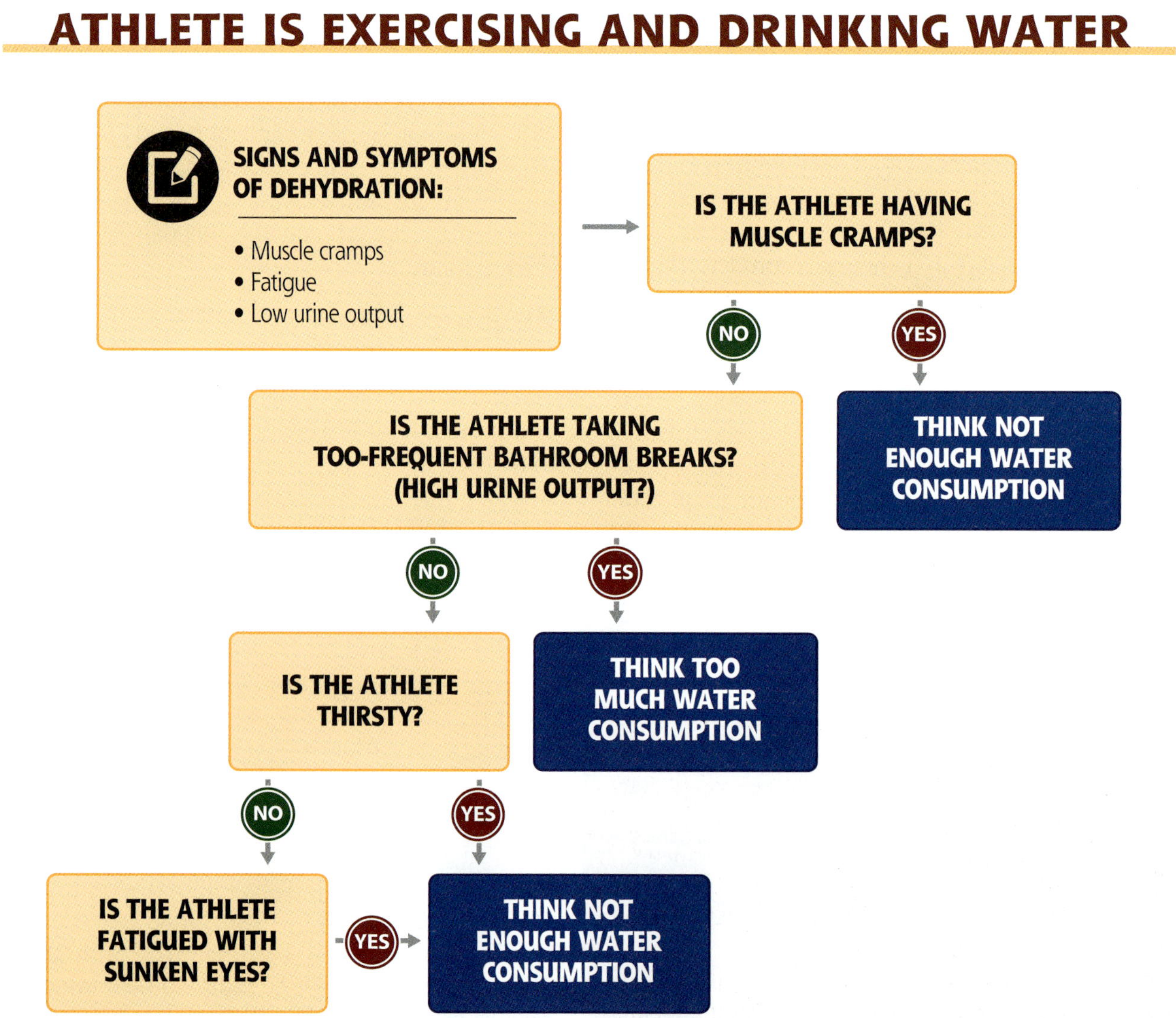
ATHLETE IS EXERCISING AND DRINKING WATER
SIGNS AND SYMPTOMS OF DEHYDRATION:
• Muscle cramps
• Fatigue
• Low urine output
IS THE ATHLETE HAVING MUSCLE CRAMPS?
NO
YES
THINK NOT ENOUGH WATER CONSUMPTION
IS THE ATHLETE TAKING TOO-FREQUENT BATHROOM BREAKS? (HIGH URINE OUTPUT?)
NO
YES
THINK TOO MUCH WATER CONSUMPTION
IS THE ATHLETE THIRSTY?
NO
YES
IS THE ATHLETE FATIGUED WITH SUNKEN EYES?
YES
THINK NOT ENOUGH WATER CONSUMPTION

Figure 34.6 Too much or too little water?

TYPES OF VEGETARIANS

- Semivegetarian: vegetable diet with occasional dairy and meats
- Lacto-ovo vegetarian: vegetable diet with dairy and eggs
- Lacto vegetarian: vegetable diet with dairy
- Vegan: vegetable diet

giving a team pizza, soda, and ice cream if they win) or as a punishment (e.g., driving the team straight home if they lose). Such actions can create an association between eating and pleasurable or miserable experiences that leads to overeating or not eating.

After the event, athletes should eat complex carbohydrates, but some protein, fat, and simple carbohydrates are also fine. Soon after practice and competitions is the best time to replenish the body's energy stores. Water replacement is necessary to compensate for sweating during competition. Several glasses of juice, water, or sport drinks are perfect choices.

Meals During All-Day Events

Many athletic competitions take place over a full day. Athletes may be asked to compete several times during the day, and a full sit-down meal is out of the question. So, what should athletes do to keep energy levels up? The answer is to eat small meals many times during the day. The meals should contain little protein and fat and a lot of complex carbohydrates and fluids (not soda). The amount of complex carbohydrates can be half a sandwich six times during the day. When the athlete eats depends on when they must compete; they must provide time to allow the food to digest as much as possible. Good all-day-event foods are bagels (no cream cheese), English muffins, bananas, baked potatoes, soup, fruit, pasta, pancakes, sport drinks, yogurt, cereal, and vegetables.

Carbohydrate Loading

Athletes who participate in endurance events (marathoners, cyclists, triathletes, long-distance swimmers) may benefit from a technique called *carbohydrate loading*. Carbohydrate loading means depleting carbohydrates for seven days and then ingesting large amounts of carbohydrates for three days before the event. The theory behind carbohydrate loading is that carbohydrate stores are used as energy during athletic competition. If the athlete has a lot of stored carbohydrates, they are less likely to run out of energy. Depleting before loading causes the body to store more carbohydrate than usual once carbohydrate consumption resumes. Remember that once carbohydrate stores are used up, the body begins to break down fat. Breaking down fat requires more energy than using readily available carbohydrate, again draining energy from the athlete. So the greater the carbohydrate stores, the better the athlete's energy.

If an athlete is involved in an endurance activity, the AT and dietitian should design a program for carbohydrate loading. The athlete's diet will change 10 days before competition. Three days before the event, 70% of what the athlete eats will be carbohydrates. During these three days, the athlete does not exercise. Foods with fat and protein are decreased as part of carbohydrate loading.

POPULAR DIETS AND FADS

Athletes are not immune to wanting to look and feel better by trying the latest diet. Some athletes struggle to keep their weight within healthy guidelines and may want to improve performance. A special diet may be the answer to feeling better, performing better, and looking better. One should not be fooled that any diet will be the answer to their weight loss. The athlete should consult with a nutritionist, who can do a comprehensive assessment of the athlete's current diet to determine the next step.

Low-Carbohydrate Diet

A low-carbohydrate diet is one in which sugars, grains, pasta, potatoes, and breads are restricted. Meat, fish, eggs, vegetables, nuts, low-glycemic fruits, and fats are included in this diet. The positive aspect of this diet is a reduction in calories, weight loss, and improved triglyceride levels.

Fruit Diet

The fruit diet is a program that primarily involves eating fresh raw fruit. Tomatoes and avocados are included in this diet (Weil 2013). People may choose this diet for religious, moral, or ethical reasons or because it is very close to the diet of their original ancestors (Capritto 2024).

Fruits are known to be high in fiber, vitamin C, antioxidants, potassium, and folate (Whelan 2017). Fruitarians may eat a limited number of vegetables, legumes, grains, root vegetables, nuts, or seeds (Whelan 2017). Those who adhere to this diet may eat one kind of fruit, wait a period of time, and eat another kind (Weil 2013). Fruit is only eaten when the person is hungry, and they eat until they are full (Weil 2013).

The fruit diet has its limitations in that it does not contain omega-3 fatty acids, iron, zinc, proteins, fat, calcium, or vitamin B_{12} (Weil 2013). The diet is high in sugar so it may not be best for those who are diabetic or prediabetic (Whelan 2017).

Ketogenic Diet

The liver makes ketones to break down fats. When a person fasts or does not have a lot of carbohydrates, ketones become the body's source of energy. The ketones burn fats, causing weight loss. This diet is low in carbohydrates and grains but allows fats and proteins. The benefit of this diet is weight loss and a reduction in blood sugar levels. For some, the lack of grains can cause constipation. Those on this diet for a long time may be prone to liver disease and kidney stones (Batch et al. 2020).

The carnivore diet is similar to the ketogenic diet. The carnivore diet is all meat (including fat), a little cream, butter, ghee, and cheese. Water is the allowed drink.

South Beach Diet

On the South Beach diet plan, a person eats 2,000 calories per day, with fewer carbohydrates than normal. Complex carbohydrates; nutrient-dense, lean protein; healthy fats; and foods high in fiber are acceptable. This diet includes an exercise plan of the individual's choice, but it must be done regularly (Mayo Clinic 2022). The positive effects include weight loss, healthier eating, and lower cholesterol (Mayo Clinic 2022). The risk is that lower carbohydrate levels may cause ketosis (see Ketogenic Diet) (Mayo Clinic 2022).

Vegan Diet

A diet that is completely plant-based is vegan. Being on a plant-based diet means that all nutrients, including those found in meat, fish, dairy, or eggs, must come from vegetables. Vegans may not get all the necessary nutrition found in a meat-based diet, so supplements may need to be considered. Areas of nutritional focus should be calcium, vitamin D, protein, essential fatty acids, zinc, iron, vitamin B_{12}, and iodine (Deckers 2016). The benefit to the vegan diet is weight loss, lower cholesterol levels, reduced risk for some cancers, reduced risk for type 2 diabetes, and reduced blood sugar levels (Healthline 2022).

POPULAR NUTRITIONAL SUPPLEMENTS

Someone is always trying to sell something. Companies hire professional athletes to hype their goods. Advertisements show a good-looking person on a beach with a beautiful companion. This makes potential customers believe that if they use the product, they, too, will be someplace warm with a beautiful companion. Some companies claim that certain nutritional items will help an athlete perform better, run faster, or have more energy. When you hear a promise but do not see independent research evidence to support the claim, keep your money in your pocket.

Herbal Supplements

Over the past several years, herbal dietary supplements derived from natural sources have become popular to reportedly curb appetite, provide energy, and burn calories. Common herbal supplements include ephedra and hydroxycitric acid. Ephe-

Understanding Diversity

Some athletes have a sensitivity or disease related to the protein gluten. It is found in wheat, barley, and rye. Some athletes have been diagnosed with celiac disease, which is an autoimmune disorder that can lead to damage of the small intestine. People who have this disease or sensitivity will eat food devoid of all wheat, barley, and rye products. Since gluten-free food does not have the same level of nutrients as foods with gluten, it is important to make sure athletes get the nutrients they need when eating a gluten-free diet (Cialdella-Kam, Kulpins, and Manore 2016). It may be necessary to refer an athlete to a dietitian to support nutrition needs with energy expenditures during physical activity.

dra was said to suppress appetite and increase metabolism. Hydroxycitric acid reportedly decreases appetite as well. Herbal supplements are officially regulated by the FDA. In 2003, the FDA banned the sale of ephedra because it is possibly associated with death of users and causes serious side effects, including high blood pressure, seizures, strokes, and irregular heartbeat. The Mayo Clinic recommends *not* taking an herbal supplement in the following cases:

- You are taking medications (prescription or over-the-counter).
- A proven medical treatment is already available to address your problem.
- You are having surgery.
- You are pregnant or breastfeeding.
- You are under age 18 or over age 65.

Creatine

Creatine is a popular nutritional supplement. This substance is found in the body in high levels right after exercise. Creatine is found in fish and meat. An athlete would have to eat 15 pounds (7 kg) of meat per day to obtain the same amount of creatine as found in a supplement. Advertisers claim that creatine is an energy source and encourages muscle growth. Athletes who take creatine supplements while strength training appear to have increased power for brief, high-intensity exercise. The long-term effects of creatine are inconclusive; thus, it should be avoided.

Amino Acids

Amino acids are the building blocks of protein. People have thought that taking daily amino acid supplements (pills or powder) would make them stronger and faster and increase protein storage. The basis for these ideas was the notion that amino acids cause the release of HGH (see chapter 33). HGH does increase muscle mass, but amino acids do not cause the release of HGH. Amino acids are sold in fitness magazines with pictures of muscular men and women holding the containers. Do not buy it. Amino acid supplements are expensive, and the athlete's daily diet should provide all necessary amino acids.

DRY SCOOPING FAD

Some athletes take powdered preworkout supplements. The supplements contain caffeine, amino acids, and other items. These supplements advise the user to use a scoop of powder and water and consume them before exercise (Johnson-Arbor 2022). Dry scooping involves consuming the powder without water. The thought behind dry scooping is that it improves the effect of the supplements (Johnson-Arbor 2022). Inhaling the scoop of powder may go into the lungs, causing choking or difficulty breathing (Johnson-Arbor 2022). If the powder is able to make it to the stomach, the large amount of caffeine can cause a rapid heart rate, anxiety, chest pain, dizziness, tremors, and heart problems (Johnson-Arbor 2022). Individuals with other health issues may find their health compromised. Those who experience life-threatening signs and symptoms should call 911 or poison control (Johnson-Arbor 2022).

Summary

An athlete's daily nutrition plays a critical role in the ability to give an optimal performance. Most athletes meet their daily requirements by eating proper portions of a balanced diet. Some athletes consistently eat foods that are high in fat and cholesterol and low in fiber. This can lead to negative health consequences. As an athlete gets older, their metabolism slows, and they must reduce the number of calories they consume, or they will gain weight. Water intake and fluid replacement are key for athletic participation. The rule for fluid replacement is 1 quart (1 L) for every 1,000 calories lost. The AT and dietitian should decide on pregame and postgame meals based on the event and the athlete's needs. Athletes are constantly looking for an edge over their opponents, and fad diets and supplements are hyped as the greatest way to improve performance. Athletes and the AT must research supplements before anyone uses them.

Key Terms

Define the following terms found in this chapter:

- amino acids
- caloric balance
- cholesterol
- fiber
- metabolism
- nutrients
- trans fat

A gymnast reports to you that her teammate is eating very little food, exercises excessively, and is vomiting daily. She has tried to talk to her, but the athlete denies having an eating disorder. As the AT, what do you do? What type of additional medical professionals can be utilized to help work with this athlete?

To access supplementary material for this chapter, including the Understanding Check worksheet, vocabulary quizzes, extension activities, and chapter-specific resources and forms, visit the web resource: http://ancillaries.humankinetics.com/FundamentalsOfAthleticTrainingAndSportsMedicine5E

chapter 35

Special Populations

Objectives

After completing this chapter, the student will be able to do the following:

- Understand the history of sport participation by people with impairments and varying ability levels.
- Understand that athletes with impairments and medical conditions can participate with or without adaptations.
- Know that there are injury-prevention programs based on the needs associated with each impairment or medical condition.

The U.S. government uses the term **disability** to encompass a range of conditions—both visible and invisible. A disability might be an impairment present from birth, an impairment caused by injury or illness, a medical condition present throughout the person's lifespan, or a medical condition that occurs for only part of the person's life. In 1990, the Americans with Disabilities Act defined disability as "a physical or mental impairment that substantially limits one or more major life activities" (U.S. Department of Justice n.d.). One of those life activities may be participation in athletics. An AT needs to understand each disability and how sport participation affects it. Supporting athletes with impairments and medical conditions is essential to the athlete's positive sport experience.

The first section of this chapter discusses the history of sport for people with impairments and medical conditions. Next, the chapter discusses various conditions and how exercise affects them as well as injuries that people with impairments and medical conditions are at higher risk for.

HISTORY OF DISABLED SPORT

After World War II, veterans with spinal cord injuries who used wheelchairs were given an opportunity to participate in the Stoke Mandeville Games in 1948 (Paralympic Movement n.d.). The games were founded by Sir Ludwig Guttmann, who considered exercise essential to the recovery of people with spinal cord injuries. Eventually the games branched off into the Paralympics, which includes athletes who have disabilities but who do not necessarily use wheelchairs.

Many organizations run programs for athletes with a specific disability, such as the Dwarf Athletic Association of America (DAAA), Second Wind Lung Transplant Association, Special Olympics, and United States Association of Blind Athletes (USABA). These groups can assist the AT in developing programming, goals, and an understanding of each disability.

Some students have a condition that makes sport participation challenging. Very few high schools provide competition exclusively for athletes with physical impairments; when athletes with impairments and medical conditions participate in high school sport, they compete against athletes without any condition. ATs have a great opportunity to work with and support those who face challenges in sport participation.

MUSCULOSKELETAL CONDITIONS

Musculoskeletal conditions are those in which the bones, joints, muscles, tendons, or ligaments are impaired. This section discusses the more common conditions that affect athletes.

Limb Deficiencies

Many athletes who have limb deficiencies were born with them. The deficiency can be an undeveloped limb or having too many or too few toes or fingers. It can also be constriction from additional webbing between fingers or toes.

The cause of the deficiency can be a birth defect caused by a drug or exposure to an illness during pregnancy. It may also result from mechanical forces placed on the limb during pregnancy, exposure to tobacco smoke, or genetic abnormalities (Stanford Medicine 2023).

An athlete with a limb deficiency can be successful playing a sport depending on the restriction of the deficiency. In some instances, no adaptation is necessary and the athlete can readily play. In other cases, an athlete may require surgery to obtain the necessary range of motion or may need to learn to adapt to the game.

It's important for the AT to learn about restrictions the athlete may have and how the athlete adapts to the game. If the athlete wears a brace or has an artificial limb, the AT needs to learn how to help the athlete stabilize the limb or brace to meet the demands of participation.

One of the most famous athletes with a limb deficiency was professional baseball player Jim Abbott. Jim played football and baseball in high school and then went on to play professional baseball. He was born without a right hand. When he played baseball, he would place his glove on his right arm, pitch the ball, and place the glove on his left hand to catch the ball.

Amputations

An amputation is the entire or partial removal of a limb or digits. Most lower-limb amputations occur from vascular disease, and others occur due to trauma (Kalapatapu 2017). Depending on the type of amputation, balance and movement may become issues.

The end of the limb is known as the residual limb. The residual limb is prone to friction, moisture, and blisters. The athlete and the AT have to watch for degradation of the residual limb. For the AT, treating a blister on the residual limb is no different than treating any other blister. The athlete needs to make care of the residual limb a part of their routine. Infection can occur if blisters are not cared for.

Phantom pain is pain felt from the amputated limb. The pain can be mild or severe. In some cases, the athlete may require medication or other therapies to control it (Mayo Clinic 2019).

Lower-extremity amputees may have an increased energy expenditure and knee joint pain. Athletes with transtibial and transfemoral amputations expend more energy (van Schaik, Geertzen, Dijkstra, and Dekker 2019). The athlete's nutrition needs need to be met based on this greater energy expenditure.

When an athlete has a lower-extremity amputation, their gait pattern changes, as does the pressure on various joints of the body. There is a greater risk of knee osteoarthritis in the normal leg if the athlete has a knee amputation (Welke 2019).

Athletes with amputations compete in many events without the aid of an artificial limb but with adaptations such as downhill ski poles, wheelchairs built for racing, and bikes for racing. In some instances, an artificial limb is designed specifically for the athlete in competition. A **prosthetic** is an artificial body part. Carbon-fiber artificial limbs provide the athlete with a prosthetic that can sustain the rigors of competition. In some instances, the constant intensity causes the artificial carbon-fiber limb to break, so more than one limb may be necessary.

Athletes with amputations can compete with those without amputations. Some people even believe that artificial limbs provide an advantage. For this reason, long jumper Markus Rehm was banned from the 2016 Olympics (Grohmann 2016). In some instances, having an amputation is a disadvantage; thus, some athletes with amputations may prefer to compete against others with the same ability level. The number of amputations and the amount of limb loss are used to place athletes with amputations into categories for competition.

People with limb amputations are classified for the sake of sport participation into the following categories:

- Lower-limb amputee levels (University of Michigan Health 1995-2022a):
    - Foot or partial foot
    - Through the ankle
    - Below the knee
    - At the knee
    - Above the knee
    - At the hip
- Upper-limb amputee levels (University of Michigan Health 1995-2022b):
    - Fingers or part of the hand
    - Through the wrist
    - Below the elbow
    - Above or through the elbow
    - At the shoulder
    - Above the shoulder

AUDITORY AND VISUAL IMPAIRMENTS

Athletes who have sensory impairments are able to adapt their other senses to accommodate. Athletes are athletes, no matter the type of adaptation. The AT should expect the athlete to be competitive and have the desire to participate, regardless of impairments. The AT should also take advantage of opportunities to learn new skills, such as sign language or using a screen reader that can read to a blind person.

Deafness

Deafness can be caused by several things, such as trauma, infection, and birth defects. Athletes may have problems with equilibrium if the semicircular canals or the vestibular apparatus are injured (Cushing and O'Reilly 2021).

Athletes with hearing loss can participate in all sports. Difficulty may come from being unable to react as quickly if the sport requires hearing. In some instances, not being able to hear the taunting of unruly fans or other distractions could be beneficial.

Some athletes with hearing loss are able to wear hearing aids. Hearing aids must be cared for to prevent sweat, rain, and water from getting into them. It is best to have extra hearing-aid batteries in case the device needs a new one. Some athletes may also have **cochlear implants**, which include an external device worn on the side of the skull behind the ear. These are permissible in all sports but do require attention to ensure proper care.

What Would You Do If . . .

You are assisting an AT who is providing medical coverage for a track meet at your school. Among the teams participating, one is from a school for students with hearing loss. An athlete from this school is injured during the long jump competition, and the AT needs to obtain a history of the injury. If you were in the AT's position, what would you do to communicate effectively with the athlete?

Blindness

People with vision impairments can be completely blind or partially blind. Each sport may have their own visual standards for participation. Paralympic athletes are classified into three categories (Sprabary 2022):

- B1: The athlete cannot see any shape at any distance and has no light perception in either eye.
- B2: The athlete has a visual field of 5° in their best eye corrected or a vision of 20/600.
- B3: The athlete has a visual field between 5° and 20° in their best eye, with vision corrected, or a visual acuity between 20/600 and 20/200.

Athletes with visual impairments are able to compete in a variety of activities, such as running, wrestling, baseball, softball, bowling, and cycling. Modifications are made to allow athletes with visual impairments to participate in sport, such as using a ball that beeps, running with another person to assist with the running path, or beginning a wrestling match in contact with the other athlete.

The AT should be aware that athletes with vision impairments are prone to falling and impact injuries. These falls can lead to typical fractures of the limbs.

In many instances, people talk louder to an athlete with a disability. It sounds obvious, but the AT should realize that talking louder will not improve the athlete's vision.

CARDIOVASCULAR DISORDERS

The cardiovascular system is made up of the heart and blood vessels. To have a normal cardiovascular system, each component must work properly. A disease or an illness may cause the system to not function properly, thus causing the athlete to struggle or even die. This section discusses fibrillation of the heart and sudden cardiac death.

Fibrillation

Fibrillation of the heart means that it is beating rapidly. The fibrillation can be in the upper chambers (atria) or lower chambers (ventricles) of the heart. A good way to visualize a fibrillating heart is as a bag filled with moving worms. The heart is not able to effectively pump blood to the body, and if fibrillation continues for a long time, it can cause death or a stroke from a blood clot.

Fibrillation in athletes can be caused by alcohol use, an overactive thyroid, a blood clot in the lungs, caffeine intake, or pneumonia. Fibrillation can also be caused by the heart itself via heart valve disease, an enlarged heart, other heart disease, high blood pressure, or a faulty electrical node (Davis 2021).

Athletes suffering from fibrillation may feel as though their heart is coming out of their chest. They may feel weak and anxious and may pass out. It is best to call for an ambulance and allow a physician to care for the athlete.

Treatment for the athlete with fibrillation can include dietary changes, medication, resolving other conditions such as high blood pressure, electrical shock to get the heart back to a regular rhythm, a pacemaker, or ablation surgery. An athlete who has fibrillation can return to participation with the permission of a physician.

Sudden Cardiac Death

Sudden cardiac death is the most serious form of a heart condition. An electrical disturbance causes the heart to stop. It is important that the AT review the preparticipation physical for risk factors of sudden cardiac death. The risk factors include a parent with cardiac history, especially death before age 50; a previous cardiac episode; high blood pressure; obesity; and diabetes. Many heart conditions may contribute to sudden cardiac death, such as an enlarged heart, coronary artery disease, an arrhythmia, or congenital heart disorder.

Signs and symptoms of a sudden cardiac episode include dizziness, lightheadedness, heart palpitations, chest pain, collapse, shortness of breath, unconsciousness, no breathing, and no heartbeat (see figure 35.1). The signs and symptoms usually occur without warning, hence the term *sudden*. For the patient to survive this condition, it is imperative that immediate care be provided. Call 911, begin CPR, and use an **automated external defibrillator (AED)**. The defibrillator will be able to administer a shock if no heartbeat is detected.

An athlete who is prone to this condition may need a defibrillator implanted (Mayo Clinic 2023). This type of defibrillator will detect the electrical

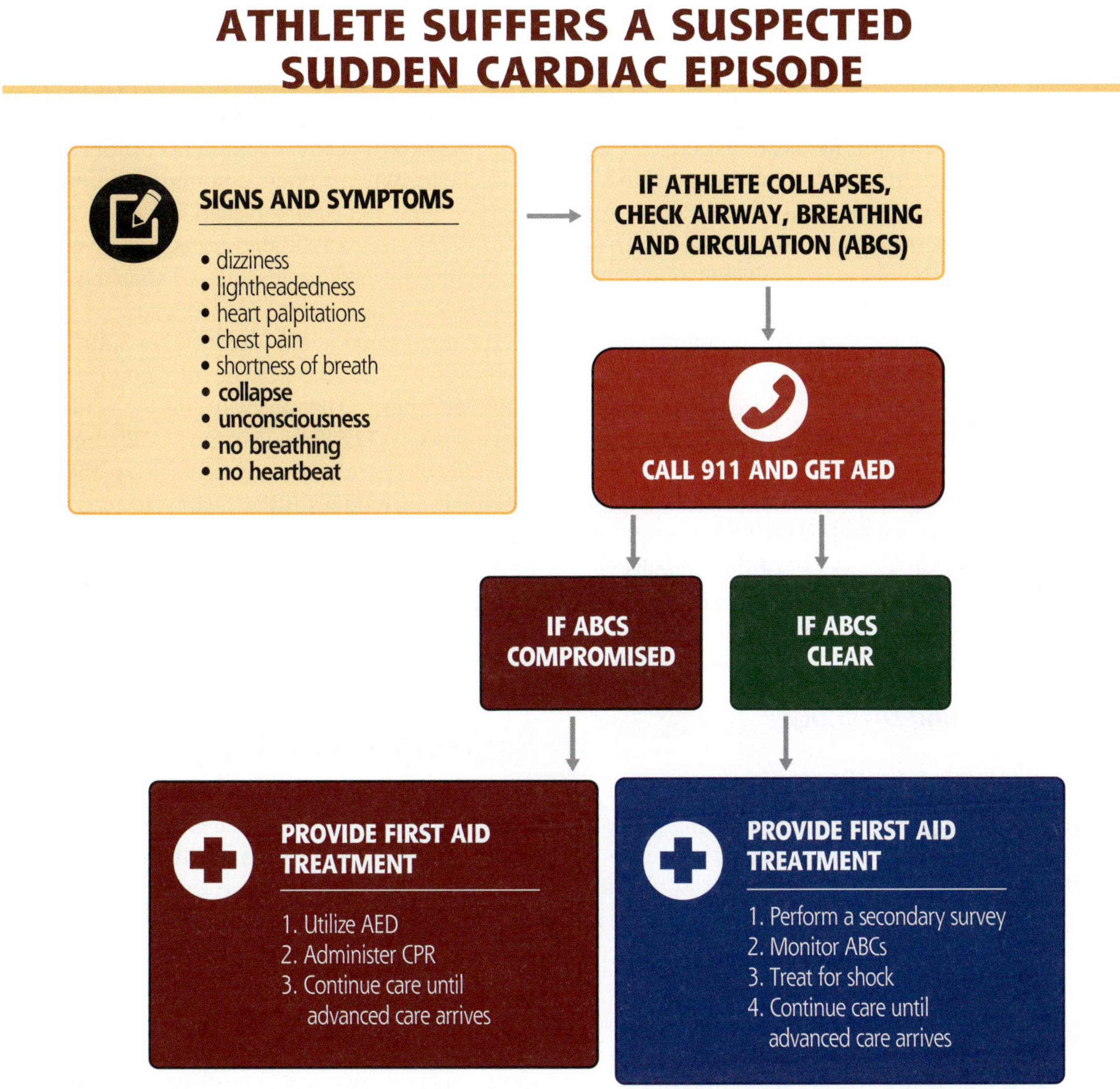

Figure 35.1 Athlete collapse algorithm.

disturbance and automatically shock the heart back into a normal rhythm. The athlete will need to monitor risk factors and maintain a healthy lifestyle, and the sports medicine team will determine if the athlete can continue to play.

TRANSPLANTS

In 2022, in the United States, there were 42,887 transplants (United Network for Organ Sharing 2023). Transplants include internal organs such as the kidney, liver, heart, lung, pancreas, and intestines. Limb transplants can be performed, but these are extremely rare. After a successful transplant, people who have received organs may participate in sports to maintain their health.

The AT must be aware of the complications associated with the organ transplantation process and conditions affiliated with pre- and postsurgical procedures. People living with end-stage organ failure can be unmotivated to exercise. Lack of exercise reduces bone density, increases muscle atrophy, and increases fatigue.

People who receive transplants are susceptible to organ rejection and thus must take antirejection medications. Antirejection medications reduce the body's ability to fight infections (Hussain and Khan 2022). The AT may work with the physician to bring about the best physical fitness state for this athlete. Following the physician's rehabilitation plan is essential for the transplant athlete to successfully return to a state of wellness. Neale, Smith, and Bishop (2017) found that transplant patients who exercised had a higher quality of health but concerns remain regarding cardiovascular and immune system function.

In 1978, the first Transplant Games were held in the United Kingdom. The purpose of the Transplant Games is to provide awareness of the benefits of transplants and resilience of life (Donate Life California 2005-2023).

Understanding Diversity

Waiting for Transplants

Sixty percent of people on the transplant list are racial/ethnic minorities; 106,000 people are on that list (VCU Health 2023). Of those 106,000, over 30,000 are African American; 22,000 are Latino; and 9,600 are Asian American and Pacific Islanders (VCU Health 2023). The greatest need is for kidneys, and African Americans need them most often. Many African American patients have been on the kidney transplant list for decades because until recently, a different calculation was used for Black patients, such that Black patients were placed lower on the waiting list than White patients with the same level of kidney dysfunction (Mayo Clinic Staff 2022).

Heart Transplant

Athletes with heart transplants can participate in athletic activities with the permission of their physician. The AT will need to be aware of the names and types of medications the athlete is using and keep an AED on hand. Accommodations may be needed for the athlete to participate, such as using a golf cart instead of carrying the golf bag and clubs.

A heart transplant is done because the athlete's heart no longer can function. An athlete who has gone through a heart transplant has likely endured a long process that may have included having an artificial pump, pacemaker, or defibrillator attached to the heart. When a donor is found, the ineffective heart is removed and replaced with the donor's heart. More than 4,100 heart transplants were performed in the United States in 2022 (United Network for Organ Sharing 2023).

The transplant patient usually takes antirejection medication so that the new heart is not rejected as a foreign object. The survival rate for adult heart transplants is 72.5% for 5 years (Wilhelm 2015). The effects of exercise that occur from the heart transplant include a resting heart rate increase by 20 beats/minute, decreased peak heart rate, delayed heart rate increase after the start of exercise, and a delayed return to resting heart rate (American College of Sports Medicine 2016).

Lung Transplant

A lung transplant is done because the lung or lungs can no longer function to keep the body oxygenated to support life. Disorders that may require a lung transplant include emphysema, high blood pressure of the arteries around the lungs, cystic fibrosis, or a congenital deformity. In the United States, 2,692 lung transplants were performed in 2022 (United Network for Organ Sharing 2023).

Before an athlete can return to physical activity, the physician must determine the rehabilitation program. Athletes who have had lung transplants are prone to hypertension, rejection of the organ, osteoporosis, diabetes, and muscle atrophy (Nassar et al. 2022; Vural and Keller 2021; Hurst et al. 2019; Oshima et al. 2020). Exercise can help improve the athlete's quality of life by reducing hypertension, osteoporosis, and muscle atrophy.

Kidney Transplant

A kidney transplant is needed when disease causes the kidney to fail to filter harmful waste products from the blood. People can receive kidney dialysis to take over the filtering process and delay transplantation.

Chronic kidney disease is commonly caused by high blood pressure and diabetes. A preventive

> **What Would You Do If . . .**
>
> A sophomore athlete approaches the AT and explains that she received a heart transplant four years earlier. She wishes to participate in basketball but isn't sure if she is at risk for heart problems if she plays. How do you think the AT should respond?

approach to the disease is to control blood pressure and maintain a healthy lifestyle. Unfortunately, 38.4 million people have diabetes, and 97.6 million are prediabetic (Centers for Disease Control and Prevention 2024), ultimately resulting in the need for kidney dialysis and transplantation. In 2022, more kidneys were transplanted in the United States than any other organ (United Network for Organ Sharing 2023).

Antirejection medications can cause high blood pressure and diabetes. The AT must regularly monitor the transplant athlete's blood pressure (Stratton, Zieve, and Conaway 2017). An athlete with a kidney transplant is more likely to develop cardiovascular disease (Birdwell and Park 2021). The five-year organ survival rate from deceased donors is 78%, while the patient survival rate from living donors is 86% (Ghelichi-Ghojogh et al. 2022).

Liver Transplant

The liver functions to detoxify various chemicals and break down nutrients before they can be circulated throughout the body. In addition, the liver secretes bile, which helps process fat. When the liver is damaged, symptoms are jaundice, diarrhea, nausea, and tiredness. The liver can be damaged by diseases such as hepatitis B and hepatitis C and behaviors such as alcohol abuse (Mayo Clinic 1998-2023). If the damage to the liver is significant, a transplant may be necessary.

An athlete who has received one of the 9,528 liver transplants performed annually in the United States (United Network for Organ Sharing 2023) may have difficulty retaining normal blood sugar levels (Pelaez-Jaramillo et al. 2018).

NEUROMUSCULAR DISORDERS

A neuromuscular disorder initiates in either the central nervous system (brain, spine) or the peripheral nervous system (nerves that originate at the spine and innervate the muscles and return to the spine). The nervous system sends messages throughout the body to cause the muscles to function. If any part of the nervous system is affected by disease or injury, the muscular system can also be compromised.

Paralympic athletes who have neuromuscular disorders are placed into one of two categories, Ataxia or Impaired Muscle Power, for the purpose of participation. Ataxia examples are those with multiple sclerosis, cerebral palsy, traumatic brain injury, stroke, and multiple sclerosis. The Impaired Muscle Power category includes athletes with spinal cord injury (complete or incomplete), muscular dystrophy, post-polio syndrome, and spina bifida (International Paralympic Committee n.d.).

The following sections explain how the nervous system affects the muscular system in various neuromuscular disorders. They also describe exercise ability and tolerance as each disorder progresses.

Multiple Sclerosis

Multiple sclerosis affects the central nervous system. The central nervous system is surrounded by a myelin sheath, a fatty substance that ensures that electrical impulses are conducted through the nervous system to the muscles and organs they are designated to serve. The conduction of the impulses is rapid and coordinated (American College of Sports Medicine 2016). With multiple sclerosis, the myelin sheath detaches from parts of the central nervous system, making the conduction of impulses erratic.

An athlete with multiple sclerosis can participate in competition but may have muscle spasms, balance issues, lack of coordination, fatigue, pain, visual problems, and numbness (WebMD 2017). The AT should be aware that as body temperature rises, sensory and cognitive issues can be exacerbated (Christogianni et al. 2018). The American College of Sports Medicine (2016) suggests selecting a supervised exercise that meet the athlete's needs.

Over time, multiple sclerosis can advance until assistive devices are needed to support the muscles. Devices may include prosthetics for the ankle joint to support foot drop.

Muscular Dystrophy

Muscular dystrophy is a group of disorders that affect the muscles by replacing muscle cells with connective tissue (American College of Sports Medicine 2016). With the progression of muscular dystrophy come cognitive deficits and memory loss. If the athlete has cognitive deficits, be sure to convey important ideas (times, place, dates) in writing. The progression of the disease also causes loss of muscle function, range of motion, and ability to perform activities of daily living.

Muscular dystrophy is genetic. Many forms of muscular dystrophy exist, but in general, muscular deficits are the commonality. The progression begins with atrophy of muscles, fatigue, muscular spasm, and weakness, and eventually leads to cardiac problems (American College of Sports Medicine 2016).

Contractures caused by muscular dystrophy can be cared for with stretching. Cardiorespiratory exercise and strength training are good ways to maintain health. In addition, helping an athlete maintain a healthy weight is supportive and has therapeutic value (Salera et al. 2017).

The Real World

I had a wrestler who had muscular dystrophy. It wasn't until his second year in our program that I was told that his teammates were carrying him up and down two flights of stairs to get to the wrestling room. His mother, who always advocated for her son, shared that she felt it was unsafe for her son to be carried in such a manner. So, I went to work on getting a lift put in so that he could freely move about the athletic area. Shortly after that, we had a ramp and another doorway built so he could lift weights with everyone else. These changes exist today for every student, a legacy of the athlete and his mother.

Anonymous

Salera and colleagues (2017) indicate that it is important to maintain bone strength. To support bone strength, athletes may add calcium and vitamin D to their diet. On the other hand, using corticosteroids can result in thinning of bone mass, thus leading to fractures.

Muscular dystrophy often results in extreme muscle tightness, especially at the ankles and hips. Surgery that releases these contractures is most often performed at the ankles as well as at the spine when scoliosis is present (National Health Service 2021; Parent Project Muscular Dystrophy 2023). Controlling body heat and maintaining fluids are essential.

Exercises that support cardiorespiratory training include walking, cycling, and swimming. If walking is the exercise of choice, a flat surface is essential to preventing falls. Strength training is also beneficial and can be accomplished using weights or therapeutic exercise bands.

Cerebral Palsy

Cerebral palsy (CP) is a disorder that affects the brain before, during, or shortly after birth. CP affects the brain by preventing normal development of the brain, and it is an irreversible condition. The patient with CP may have poor balance, lack of muscle tone, loss of control over bodily movements, speech impairment, seizures, and lack of control of posture (American College of Sports Medicine 2016).

The level of CP is based on the extent and location of damage in the brain. CP can be severe enough that the patient needs a wheelchair and an assistant, and it can be mild to the point where the person has movement problems but for the most part can get around without assistance.

Maintaining a level of fitness is important for people with CP. Watch for fatigue and increased muscle spasms. The American College of Sports Medicine (2016) indicates that people with CP who participate in regular exercise are able to reduce their antispasm medication.

Athletes with CP have difficulty with regulating body heat, so the AT needs to anticipate keeping the athlete warm in cool weather and cool in hot weather.

During exercise, the athlete with CP may require spotting. An athlete who is in a wheelchair may require restraints, so the AT needs to watch for blisters or pain (American College of Sports Medicine 2016).

COGNITIVE CONDITIONS

When an individual has decreased cognitive function, they are known to have a cognitive condition. Some conditions involve genetic disorders, brain development issues, decreased brain function, injury, and memory loss. In this section, Down syndrome and closed head trauma are discussed.

Down Syndrome

Down syndrome is a genetic disorder that is associated with cognitive delays, delayed growth, and intellectual disabilities (MedlinePlus 2020). Facial features include a flatter face with slanting eyes (Jacob 2018). Athletes with Down syndrome generally have overall muscular weakness, poor cardiorespiratory fitness, less than normal coordination, and shorter spans of exercise tolerance (Jacob 2018). So, athletes with Down syndrome need individualized exercise programs to increase strength, endurance, and coordination. Sweat glands can be affected by heat, so the AT must be aware of environmental conditions.

Closed Head Trauma

A closed head injury is caused by an impact to the head that does not fracture the skull. The impact may cause bleeding and swelling in the brain that can lead to brain damage or even death. For those who survive the trauma, there may be permanent damage to the brain. The damage can be minimal or severe.

The impairment from the trauma will correlate to the portion of the brain that was damaged. Some people may experience memory deficits, cognitive deficits, mood swings, an inability to move arms and legs on one or both sides, and losing the ability to speak.

If an athlete with a closed head trauma chooses to participate in sport, the sport may need to be one where falling or head trauma is not possible. In some instances, headgear may be worn to protect the head, regardless of the sport.

Disabled Sports USA is a group dedicated to helping people with disabilities, including those with head injuries. The sports offered are vast but may require that the athlete use adaptive equipment to participate.

TEMPORARY MEDICAL CONDITIONS

Some conditions are classified as temporary disability because they affect the individual for a shorter period of time. Under U.S. law, pregnancy is considered a temporary disability, and schools must accommodate pregnant student-athletes in the same way that they would make accommodations for other student-athletes with a temporary disability (U.S. Department of Education Office for Civil Rights 2022).

Pregnancy

Physically active pregnant individuals who continue their exercise regimen can maintain fitness, manage weight, and reduce the risk of pregnancy-related diabetes (Jacobs 2018). The Department of Health and Human Services (2018) recommends 2 hours and 30 minutes of moderate-intensity aerobic activity per week during pregnancy and postpartum. The obstetrician should be involved in the care of the athlete and in determining whether any medical conditions exist that would complicate exercising.

! RED FLAGS

Causes of concern in athletes with decreased neurological function include the following:

- Blisters
- Sprains and strains
- Bladder infections
- Constipation
- Headaches
- Visual impairment
- Hearing impairment
- Balance issues
- Heat illnesses
- Skin infections or ulcerations

What Would You Do If . . .

An athlete playing in a wheelchair basketball competition reports to you with a severe blister on his right hand. He wishes to continue playing, but the tape he used to cover the wound does not stay in place well.

ASSESSING PARTICIPATION CONDITIONS

The AT needs an overview of each athlete's abilities or lack thereof. It is useful to have an adjustable table that will allow the athlete to get on it comfortably so the AT can adjust its height based on their needs. During the physical examination of an athlete with an impairment or medical condition, the AT will want to know the following:

- Athlete's strength
- Range of motion at each joint
- Medications used
- Ability to balance
- Appliances worn
- Visual acuity
- Auditory acuity
- Physical reaction to exercise
- Coordination
- Ability to understand direction
- Reaction time

The assessment will assist the AT and coach in establishing realistic goals and expectations for participation. Participation should be a positive experience so that the athlete can pursue the activity throughout a lifetime.

COMMON INJURIES

Competitive athletes with impairments and medical conditions are similar to other athletes in that they can and do get injured. Some of these are the same injuries as those suffered by athletes without these conditions, such as a muscle sprain. However, some injuries and medical emergencies are more likely for an athlete who has an impairment or medical condition. The AT should be watchful for the following injuries, illnesses, and medical emergencies:

- Amputations: abrasions, blisters, and skin rash (Patel and Greydan 2010); ankle injuries (Willick 2018); low back injuries for lower limb amputations (Willick 2018); and cervical and thoracic injuries for upper extremity amputations (Willick 2018)
- Fibrillation: stroke, heart attack
- Heart transplant: heart attack, heart failure, arrhythmias, sudden cardiac death (Mayo Clinic Staff 2024)
- Muscular dystrophy: fractures (Liaw et al. 2023)
- Cerebral palsy: seizures, bowel obstruction, fall injuries, osteoporosis (Penn Medicine 2023)
- Closed head trauma: additional head injuries
- Visual impairment: fractures, sprains, lower extremity injuries (Ferrera and Peterson 2000)

The Real World

I had a swimmer who had autism. He was about 280 pounds (127 kg) and loved to swim, but the swim coach was afraid he would drown. She could not save him because of her slight frame and weight of 125 pounds (57 kg). There was an obvious potential for liability and danger but also an obligation to allow the young man to swim. In talking with the parents, we found a compromise. We hired a lifeguard who was designated to be the young man's personal supervisor. The young man enjoyed swimming the entire season and never had any difficulty. The coach felt relieved, and the young man had a blast.

Anonymous

- Wheelchair use: blisters, ulcers (Alkhalifah et al. 2023); autonomic dysreflexia (the sympathetic nervous system is uncontrolled) causing a rise in blood pressure, headache, and sweating (Lexell 2018; Fitzpatrick, De Luigi, and Pasquina 2012); upper extremity overuse injuries, urinary tract infections, heat regulation, high blood pressure (Lexell 2018)

When working with an athlete with an impairment or medical condition, the AT should use the standard of care for injuries. This means that a sprain or strain should be treated with PRICES, fractures should be splinted, and all emergency parameters should be used as necessary. Modifications in treatment arise in how an AT communicates with an athlete or how bandages are applied. (Consider a limb deficiency, for example; taping or wrapping may not contour itself the way it does on a typical limb.)

Summary

Athletes with impairments or medical conditions deserve an opportunity to participate in sport. The AT needs to know as much as possible about the athlete and the disability to ensure safe participation. Each condition brings its own concerns, such as blisters, ulcers, or possibility of falls. The AT and coach should work together to help the athletes obtain their personal goals. Athletes with impairments or medical conditions can participate in many sports with modification of the game, specialized equipment, or prosthetics.

Key Terms

Define the following terms found in this chapter:

- antirejection medications
- automated external defibrillator (AED)
- cerebral palsy (CP)
- cochlear implant
- disability
- fibrillation
- multiple sclerosis
- muscular dystrophy
- prosthetic

An athlete reports blisters and painful lesions on their residual limb after athletic participation. What is your advice to this athlete to help prevent the blisters?

To access supplementary material for this chapter, including the Understanding Check worksheet, vocabulary quizzes, extension activities, and chapter-specific resources and forms, visit the web resource: http://ancillaries.humankinetics.com/FundamentalsOfAthleticTrainingAndSportsMedicine5E

GLOSSARY

ABCs—Acronym standing for airway, breathing, and circulation. These are the first three things to check after determining that a person is unresponsive.

abduction—Movement away from the midline of the body.

acetabulum—The bones that form the hip socket.

Achilles tendon—Structure that attaches the gastrocnemius muscle to the calcaneus bone of the foot.

acne—When numerous hair follicles are plugged with sebum and then create pustules.

active range of motion (AROM)—The range through which the athlete can move a limb unassisted.

active-assistive range of motion (AAROM)—The range of motion through which the athlete can move a limb with the help of the AT.

acupuncture—An ancient Chinese medical practice of inserting needles into the body at specific points to transform energy.

adduction—Movement toward the midline of the body.

agonist—Prime mover in muscle action; biceps in elbow flexion.

air embolism—A blockage of blood flow to an area when air enters the bloodstream.

allergist—A physician who specializes in determining the substances to which a person is allergic and treating such allergies.

allergy—A condition in which a person has a low tolerance for pollen, ragweed, dogs, cats, specific foods, and so on. These often trigger an allergic reaction, typically a sudden runny nose; congestion; red, itchy eyes; and sneezing.

alternating current (AC)—An electrical current that changes direction as it moves back and forth between electrodes.

alveoli—The lung tissue where the gas exchange of oxygen and carbon dioxide occurs.

ambulatory—Able to walk independently or with light support.

amenorrhea—Absence of a menstrual cycle for three or more months.

American Red Cross—A national organization that certifies people in first aid and CPR. The American Red Cross also sponsors services such as disaster relief for communities throughout the world.

amino acid—The basic component of protein.

amnesia—Loss of memory, usually due to a head injury.

amphiarthrodial joint—A joint of cartilage that links bones that don't move much, such as where the ribs join the sternum.

anabolic steroids—A group of synthetic male hormones. Athletes use anabolic steroids to build muscle and recover from workouts more quickly, which allows them to increase their workload.

anatomical position—A standing posture with the arms at the sides and palms facing forward.

anatomy—The science of how the body is organized, concentrating on bones, joints, muscles, and organs and their arrangements.

androstenedione—A steroid that increases one's testosterone level.

anemia—A condition in which fewer red blood cells than normal are in the circulatory system. May be caused by bleeding.

aneurysm—A bulge in a blood vessel that can rupture.

angina pectoris—Pain commonly felt around the heart and chest cavity caused by lack of oxygen to the heart muscle.

annulus fibrosus—The rings of tissue that surround the nucleus pulposus of an intervertebral disc.

anorexia nervosa—A serious eating disorder marked by a pathological fear of weight gain and a loss of appetite. The anorexic has a low body weight and low body fat but may exercise excessively and avoid eating.

antagonist—The muscle that works opposite or against the prime mover in an action. The triceps is the antagonist in elbow flexion.

anterior cruciate ligament (ACL)—A knee ligament that keeps the tibia from moving forward on the femur.

anterior—Pertaining to the front of the body.

antirejection medications—Medications that help reduce the chance that a transplanted organ will be rejected by the body.

apnea—The temporary cessation of breathing.

appendicular skeleton—The bones of the extremities (shoulders, arms, hands, legs, feet, and pelvis).

arrhythmia—An irregular heartbeat rhythm.

arthroscopic surgery—A type of surgery performed on a joint using only small puncture holes to insert instruments, including a camera, to observe and fix injured structures.

articulate—The coming together of two bones to form a joint.

aseptic meningitis—A viral inflammation of the coverings of the brain.

assessment—Determining a diagnosis and determining how to prioritize issues.

assumption of risk—When an athlete fully understands that they may be injured by participating in sport.

asthma—A condition in which the air passages contract in response to an allergy. The contraction may close the air passage entirely.

ATC—A credential awarded by the Board of Certification (BOC) after a person has met the AT education requirements and passed the BOC national examination.

athletic training facility—The place in which athletic training services are provided.

athletic training strategic alliance—The professional organizations that work collaboratively on athletic training education, including the CAATE, BOC, NATA, and REF.

atrioventricular node—The node that communicates with the SA node in the heart to regulate heart rate.

atrium—One of two upper chambers of the heart that receive blood from the veins and force it into the ventricles.

attention-deficit hyperactivity disorder (ADHD)—A brain development disorder characterized by the athlete having inattentive issues or hyperactivity, or both.

automated external defibrillator (AED)—A device that administers a shock if no heartbeat is detected.

avascular necrosis—The death of body tissue from lack of blood.

axial load—End-to-end loading of a bone or series of vertebrae. This term is commonly used to denote the loading of the cervical spine when a player makes contact with the top of his head.

axial skeleton—The bones of the body that compose the spine, chest, and head.

backboarding—The process of securing an athlete to a spine board in order to stabilize the victim when a spine injury is suspected.

ball-and-socket joint—A joint in which a rounded bone fits into a cuplike socket and swivels. Examples include the hip and shoulder joints. Also called a *multiaxial joint.*

ballistic stretching—A bouncing movement used to lengthen or stretch tissue. Ballistic stretching is not recommended and may cause injury.

battle sign—A discoloration behind the ear resulting from a skull fracture.

Bell's palsy—A temporary paralysis of the face resulting from a virus causing eyelid and facial drooping.

benign paroxysmal positional vertigo—This is vertigo that is caused by idiopathic means or by head impact. Calcium crystals found in the semicircular canals move and the vestibular system does not function properly.

beta-adrenergic drugs—Drugs used to control the release of chemicals during an asthma attack by maintaining the airway.

bile—A substance produced by the liver and stored in the gallbladder that assists in the digestion of fat in the small intestine.

biomechanics—The study of the movement of living creatures.

biometric—An instrument or device that measures body functions through technology.

blister—A skin wound characterized by a fluid-filled lesion caused by friction.

blowout—A type of fracture caused when the thin bones beneath the eye absorb the sudden increase in pressure from an impact.

Board of Certification (BOC)—The national organization that examines and certifies athletic trainers so they can practice as ATs.

body temperature—The temperature at which bodily processes take place, normally 98.6 °F (37 °C).

bone scan—A radiological test in which the patient receives an injection containing low-level radioactive tracers; used to focus on injuries and conditions of bony tissue.

boutonniere deformity—A structural irregularity that occurs at the PIP joint of the fingers. A hard impact over the PIP joint can cause a tear in the joint capsule, which will allow the extensor tendons to fall laterally. When the tendons are in the lateral position, they contract and force flexion of the distal interphalangeal joint.

boxer's fracture—A fracture to the metacarpal region, specifically to the fourth or fifth metacarpal as a result of punching.

breathing rate—The number of breaths taken per minute. Normal breathing rate is 12 to 20 breaths per minute.

bronchitis—An inflammation of the bronchial passages, which can be caused by an infection or an allergy.

budgeting—The process of determining the amount of revenue and expenditures as well as the categories in which each belongs.

bulimia nervosa—An eating disorder characterized by bouts of bingeing and self-induced vomiting.

bunion—Excessive deviation or valgus stress at the great toe. Also known as hallux valgus.

burner—A group of symptoms including burning, numbness, tingling, and pain down the arm that results from stretching a group of nerves called the *brachial plexus*. This condition is also called a *stinger*.

burnout—A syndrome of continual training and sport-specific stress, resulting in staleness and overtraining, causing the athlete to no longer desire to participate in that sport.

bursa—A fluid-filled sac between a tendon and a bone that eases the friction of muscle movement.

bursitis—Inflammation of a bursa sac often characterized by swelling.

calcaneus—The heel bone of the foot.

calibration—A method to ensure safe and appropriate function of the modality.

callus—A mass of connective tissue that forms at the site of a fracture and is converted into bone or a thickening of skin in response to repeated stress.

caloric balance—The relationship between calories ingested and calories expended.

Canadian Standards Association (CSA)—The committee that sets the standards for eye guards and ice hockey helmets.

capillary refill—Blood moving back into the end of a finger or toe after it has been pinched for a moment.

capital femoral epiphysis—The growth plate located between the head and the neck of the femur. It can be fractured, especially in young athletes.

carbuncles—A cluster of boils on the skin caused by a bacterial infection.

cardiac arrest—When the heart stops beating.

cardiac tamponade—A critical injury whereby fluid fills the sac surrounding the heart.

cardiologist—A physician with specialized knowledge of the cardiovascular system.

cardiomyopathy—A condition in which the heart muscle thickens causing a dangerous cardiac condition.

cardiopulmonary resuscitation (CPR)—Used when the heart stops. One CPR cycle for an adult is 30 chest compressions and two slow breaths.

cardiorespiratory endurance—The ability to sustain exercise over a long time.

carotid artery—One of two vessels that run from the aorta through the neck and supply the head with oxygenated blood.

carpal tunnel syndrome—A chronic condition caused by compression of the medial nerve where it runs through the carpal tunnel at the anterior aspect of the wrist.

casting—The complete immobilization of a body part with a hard cast that is made with either plaster or fiberglass.

catastrophic policy—Insurance policy purchased by organizations in the event of a fatality or catastrophic injury.

caudal—A point that is lower than another; synonymous with *inferior.*

cauliflower ear—A condition that occurs when the pinna (the projecting portion of the external ear) begins to bleed internally after an impact, causing swelling, redness, and pain. As the ear heals, an excessive growth of reparative tissue distorts the pinna, making it look like a piece of cauliflower.

cephalgia—This term means *headache*; they are classified by the location of the pain, called zones.

cephalic—Toward the head; synonymous with *superior.*

cerebral palsy (CP)—A disorder that affects the brain before, during, or shortly after birth and inhibits normal brain development.

cerebrospinal fluid—A liquid from the blood that maintains uniform pressure within the brain, bathes the brain in chemicals for proper functioning, and protects the brain from impacts.

certification—An acknowledgment by an organization or certification board stating that a person possesses specific skills and competencies.

certified athletic trainer (AT)—A person who is concerned with the health and well-being of the physically active and athletic population. The AT's credentials are *ATC.*

cervical spine—The seven vertebrae that compose the uppermost region of the spine.

checkrein—A taping procedure whereby a piece of tape is looped around the thumb and index finger to prevent the thumb from being forcefully abducted.

chicken pox (varicella)—A childhood disease characterized by flulike symptoms and a spotted rash.

chiropractor—Medical personnel who treats mainly musculoskeletal disorders and restores normal function by manipulating bones, specifically at the spinal column.

cholesterol—A fatlike substance produced within the body to perform essential cellular functions.

chondromalacia—The softening or wearing away of the cartilage that lies on the back of the patella.

chronic obstructive pulmonary disease (COPD)—A medical condition in which the lung tissue is compromised by disease and is unable to effectively exchange air.

chronic traumatic encephalopathy (CTE)—A condition that most often occurs in athletes who participate in contact or collision sports, where repeated impact to the head causes degenerative brain damage.

circuit training—A weight training method whereby a person rotates through a series of 8 to 20 exercises. It is a full-body workout that elevates the heart rate.

circumduction—The movement of a limb in a circular pattern. Occurs when a ball-and-socket joint (shoulder or hip) encompasses several directions with one motion.

closed kinetic chain—When a segment, such as the foot or hand, is in contact with the ground and bearing weight.

cochlear implant—A device implanted on the side of the skull that provides a sense of sound to a person who is deaf or hard of hearing.

code of ethics—A series of behaviors and beliefs that articulate how professionals are to act.

cognitive behavioral therapy—Learning to recognize thought patterns that are not based in fact and can manifest in anxiety and stress. Then utilizing skills to manage and refute those thinking patterns.

Colles' fracture—A fracture of the radius and ulna whereby the limb bends into extension at the fracture site.

Commission on Accreditation of Athletic Training Education (CAATE)—The accrediting body for athletic training education programs in the United States.

common cold (coryza)—An illness caused by many common viruses and characterized by runny nose, sneezing, and coughing.

complete blood count (CBC)—A check of the blood that can detect conditions such as anemia (low iron count), infections, clotting problems, and other disorders.

compression—To apply pressure on a structure.

computerized tomography (CT) scan—Uses X-ray technology to produce images or slices of tissue in the body tissue.

concussion—Temporarily impaired brain function caused by a jarring impact to the head or by a rotational force of the head.

conduction—The transfer of heat between two objects in contact with one another.

conjunctiva—The membrane lining of the eye.

conjunctivitis—An infection and inflammatory response affecting the conjunctiva. Often called *pink eye*.

constipation—A condition in which it is difficult to perform a bowel movement due to lack of fiber, dehydration, or other medical conditions.

constrict—To narrow an opening or a blood vessel.

contrecoup—An injury that occurs when the head is moving and hits an unyielding surface or object. On impact, the brain is forced to the side opposite the blow.

convection—The transfer of heat from the movement of a medium. An example of a medium is water.

copay—The amount that the insured is responsible for paying at the time of service through insurance company standards.

corneal abrasion—An abrasion or laceration caused by a poke in the eye by a foreign object or by wearing contact lenses too long.

coronavirus—A virus that is spread through droplets. The droplets are released through the air when a person breathes, talks, coughs, sneezes, or sings. A person may suffer breathing or heart problems as a long-term effect.

crepitus—A grinding sound that is heard by the athlete, AT, or both. Crepitus can indicate a fracture, cartilage wear, or severe joint inflammation.

Crohn's disease—An autoimmune disorder that affects the gastrointestinal tract causing weight loss, fatigue, and fever.

CrossFit—A branded fitness program adopted by fitness gyms across the country. The program began in 2000 and is considered a high intensity interval program and nutrition regimen.

cryotherapy—The use of cold on a body part during treatment or rehabilitation.

cupping—An ancient form of Chinese therapy that causes the skin and tissue to be drawn upward by a suction cup.

de Quervain's tendinitis—An inflammation that affects the abductor pollicis longus and extensor pollicis brevis as they pass through the wrist.

deep—Away from the body's surface.

deep vein thrombosis—A medical condition where a clot forms in the vein causing pain.

DeLorme method—A weight training regimen consisting of three sets of 10 repetitions performed at successively greater intensities.

dental caries—The medical term for cavities that result from tooth decay.

dentist—A medical specialist who treats primarily teeth and gums.

depression (anatomical)—When a bony segment is moved in an inferior direction.

depression (psychological)—A feeling of hopelessness. Severe depression may need to be observed and treated by a physician, in which case it is referred to as *clinical depression*.

dermis—A layer that helps hold the skin to underlying bone and muscle tissue.

detached retina—A condition in which the retina of the eye is torn from its normal position. An athlete with a detached retina will have difficulty seeing and requires a physician's care.

diabetes—A disease whereby the pancreas does not secrete insulin effectively or the body is resistant to insulin.

diabetic coma—A condition that occurs when there is not enough insulin to control the sugar in the blood.

diaphragm—The muscle located between the chest and the abdomen that contracts and relaxes to assist with breathing.

diarrhea—A condition resulting in watery stool that can quickly result in dehydration and other medical complications.

diarthrodial joint—A freely movable joint, such as the shoulder. This kind of joint has a joint capsule, a synovial membrane, cartilage, and ligaments.

diastolic pressure—The pressure in the arteries when the heart is resting. Normal diastolic pressure is 80 mmHg.

dietitian (registered)—A specialist concerned with the dietary needs of people.

dilate—To widen an opening or a blood vessel.

dimethyl sulfoxide (DMSO)—A veterinary medicine used to enhance tissue healing. Animal research found that DMSO decreased healing time and wound swelling. Though used by some athletes, there is no indication that it works on humans.

direct current (DC)—Electricity that moves in one direction as it passes through the circuit.

direct pressure—External pressure applied to an open bleeding wound.

disability—A physical or mental impairment that substantially limits one or more major life activities.

disablement model—A model designed as the international classification of functioning, disability, and health by the World Health Organization that addresses the multiple facets of health.

dislocation—An injury that disrupts the alignment of bones at a joint, resulting in obvious deformity.

disordered eating—Abnormal eating patterns, often either bulimia or anorexia.

distal—Away from the attachment of a limb.

diverticulitis—A gastrointestinal condition resulting in outpouching in the bowel, resulting in pain and infection.

documentation—The permanent record of what happened in an athlete's injury, illness, or rehabilitation.

dorsal—The posterior aspect (back) of a structure.

drug—Any substance other than food or water that changes the body's chemistry when it is ingested or applied topically.

dual-energy X-ray absorptiometry (DEXA) scan—A test with a diagnostic machine that determines the density of bones.

duty of care—Having a responsibility to care for an injured person.

dynamic stabilization—A method of spinal exercises that establishes a strong core by using the principles of balancing stretching and strengthening of the anterior, posterior, inferior, and superior regions of the spine to allow for functional, pain-free movements.

dynamic stretching—Moving a limb or part of the body through its range of motion. Swinging the leg forward and backward is an example.

dysmenorrhea—Painful menstrual cycles.

dyspnea—Difficult or labored breathing.

ECG—Electrocardiogram, a recording of the heart's rhythm that will reflect patterns and pace of the heartbeats.

ectopic—A pregnancy where the embryo develops in the fallopian tubes rather than the uterus.

edema—Tissue swelling caused by high levels of protein-based fluid.

effective dose—The amount of the drug needed to achieve the desired effect.

effleurage—Massage that involves stroking the tissue with the palm of the hand in a smooth, rhythmical manner.

elastic tape—A flexible tape made of stretchy nylon fibers.

elastic wraps—Stretchy strips of cloth that come in various widths. They are most commonly applied to the body to provide compression around a joint or injured area.

electronic medical record (EMR)—A medical record created and stored electronically in a patient management system that allows doctors to share information throughout the healthcare system.

elevation mask—A training tool worn on the face that mimics training at high elevation.

elevation—When a bony segment is moved in a superior direction.

embolism—A blood clot or air mass that moves to regions of the body causing disability or death.

emergency action plan (EAP)—The organized action that people should take if an emergency arises.

emergency medical technician (EMT)—Someone who is certified to treat and transport people who are ill or injured.

emphysema—A chronic lung condition where the airways are congested with phlegm, causing a poor exchange of air.

endurance—The ability to withstand fatigue and tolerate prolonged activity.

ephedra—A drug used for weight loss that has been banned by the FDA.

epidermis—The most superficial layer of skin.

epidural hematoma—A blood clot that forms between the skull and the outermost protective membrane of the brain called the dura mater.

epilepsy—A disorder marked by disturbed electrical rhythms of the central nervous system.

epiphysis (growth plate)—The area of the bone where growth occurs.

epistaxis—A bloody nose.

Epley maneuver—A series of movements used to determine in which ear the crystals are not aligned, as well as to move them back into their proper place.

equipment manager—The person responsible for assigning and fitting appropriate playing equipment to athletes.

ergonomics specialist—A person who measures, modifies, and adapts a work environment to prevent injuries.

ergonomics—Adapting the athletic training environment to prevent injuries to the AT from repetitive strain on all parts of her body.

esophagus—The passage at the back of the throat that carries food from the mouth to the stomach.

evaporation—The process that cools the body.

eversion—A movement that turns the sole of the foot outward, away from the midline of the body.

extension—A straightening movement around a joint to restore it to anatomical position. The anatomical position of the knee, for example, is straight.

extrication—The removal of an injured person from a dangerous situation in order to provide further care without causing more harm.

failure point—The amount of force required to cause a fracture.

fallopian tubes—The anatomical structure in the female reproductive system that connects the ovary to the uterus.

Family Educational Rights and Privacy Act (FERPA)—Law that protects a student's right to privacy connected with his education records and gives him the right to access his records. If an athlete wants ATs and other personnel to be able to view his educational records, the athlete or a parent or guardian must first provide written consent.

fasciitis—Chronic inflammation of the fascia, the tissue that surrounds muscle tissue and binds skin to the underlying fat and muscle tissue.

fat pad syndrome—A condition whereby the fat pad of the knee becomes trapped between the patella and the femur. Often referred to as *Hoffa's syndrome.*

female athlete triad syndrome—A collection of symptoms and decreased bone health caused by disordered eating, amenorrhea, and osteoporosis.

fiber—Indigestible material found in foods high in carbohydrate.

fibrillation—When the heart beats in an extremely rapid fashion and fails to contract properly.

fibroblasts—Connective tissue cells that begin building fibers across an area of injury. They form the scar and take about six weeks to accomplish their task.

fibrous joint—A synarthrodial joint.

fixed budget—A month-to-month budget summed together to reflect the annual expenditures and income.

flail chest—An injury whereby several consecutive ribs are fractured in two or more places.

flexibility—The ability to move a joint through a full range of motion without restriction.

flexion—A bending movement around a joint in a limb away from its straightened position.

folliculitis—An inflammation of a follicle, especially of a hair follicle.

foramen—An opening; in the spine, there are vertebral foramen where the spinal cord proper passes through the vertebrae and the intervertebral foramen where the nerve roots extend in the openings between where two vertebrae come together.

forward head posture—When the head juts forward so that the athlete's ears are not lined up with the shoulders.

fracture—A break in a bone.

friction massage—Massage using deep, penetrating pressure into the tissue with movement of the finger, thumb, or elbow.

frontal plane—The plane that separates the body into front and back halves.

furuncle—An infection in a skin gland that forms a bright red lump that hurts when touched. It is also known as a boil.

gamekeeper's thumb—An injury to the MCL of the thumb.

gamma hydroxybutyrate (GHB)—A central nervous system depressant also known as a club drug.

ganglion cyst—A pocket of fluid within the sheath of the wrist.

gastrocnemius—A large muscle at the back of the lower leg responsible for pointing the toes.

gastroesophageal reflux disease (GERD)—A condition in which the acid from the stomach regurgitates into the throat causing pain, discomfort, and sour taste.

generic name drug—A medication produced and put in the marketplace in competition with the trade drug.

girth—The distance around a body part.

glenoid labrum—A cartilage disc that surrounds the edge of the scapular fossa and deepens the socket in which the head of the humerus inserts.

goniometer—A device that measures range of motion at joints.

gross negligence—A step beyond negligence whereby a person fails to provide even minimal care when needed.

ground fault interrupter—Known as GFI; an electrical outlet placed near water to prevent electrocution.

gynecologist—A physician who specializes in the diagnosis and treatment of diseases of the female reproductive system.

half-life—The time it takes for only half the initial amount of a drug to be remaining in a person's system.

hallux valgus—Excessive valgus stress at the great toe, also known as a bunion.

hammertoe—A deformity in which the middle joint of the toe is flexed and the metatarsophalangeal and distal phalangeal joints are hyperextended.

hamstrings—The name given collectively to the semimembranosus, semitendinosus, and biceps femoris muscles, which are responsible for flexing the knee and extending the hip.

Health Insurance Portability and Accountability Act (HIPAA)—Defines what can be shared with others about a medical record of a patient being treated.

heart attack—A injury to the heart that occurs when a blocked vessel to the heart, a clot, stress over time, or an injury to the heart muscle itself creates an insufficient blood supply.

heart rate—The number of times the heart beats in a minute; often measured as the pulse in a superficial artery. The normal pulse rate for a teenager is between 60 and 80 beats per minute.

heat cramps—A mild heat-related illness marked by sudden muscular contractions that will not release because the necessary minerals and water are not available.

heat exhaustion—A moderate heat-related illness caused by exercising in a hot, humid environment. Effects are weakness, nausea, dizziness, and profuse sweating, causing dehydration with excessive sodium loss through sweat.

heat index—The measure of the temperature the body feels when air temperature and relative humidity are combined. It indicates how safe it is to participate in activities and the body's ability to dissipate heat on a particular day.

heat syncope—Fainting due to heat exposure.

heatstroke—A severe heat-related illness caused by prolonged exposure to high temperature and humidity and marked by the hypothalamus shutting down, which causes body temperature to rise dangerously. Secondary causes of heatstroke include dehydration, excessive weight loss, obesity, alcoholism, CP, and diabetes.

heel spur—A small, pointy, bony growth at the bottom of the calcaneus; often caused by plantar fasciitis.

hematoma—A collection of blood at an anatomical site.

hematuria—Blood found in urine that can be caused by several things.

hemiplegia—The loss of sensation and muscular function on one side of the body that results from injury to or disease of the motor processes of the brain.

hemophilia—A hereditary blood disorder characterized by delayed clotting of the blood.

hemothorax—Blood in the chest cavity.

hepatitis A virus (HAV)—A form of hepatitis that is rarely chronic.

hepatitis B virus (HBV)—A virus that tends to persist in the blood and causes an infection in the liver.

hepatitis C virus (HCV)—A form of hepatitis that does not show signs and symptoms until the diseased has progressed, causing permanent damage to the liver; may lead to death.

hepatitis D virus (HDV)—A form of hepatitis that can infect a person if they have had hepatitis B. Essentially it is a second bout of hepatitis or it can be a coinfection.

hepatitis E virus (HEV)—A form of hepatitis usually in places without clean water. In the United States hepatitis E can be transmitted by undercooked meat.

hepatitis—A viral illness that affects the liver.

hernia—A lump of tissue, usually the intestine, that bulges through a weakness in the abdominal wall.

herpes—A highly contagious skin condition caused by a virus.

hidradenitis suppurativa—This is a skin disease that appears similar to acne in the early phases, but as it progresses the lesion looks more like oval lumps and in later stages appears tubular. HS in the later stages tunnels to connect each of the lesions.

hinge joint—An articulation whereby the joint can move primarily in flexion and extension. An example of a hinge joint is the knee or elbow.

hip pointer—A contusion to the iliac crest.

history—The portion of the assessment process consisting of understanding the injured athlete's chief complaint, determining exactly how the injury occurred, assessing functional problems that exist, noting signs and symptoms, and determining preexisting medical conditions.

HIT—An injury assessment process that follows this sequence: **h**istory, **i**nspection, and **t**esting.

Hoffa's syndrome—A condition whereby the fat pad of the knee becomes trapped between the patella and the femur. Often referred to as *fat pad syndrome*.

human growth hormone (HGH)—Protein-based hormone used to stimulate muscle growth.

human immunodeficiency virus (HIV)—A virus known to cause AIDS, which affects the body's ability to fight infection and disease.

humidity—The amount of moisture in the air.

hyaline cartilage—A thin layer of cartilage that covers the ends of a bone where it articulates with another bone.

hybrid tape—Tape made from both linen and elastic.

hydrocele—The formation of a water cyst in the scrotum that causes pressure on the testicles.

hyperglycemia—A condition in which the blood sugar level is too high.

hypertension—Abnormally high blood pressure, especially arterial pressure.

hyperthermia—Excessive buildup of heat within the body; an exceptionally high fever.

hyphema—An injury to the eye that causes blood to flow into the anterior chamber.

hypoglycemia—A condition in which the blood sugar level is too low.

hyponatremia—Low blood sodium level.

hypotension—Abnormally low blood pressure.

hypothermia—Subnormal body temperature from prolonged exposure to damp cold.

iliopsoas syndrome—A syndrome attributed to the movement of the iliopsoas tendon over bony prominence of the hip which causes pain.

immune system—The internal defense mechanisms of the body.

impetigo—A skin disease characterized by itching and the development of a yellow crusted exterior.

impingement syndrome—A collection of symptoms caused by compression of either the biceps tendon or supraspinatus tendon below the acromion of the shoulder.

infectious mononucleosis—A viral disease, often referred to as *mono*, characterized by headache, extreme fatigue, fever, and body aches. It can result in enlargement of the spleen.

inferior—One point, or structure, being lower than another.

influenza—The medical name for the flu.

informed consent—Permission by parents, after being informed of the possible dangers of participation in athletic activities, for medical staff to treat their child if he is injured.

ingrown toenail—An injury whereby the nail grows into the surrounding soft tissue.

insertion—The location where a muscle ends or attaches at the distal point.

insulin shock—A condition resulting in low blood sugar levels caused by too much insulin.

intermittent compression—A device with a built-in sleeve that fits over a body part. The sleeve periodically fills with air and applies compression to the area to reduce swelling.

intervertebral discs—Structures between the vertebrae that cushion them.

intracranial hematoma—Severe bleeding within the brain caused by a blow to the head.

intravenous therapy—Adding fluid via a vein in the hope to increase the blood volume and oxygen carrying capacity depending on the type of shock.

inversion—A movement that turns the sole of the foot inward toward the midline of the body.

irritable bowel syndrome—A condition where the gastrointestinal tract is irritated by food, stress, or medications causing episodes of diarrhea followed by constipation and pain.

isokinetic contraction—The muscular force applied against a machine that allows the joint to move only at a specific speed.

isometric contraction—A movement that causes the muscle to contract against resistance without changing its length.

isotonic contraction—A movement that causes the muscle fibers to shorten and lengthen against resistance when lifting and lowering a weight.

jersey finger—An injury of the finger in which the flexor tendon tears from the fingertip.

joint capsule—A sac or sleevelike structure that covers a joint. The capsule has a synovial membrane containing synovial fluid to ease joint movement.

Jones fracture—A fracture occurring at the base of the fifth metatarsal bone.

jugular vein—One of two vessels that takes unoxygenated blood from the head to the heart.

Kehr's sign—Pain in the abdomen and the left shoulder that most often indicates injury to the spleen.

kidney—A set of organs designed to filter waste products from the human body.

kinesiology tape—Tape that stretches only lengthwise; used to allow range of motion and normal movement of fluids, reduce pain, and take pressure off underlying tissues.

kinesiology—The study of human movement.

kyphosis—Excessive roundedness that can occur at the thoracic spine.

labrum—Cartilaginous tissue that deepens the sockets at the hip and shoulder joints.

laryngitis—Inflammation of the larynx.

larynx—An enlarged tube at the top of the trachea made of cartilage and muscle. The voice is created by air passing through the vocal cords in the larynx.

lateral collateral ligament (LCL)—This is the ligament that attaches the femur to the tibia on the lateral aspect of the knee.

lateral malleolus—The most prominent aspect of the fibula; located on the lateral aspect of the ankle.

lateral—Away from the midline of the body.

Legg-Calvé-Perthes disease—A condition found in some children that is characterized by a disruption of blood flow to the head of the femur, which causes the tissue at the head of the femur to die.

leukocytes—Infection-fighting white blood cells that go to the site of an injury.

leukoplakia—Precancerous cells often found on the cheek, tongue, and gums of those who use smokeless tobacco.

licensure—A state act that specifies who is allowed to practice athletic training and what duties they are allowed to perform.

ligaments—Tissues in the body that connect bone to bone.

line-item budget—This budget model divides expenditures into categories such as expendable supplies, equipment, insurance, and personnel resources.

linen tape—Tape made from cotton fibers.

Little League elbow—An injury to the medial aspect of the elbow in young throwing athletes, usually from overuse.

local steroid—A drug that is applied to the skin or injected in a joint to reduce swelling and pain; it should not be confused with anabolic steroids.

lordosis—Excessive curvature at the lumbar spine.

lumbar spine—The five vertebrae that compose the low back; located just above the sacrum.

lump-sum budget—This budget model revolves around one lump sum of money that is spent at the discretion of the budget director.

lunate dislocation—A condition in which the carpal bone called the lunate dislocates through injury to the wrist complex.

magnetic resonance imaging (MRI)—Uses radio waves and a magnetic field to make a picture of the body.

mallet finger—An injury to the fingertip caused by impact that tears the extensor tendon from the bone. Fingertip flexion is the distinguishing feature of this injury.

malpractice—When the AT causes an injury to an athlete by an act of omission or commission.

massage therapist—A person who administers massage for therapeutic purposes.

massage—Kneading and stroking of muscles and other soft tissue by the AT or massage therapist for therapeutic purposes.

McBurney's point—The area between the navel and the hip that becomes painful when the appendix becomes inflamed.

medial collateral ligament (MCL)—The ligament that attaches the femur to the tibia on the medial aspect of the knee.

medial malleolus—The end of the tibia on the medial side.

medial—Toward the midline of the body.

meniscectomy—A surgical procedure to remove the meniscus from the knee joint.

meniscus—A piece of cartilage within a joint, especially those pieces known as the medial and lateral menisci, which lie between the femur and the tibia.

metabolism—The body's energy system.

metatarsals—The five longest bones of the foot.

microorganism—An organism of microscopic or submicroscopic size such as a virus or bacteria.

mitral valve prolapse (MVP)—A condition in which the bicuspid (mitral) valve of the heart becomes weakened or less effective causing a regurgitation of blood between the chambers of the heart. A heart murmur.

moleskin—A thick, soft sticky tape that cannot be torn by hand.

molluscum contagiosum—A skin condition caused by a virus. It is characterized by the formation of pink lumps.

MRSA—Methicillin-resistant *Staphylococcus aureus* bacterial infection.

multiaxial joint—A joint that has a large range of movement because it can move in a variety of planes.

multiple sclerosis—A condition whereby the myelin sheath detaches from parts of the central nervous system, leading to erratic conduction of electrical impulses.

mumps—A viral illness characterized by swelling around the jawline.

muscular dystrophy—A group of disorders that affect the muscles by replacing muscle cells with connective tissue.

muscular endurance—The ability of a muscle to perform repetitive movements for an extended period. It can be developed by using a high number of repetitions and a small amount of weight.

muscular power—The ability to exert force quickly.

muscular strength—The ability to exert force against a resistance. It can be developed by using a low number of repetitions and heavy weight.

myocarditis—a condition where the cardiac muscle is inflamed.

myofascial release—A massage technique where the AT applies manual pressure to the muscle to lengthen the tissue.

myositis ossificans—The buildup of bone tissue in a muscle following an injury.

myositis—A chronic inflammation of the muscle tissue.

National Athletic Trainers' Association (NATA)—The professional association that recognizes ATs as its primary members and establishes codes of professional conduct.

National Operating Committee on Standards for Athletic Equipment (NOCSAE)—A committee that sets the standards for football, baseball, and softball helmets.

National Safety Council—An organization that certifies people in first aid and CPR procedures.

neck roll—Protective padding that keeps the head within a safe range of motion.

needs assessment—Defines the important elements of an athletic training program to help determine a budget.

negligence—A legal wrong characterized by the failure to act as a reasonably prudent person would act in a similar situation.

neurocognitive testing—Systematic, objective procedures used to examine the function of the brain. These tests are often computer based and used to create baseline performance measures that are then compared with postconcussion performance to determine if an athlete can return to play.

neurologist—A physician who specializes in the diagnosis and treatment of diseases of the nervous system.

neurosis—A mild form of mental health disorder such as anxiety, fears, depression, anger issues, compulsive disorders, obsessions, and low self-worth.

neutral spine—Normal cervical, thoracic, and lumbar curvature having neither too much flexion nor too much extension in a position that is comfortable for the athlete.

No HARM—An acronym that denotes using **no** **h**eat, **a**lcohol, **r**unning, or **m**assage to an injury.

nonsteroidal anti-inflammatory drug (NSAID)—A drug used to reduce tissue swelling after an injury.

nonunion—A fracture that does not heal, leaving two pieces of bone where there was one before.

nucleus pulposus—The soft structure at the center of an intervertebral disc.

nutrients—Substances in food that the body uses in metabolism.

nutrition—The processes that use food to fulfill the metabolic needs of the body.

objective—The things the AT can see or measure regarding an injury or illness.

observation—What the AT can see when assessing an injury, such as discoloration or swelling.

Occupational Safety and Health Administration (OSHA)—A national organization that makes sure work environments are safe by preventing injuries.

oncologist—A physician who treats patients with cancer.

one-repetition maximum (1RM)—The amount of weight an athlete can lift for only one repetition.

open kinetic chain—When a segment, such as the foot or hand, is moving freely in space (not in contact with the ground) and not bearing weight.

ophthalmologist—A physician who treats medical conditions of the eye.

opposition—Occurs when you move your thumb across your hand to meet your smallest finger, or fifth digit.

origin—The point at which a muscle begins; the proximal attachment.

orthopedist—A physician who deals primarily with conditions and injuries of the musculoskeletal system.

Osgood-Schlatter disorder—A condition characterized by an irritation or loosening of the patellar tendon at its attachment at the top anterior aspect of the tibia, usually seen in younger athletes who perform a great deal of running and jumping.

osteitis pubis—When the pubic symphysis is subject to repeated stress, it can become inflamed and painful.

osteoarthritis—An arthritis of the hip caused by the wearing away of the articular surface of the head of the femur and degradation of the labrum of the acetabulum.

osteomyelitis—An infection of the bone caused by a traumatic injury, open wound, or general infection.

osteoporosis—The loss of calcium from the bones creating porous, weak bones. Osteopenia is the precursor to osteoporosis.

ovary—The female reproductive organs that produce eggs.

overload principle—A strength and conditioning principle based on the idea that in order for muscles to get stronger, they must be challenged to lift more than they are used to lifting.

over-the-counter (OTC) drug—Can be purchased at a store without a prescription.

palpation—Examination of an injured area by touch to determine the type of injury, such as fracture, swelling, muscle ruptures, and tendinitis.

Palpation also gives an indication of the athlete's pain level.

pandemic—When a disease, infection, or virus occurs, and most people do not have immunity. Healthy people are at risk for complications, health care providers and hospitals are overwhelmed, and medication supply is inadequate. There's an increase in medical visits, more complications from the disease and high death rates, and an impact to the public and business and world economies.

paraffin bath—Heated wax that is used to warm a body area, such as a hand or foot.

paralysis—The inability to move.

paraplegia—The loss of sensation and muscular function in the lower extremities caused by an injury of the spinal cord.

parotid—A gland in the mouth that produces saliva; one of three oral glands.

partial airway obstruction—When a portion of the airway is closed off by an object in the throat.

passive range of motion (PROM)—The extent to which an injured body part can be moved by the AT without pain or exertion from the athlete.

patellar tendinitis—Inflammation of the patellar tendon; often called *jumper's knee*.

peak flow meter—A medical device used to determine the amount of airflow produced with exhalation.

pediatrician—A specialist in the medical treatment of children.

pelvic inflammatory disease—A condition resulting in scarring and infertility from infections or other medical conditions.

percussion—The tapping on an organ as part of a medical assessment.

percussion massage—Massage using light chopping motions to the tissue.

petrissage—A massage stroke that squeezes the skin, muscles, and fasciae between the hands; it is often described as kneading the tissue.

phagocytes—Specialized white blood cells that clear dead cells from the site of an injury.

phalanges—The small bones that make up the fingers and toes.

pharyngitis—Inflammation of the pharynx.

physical therapist—An allied medical professional who specializes in rehabilitation of orthopedic and nonorthopedic conditions.

physician assistant—An allied medical professional who works directly under the supervision of a physician and conducts examinations, orders diagnostic tests, writes prescriptions, and diagnoses and treats injuries and illnesses.

piriformis syndrome—This syndrome occurs when the sciatic nerve is entrapped between the piriformis muscle and the tissue around the ischial tuberosity.

plan—The AT decides what to do with the issue that has been presented. Some examples are getting an X-ray, deciding how to remove an athlete from the field, or deciding when to progress an athlete in rehabilitation.

plantar fasciitis—Inflammation of the plantar fascia of the foot.

plantar surface—The bottom of the foot.

plantar warts—A skin disorder caused by HPV that commonly affects weight-bearing portions of the foot.

platelets—Blood cells that carry blood-clotting materials.

pleurisy—A medical condition where the lining of the lungs is inflamed, causing pain.

plyometric—Movements that stretch muscles, then go through eccentric contraction, amortization, and then to concentric contraction.

pneumonia—A bacterial or viral infection of the lungs causing fever, shortness of breath, and fatigue.

pneumothorax—Air in the chest cavity, commonly referred to as a *collapsed lung*.

podiatrist—A specialist in foot disorders.

positional release—A massage technique where the AT finds a muscle spasm and applies pressure. With the athlete relaxed, the AT takes the body part and moves it into a position where the athlete is comfortable, then holds this position for 90 seconds.

positron emission tomography (PET) scan—A nuclear medicine test that focuses on the metabolism of specific tissues or organs.

posterior—The back of the body.

posterior cruciate ligament (PCL)—A knee ligament that prevents the tibia from moving posteriorly on the femur.

post-traumatic response—An emotional disorder resulting from a traumatic experience.

PREMIER model—A framework for thinking about being a professional: **P**romote a professional image. **R**emember your vision. **E**ngage in learning. **M**aximize your strengths. **I**nnovate and create. **E**nlist the help of others. **R**eflect on your actions.

pressure point—A place on the body where arteries, such as the brachial artery and the femoral artery, are easily accessed and pressure can be applied with the hand to slow the blood flow to a body part.

PRICES—An acronym for **p**rotection, **r**est, **i**ce, **c**ompression, **e**levation, and **s**upport of an injured body part that represents the initial steps of care for musculoskeletal injuries such as ligament sprains or muscle strains.

primary assessment—The aspect of assessment devoted to determining if an athlete has a clear airway, is breathing, and has a pulse.

primary care physician—The athlete's primary doctor. She must be notified after an athlete is injured.

progression—The advancement of an exercise or activity from simple to complex, slow to fast, and less aggressive to more aggressive.

progressive resistive exercise (PRE)—The gradual progression of an exercise from easy to more difficult from one set to the next and over time.

pronation—A movement that turns the palm of the hand down as if it were emptying a bowl of soup.

proprioception—The ability of the body to give information to the brain regarding the body's position, movements being performed, and forces acting on it.

prosthetic—An artificial body part.

protraction—Movement of the scapulas away from one another; the opposite of retraction.

proximal—Toward the attachment of the limb to the trunk.

proximate cause—A close connection between the act of a certified AT and resulting injury to an athlete.

psychosis—A significant form of mental illness when a person may lose touch with reality. Some psychotic forms of illness include bipolar disorder, schizophrenia, or severe depression.

pulse points—Areas where arteries lie close to the skin.

pulse pressure—The difference between the diastolic and systolic pressures.

pulse rate—The number of times the heart beats per minute, normally 60 to 80 per minute, taken at the wrist or neck.

purchase order—The order that is sent to the vendor that defines the terms and conditions of the purchase.

pyramid method—A strength-training regimen that involves multiple sets. The first set is low intensity, the second set is moderate intensity, the third set is intense, the fourth set returns to moderate intensity, and the fifth set is low intensity.

quadriplegia—The inability to move the arms and legs.

radiologist—A physician who specializes in reading medical imaging such as X-rays, CT scans, and bone scans.

reconditioning—Getting the athlete back into shape for athletic participation.

recreational drug—A drug that has no medical purpose.

red blood cells (RBC)—The cells in the blood that carry oxygen.

referral point—The place in another part of the body where an injured or diseased abdominal organ refers pain.

registration—The step of contacting state authorities before acting in the capacity of an AT. It is required by law in some states.

rehabilitation—The process or means of getting a person back to his normal level of function following an injury or illness.

reimbursement—A process in which a health care provider is given money for the services provided to a patient.

remodeling—The body's way of building tissue strength in the tendons, ligaments, and muscles to withstand the stress applied to the body during activity.

reposition—Returning your thumb and fifth digit to their starting positions.

resistance training—An organized program to work the muscles, usually by lifting weights.

retraction—When the scapulas are moved, or pulled, together.

rhabdomyolysis—A serious muscle injury that can be caused by a blow to the muscle or by overworking the muscle, which causes death of muscle fibers.

rhinitis—Inflammation of the nasal passages.

rigid tape—Tape used to improvement joint movement by slightly changing alignment or stabilizing a joint; has no stretch in the material.

rotation—The spinning or turning movement of a bony segment around an axis.

rotator cuff—A group of muscles around the shoulder joint. The muscles of the rotator cuff are the supraspinatus, infraspinatus, teres minor, and subscapularis.

rubella—A form of measles often referred to as *German measles*. It is characterized by a rash and itching.

rubeola—A form of measles characterized by high fever, chills, rash (even inside the mouth), and coughing.

ruptured eardrum—A tear of the tympanic membrane.

sacrum—The bottommost segment of the spine, which consists of bones that are fused.

sagittal plane—A plane that divides the body into left and right halves.

school nurse—A licensed nurse who provides services to a school or school district.

sciatica—A back condition that occurs when a disc bulges or there is a bone spur or a stenosis of the spine. Typical symptoms include shooting pain down the hip and into the leg and muscular weakness.

scoliosis—Excessive side-to-side curvature of the spine.

scrotum—The sac surrounding the testicles.

sebaceous cyst—This is a cyst that develops when the opening of a skin gland becomes blocked, or the gland is misshaped.

second-impact syndrome—A set of symptoms resulting from more than one concussion or blow to the head in a relatively short time.

seizure—Uncontrollable shaking resulting from a brain chemical imbalance or head injury.

septic arthritis—An infection within the synovial fluid.

shared professional values—The foundation upon which ethical and legal practice is guided in the profession of athletic training; CIRCA.

shin splints—A term for pain of the lower leg, often along the tibia. It is often called *medial tibial stress syndrome*.

shingles (herpes zoster)—The same virus that causes chickenpox that can remain dormant until adulthood.

shoulder separation—A sprain of the acromioclavicular joint.

sickle cell anemia—An inherited disease in which the red blood cells become shaped like sickles with points on each end, which causes the cells to hook onto the sides of the blood vessels, creating a logjam of cells in a particular area. The result is that oxygen is not carried efficiently to all parts of the body.

sign—Objective evidence that a rescuer can measure or sense, such as sweating, breath odor, temperature, blood pressure, breathing rate, or heart rate.

sinusitis—Inflammation of the sinuses.

SITS—An acronym for the muscles of the rotator cuff: **s**upraspinatus, **i**nfraspinatus, **t**eres minor, and **s**ubscapularis.

SLAP lesion—Superior labrum anterior and posterior; a type of tear in the shoulder labrum, resulting in instability and pain.

SOAP note—A document outlining the findings of an injury assessment using **s**ubjective, **o**bjective, **a**ssessment, and **p**lan-of-action components.

soleus—A posterior lower-leg muscle that plantar flexes the foot.

special tests—The tests performed to determine the severity of an injury or illness.

specificity—The principle stating that the type of activity a person performs in training is the type of activity she will get better at performing.

sphygmomanometer—Another name for blood pressure cuff.

spinal stenosis—A condition in which there is a narrowing of the spinal canal or the intervertebral foramen.

splinting—The immobilization of a body part with a splint, which is usually made of wood, plastic, cloth, or aluminum and taped into place.

spondylolisthesis—A degeneration of a vertebra that fails to heal, therefore separating and causing the spine to become unstable. The resulting instability allows a vertebra to shunt, or slip, forward on the vertebra below it.

spondylolysis—A stress fracture or bone degeneration of the vertebrae.

sport psychologist—A professional who works with athletes who may need help with goal setting, anxiety, frustration, self-esteem, or family issues.

sport psychology—The science of how variables such as life stress, mood, and motivation affect sport performance and sport-related injury.

sports medicine team—All the people who might work with and care for an athlete at one point or another during their participation in athletics.

sport-specific function—Specific exercises and activities that are similar to the activities that the athlete will face on return to participation.

sprain—Injury to a ligament.

standards of professional practice—The way an AT is expected to act while doing their job.

static stretching—Holding a stretched muscle in one position for a short length of time.

steady state—When the amount of a drug in the body is equal to its removal from the body.

stinger—A group of symptoms including burning, numbness, tingling, and pain down the arm that result from stretching a group of nerves called the *brachial plexus*. This condition is also called a *burner*.

strain—An injury that occurs to a muscle or tendon.

strength and conditioning coach—A person who works with athletes to ensure that each is in shape to meet the demands of athletic competition.

student assistant—A student who volunteers to observe (and assist when deemed appropriate) a certified AT in order to learn more about the profession.

subconjunctival hemorrhage—An athlete may cough hard repeatedly, which causes the small vessels in the eye to rupture, turning the conjunctiva red. An athlete may also get poked in the conjunctiva or hit by a ball, which causes the same result.

subdural hematoma—A condition where blood collects between the skull and the surface of the brain.

subjective—Anything an athlete shares about an injury or illness that may not be visual.

sublingual—One of three glands of the mouth; produce saliva.

submandibular—Saliva producing gland in the mouth; one of three glands.

subungual hematoma—Bleeding under the fingernail, often caused by a direct impact to the tip of the finger.

superficial—Close to the body's surface.

superior—One point, or structure, being higher than another.

supination—A movement that turns the palm of the hand up as if it were holding a bowl of soup.

suture—A synthetic material, either dissolvable or nondissolvable, used to close a wound.

swimmer's ear—An infection that results from water in the ear.

SWOT analysis—SWOT is an acronym for **s**trengths, **w**eaknesses, **o**pportunities, and **t**hreats.

symptom—What the athlete feels but cannot see, smell, or hear, such as pain, nausea, or anxiousness.

synarthrodial joint—A type of joint in which bones are held together by tough connective tissue, making the joint essentially immovable.

syncope—Fainting caused by a lack of blood flow to the brain, such as from standing up quickly.

syndesmosis—The soft tissue that binds the distal ends of the tibia and fibula together.

synovial membrane—A tissue that surrounds diarthrodial joints and secretes a slippery fluid.

synovitis—Inflammation of the synovial lining of diarthrodial joints.

systolic pressure—The pressure in the arteries when the heart is beating. Normal systolic pressure is 120 mmHg.

talus—Ankle bone located directly above the calcaneus.

tarsal tunnel syndrome—A compromise of the tarsal tunnel can compress the tendons, nerve, or blood supply.

team physician—The medical authority of the sports medicine team whose role is to work with the AT to oversee the entire sports medicine team.

temporomandibular joint (TMJ) dysfunction—A condition in which the muscles surrounding the joint spasm.

tendinitis—Chronic inflammation of a tendon.

tendons—Tissues in the body that connect a muscle to a bone.

tennis elbow—Inflammation of the lateral epicondyle of the elbow, usually from overuse of the wrist extensor muscles.

testicular torsion—A condition in which the testicle rotates or twists and occludes the blood flow to the testicle creating a medical emergency.

therapeutic drug—A drug that has a medical purpose.

thermometry—The use of a thermometer to establish one's body temperature.

thoracic spine—The middle portion of the spine which includes 12 vertebrae.

Throwers' Ten—A shoulder rehabilitation program established by Dr. James Andrews and Kevin Wilk, PT, to help throwing athletes keep all-around shoulder strength and function.

tinea corporis—A red, scaly, ring-shaped abnormality that appears on the skin. It is a fungal skin condition commonly called *ringworm*.

tinea cruris—Also known as *jock itch*. It is caused by a fungal infection that causes a red, itchy rash in moist areas of the body such as the groin and inner thighs.

tinea pedis—A fungal infection of the foot commonly called *athlete's foot*.

tinnitus—Ringing in the ears.

Tommy John surgery—A surgical procedure used to repair ulnar collateral ligament ruptures caused from excessive throwing or overuse.

tonsillitis—An inflammation of the tonsils causing pain and infection.

torticollis—A condition of the neck in which the head is tilted toward the shoulder where a muscle strain or sprain has occurred.

total airway obstruction—Complete blockage of the airway by an object that prevents the athlete from speaking, coughing, or breathing.

trachea—A cartilage tube that allows passage of air from the larynx in the throat to the bronchial tube of the lungs.

traction—A pulling force used deliberately to separate joints of the body that have been compressed or gotten stiff.

trade name—A patented drug name given by a pharmaceutical company.

trans fat—Fatty acids that are created when hydrogen is added to vegetable oil so they are more solid.

transcutaneous electrical nerve stimulation (TENS)—The application of an electrical current to the surface of the skin to stimulate the region.

transverse plane—The plane that divides the body into top and bottom halves.

triage—The determination of the order in which to send injured patients to the hospital; the most seriously hurt go first.

triangular fibrocartilage complex (TFCC)—An anatomical structure located at the medial aspect of the wrist that supports the carpal bones.

tricompartment failure—When there is osteoarthritis of the knee (medial, lateral, and anterior).

trigger-point therapy—A massage technique where the AT finds the trigger point within the muscle and treats this area by applying pressure on a scale of 1 to 10 and then holding pressure at a 5 to relieve the pain.

trochanteric bursitis—Irritation of the greater trochanteric bursa of the hip, often caused by rubbing of the musculature.

ulnar nerve relocation—A procedure by which the ulnar nerve is transposed to eliminate pressure on the nerve.

ultrasound—This is considered a thermal modality because it can produce a deep-heating effect, break down tissues, or image soft tissues on a screen (used to determine the sex of an unborn baby, for example).

universal choking sign—Grabbing the throat with both hands to indicate choking. People who are choking instinctively do this, no matter what their nationality.

universal precautions—A set of procedures designed to prevent the spread of blood-borne diseases.

ureter—The anatomical structure that carries urine from the kidney to the bladder.

urethra—The anatomical structure that carries urine from the bladder to the outside of the body.

urologist—A physician who deals with problems of the urinary tract such as painful urination.

urticaria (hives)—A rash that can be contained in one body part or can cover the entire body caused when an irritant enters the body and histamine is released.

vaccination—Injection of tiny amounts of viruses (sometimes live and sometimes dead) into the body to create an immunity to specific viruses.

valgus—An outward deviation of a body segment.

variable budget—This model allows for adjustments throughout the year based on the ebb and flow of the expenditures.

ventral—The anterior aspect of a structure.

ventricle—A chamber of the heart that receives blood from a corresponding atrium and from which blood is forced into the arteries.

vestibular ocular motor screening—A series of tests is used to determine the significance of a concussion. Areas tested are vision, balance, and movement.

vibration massage—A massage stroke that causes the tissue to tremble or shake vigorously.

vital signs—Signs of life observed and measured during the secondary assessment to determine the seriousness of an injury, including body temperature, skin color, breathing rate, heart rate, response to pain, pupillary reaction, ability to move, and capillary refill.

whirlpool—A tub in which jets of air circulate hot or cold water.

white blood cells (WBC)—These cells in the blood help fight infection.

work–life balance—A way of life where professionals such as athletic trainers find time to enjoy both work and personal life activities to prevent burnout.

X-ray—Electromagnetic waves used to make a picture to aid in diagnosing injuries to bones and joints.

zero-based budget—This budget process essentially starts at zero each year; no money is rolled over from a previous year.

REFERENCES

Preface

Black, L.I., E.P. Terlizzi, and A. Vahratian. 2022. "Organized Sport Participation among Children Aged 6–17 Years: United States, 2020." www.cdc.gov/nchs/products/databriefs/db441.htm. Accessed June 6, 2024.

Stanford Medicine. 2024. "Sports Injury Statistics." www.stanfordchildrens.org/en/topic/default%3Fid%3Dsports-injury-statistics-90-P02787#:~:text=How%20frequently%20do%20sports%20injuries,are%20experienced%20by%20the%20participants. Accessed June 4, 2024.

Chapter 1

American Medical Association. 2016. "AMA Principles of Medical Ethics." www.ama-assn.org/delivering-care/ama-principles-medical-ethics. Accessed June 6, 2024.

Board of Certification. 2022. *Practice Analysis.* 8th ed.

Bureau of Labor Statistics, U.S. Department of Labor, *Occupational Outlook Handbook*, Athletic Trainers. Accessed July 9, 2022. www.bls.gov/ooh/healthcare/athletic-trainers.htm.

Commission on Accreditation of Athletic Training Education (CAATE). 2020. "Standards." https://caate.net/pp-standards. Accessed June 4, 2024.

National Athletic Trainers' Association. n.d. "Position Statements." www.nata.org/news-publications/pressroom/statements/position. Accessed June 12, 2024.

National Athletic Trainers' Association. 2021. "Salary Survey." www.nata.org/nata-salary-survey-resources. Accessed June 12, 2024.

National Athletic Trainers' Association. 2022. *Code of Ethics.* www.nata.org/sites/default/files/nata_code_of_ethics_2022.pdf.

National Registry of Emergency Medical Technicians. 2023. "Certification." www.nremt.org/EMT/Certification. Accessed June 12, 2024.

Chapter 2

Board of Certification. 2022. *Standards of Professional Practice.* www.bocatc.org/system/document_versions/versions/154/original/boc-standards-of-professional-practice-2018-20180619.pdf?1529433022. Accessed June 12, 2024.

Board of Certification. n.d.a. "Maintaining Certification." https://bocatc.org/athletic-trainers/maintain-certification/continuing-education/continuing-education. Accessed June 12, 2024.

Board of Certification. n.d.b. "State Regulation." https://bocatc.org/state-regulation/state-regulation. Accessed June 12, 2024.

Briscoe, B. 2015. "Understanding Health Plan Types: What's in a Name?" *Beyond the Numbers: Pay & Benefits* 4 (2) (U.S. Bureau of Labor Statistics, January 2015). www.bls.gov/opub/btn/volume-4/understanding_health_plan_types.htm. Accessed June 12, 2024.

Konin, J.G., and R. Ray. 2019. *Management Strategies in Athletic Training.* Champaign, IL: Human Kinetics.

National Athletic Trainers' Association. n.d. "Volunteer Opportunities." https://gather.nata.org/participate/volunteeropportunities/i-volunteer. Accessed June 12, 2024.

National Athletic Trainers' Association. 2022. "Code of Ethics." www.nata.org/sites/default/files/nata_code_of_ethics_2022.pdf. Accessed June 12, 2024.

Chapter 3

Board of Certification. 2020. "BOC Facility Principles." https://7f6907b2.flowpaper.com/BOCFacilityPrinciples/#page=1. Accessed June 12, 2024.

Konin, J.G., and R. Ray. 2019. *Management Strategies in Athletic Training.* Champaign, IL: Human Kinetics.

National Athletic Trainers' Association. n.d. "Inclusion and Wellness." www.nata.org/professional-interests/inclusion. Accessed June 12, 2024.

Occupational Safety and Health Administration. n.d. *Material Safety.* www.osha.gov/sites/default/files/publications/OSHA3493QuickCardSafetyDataSheet.pdf. Accessed June 12, 2024.

Chapter 4

Harvard. n.d. *Recruiting for Diversity.* https://hr.fas.harvard.edu/files/fas-hr/files/recruiting_for_diversity_9.17.13_0.pdf. Accessed June 12, 2024.

National Athletic Trainers' Association. 2016. "ICF Model: A Framework for Athletic Training Practice." www.nata.org/blog/beth-sitzler/icf-model-framework-athletic-training-practice . Accessed June 12, 2024.

Chapter 5

Harrelson, G., G. Gardner, and A. Winterstein, A. 2016. *Administrative Topics in Athletic Training: Concepts to Practice.* 2nd ed. Thorofare, NJ: Slack Inc.

Konin, J.G., and R. Ray. 2019. *Management Strategies in Athletic Training.* Champaign, IL: Human Kinetics.

Chapter 6

American Academy of Pediatrics. n.d. "Preparticipation Physical Evaluation." www.aap.org/en/patient-care/preparticipation-physical-evaluation. Accessed June 12, 2024.

Cleary, M.A., and K. Walsh Flanagan. 2020. *Acute and Emergency Care in Athletic Training.* Champaign, IL: Human Kinetics.

Conley, K.M., D.J. Bolin, P.J. Carek, J.G. Konin, T.L. Neal, and D. Violette. 2014. "NATA Position Statement: Preparticipation Physical Examinations and Disqualifying Conditions." *Journal of Athletic Training* 49 (1): 102-120. https://pubmed.ncbi.nlm.nih.gov/24499039.

Haff, G.G., and N.T. Triplett, eds. 2016. *Essentials of Strength Training and Conditioning.* 4th ed. Champaign, IL: Human Kinetics.

Houglum, P.A. 2016. *Therapeutic Exercise for Musculoskeletal Injuries.* 4th ed. Champaign, IL: Human Kinetics.

Houglum, P.A., K.L. Boyle-Walker, and D.E. Houglum. 2023. *Rehabilitation of Musculoskeletal Injuries.* 5th ed. Champaign, IL: Human Kinetics.

Kahanov, L., and E.K. Payne. 2022. *Athletic Training and Therapy Foundation of Behavior and Practice.* Champaign, IL: Human Kinetics.

National Athletic Trainers' Association. n.d. "Position Statements." www.nata.org/news-publications/pressroom/statements/position. Accessed June 12, 2024.

National Heart, Lung, and Blood Institute. n.d. "BMI Categories." www.nhlbi.nih.gov/. Accessed June 12, 2024.

Prentice, W.E. 2021. *Principles of Athletic Training: A Guide to Evidence Based Clinical Practice.* 17th ed. Boston: McGraw-Hill.

Reiman, M.P. 2016. *Orthopedic Clinical Examination.* Champaign, IL: Human Kinetics.

Chapter 7

Flanagan, K.W., and M. Cuppett. 2017. *General Medical Conditions in the Athlete.* 3rd ed. Champaign, IL: Human Kinetics.

Griffin, J. 2015. *Client-Centered Exercise Prescription.* 3rd ed. Champaign, IL: Human Kinetics.

Masaracchio, M., and C. Frommer. 2022. *A Clinical Guide to Surface Palpation: The Art and Science of the Perfect Touch.* Champaign, IL: Human Kinetics.

MedlinePlus. 2017. "Fat Layer in Skin." https://medlineplus.gov/ency/imagepages/19490.htm. Accessed June 12, 2024.

Chapter 8

Boyd, A.S., H.J. Benjamin, and C. Asplund. 2009. "Principles of Splinting." *American Family Physician* Jan. 1; 79 (1): 16-22.

Cartwright, L.A., and R.R. Shingles. 2011. *Cultural Competence in Sports Medicine.* Champaign, IL: Human Kinetics.

Cleary, M.A., and K. Walsh Flanagan. 2020. *Acute and Emergency Care in Athletic Training.* Champaign, IL: Human Kinetics.

Haff, G.G., and N.T. Triplett, eds. 2016. *Essentials of Strength Training and Conditioning.* 4th ed. Champaign, IL: Human Kinetics.

Kahanov, L, and E.K. Payne. 2022. *Athletic Training and Therapy Foundation of Behavior and Practice.* Champaign, IL: Human Kinetics.

Mayo Clinic. 2024. "Keloid Scar Formation." https://mayoclinic.org/diseases-conditions/keloid-scar/symptoms-causes/syc-20520901. Accessed June 12, 2024.

Prentice, W.E. 2021. *Principles of Athletic Training: A Guide to Evidence-Based Clinical Practice.* 17th ed. Boston: McGraw-Hill.

Chapter 9

American Academy of Neurology. 2020. www.aan.com/advocacy/sports-concussion-position-statement#:~:text=The%20AAN%20supports%20removal%20from,as%20defined%20by%20state%20law. Accessed June 12, 2024.

Centers for Disease Control and Prevention. 2024a. "HEADSUP." www.cdc.gov/heads-up/communication-resources/training.html. Accessed June 12, 2024.

Centers for Disease Control and Prevention. 2024b. "What to Do After a Mild TBI or Concussion." www.cdc.gov/traumatic-brain-injury/response/. Accessed June 12, 2024.

Cleary, M.A., and K. Walsh Flanagan. 2020. *Acute and Emergency Care in Athletic Training.* Champaign, IL: Human Kinetics.

Fuller, P. 2018. "The Narratives of Ethnocentric Buddhist Identity." *Journal of the British Association for the Study of Religions* 20: 19-44. https://doi.org/10.18792/jbasr.v20i0.25.

Mayo Clinic. n.d. "Bell's Palsy." www.mayoclinic.org/diseases-conditions/bells-palsy/symptoms-causes/syc-20370028. Accessed June 12, 2024.

Mayo Clinic. 2017. "Chronic Traumatic Encephalopathy." www.mayoclinic.org/diseases-conditions/chronic-traumatic-encephalopathy/symptoms-causes/syc-20370921. Accessed June 12, 2024.

McGrath, N. 2010. "Supporting the Student Athlete's Return to the Classroom after a Sport-Related Concussion." *Journal of Athletic Training* Sept-Oct; 45 (5): 492-498. doi: 10.4085/1062-6050-45.5.492.

Swartz, E.E., J.K. Register-Mihalik, S.P. Broglio, J.P. Mihalik, J.L. Myers, K.M. Guskiewicz, and J. Bailes. 2022. *NATA Position Statement: Reducing Intentional Head-First Contact Behavior in American Football Players.* www.nata.org/sites/default/files/reducing_intentional_head-first_contact_behavior_in_american_football_players.pdf. Accessed June 12, 2024.

Teasdale, G., and B. Jennett. 1974. "Assessment of Coma and Impaired Consciousness: A Practical Scale." *Lancet* 2: 81-84.

Chapter 10

American Academy of Ophthalmology. 2013. www.aao.org.

American Academy of Pediatric Dentistry. 2023. "Policy on Prevention of Sports-Related Orofacial Injuries." *The Reference Manual of Pediatric Dentistry* 110-115.

American Association of Orthodontists. n.d. *Handling Orthodontic Emergencies.* www.atsu.edu/asdoh/programs/orthodontics/pdfs/Orthodontic_Emergencies.pdf.

American Association of Otolaryngology. n.d. "Clinical Practice Guidelines: Ear Wax Impaction." www.entnet.org/quality-practice/quality-products/clinical-practice-guidelines/cerumen-impaction/. Accessed June 12, 2024.

California Dental Association. 2017. "Oral Piercing: What You Should Know." www.cda.org/wp-content/uploads/oral_piercing_english.pdf. Accessed June 12, 2024.

Colorblind Guide. n.d. www.colorblindguide.com/. Accessed June 12, 2024.

Dain, S.J. 2016. "Sports Eyewear Protective Standards." *Clinical Experimental Optometry* 99: 4-23.

Flanagan, K.W., and M. Cuppett. 2017. *General Medical Conditions in the Athlete.* 3rd ed. Champaign, IL: Human Kinetics.

Johns Hopkins Medicine. n.d. "Kaposi's Sarcoma." www.hopkinsmedicine.org/health/conditions-and-diseases/sarcoma/kaposi-sarcoma#:~:text=Kaposi%20sarcoma%20is%20a%20disease,to%20lymph%20nodes%20and%20lungs. Accessed June 12, 2024.

National Institutes of Health. National Eye Institute. 2019. "Colorblindness." www.nei.nih.gov/learn-about-eye-health/eye-conditions-and-diseases/color-blindness. Accessed June 12, 2024.

U.S. Lacrosse. 2017. "Approved Eyewear List." www.uslacrosse.rg/safety/equipment/approved-eyewear-list. Accessed June 12, 2024.

Chapter 11

Behnke, R.S., and J.L. Plant. 2022. *Kinetic Anatomy.* 4th ed. Champaign, IL: Human Kinetics.

Cleary, M.A., and K. Walsh Flanagan. 2020. *Acute and Emergency Care in Athletic Training.* Champaign, IL: Human Kinetics.

Cleveland Clinic Foundation. 2022. "Situs Inversus." https://my.clevelandclinic.org/health/diseases/23486-situs-inversus. Accessed June 12, 2024.

Johns Hopkins Medicine. n.d. "Mammography." www.hopkinsmedicine.org/imaging/exams-and-procedures/breast-imaging-procedures/3dmammography.html. Accessed June 12, 2024.

National Heart, Lung, and Blood Institute. n.d. "Low Blood Pressure." www.nhlbi.nih.gov/health/low-blood-pressure. Accessed June 12, 2024.

Wilmore, J., and D. Costill. 2007. *Physiology of Sport and Exercise.* 4th ed. Champaign, IL: Human Kinetics.

Chapter 12

Cleary, M.A., and K. Walsh Flanagan. 2020. *Acute and Emergency Care in Athletic Training.* Champaign, IL: Human Kinetics.

Cleveland Clinic. n.d. "Diverticulitis." https://my.clevelandclinic.org/health/diseases/10352-diverticular-disease. Accessed June 12, 2024.

Johns Hopkins Medicine. n.d. "Cholecystitis." www.hopkinsmedicine.org/health/conditions-and-diseases/cholecystitis. Accessed June 12, 2024.

Mayo Clinic. 2017a. "Blood in Urine (Hematuria)." www.mayoclinic.org/diseases-conditions/blood-in-urine/symptoms-causes/dxc-20346636?p=1. Accessed June 12, 2024.

Mayo Clinic. 2023. "Appendicitis." https://www.mayoclinic.org/diseases-conditions/appendicitis/symptoms-causes/syc-20369543. Accessed June 12, 2024.

Parker, R. 2017. "Parasitic Infections." https://humankinetics.me/2017/07/20/common-medical-conditions-in-athletes/. Accessed June 12, 2024.

Stanford Medicine. 2016. "Shoulder Pain and Shortness of Breath. Shoulder Exam Is Normal. Diagnosis?" www.stanfordmedicine25.stanford.edu/blog/archive/2016/Shoulder-pain-and-shortness-of-breath.html. Accessed June 12, 2024.

World Health Organization. 2023. "Obesity and Overweight." www.who.int/news-room/fact-sheets/detail/obesity-and-overweight. Accessed June 12, 2024.

Chapter 13

Cleary, M.A., and K. Walsh Flanagan. 2020. *Acute and Emergency Care in Athletic Training.* Champaign, IL: Human Kinetics.

Gao, Y., C. Wang, K. Wang, C. He, K. Hu, and M. Liang. 2022. "The Effects and Molecular Mechanism of Heat Stress on Spermatogenesis and the Mitigation Measures." *Systems Biology in Reproductive Medicine* 68 (5-6): 331-347. doi:10.1080/19396368.2022.2074325.

Kahanov, L., and E.K. Payne. 2022. *Athletic Training and Therapy Foundation of Behavior and Practice.* Champaign, IL: Human Kinetics.

Mayo Clinic. n.d.a. "Hydrocele and Varicocele." www.mayoclinic.org/diseases-conditions/varicocele/diagnosis-treatment/drc-20378772. Accessed June 12, 2024.

Mayo Clinic. n.d.b. "Vaginitis." www.mayoclinic.org/diseases-conditions/vaginitis/symptoms-causes/syc-20354707. Accessed June 12, 2024.

The Williams Institute. 2021. "We Are LA! What LGBTQ People Contribute to Los Angeles." https://williamsinstitute.law.ucla.edu. Accessed June 12, 2024.

Chapter 14

Behnke, R.S., and J.L. Plant. 2022. *Kinetic Anatomy.* 4th ed. Champaign, IL: Human Kinetics.

Cleary, M.A., and K. Walsh Flanagan. 2020. *Acute and Emergency Care in Athletic Training.* Champaign, IL: Human Kinetics.

Kisner, C., and L.A. Colby. 2007. *Therapeutic Exercise.* 5th ed. Philadelphia: Davis.

National Heart, Lung, and Blood Institute. n.d. "Low Blood Pressure." www.nhlbi.nih.gov/health/low-blood-pressure. Accessed June 12, 2024.

Porterfield, J.A., and C. DeRosa. 1991. *Mechanical Low Back Pain.* Philadelphia: Saunders.

Chapter 15

National Athletic Trainers' Association. n.d. "Position Statements." www.nata.org/news-publications/pressroom/statements/position. Accessed June 12, 2024.

OrthoInfo. n.d. "SLAP Tears." https://orthoinfo.aaos.org/en/diseases--conditions/slap-tears. Accessed June 12, 2024.

Chapter 16

Behnke, R.S., and J.L. Plant. 2022. *Kinetic Anatomy.* 4th ed. Champaign, IL: Human Kinetics.

Shultz, S.J., P.A. Houglum, and D.H. Perrin. 2016. *Examination of Musculoskeletal Injuries.* 4th ed. Champaign, IL: Human Kinetics.

Treuer, N. 2012. *Everything You Wanted to Know About Indians but Were Afraid to Ask.* Nepean, ON: Borealis Books.

Chapter 17

Ioannis, D., K. Anastosios, N. Konstantinos, K. Lazaros, and N. Georgios. 2015. "Palmaris Longus Muscle's Prevalence in Different Nations and Interesting Anatomical Variations: Review of Literature." *Journal of Clinical Medical Research* 7 (1): 825-830. doi: 10.14740/jocmr2243w.

Chapter 18

Miller, K., T. Frech, T. Greene, K.N. Ma, M. McFadden, L. Tom-Orme, M.L. Slattery, and M.A. Murtaugh. 2016. "Bone Mineral Density in Navajo Men and Women and Comparison to Non-Hispanic Whites from NHANES (2005-2008)." *Journal of Health Care for the Poor and Underserved* 27 (2): 644-662.

Chapter 19

Lee, W.Q., J.Z. Gan, and D.T.T. Lie. 2019. "Save the Meniscus—Clinical Outcomes of Meniscectomy Versus Meniscal Repair." *Journal of Orthopaedic Surgery* 27 (2).

Chapter 20

Patel, R.K., and V.D. Patel. 2021. "Peroneus Tertius: Variations and Clinical Application in Gujarati Population." *National Journal of Medical Research* 11 (02): 43-45. https://njmr.in/index.php/file/article/view/15.

Stanford Medicine. 2024. "Reflex Sympathetic Dystrophy Syndrome and Complex Regional Pain Syndrome." https://stanfordhealthcare.org/medical-conditions/brain-and-nerves/chronic-pain/types/rsds.html. Accessed June 3, 2024.

University of Rochester Medical Center. 2024. "Reflex Sympathetic Dystrophy Syndrome." www.urmc.rochester.edu/encyclopedia/content.aspx?contenttypeid=22&contentid=reflexsympatheticdystrophysyndrome. Accessed June 3, 2024.

Chapter 21

Abaïdia, A.E., J. Lamblin, B. Delecroix, C. Leduc, A. McCall, M. Nédélec, B. Dawson, G. Baquet, and G. Dupont. 2017. "Recovery From Exercise-Induced Muscle Damage: Cold-Water Immersion Versus Whole-Body Cryotherapy." *International Journal of Sports Physiology and Performance* Mar; 12 (3): 402-409.

Anderson, M.K., and M.G. Barnum. 2022. *Foundations of Athletic Training Prevention, Assessment, and Management.* 7th ed. Philadelphia: Wolters Kluwer.

Cheatham, S.W., E. Kreiswirth, and R. Baker. 2019. "Does a Light Pressure Instrument-Assisted Soft-Tissue Mobilization Technique Modulate Tactile Discrimination and Perceived Pain in Healthy Individuals with DOMS?" *Journal of the Canadian Chiropractor Association* Apr; 63 (1): 18-25.

Denegar, C.R., E. Saliba, and S. Saliba. 2016. *Therapeutic Modalities for Musculoskeletal Injuries.* 3rd ed. Champaign, IL: Human Kinetics.

Gulick, D.T. 2018. "Instrument-Assisted Soft Tissue Mobilization Increases Myofascial Trigger Point Pain Threshold." *Journal of Bodywork and Movement Therapies* Apr; 22 (2): 341-345.

Higgins T.R., D.A. Greene, and M.K. Baker. 2017. "Effects of Cold-Water Immersion and Contrast Water Therapy for Recovery From Team Sport: A Systematic Review and Meta-Analysis." *Journal of Strength and Conditioning Research* May; 31 (5): 1443-1460.

Kahanov, L., and E.K. Payne. 2022. *Athletic Training and Therapy Foundation of Behavior and Practice.* Champaign, IL: Human Kinetics.

Machado, A.F., P.H. Ferreira, J.K. Micheletti, A.C. de Almeida, I.R. Lemes, F.M. Vanderlei, J. Netto Junior, and C.M. Pastre. 2016. "Can Water Temperature and Immersion Time Influence the Effect of Cold-Water Immersion on Muscle Soreness? A Systematic Review and Meta-Analysis." *Sports Medicine* Apr; 46 (4): 503-514.

Markovic, G. 2015. "Acute Effects of Instrument-Assisted Soft-Tissue Mobilization vs. Foam Rolling on Knee and Hip Range of Motion in Soccer Players." *Journal of Bodywork and Movement Therapies* Oct; 19 (4): 690-696.

Mehta, P., and V. Dhapte. 2015. "Cupping Therapy: A Prudent Remedy for a Plethora of Medical Ailments." *Journal of Traditional and Complementary Medicine* 5 (3): 127-134.

Rehman, R., A. Chabaan, I. Hamzavi, F. Fahs, and T.F. Mohammad. 2022. "The Etiquette of Hijab: Recommendations to Improve Care in Dermatology Clinics." *British Journal of Dermatology* 186: 176-177. https://doi.org/10.1111/bjd.20665.

Rushall, K. 2014. "The Many Benefits of Chinese Cupping." www.pacificcollege.edu/new/blog/2014/09/20/many-benefits-chinese-cupping. Accessed June 5, 2024.

UC San Diego School of Medicine. 2017. "How Acupuncture Can Relieve Pain and Improve Sleep, Digestion, and Emotional Well-Being." cim.ucsd.edu/clinical-care/acupuncture.shtml. Accessed June 5, 2024.

Unverzagt, C., K. Berglund, and J.J. Thomas. 2015. "Dry Needling for Myofascial Trigger Point: A Clinical Commentary." *International Journal of Sports Physical Therapy* Jun; 10 (3): 402-418.

Vardiman, J.P., J. Siedlik, T. Herda, W. Hawkins, M. Cooper, Z.A. Graham, J. Deckert, and P. Gallagher. 2015. "Instrument-Assisted Soft Tissue Mobilization: Effects on the Properties of Human Plantar Flexors." *International Journal of Sports Medicine* Mar; 36 (3): 197-203.

WebMD. n.d. "Cupping Therapy." www.webmd.com/balance/guide/cupping-therapy?print=true. Accessed June 5, 2024.

Chapter 22

ACSM. n.d. "ACSM Cardiorespiratory Training." mkrt.hu/doc/acsm%20cardiorespiratory%20training%20guidelines.pdf.

ACSM. 2013. "ACSM Information on Resistance Training for Health and Fitness." www.prescriptiontogetactive.com/static/pdfs/resistance-training-ACSM.pdf.

Antony, B., M.U. Maheswri, and A. Palanisamy. 2015. "Effect of Battle Rope Training on Selected Physical and Physiological Variables Among College-Level Athletes." *Indian Journal of Applied Research* 5: 19-22.

Anzalone, A.J., D. Blueitt, T. Case, T. McGuffin, K. Pollard, J.C. Garrison, M.T. Jones, et al. 2017. "A Positive Vestibular/Ocular Motor Screening (VOMS) Is Associated With Increased Recovery Time after Sports-Related Concussion in Youth and Adolescent Athletes." *The American Journal of Sports Medicine* 45 (2): 474-479.

Bornath, D., and K. Kenno. 2022. "Physiological Responses to Increasing Battling Rope Weight During Two 3-Week High-Intensity Interval Training Programs." *Journal of Strength and Conditioning Research* 36 (2): 352-358.

Clark, J., K. Hasselfeld, K. Bigsby, and J. Divine. 2017. "Colored Glasses to Mitigate Photophobia Symptoms Posttraumatic Brain Injury." *Journal of Athletic Training* 52 (8): 725-729.

Commisceo Global. 2022. "What Behaviours are Rude in the Middle East?" www.commisceo-global.com/blog/what-behaviours-are-rude-in-the-middle-east. Accessed June 4, 2024.

CrossFit. 2002-2020. "CrossFit Certificate Course L1." http://library.crossfit.com/free/pdf/CFJ_English_Level1_TrainingGuide.pdf.

Fackrell, K., I. Potgieter, G.S. Shekhawat, D.M. Baguley, M. Sereda, and D.J. Hoare. 2017. "Clinical Interventions for Hyperacusis in Adults: A Scoping Review to Assess the Current Position and Determine Priorities for Research." www.ncbi.nlm.nih.gov/pmc/articles/PMC5654244/. Accessed June 4, 2024.

Haff, G., and N.T. Triplett. 2016. *Essentials of Strength Training and Conditioning.* 4th ed. Champaign, IL: Human Kinetics.

Healthline. 2019. "How to Do 8 Different Plyometric Exercises." www.healthline.com/health/exercise-fitness/plyometric-exercises. Accessed June 4, 2024.

Kuklick, C.R., M.A. Martino, and C.D. Black. 2013. "Throwing Velocity and Stamina in Baseball Pitchers as a Function of Training Methods." *Journal of Australian Strength and Conditioning Research* 21: 13.

Mosti, C., M.V. Spiers, and J.D. Kloss. 2016. "A Practical Guide to Evaluating Sleep Disturbance in Concussion Patients." *Neurology: Clinical Practice* 6 (2): 129-137.

Nelson, B.W., and N.B. Allen. 2019. "Accuracy of Consumer Wearable Heart Rate Measurement During an Ecologically Valid 24-Hour Period: Intraindividual Validation Study." *JMIR mHealth and uHealth* 7 (3): e10828.

Otto, W.H. III, J.W. Coburn, L.E. Brown, and B.A. Spiering. 2012. "Effects of Weightlifting vs. Kettlebell Training on Vertical Jump, Strength, and Body Composition." *Journal of Strength and Conditioning Research* 26: 1199-1202.

Porcari, J.P., L. Probst, K. Forrester, S. Doberstein, C. Foster, M.L. Cress, and K. Schmidt. 2016. "Effect of Wearing the Elevation Training Mask on Aerobic Capacity, Lung Function, and Hematological Variables." *Journal of Sports Science & Medicine* 15 (2): 379-386.

Tison, G.H., J.M. Sanchez, B. Ballinger, A. Singh, J.E. Olgin, M.J. Pletcher, E. Vittinghoff, et al. 2018. "Passive Detection of Atrial Fibrillation Using a Commercially Available Smartwatch." *Journal of the American Medical Association Cardiology* May 1; 3 (5): 409-416.

Chapter 23

American Psychiatric Association. 2023. "Warning Signs of Mental Illness." www.psychiatry.org/patients-families/warning-signs-of-mental-illness. Accessed June 4, 2024.

American Psychological Association. 2022. "What Is Cognitive Behavioral Therapy?" www.apa.org/ptsd-guideline/patients-and-families/cognitive-behavioral. Accessed June 4, 2024.

Crane, M. 2019. "How Coaches Impact a Female Athlete's Body Image." www.climbingpsychology.com/blog/coaches-influence-body-image. Accessed June 4, 2024.

Hedegaard, H., S.C. Curtin, and M. Warner. 2018. *Suicide Mortality in the United States, 1999-2017.* Hyattsville, MD: National Center for Health Statistics.

Hesler, B. 2023. "5 Tips to Stress Management." www.mayoclinichealthsystem.org/hometown-health/speaking-of-health/5-tips-to-manage-stress. Accessed June 4, 2024.

Hyun Han, D., D. McDuff, D. Thompson, M.E. Hitchcock, D.L. Reardon, and B. Hainline. 2019. "Attention-Deficit Hyperactivity Disorder." bjsm.bmj.com/content/bjsports/53/12/741.full.pdf.

Johns Hopkins. 2023. "Body Dysmorphic Disorder." www.hopkinsmedicine.org/health/conditions-and-diseases/body-dysmorphic-disorder. Accessed June 4, 2024.

Kahanov, L., and E.K. Payne. 2022. *Athletic Training and Therapy Foundation of Behavior and Practice.* Champaign, IL: Human Kinetics.

Kratina, K., and M. Albers. 2015. *Nutrition for Eating Disorders.* Tallahassee: Florida Academy of Nutrition and Dietetics.

Mayo Clinic. 2022a. "Body Dysmorphic Disorder." www.mayoclinic.org/diseases-conditions/body-dysmorphic-disorder/symptoms-causes/syc-20353938. Accessed June 4, 2024.

Mayo Clinic. 2022b. "Mental Health." www.mayoclinic.org/diseases-conditions/mental-illness/symptoms-causes/syc-20374968. Accessed June 4, 2024.

Mayo Clinic. 2022c. "Obsessive-Compulsive Disorder." www.mayoclinic.org/diseases-conditions/obsessive-compulsive-disorder/diagnosis-treatment/drc-20354438. Accessed June 4, 2024.

Mayo Clinic. 2022d. "Panic Attacks." www.mayoclinic.org/diseases-conditions/panic-attacks/diagnosis-treatment/drc-20376027. Accessed June 4, 2024.

Mayo Clinic. 2023. "Eating Disorders." www.mayoclinic.org/diseases-conditions/eating-disorders/symptoms-causes/syc-20353603. Accessed June 4, 2024.

National Institute of Mental Health. n.d. "Understanding Psychosis?" www.nimh.nih.gov/health/publications/understanding-psychosis. Accessed June 4, 2024.

National Institute of Mental Health. 2018. "Anxiety Disorders." www.nimh.nih.gov/health/topics/anxiety-disorders. Accessed June 4, 2024.

National Institute of Mental Health. 2022. "Mental Illness." www.nimh.nih.gov/health/statistics/mental-illness. Accessed June 4, 2024.

Neal, T. 2016. "Burnout in Athletes." www.nata.org/blog/beth-sitzler/burnout-athletes. Accessed June 4, 2024.

Quinn, E. 2020. "Assisting Athletes With Anxiety on Game Day." www.nata.org/blog/elizabeth-quinn/assisting-athletes-anxiety-game-day. Accessed June 4, 2024.

St. Bonaventure University. 2022. "Strategies for Reframing Negative Thoughts." https://online.sbu.edu/news/strategies-reframing-negative-thoughts. Accessed June 4, 2024.

Weinberg, R.S., and D. Gould. 2024. *Foundation of Sport and Exercise Psychology.* 8th ed. Champaign, IL: Human Kinetics.

Yang, J., J.T. Schaefer, N. Zhang, T. Covassin, K. Ding, and E. Heiden. 2014. "Social Support from the Athletic Trainer and Symptoms of Depression and Anxiety at Return to Play." *Journal of Athletic Training* Nov-Dec; 49 (6): 773-779.

Chapter 24

Centers for Disease Control and Prevention. 2019. "How Is Pandemic Flu Different From Seasonal Flu?" www.cdc.gov/flu/pandemic-resources/basics/about.html. Accessed June 5, 2024.

Centers for Disease Control and Prevention. 2020. "Prepare Your Health. Plan Ahead." www.cdc.gov/prepare-your-health/plan-ahead/?CDC_AAref_Val=https://www.cdc.gov/prepyourhealth/planahead/index.htm. Accessed June 4, 2024.

Drezner, J.A., B.G. Toresdahl, A.L. Rao, E. Huszti, and K.G. Harmon. 2013. "Outcomes from Sudden Cardiac Arrest in U.S. High Schools: A 2-year Prospective Study from the National Registry for AED Use in Sports." *British Journal of Sports Medicine* 47 (18): 1179-1183.

FEMA. 2020. "Be Prepared for a Novel Pandemic." www.ready.gov/sites/default/files/2020-11/novel-pandemic_hazard-sheet.pdf.

Chapter 25

American Red Cross. 2021. *First Aid/CPR/AED Participant's Manual.*

Anderson, M.K., and M.G. Barnum. 2022. *Foundations of Athletic Training prevention, Assessment and Management.* 7th ed. Philadelphia: Wolters Kluwer.

British Heart Foundation. 2019. "Cardiac Arrest." www.bhf.org.uk/informationsupport/conditions/cardiac-arrest. Accessed June 4, 2024.

Cleary, M.A., and K. Walsh Flanagan. 2020. *Acute and Emergency Care in Athletic Training.* Champaign, IL: Human Kinetics.

Fowler, P. 2023. "Pediatric Vital Signs." www.webmd.com/children/children-vital-signs. Accessed June 4, 2024.

Heritage Urgent & Primary Care. n.d. "When Should Stiches or Sutures Be Removed?" www.heritageucpc.com/when-should-stitches-or-sutures-be-removed. Accessed June 4, 2024.

National Center for Early Defibrillation. n.d. "National Center for Early Defibrillation, Fast Facts for Sudden Cardiac Arrest." www.early-defib.org. Accessed June 4, 2024.

Pollack, A.N. 2022. *Emergency Medical Responder.* 7th ed. Park Ridge, IL: American Academy of Orthopaedic Surgeons.

Purnell, L., and E.A. Fenkl. 2019. *Handbook for Culturally Competent Care.* Cham, Switzerland: Springer International Publishing AG.

Ratner, D. 2020. "When Should Sutures Be Removed?" www.medscape.com/answers/1824895-34809/when-should-sutures-be-removed. Accessed June 4, 2024.

Seattle Children's. 2022. "Suture Questions." www.seattlechildrens.org/conditions/a-z/suture-questions. Accessed June 4, 2024.

Weekley, M.S., and L.E. Bland. 2023. "Oxygen Administration." www.ncbi.nlm.nih.gov/books/NBK551617/.

Chapter 26

Affiliated Community Medical Centers. n.d. "Hydration for Athletes: Coaches Toolkit." www.acmc.com/sportsMedicine/pdf/04_hydrationForAthletes.pdf.

Army Public Health Center. n.d. *Injury Prevention: Just the Facts. Cold Weather Injuries.* https://phc.amedd.army.mil/PHC%20Resource%20Library/ColdWeatherInjuries_FS_12-004-0915.pdf.

Bedford, M. 2019. "6 Culturally Sensitive Ways to Approach Mental Health." www.qualityinteractions.com/blog/6-culturally-sensitive-ways-to-approach-mental-health.

Casa, D.J., J.K. DeMartini, M.F. Bergeron, D. Csillan, E.R. Eichner, R.M. Lopez, M.S. Ferrara, et al. 2015. "National Athletic Trainers' Association Position Statement: Exertional Heat Illnesses." *Journal of Athletic Training* 50 (9): 989-1000.

Centers for Disease Control and Prevention. 2016. "Venomous Snakes." www.cdc.gov/niosh/topics/snakes/symptoms.html. Accessed June 4, 2024.

Centers for Disease Control and Prevention. 2018. "Zika Virus." www.cdc.gov/zika/index.html. Accessed June 4, 2024.

Centers for Disease Control and Prevention. 2020. "Fleas." www.cdc.gov/fleas/index.html. Accessed June 4, 2024.

Centers for Disease Control and Prevention. 2021. "Lyme Disease." www.cdc.gov/lyme/index.html. June 4, 2024.

Centers for Disease Control and Prevention. 2022. "Scabies." wwwnc.cdc.gov/travel/diseases/scabies. Accessed June 4, 2024.

Centers for Disease Control and Prevention. 2024. "About Body Lice." www.cdc.gov/lice/about/body-lice.html. Accessed June 4, 2024.

Cleveland Clinic. 2021. "Heat Illness." https://my.clevelandclinic.org/health/diseases/16425-heat-illness. Accessed June 4, 2024.

Kenney, W.L., J.H. Wilmore, and D.L. Costill. 2022. *Physiology of Sport and Exercise.* 8th ed. Champaign, IL: Human Kinetics.

Luhring, K.E., C.L. Butts, C.R. Smith, J.A. Bonacci, R.C. Ylanan, M.S. Ganio, and B.P. McDermott. 2016. "Cooling Effectiveness of a Modified Cold-Water Immersion Method After Exercise-Induced Hyperthermia." *Journal of Athletic Training* 51 (11): 946-951.

Mayo Clinic Staff. 1998-2023. "Heat Exhaustion." www.mayoclinic.org/diseases-conditions/heat-exhaustion/symptoms-causes/syc-20373250. Accessed June 4, 2024.

McDermott, B.P., S.A. Anderson, L.E. Armstrong, D.J. Casa, S.N. Cheuvront, L. Cooper, W.L Kenney, F.G. O'Connor, and W.O. Roberts. 2017. "National Athletic Trainers' Association Position Statement: Fluid Replacement for the Physically Active." *Journal of Athletic Training* 52 (9): 877-895.

National Weather Service. n.d. "Lightning Safety." www.weather.gov/safety/lightning-safety. Accessed June 4, 2024.

National Weather Service. 2024. "What Is the Heat Index?" www.weather.gov/ama/heatindex#:~:text=The%20heat%20index%2C%20also%20known,for%20the%20human%20body's%20comfort. Accessed June 4, 2024.

WebMD. 2023. "Bedbugs." www.webmd.com/skin-problems-and-treatments/guide/bedbugs-infestation. Accessed June 4, 2024.

Chapter 27

Editors of Encyclopedia Britannica. 2024, April 19. "evil eye." *Encyclopedia Britannica.* www.britannica.com/topic/evil-eye. Accessed June 4, 2024.

Cleary, M.A., and K. Walsh Flanagan. 2020. *Acute and Emergency Care in Athletic Training.* Champaign, IL: Human Kinetics.

Courson, R., J. Ellis, S.A. Herring, B.P. Boden, G. Henry, D. Conway, L. McNamara, et al. 2020. "Best Practices and Current Concepts in Prehospital Care of the Spine-Injured Athlete in American Tackle Football." *Journal of Athletic Training* 55 (6): 545-562.

Pew Research Center. 2018. "Eastern and Western Europeans Differ on Importance of Religion, Views of Minorities, and Key Social Issues." www.pewresearch.org/religion/2018/10/29/eastern-and-western-europeans-differ-on-importance-of-religion-views-of-minorities-and-key-social-issues. Accessed June 4, 2024.

Chapter 28

Quality Interactions. 2023. "Cultural Competency in Telemedicine." https://2948922.fs1.hubspotusercontent-na1.net/hubfs/2948922/QI%20Checklist%20-%20Telemedicine.pdf.

Chapter 29

Canadian Ski Council. 2018. "How to Choose a Helmet." www.skicanada.org/safety/how-to-choose-a-helmet. Accessed June 4, 2024.

Centers for Disease Control and Prevention. n.d. "Get a Heads-Up on Ski Helmet Safety." www.cdc.gov/headsup/pdfs/helmets/headsup_helmetfactsheet_ski_508.pdf.

Consumers Product Safety Commission. n.d. "Which Helmet for Which Activity?" www.cpsc.gov/safety-education/safety-guides/sports-fitness-and-recreation-bicycles/which-helmet-which-activity. Accessed June 4, 2024.

Engel, F.A., H.C. Holmberg, and B. Sperlich. 2016. "Is There Evidence that Runners Can Benefit from Wearing Compression Clothing?" *Sports Med* Dec; 46 (12): 1939-1952.

EVO. 2020-2021. "How to Choose a Ski and Snowboard Helmet and Size Chart." www.evo.com/guides/ski-snowboard-helmet-size-fit. Accessed June 5, 2024.

Fair Play for Women. 2017. "Biological Sex Differences: Bones & Muscles." https://fairplayforwomen.com/biological-sex-differences. Accessed June 4, 2024.

Hettchen, M., K. Glöckler, S. von Stengel, A. Piechele, H. Lötzerich, M. Kohl, and W. Kemmler. 2019. "Effects of Compression Tights on Recovery Parameters After Exercise-Induced Muscle Damage: A Randomized Controlled Crossover Study." *Evidence-Based Complementary and Alternative Medicine: eCAM.*

Riddell. 2014. "New Riddell SpeedFlex Highlights the Future of Football Helmet Design and Innovation." https://news.riddell.com/info/releases/new-riddell-speedflex-highlights-the-future-of-football-helmet-design-and-innovation. Accessed June 4, 2024.

Schutt. 2023. "F7 2.0 Collegiate Helmet." https://schutt-sports.com/products/f7-2-0-collegiate-helmet. Accessed June 4, 2024.

Chapter 30

Cleveland Clinic. 2021. "Lipid Panel." https://my.clevelandclinic.org/health/diagnostics/17176-lipid-panel. Accessed June 4, 2024.

Mayo Clinic.org. 2023. "Complete Blood Count." www.mayoclinic.org/tests-procedures/complete-blood-count/about/pac-20384919. Accessed June 5, 2024.

Medical News Today. 2023. "Blood Type by Race." www.medicalnewstoday.com/articles/most-common-blood-type-by-race#summary. Accessed June 4, 2024.

MedlinePlus. 2021. "Basic Metabolic Panel." https://medlineplus.gov/ency/article/003462.htm. Accessed June 4, 2024.

Statista. 2023. "Distribution of Blood Types in the United States as of 2021, by Diversity." www.statista.com/statistics/1203831/blood-type-distribution-us-by-ethnicity. Accessed June 4, 2024.

Chapter 31

American Cancer Society. 2022. "About Non-Hodgkin Lymphoma." www.cancer.org/cancer/non-hodgkin-lymphoma/about.html. Accessed June 4, 2024.

American Diabetes Association. 2022. "The Big Picture: Checking Your Blood Sugar." www.diabetes.org/healthy-living/medication-treatments/blood-glucose-testing-and-control/checking-your-blood-sugar. Accessed June 4, 2024.

Britannica, The Editors of Encyclopedia. 2024, May 10. "Myalgic Encephalomyelitis/Chronic Fatigue Syndrome." *Encyclopedia Britannica.* www.britannica.com/science/chronic-fatigue-syndrome. Accessed June 4, 2024.

Centers for Disease Control and Prevention. 2018. "Myalgic Encephalomyelitis/Chronic Fatigue Syndrome." www.cdc.gov/me-cfs/index.html. Accessed June 4, 2024.

Centers for Disease Control and Prevention. 2022. "Your Diabetes Care Schedule." https://www.cdc.gov/diabetes/treatment/your-diabetes-care-schedule.html. Accessed June 8, 2024.

Cleveland Clinic. 2022. "Immune System." https://my.clevelandclinic.org/health/articles/21196-immune-system. Accessed June 4, 2024.

Coviser, J.H., A. Schlitzer Tierney, and R. Nickols. 2018. "Essentials for Best Practice: Treatment Approaches for Athletes With Eating Disorders." *Journal of Clinical Sport Psychology* 12: 495-507.

Johns Hopkins Medicine. 2022. "Lupus." www.hopkinsmedicine.org/health/conditions-and-diseases/lupus. Accessed June 4, 2024.

Johns Hopkins Medicine. 2024. "Raynaud's Phenomenon." www.hopkinsmedicine.org/health/conditions-and-diseases/raynauds-phenomenon. Accessed June 5, 2024.

Lupus Foundation of America. 2021. "What Is Lupus?" www.lupus.org/resources/what-is-lupus. Accessed June 4, 2024.

Mayo Clinic. 1998-2023a. "Hypothyroidism (Underactive Thyroid)." www.mayoclinic.org/diseases-conditions/hypothyroidism/symptoms-causes/syc-20350284. Accessed June 5, 2024.

Mayo Clinic. 1998-2023b. "Hyperthyroidism (Overactive Thyroid)." www.mayoclinic.org/diseases-conditions/hyperthyroidism/symptoms-causes/syc-20373659. Accessed June 4, 2024.

Mayo Clinic. 2022a. "Chronic Fatigue Syndrome." www.mayoclinic.org/diseases-conditions/chronic-fatigue-syndrome/symptoms-causes/syc-20360490. Accessed June 5, 2024.

Mayo Clinic. 2022b. "Hodgkin's Lymphoma (Hodgkin's Disease)." www.mayoclinic.org/diseases-conditions/hodgkins-lymphoma/symptoms-causes/syc-20352646. Accessed June 4, 2024.

National Cancer Institute. 2022. "Lymph Node." www.cancer.gov/publications/dictionaries/cancer-terms/def/lymph-node. Accessed June 4, 2024.

Nationwide Children's Hospital. 2023. "About Cleft Lip and Palate." www.nationwidechildrens.org/specialties/cleft-lip-and-palate-center/about-cleft-lip-and-palate. Accessed June 5, 2024.

Nolan, E., L. Bunting, C. McCartan, G. Davidson, A. Grant, D. Schubotz, C. Mulholland, et al. 2022. "Prevalence of Probable Eating Disorders and Associated Risk Factors: An Analysis of the Northern Ireland Youth Wellbeing Survey Using the SCOFF." *British Journal of Clinical Psychology* 62 (1): 180-195.

Rawson, E.S., P.M. Clarkson, and M.A. Tarnopolsky. 2017. "Perspectives on Exertional Rhabdomyolysis." *Sports Med* Mar; 47 (1): 33-49.

Sotzny, F., J. Blanco, E. Capelli, J. Castro-Marrero, S. Steiner, M. Murovska, and C. Scheibenbogen. 2018. "Myalgic Encephalomyelitis/Chronic Fatigue Syndrome—Evidence for an Autoimmune Disease." *Autoimmunity Reviews* 17 (6): 601-609.

Stuart, A., S. Amandolare, and A. Gopal. 2024. "Rhabdomyolysis: What Is It?" www.webmd.com/a-to-z-guides/rhabdomyolysis-symptoms-causes-treatments. Accessed June 5, 2024.

US Preventive Services Task Force. 2022. "Screening for Eating Disorders in Adolescents and Adults: US Preventive Services Task Force Recommendation Statement." *JAMA* 327 (11): 1061-1067.

Chapter 32

Centers for Disease Control and Prevention. 2019. "Shingles (Herpes Zoster)." www.cdc.gov/shingles/index.html. Accessed June 4, 2024.

Centers for Disease Control and Prevention. 2020. "Hepatitis E." www.cdc.gov/hepatitis/hev/index.htm. Accessed June 4, 2024.

Centers for Disease Control and Prevention. 2021a. "How HIV Spreads." Last modified April 21, 2021. www.cdc.gov/hiv/causes/?CDC_AAref_Val=https://www.cdc.gov/hiv/basics/hiv-transmission/body-fluids.html%20l. Accessed June 5, 2024.

Centers for Disease Control and Prevention. 2021b. "Ways HIV Is Not Transmitted." Last modified April 21, 2021. www.cdc.gov/hiv/causes/?CDC_AAref_Val=https://www.cdc.gov/hiv/basics/hiv-transmission/not-transmitted.html. Accessed June 5, 2024.

Centers for Disease Control and Prevention. 2022. "About HIV." Last modified July 30, 2022. www.cdc.gov/hiv/about/?CDC_AAref_Val=https://www.cdc.gov/hiv/basics/whatishiv.html. Accessed June 4, 2024.

Centers for Disease Control and Prevention. 2023. "Living With HIV." Last modified January 31, 2023. www.cdc.gov/hiv/living-with/?CDC_AAref_Val=https://www.cdc.gov/hiv/basics/livingwithhiv/protecting-others.html. Accessed June 5, 2024.

Centers for Disease Control and Prevention. 2024a. "Methicillin-Resistant Staphylococcus Aureus (MRSA) Basics." www.cdc.gov/mrsa/about/?CDC_AAref_Val=https://www.cdc.gov/mrsa/community/. Accessed June 8, 2024.

Centers for Disease Control and Prevention. 2024b. "Preventing HIV with PReP." www.cdc.gov/hiv/prevention/prep.html. Accessed June 8, 2024.

Centers for Disease Control and Prevention. 2024c. "Preventing HIV with PEP." www.cdc.gov/hiv/prevention/pep.html. Accessed June 9, 2024.

Centers for Disease Control and Prevention. 2024d. "Understanding a Positive Result." Last modified February 7, 2024. www.cdc.gov/hiv/causes/?CDC_AAref_Val=https://www.cdc.gov/hiv/basics/hiv-transmission/ways-people-get-hiv.html. Accessed June 5, 2024.

Cleveland Clinic. 2020. "Psoriasis." https://my.clevelandclinic.org/health/diseases/6866-psoriasis#management-and-treatment. Accessed June 4, 2024.

Cleveland Clinic. 2021. "Sebaceous Cysts." https://my.clevelandclinic.org/health/diseases/14165-sebaceous-cysts. Accessed June 5, 2024.

Cox, R. 2017. "Hepatitis C." www.emedicinehealth.com/hepatitis_c/page12_em.htm#can_hepatitis_c_be_prevented. Accessed June 5, 2024.

Davis, C.P. 2017. "Hepatitis A." www.emedicinehealth.com/hepatitis_a/page5_em.htm#hepatitis_a_medical_treatment. Accessed June 5, 2024.

Dulski, A., and C.W. Edwards. 2022. "Paronychia". [Updated 2022 Apr 30]. www.ncbi.nlm.nih.gov/books/NBK544307. Accessed June 5, 2024.

Holland, K. 2021. "Everything You Need to Know About Psoriasis." www.healthline.com/health/psoriasis. Accessed June 5, 2024.

Johns Hopkins. 2022. "What Is Coronavirus?" www.hopkinsmedicine.org/health/conditions-and-diseases/coronavirus. Accessed June 5, 2024.

Mayo Clinic. 1998-2023. "Boils and Carbuncles." www.mayoclinic.org/diseases-conditions/boils-and-carbuncles/symptoms-causes/syc-20353770. Accessed June 5, 2024.

Mayo Clinic. 2022a. "Hives and Angioedema." www.mayoclinic.org/diseases-conditions/hives-and-angioedema/symptoms-causes/syc-20354908. Accessed June 5, 2024.

Mayo Clinic. 2022b. "Dermatitis." www.mayoclinic.org/diseases-conditions/dermatitis-eczema/diagnosis-treatment/drc-20352386. Accessed June 5, 2024.

Mayo Clinic. 2022c. "Hidradenitis Suppurativa." www.mayoclinic.org/diseases-conditions/hidradenitis-suppurativa/symptoms-causes/syc-20352306. Accessed June 5, 2024.

National Health Service. 2021. "Cellulitis." www.nhs.uk/conditions/cellulitis. Accessed June 5, 2024.

National Institute of Arthritis and Musculoskeletal and Skin Diseases. 2020. "Acne Basics: Diagnosis, Treatment, and Steps to Take." www.niams.nih.gov/health-topics/acne/basics/diagnosis-treatment-and-steps-to-take. Accessed June 5, 2024.

National Institute of Health. 2017. "Hepatitis D." www.niddk.nih.gov/health-information/liver-disease/viral-hepatitis/hepatitis-d#whatis. Accessed June 5, 2024.

Nobles, T., M.E. Muse, and G.J. Schmieder. 2022. *Dermatographism.* [Updated 2022 Feb 23]. Treasure Island, FL: StatPearls Publishing. www.ncbi.nlm.nih.gov/books/NBK531496.

Scala, E., S. Cacciapuoti, N. Garzorz-Stark, M. Megna, C. Marasca, P. Seiringer, T. Volz, K. Eyerich, and G. Fabbrocini. 2021. "Hidradenitis Suppurativa: Where We Are and Where We Are Going." *Cells* 10 (8): 2094.

Stanford Medicine. n.d. "Symptoms of HIV and AIDS." https://stanfordhealthcare.org/medical-conditions/sexual-and-reproductive-health/hiv-aids/symptoms.html. Accessed June 5, 2024.

Wang, Y., and L. Bourouiba. 2017. "Drop Impact on Small Surfaces: Thickness and Velocity Profiles of the Expanding Sheet in the Air." *Journal of Fluid Mechanics* 814: 510-534.

Chapter 33

American College of Sports Medicine. 2016. *ACSM's Exercise Management for Persons With Chronic Diseases and Disabilities.* 4th ed. Champaign, IL: Human Kinetics.

Anderson, L.A. 2022. "Drug and Substance Abuse." www.drugs.com/article/drug-substance-abuse.html. Accessed June 5, 2024.

Cleary, M.A., Abdenour, T., and M. Pavlovich. 2022. *Clinical Pharmacology in Athletic Training.* Champaign, IL: Human Kinetics.

Cleveland Clinic. 2024. "Antivirals." https://my.clevelandclinic.org/health/drugs/21531-antivirals. Accessed June 5, 2024.

Drug Enforcement Agency. 2019. "Desomorphine." www.deadiversion.usdoj.gov/drug_chem_info/desomorphine.pdf.

Drug Enforcement Agency. 2020a. "LSD." www.dea.gov/sites/default/files/2020-06/LSD-2020.pdf.

Drug Enforcement Agency. 2020b. "Salvia Divinorum." www.dea.gov/sites/default/files/2020-06/Salvia%20Divinorum-2020_0.pdf.

Drug Enforcement Agency. 2022. "Drugs of Abuse." www.campusdrugprevention.gov/sites/default/files/2022-11/2022_DOA_eBook_File_Final.pdf. Accessed June 5, 2024.

Food and Drug Administration. 2018a. "Drug Disposal: Dispose 'Non-Flush List.' Medicine in Trash." www.fda.gov/drugs/disposal-unused-medicines-what-you-should-know/drug-disposal-dispose-non-flush-list-medicine-trash. Accessed June 5, 2024.

Food and Drug Administration. 2018b. "Disposal of Unused Medicines: What You Should Know." www.fda.gov/Drugs/ResourcesForYou/Consumers/BuyingUsingMedicineSafely/EnsuringSafeUseofMedicine/SafeDisposalofMedicines/ucm186187.htm. Accessed June 5, 2024.

Food and Drug Administration. 2022. "Development and Approval Process: Drugs." www.fda.gov/drugs/development-approval-process-drugs. Accessed June 5, 2024.

Fookes, D. 2022. "Drug Half-Life Explained." www.drugs.com/article/drug-half-life.html. Accessed June 5, 2024.

Gill, K.G. 2017. "Performance-Enhancing Drugs: A Review." digitalrepository.unm.edu/cgi/viewcontent.cgi?article=1164&context=unm_jor. Accessed June 5, 2024.

Johns Hopkins. 2022. "5 Vaping Facts You Need to Know." www.hopkinsmedicine.org/health/wellness-and-prevention/5-truths-you-need-to-know-about-vaping. Accessed June 5, 2024.

Johns Hopkins. 2023. "What Does Vaping Do to Your Lungs?" www.hopkinsmedicine.org/health/wellness-and-prevention/what-does-vaping-do-to-your-lungs. Accessed June 5, 2024.

MedicineNet. 2021. "Medical Definition of Effective Dose." www.medicinenet.com/effective_dose/definition.htm. Accessed June 5, 2024.

National Institute on Drug Abuse (NIDA). 2020. "Commonly Used Drug Charts." https://nida.nih.gov/research-topics/commonly-used-drugs-charts#ghb. Accessed June 5, 2024.

Puckey, M. 2022. "Bath Salts Drugs." www.drugs.com/illicit/bath-salts.html. Accessed June 5, 2024.

Substance Abuse and Mental Health Services Administration. 2018. "Tips for Teens: Methamphetamine." https://store.samhsa.gov/product/Tips-for-Teens-The-Truth-About-Methamphetamine/PEP18-03. Accessed June 5, 2024.

Wadhwa, R.R., and M. Cascella. 2022. "Steady State Concentration." [Updated 2022 Mar 9]. Treasure Island, FL: StatPearls Publishing. www.ncbi.nlm.nih.gov/books/NBK553132.

WebMD. 2005-2022. "Cannabidiol (CBD) Uses, Side Effects, and More." www.webmd.com/vitamins/ai/ingredientmono-1439/cannabidiol-cbd. Accessed June 5, 2024.

Chapter 34

Batch, J.T., S.P. Lamsal, M. Adkins, S. Sultan, and M.N. Ramirez. 2020. "Advantages and Disadvantages of the Ketogenic Diet: A Review Article." *Cureus* 12 (8): e9639.

Capritto, A. 2024. "What Is the Fruitarian Diet?" www.verywellfit.com/the-fruitarian-diet-4682619. Accessed June 4, 2024.

Cialdella-Kam, L., D. Kulpins, and M.M. Manore. 2016. "Vegetarian, Gluten-Free, and Energy-Restricted Diets in Female Athletes." *Sports* 4: 50.

Cleveland Clinic. 2022. "Strategies for Successful Weight Loss." https://health.clevelandclinic.org/how-to-lose-weight. Accessed June 9, 2024.

Deckers, J. 2016. "Animal (De)liberation: Should the Consumption of Animal Products Be Banned? Might a Vegan Diet Be Healthy, or Even Healthier?" www.ncbi.nlm.nih.gov/books/NBK396513. Accessed June 9, 2024.

Garnet Health. 2016. "Basal Metabolic Rate Calculator." www.garnethealth.org/news/basal-metabolic-rate-calculator. Accessed June 5, 2024.

Healthline. 2022. "6 Science-Based Health Benefit of Eating Vegan." www.healthline.com/nutrition/vegan-diet-benefits#lose-excess-weight. Accessed June 5, 2024.

Johnson-Arbor, K. 2022. "Dry Scooping Can Be Life-Threatening." www.poison.org/articles/dry-scooping-can-be-life-threatening. Accessed June 5, 2024.

Korey Stringer Institute. 2019. "Hydration." https://ksi.uconn.edu/prevention/hydration. Accessed June 5, 2024.

Mayo Clinic. 2022. "South Beach Diet." www.mayoclinic.org/healthy-lifestyle/weight-loss/in-depth/south-beach-diet/art-20048491. Accessed June 5, 2024.

Rowlands, D.S., B.H. Kopetschny, and C.E. Badenhorst. 2022. "The Hydrating Effects of Hypertonic, Isotonic and Hypotonic Sports Drinks and Waters on Central Hydration During Continuous Exercise: A Systematic Meta-Analysis and Perspective." *Sports Medicine* Feb; 52 (2): 349-375.

U.S. Department of Health and Human Services & U.S. Department of Agriculture. 2020-2025. "Dietary Guidelines for Americans." www.dietaryguidelines.gov/sites/default/files/2021-03/Dietary_Guidelines_for_Americans-2020-2025.pdf.

WebMD. 2020. "What Your Poop Type and Color Mean." www.webmd.com/digestive-disorders/ss/slideshow-poop-type-color. Accessed June 5, 2024.

Weil, A. 2013. "What Is Fruitarianism?" www.drweil.com/diet-nutrition/diets-weight-loss/what-is-fruitarianism/. Accessed June 4, 2024.

Whelan, C. 2017. "Everything You Need to Know About the Fruitarian Diet." www.healthline.com/health/food-nutrition/fruit-diet. Accessed June 4, 2024.

Chapter 35

Alkhalifah, A., M. Aljohani, W. Almasaud, R. Alsalamah, A. Alhomili, A. Almasaud, and F.H. Tobeigei. 2023. "Skin Problems Among the Wheelchair Users: A Prospective Cross-Sectional Study." *Ann Med Surg (Lond)* Mar 27; 85 (4): 655-658.

Birdwell, K.A., and M. Park. 2021. "Post-Transplant Cardiovascular Disease." *Clinical Journal of the American Society of Nephrology* 16 (12): 1878-1889.

Centers for Disease Control and Prevention. 2024. "National Diabetes Statistics Report." www.cdc.gov/diabetes/php/data-research/. Accessed June 5, 2024.

Christogianni, A., R. Bibb, S.L. Davis, O. Jay, M. Barnett, N. Evangelou, and D. Filingeri. 2018. "Temperature Sensitivity in Multiple Sclerosis: An Overview of Its Impact on Sensory and Cognitive Symptoms." *Temperature (Austin)* 5 (3): 208-223.

Cushing, S.L., and R.C. O'Reilly. 2021. "Out of Committee: Equilibrium Vestibular and Balance Dysfunction in Children with Hearing Loss." https://bulletin.entnet.org/aao-hnsf-2021/article/21259156/out-of-committee-equilibrium-vestibular-and-balance-dysfunction-in-children-with-sensorineural-hearing-loss. Accessed June 5, 2024.

Davis, C.P. 2021. "Atrial Fibrillation." www.emedicinehealth.com/atrial_fibrillation/article_em.htm. Accessed June 5, 2024.

Donate Life California. 2005-2023. "Transplant Games of America." https://donatelifecalifornia.org/transplant-games-of-america. Accessed June 5, 2024.

Ferrera, M.S., and C.L. Peterson. 2000. "Injuries to Athletes with Disabilities: Identifying Injury Patterns." *Sports Med* Aug; 30 (2): 137-143.

Fitzpatrick, K., A.J. De Luigi, and P.F. Pasquina. 2012. "The Disabled Athlete." In F. O'Connor, ed., *ACSM's Sports Medicine: A Comprehensive Review.* Philadelphia: Lippincott Williams & Wilkins.

Ghelichi-Ghojogh, M., F. Mohammadizadeh, F. Jafari, M. Vali, S. Jahanian, M. Mohammadi, A. Jafari, R. Khezri, H.A. Nikbakht, M. Daliri, and A. Rajabi. 2022. "The Global Survival Rate of Graft and Patient in Kidney Transplantation of Children: A Systematic Review and Meta-analysis." *BMC Pediatrics* Aug 24; 22 (1): 503.

Grohmann, K. 2016. "'Blade Jumper' Turns to Science to Earn Rio Games Place." www.reuters.com/article/us-olympics-rehm/blade-jumper-turns-to-science-to-earn-rio-games-place-idUSKCN0XG0QK. Accessed June 5, 2024.

Hurst, T.E., L.J. Fitzgerald, K.M. Chan, C. DeGeorge, P. Patil, and R. Gianchandani. 2019. "Post-Transplant Diabetes Mellitus (PTDM) in Lung Transplant Recipients: Prevalence and Outcomes." *Trends in Transplant* 12: 1-4.

Hussain, Y., and H. Khan. 2022. "Immunosuppressive Drugs." *Encyclopedia of Infection and Immunity* 726-740.

International Paralympic Committee. n.d. "IPC Classification." www.paralympic.org/classification. Accessed June 5, 2024.

Jacobs, P.L., ed. 2018. *NSCA's Essentials of Training Special Populations.* Champaign, IL: Human Kinetics.

Kalapatapu, V. 2017. "Lower Extremity Amputation." www.uptodate.com/contents/lower-extremity-amputation. Accessed June 5, 2024.

Lexell, J. 2018. "The Athlete with Spinal Cord Injury." *Aspetar Sports Medicine Journal* Jan; 7: 126-131.

Liaw, J., N. Billich, K. Carroll, J. Adams, M.M. Ryan, E.M. Yiu, M. Zacharin, P. Simm, and Z.E. Davidson. 2023. "Fracture Risk and Impact in Boys with Duchenne Muscular Dystrophy: A Retrospective Cohort Study." *Muscle Nerve* June; 67 (6): 489-496.

Mayo Clinic Staff. 1998-2023. "Liver Transplant." www.mayoclinic.org/tests-procedures/liver-transplant/about/pac-20384842. Accessed June 4, 2024.

Mayo Clinic Staff. 2019. "Residual Limb Pain." www.mayoclinic.org/diseases-conditions/residual-limb-pain/symptoms-causes/syc-20541403. Accessed June 9, 2024.

Mayo Clinic Staff. 2022. "Mayo Clinic Experts Hope New Race-Neutral Kidney Transplant Listing Criteria Improve Access for Black Individuals." www.mayoclinic.org/medical-professionals/transplant-medicine/news/mayo-clinic-experts-hope-new-race-neutral-kidney-transplant-listing-criteria-improve-access-for-black-individuals/mac-20540334. Accessed July 10, 2024.

Mayo Clinic Staff. 2023. "Sudden Cardiac Arrest." www.mayoclinic.org/diseases-conditions/sudden-cardiac-arrest/diagnosis-treatment/drc-20350640. Accessed June 4, 2024.

Mayo Clinic Staff. 2024. "Heart Transplant." www.mayoclinic.org/tests-procedures/heart-transplant/about/pac-20384750. Accessed June 4, 2024.

MedlinePlus. 2020. "Down Syndrome." medlineplus.gov/genetics/condition/down-syndrome. Accessed June 5, 2024.

Nassar, M., N. Nso, S. Lakhdar, R. Kondaveeti, C. Buttar, H. Bhangoo, M. Awad, et al. 2022. "New Onset Hypertension After Transplantation." *World Journal of Transplantation* Mar 18; 12 (3): 42-54.

National Health Service. 2021. "Muscular Dystrophy Treatment." www.nhs.uk/conditions/muscular-dystrophy/treatment. Accessed June 5, 2024.

Neale, J., A.C. Smith, and N.C. Bishop. 2017. "Effects of Exercise and Sport in Solid Organ Transplant Recipients: A Review." *American Journal of Physical Medicine & Rehabilitation* 96 (4): 273-288.

Oshima Y., S. Sato, T.F. Chen-Yoshikawa, Y. Yoshioka, N. Shimamura, R. Hamada, M. Nankaku, et al. 2020. "Quantity and Quality of Antigravity Muscles in Patients Undergoing Living-Donor Lobar Lung Transplantation: 1-Year Longitudinal Analysis Using Chest-Computed Tomography Images." *ERJ Open Research* Apr; 6 (2): 205-2019.

Paralympic Movement. n.d. "Paralympics—History of the Movement." www.paralympic.org/the-ipc/history-of-the-movement. Accessed June 5, 2024.

Parent Project Muscular Dystrophy. 2023. "Contractures and Scoliosis." www.parentprojectmd.org/care/care-guidelines/by-area/bone-and-joint-care/orthopedic-issues. Accessed June 5, 2024.

Patel, D.R., and D.E. Greydan. 2010. "Sport Participation by Physically and Cognitively Challenged Young Athletes." *Pediatric Clinics of North America* 57 (3): 795-817. doi:10.1016/j.pcl.2010.03.002.

Peláez-Jaramillo, M.J., A.A. Cárdenas-Mojica, P.V. Gaete, and C.O. Mendivil. 2018. "Post-Liver Transplantation Diabetes Mellitus: A Review of Relevance and Approach to Treatment." *Diabetes Therapy* Apr; 9 (2): 521-543.

Penn Medicine. 2023. "Cerebral Palsy." www.pennmedicine.org/for-patients-and-visitors/patient-information/conditions-treated-a-to-z/cerebral-palsy-complications. Accessed June 5, 2024.

Salera, S., F. Menni, M. Moggio, S. Guez, M. Sciacco, and S. Esposito. 2017. "Nutritional Challenges in Duchenne Muscular Dystrophy." *Nutrients* 9 (6): 594. https://doi.org/10.3390/nu9060594.

Sprabary, A. 2022. "The Paralympics and Olympic Games: How Visually Impaired Athletes Can Compete." www.allaboutvision.com/resources/human-interest/visually-impaired-athletes-olympics. Accessed June 5, 2024.

Stanford Medicine. 2023. "Congenital Limb Defect in Children." www.stanfordchildrens.org/en/topic/default?id=congenital-limb-defect-in-children-90-P02752. Accessed June 5, 2024.

Stratton, K.L., D. Zieve, and B. Conaway. MedlinePlus. 2017. "Kidney Transplant." https://medlineplus.gov/ency/article/003005.htm. Accessed June 5, 2024.

U.S. Department of Education Office for Civil Rights. 2022. "Discrimination Based on Pregnancy and Related Conditions." www2.ed.gov/about/offices/list/ocr/docs/ocr-pregnancy-resource.pdf. Accessed June 21, 2024.

U.S. Department of Health and Human Services. 2018. *Physical Activity Guidelines for Americans.* 2nd ed. Washington, DC: U.S. Department of Health and Human Services.

U.S. Department of Justice. n.d. "Introduction to the Americans with Disabilities Act." www.ada.gov/topics/intro-to-ada. Accessed June 5, 2024.

United Network for Organ Sharing. 2023. "2022 Organ Transplants Again Set Annual Records. https://unos.org/news/2022-organ-transplants-again-set-annual-records. Accessed June 5, 2024.

University of Michigan Health. 1995-2022a. "Lower-Extremity Amputation." www.uofmhealth.org/conditions-treatments/rehabilitation/lower-extremity-amputation. Accessed June 5, 2024.

University of Michigan Health. 1995-2022b. "Upper-Extremity Amputation." www.uofmhealth.org/conditions-treatments/rehabilitation/upper-extremity-amputation. Accessed June 5, 2024.

Van Schaik, L., J.H.B. Geertzen, P.U. Dijkstra, and R. Dekker. 2019. "Metabolic Costs of Activities of Daily Living in Person with a Lower Limb Amputation: A Systemic Review and Meta-Analysis." *PLoS One* 14 (3): e0213256. https://doi.org/10.1371/journal.pone.0213256.

VCU Health. 2023. "Race, Ethnicity and Living Donor Organ Transplantation." www.vcuhealth.org/news/race-ethnicity-and-living-donor-organ-transplantation. Accessed June 5, 2024.

Vural, A., and S.F. Keller. 2021. "Lung Transplantation and Metabolic Bone Disease." https://consultqd.clevelandclinic.org/lung-transplantation-and-metabolic-bone-disease. Accessed June 5, 2024.

WebMD. 2017. "Multiple Sclerosis." www.webmd.com/multiple-sclerosis/what-is-multiple-sclerosis#1. Accessed June 5, 2024.

Welke, B., E. Jakubowitz, F. Seehaus, K. Daniilidis, M. Timpner, N. Tremer, C. Hurschler, and M. Schwarze. 2019. "The Prevalence of Osteoarthritis: Higher Risk After Transfemoral Amputation—A Database Analysis with 1,569 Amputees and Matched Controls." *PLoS One* Jan 22; 14 (1): e0210868.

Wilhelm, M.J. 2015. "Long-Term Outcome Following Heart Transplantation: Current Perspective." *Journal of Thoracic Disease* 7 (3): 549-551.

Willick, S.E. 2018. "The Athlete with Limb Deficiency." *Aspetar Sports Medicine Journal* Jan; 7: 132-137.

INDEX

Note: Page numbers followed by an italicized *f* or *t* indicate figures or tables on that page.

N

O

ABOUT THE AUTHORS

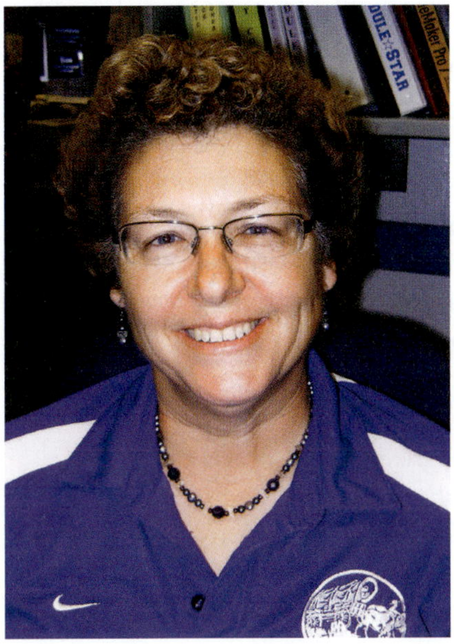

Lorin A. Cartwright, MS, ATC, has extensive experience in all aspects of instruction of student athletic trainers. She was the first woman to graduate from Grand Valley State University with a degree in athletic training, and she went on to earn a master's degree in education from the University of Michigan. She was the head athletic trainer, assistant principal, and athletic director at Pioneer High School in Ann Arbor, Michigan, where she served for more than 32 years. She was an adjunct professor in athletic training at the University of Michigan for three years and also taught at Eastern Michigan University and Concordia University.

Cartwright was also the first woman to serve as president of the Great Lakes Athletic Trainers Association (GLATA). She was appointed by the governor of Michigan to the Michigan Board of Athletic Trainers and the state's Task Force on Women in Sports. She has been an active member of the National Athletic Trainers' Association (NATA) LGBTQ+ Advisory Committee, recent cochair of the Michigan Athletic Trainers' Society Diversity, Equity, and Inclusion Committee, and is currently working on the NATA Honors and Awards Committee.

Highly regarded in her field, Cartwright received NATA's Gail Weldon Award of Excellence in 2022. She was also the recipient of NATA's Most Distinguished Athletic Trainer Award in 2018, GLATA's Golden Pinnacle Award in 2016, and GLATA's Outstanding Educator Award in 2010. She has been inducted into the Ann Arbor Pioneer High School Hall of Fame, the Michigan Athletic Trainers' Society Hall of Fame, the Great Lakes Athletic Trainers Association Hall of Fame, and the National Athletic Trainers' Association Hall of Fame.

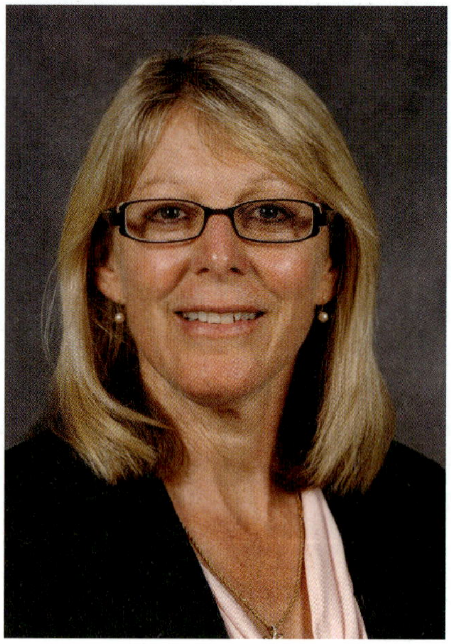

Kimberly S. Peer, EdD, ATC, FNATA, FNAP, is a full professor in the athletic training department at Kent State University in Kent, Ohio. She holds a doctorate in higher education administration with a cognate in health care management from the University of Akron. She teaches in the areas of professional development, ethics for health care providers, education and supervision, and scientific writing. Before coming to Kent State University, Peer was on the faculty of University of Mount Union (formerly Mount Union College) and served as the director of the Academy for Health and Sport Science and as coordinator for sports medicine at the Rehabilitation and Health Center. Prior to beginning her clinical and academic positions, Peer received her master's degree in athletic training from Western Michigan University and her bachelor's degree from Kent State University.

In addition to having served as the editor in chief for the *Athletic Training Education Journal*, Peer serves on the National Athletic Trainers' Association (NATA) Executive Council for Education and the NATA Committee on Professional Ethics. She also serves on the Board of Certification (BOC) Standards Committee. Her statewide service includes the governor's appointment to the Ohio licensure board and over 12 years of leadership service, including as president of the Ohio Athletic Trainers' Association (OATA).

Peer is a fellow of the NATA and a distinguished scholar fellow of the National Academies of Practice (NAP). She is a member of the NATA Hall of Fame (2024 class), was awarded NATA's Gail Weldon Award of Excellence in 2023, and received NATA's Most Distinguished Athletic Trainer Award. In addition, she was inducted into the OATA Hall of Fame in 2012 and earned the Dan Libera Service Award from the BOC in 2014. She has also been lauded with other national, regional, and state-level awards for her contributions to the profession and to athletic training education, including NATA's Sayers "Bud" Miller Distinguished Educator Award, GLATA's Outstanding Educator Award, and OATA's Linda Weber Daniel Outstanding Mentor Award. She has published and presented extensively on ethics education and pedagogy, and she has coauthored textbooks on professional ethics and fundamentals in athletic training.